MOSBY'S
EMT – BASIC
TEXTBOOK

Walt A. Stoy, PhD
and the
Center for Emergency Medicine

with 622 illustrations

Mosby
Lifeline

St. Louis Baltimore Boston Carlsbad Chicago Naples New York Philadelphia Portland
London Madrid Mexico City Singapore Sydney Tokyo Toronto Wiesbaden

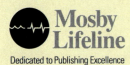

Dedicated to Publishing Excellence

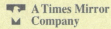

A Times Mirror
Company

Senior Vice President: David T. Culverwell
Publisher: David Dusthimer
Executive Editor: Claire Merrick
Editor: Julie Scardiglia
Assistant Editors: Lisa Esposito
                   John Goucher

Editorial Assistant: Lisa Benson
Project Manager: Chris Baumle
Production Editor: Michelle R. Fitzgerald
Production Assistant: Susie Coladonato
Design Manager: Nancy J. McDonald
Designer: Carolyn O'Brien

Printed in the United States of America

Mosby–Year Book, Inc.
11830 Westline Industrial Drive
St. Louis, Missouri 63146

Library of Congress Cataloging in Publication Data

Stoy, Walt A.
    Mosby's EMT–basic textbook / Walt A. Stoy and the Center for Emergency Medicine.
        p.   cm.
    Includes bibliographical references and index.
    ISBN 0-8151-7958-8
    1. Emergency medicine.   2. Emergency medical technicians.
I. Center for Emergency Medicine (Pittsburgh, Pa.)   II. Title.
    [DNLM: 1. Emergency Medical Technicians—education.   2. Emergency Medical
Technicians—education—examination questions.   3. Emergency Medicine—
education.   4. Curriculum—standards.   5. Emergency Medical Services—
methods.   WB 18 S893m 1996]
RC86.7.S76   1996
616.02'5—dc20
DNLM/DLC
for Library of Congress   95-24140
                                                                    CIP

This textbook is dedicated to each and
every one of you for accepting the calling
into the field of EMS.

NOTE TO THE READER

The author and publisher have made every attempt to ensure that the drug dosages and patient care procedures presented in this text are accurate and represent accepted practices in the United States. They are not provided as a standard of care. It is the Emergency Medical Technician – Basic's responsibility to follow patient care protocols established by a medical direction physician and to remain current in the delivery of emergency care.

Infection control practices may vary from agency to agency and may be updated periodically. It is the Emergency Medical Technician – Basic's responsibility to follow their local protocols regarding infection control and personal protective equipment.

The scene photographs in this text were taken during past emergency responses. There they may depict some patient care activities that do not accurately represent the current practice in prehospital emergency care.

Primary Author and Editor
WALT ALAN STOY, PHD, EMT-P

Walt Stoy, Director of the Office of Education at the Center for Emergency Medicine, has more than 20 years experience in prehospital emergency medicine and is internationally known for his expertise in prehospital education. Dr. Stoy is also a Research Assistant Professor of Medicine at the University of Pittsburgh School of Medicine, Division of Emergency Medicine, and is a flight paramedic for the STAT MedEvac flight program. Dr. Stoy served as the Principal Investigator for the 1994 EMT–Basic: National Standard Curriculum and as Project Director of the 1995 First Responder: National Standard Curriculum.

As the Director of the Office of Education at the Center for Emergency Medicine, Dr. Stoy is responsible for all the education programs offered by the Center including education for EMTs, paramedics, and continuing education in cardiac and trauma life support for all levels of healthcare professionals and the lay public.

Dr. Stoy is also the author of many instructional video guides for American Safety Video Publishers. These videos are used in educating prehospital professionals across the country. In addition, Dr. Stoy has lectured extensively on prehospital patient care at professional meetings across the United States. He serves on committees of numerous organizations committed to excellence in the practice and education of prehospital emergency medicine. Dr. Stoy has conducted research and has been published in professional emergency medicine journals.

Author and Contributing Editor
DEBRA A. BARCLAY, NREMT-P

Debra Barclay is the Coordinator of Publishing at the Center for Emergency Medicine and oversees all aspects of publishing including textbooks, videos, and other productions. Ms. Barclay joined the Center for Emergency Medicine in 1991.

Ms. Barclay is pursuing her Bachelor of Science degree at the University of Pittsburgh, and obtained her paramedic education at the Center for Emergency Medicine in 1991. She is also a flight paramedic for the STAT MedEvac flight program.

Authors
GREGG S. MARGOLIS, MS, NREMT-P

Gregg Margolis is the Associate Director of Education at the Center for Emergency Medicine. He is responsible for the development, coordination, management, and supervision of all levels of emergency medical education.

Mr. Margolis obtained his Bachelor of Science and his Masters Degree in Healthcare Management and Supervision with an emphasis in Education from the University of Pittsburgh. Mr. Margolis is a flight paramedic with the STAT MedEvac flight program.

THOMAS E. PLATT, NREMT-P

Thomas Platt is the Coordinator of EMS Education at the Center for Emergency Medicine. He is responsible for the development and implementation of basic life support training. In addition, Mr. Platt has worked on the 1994 EMT–Basic: National Standard Curriculum. Mr. Platt also served as Co-Principal Investigator for the First Responder: National Standard Curriculum.

Mr. Platt is working toward his bachelor's degree in Public Administration at the University of Pittsburgh. He is an active volunteer paramedic with a community ambulance service, and he works part time as a flight paramedic with the STAT MedEvac flight program.

AMY M. TREMEL, BS, NREMT-P

Amy Tremel is the Coordinator of EMS Education at the Center for Emergency Medicine, which she joined in 1989. Ms. Tremel oversees paramedic education at the Center.

Ms. Tremel obtained her Bachelor of Science degree in 1989 from the University of Pittsburgh and received her teaching certificate in 1990. She currently is an active volunteer paramedic at a local EMS agency.

BRIAN D. CHECK, BS, NREMT-P

Brian Check is the Coordinator of Medical Education at the Center for Emergency Medicine. Mr. Check oversees various programs for continuing education for EMS personnel and primary education for medical students at the University of Pittsburgh.

Mr. Check obtained his Bachelor of Science degree from the University of Pittsburgh. Mr. Check is a flight paramedic with the STAT MedEvac flight program.

WILLIAM R. MILLER, NREMT-P

William Miller is the Education Specialist for the Office of Prehospital Services at the Mercy Hospital of Pittsburgh. Mr. Miller is responsible for coordinating various continuing education courses for healthcare professionals including Advanced Cardiac Life Support, Pediatric Advanced Life Support, Advanced Trauma Life Support, and EMS Grand Rounds.

Mr. Miller has been involved in EMS for more than 20 years, including 15 years with the City of Pittsburgh Emergency Medical Services. Mr. Miller served as Training Division Supervisor for the City of Pittsburgh EMS for 7 years, and he has an extensive background in the delivery of patient care and rescue services.

Physician Advisor
PAUL M. PARIS, MD, FACEP

Paul M. Paris, MD, is the Medical Director at the Center for Emergency Medicine and acted as advisor for this textbook.

ABOUT THE CENTER FOR EMERGENCY MEDICINE

The Center for Emergency Medicine is a multihospital consortium dedicated to the advancement of emergency medicine through research, education, air medical transport, and quality care.

Office of Education

The Center's Office of Education provides educational programs to thousands of students each year, including EMTs, paramedics, nurses, physicians, medical students, and the lay public. Courses include Cardiopulmonary Resuscitation (CPR); Advanced Cardiac Life Support (ACLS); First Responder; Basic Trauma Life Support (BTLS); Emergency Medical Technician–Basic, Emergency Medical Technician–Paramedic; EMS Computer Learning Center; First Aid; and Wilderness Emergency Medicine. The Center revised the EMT–Basic National Standard Curriculum for the United States Department of Transportation National Highway Traffic Safety Administration.

Office of Research

The Center is known internationally for its research in emergency medicine. The Center researchers have helped to shape current emergency medicine protocols through ground-breaking studies in many important areas, including resuscitation from cardiac arrest, airway control, automated external defibrillation, pediatric emergencies, and pain management. The Center and its research affiliates have been responsible for more published studies in emergency medicine than any other facility in the world.

STAT MedEvac

STAT MedEvac is the region's leader in air medical transport. The program provides medical transport of critically ill or injured patients regionally and nationally. In 1994, the program transported nearly 3500 patients, making it one of the busiest air medical programs in the country. The fleet now includes seven helicopters, one dedicated medically-configured turbo prop airplane, and a Learjet. An instrument-rated Dauphin AS-365N helicopter makes flying in adverse weather conditions possible. STAT MedEvac is the only provider in the region for international medevac missions.

Residency Programs

The Center is also home to the University of Pittsburgh Affiliated Residency in Emergency Medicine. This is one of the leading emergency medicine residency programs in the nation.

National Association of EMS Physicians (NAEMSP)

The National Association of EMS Physicians is based at the Center for Emergency Medicine. With a membership of more than 1500 EMS professionals, this organization fosters excellence and provides medical leadership with the goal that all individuals and communities receive high quality prehospital emergency medical care.

Emergency Medical Services is a unique field of healthcare. Those of us who have been privileged to work in the streets have recognized this fact from the very first day we stepped out of an ambulance. We may have begun our careers as volunteers — young, eager, idealistic, and often plain frightened at the prospect of taking care of the needs of others. Much of the time we have spent in the field proves to be ordinary and even boring. But then a call comes in that makes it all worthwhile, exciting, interesting, and rewarding. It is perhaps this EMS "roller coaster" that makes prehospital care both exhilarating and unique.

This career is also unique in that EMS represents, for many, access to healthcare. No matter what the design of our healthcare system, prehospital care is often the open door for many patients to gain access to care. We treat all comers, regardless of payment mechanism, socioeconomic status, or level of blood alcohol. In some cases, EMS represents the only reasonably accessible portal of entry to the healthcare system. This is not always how we want it, but a better system has not yet been developed.

The system of emergency prehospital care is unique as well in that those using it have no choice. Citizens usually come into contact with us unexpectedly, often due to a sudden and unfortunate turn of fate. In this situation, they have little or no choice in who takes care of them. People can choose their own physician, hire their own nurse, or choose their physiotherapist. However, in an emergency, people cannot usually select their own EMS system. Dialing "911" sets in motion a series of events over which an individual has little control. Because of this, it is essential that the community ensures a standard of care that is uniformly high, predictable, and consistent across the entire system. Achieving this requires instituting programs of training, retraining, quality assurance, and outcome measurement.

This curriculum represents a compendium of many years' experience in the field of EMS. It combines clinical experience with a solid approach to educational methods. In fact, it sets the standard. It is a tool which, in the hands of dedicated instructors and students of prehospital care, can be as life-saving as the nearest airway or defibrillator. In many respects, this curriculum marks the "coming of age" of field practice. One of the most exciting aspects of the curriculum is the fact that it was created by a generation of *prehospital care clinicians* — EMTs, nurses, physicians — all with an interest and experience in field care; many educated in sound educational theory, and most of whom are still "in the trenches."

EMS is also unique because we often learn from each other. We work in teams; we depend on each other. These elements of prehospital care are woven throughout the curriculum. A few of us were privileged to have been there in early days of EMS. The technology, the faces, and the vision have changed, but one thing has not. This is the fact that, when all is said and done, we still have a single focus — the person we are caring for. No amount of bells or whistles, gadgets, or griping can dim that light. As you experience this curriculum and become immersed in the demands of training, never forget that focus. That is the core of this text and the reason for its content.

To paraphrase Sir Isaac Newton, if you see further with the help of this curriculum, it is because you are standing on the shoulders of giants. Those giants are those who have come before you and who have worked so diligently to improve the field of prehospital care. Some of these people have contributed to this text. Some you will know; most you will not. In your learning, always keep in mind that our best "giants" are those we care for and try to serve; they are indeed our best teachers.

Ronald D. Stewart, OC, MD, FACEP, FRCPC, Dsc (Honorary)
Minister of Health, Providence of Nova Scotia
Former Director of Paramedic Training, Los Angeles County
Former Medical Director, City of Pittsburgh Emergency Medical Services

Welcome to the beginning of your study to become an EMT–Basic!

This textbook is an instrument for your use along with the classroom study of the 1994 EMT–Basic: National Standard Curriculum.

The goal of the authors and reviewers involved in this project is to provide you with a basic textbook for easy and quick reference to the information necessary to succeed in your EMT–Basic program. As EMS educators, we wanted to provide a text to meet the needs of both instructors and students with different learning styles. Using many illustrations, we wanted to provide a visually appealing book complete with easy-to-read text and graphically displayed information. We also planned this textbook to offer flexibility for students and instructors as EMS education and the EMS community continue to evolve.

The Approach

This text focuses, quite simply, on what EMT–Basics *need to know.* One of the problems in providing too much information is that students are forced to determine what content is really important—where to focus attention. Therefore, the topics covered in this text are more concise and focused than that of similar texts. Nonetheless, all of the information in the National Curriculum and all EMT–Basics must know to provide quality emergency medical care is covered with as much background information and explanation as necessary for students to learn and become excellent prehospital providers.

The Author–Reviewer Team

This textbook is the result of many individuals contributing their time and energy to see it through to successful completion. In addition to the principal writers, countless reviewers, outside consultants, and treatment specialists contributed to this project in numerous ways to ensure not only its technical accuracy and completeness, but also its effectiveness as a teaching and learning tool.

The National Standard Curriculum

In 1994, the United States Department of Transportation National Highway Traffic Safety Administration released the EMT–Basic: National Standard Curriculum, replacing the former 10-year-old curriculum. Walt A. Stoy, PhD, of the Center for Emergency Medicine, was the Principal Investigator for this new curriculum.

Previously, the curriculum and education of EMTs had been based on a diagnostic approach. With this approach, EMTs attempted to diagnose a patient's medical problem and then provide the care appropriate for that diagnosis. The new curriculum replaces this approach with an emphasis on assessment which allows the EMT to quickly assess the patient and provide care based on the assessment findings. This approach has been found to be much more effective in providing medical care in prehospital settings.

For example, if the EMT's assessment reveals the patient is having difficulty breathing, then the EMT provides oxygen and other care for the breathing problem, regardless of the underlying cause. This method gives EMTs a consistent and appropriate approach to every patient so that the best prehospital care can be given rapidly—in situations where often minutes or seconds count.

This textbook follows the new National Standard Curriculum content. In it, you will learn the different patient assessments exactly as outlined in the Curriculum, and in later chapters on specific patient problems, you will continue to apply the same assessments to new situations. This integrated approach to patient assessment and care developed from many years of EMT experience and has been thoroughly tested and found effective. It is now the cornerstone of EMT emergency care.

Organization of Content

This textbook, like the National Curriculum, is divided into eight divisions. Division One, Preparatory, is designed to help students understand emergency medical services. It also includes material on the well-being of EMT–Basics; medical/legal and ethical issues; the human body; baseline vital signs and patient history; and lifting and moving patients. Division Two focuses on the airway and basic airway skills. Division Three contains the patient assessment section and concerns the very essence of EMS practice: patient assessment. Patient assessment includes the scene size-up; the initial assessment; the focused history and physical examination (for trauma and medical patients); the detailed physical examination; and the ongoing assessment. This module also includes communication and documentation skills. Division Four focuses on medical problems and includes chapters on general pharmacology; respiratory emergencies; cardiac emergencies; diabetes and altered mental status; allergies; poisoning and overdose; environmental emergencies; behavioral emergencies; and obstetrics and gynecology situations. Division Five focuses on trauma (injuries). This module includes bleeding and shock; soft-tissue injuries; musculoskeletal care; and injuries to the head and spine. Division Six focuses on the emergency care for infants and children. Division Seven covers issues of EMS operations, such as ambulance operations, gaining access, and overviews of related topics (eg, triage and hazardous materials). Division Eight is elective content on advanced airway management. This module is designed for those EMTs who will be able to provide advanced airway procedures for patients in prehospital settings.

The design of individual chapters within this text reflects the same focus on helping you learn this essential material in the most timely and effective manner. The following chapter elements enhance both your learning and review of each chapter's content.

Chapter Outline
Each chapter begins with an outline of the material included within. This affords the student an opportunity to see how the information fits together at a glance. This outline is also useful for reviewing material later.

Key Terms
The key terms highlighted in the chapter are defined at the beginning to help focus and prepare you for the chapter content. These definitions are also helpful when reviewing the material later.

In the Field Scenario
Each chapter opens with a short story of EMT patient care in a realistic prehospital situation. The patient's problem described in the scenarios relates to the chapter topic. These scenarios help you focus on the material covered in the chapter and on the real-life context in which you will use your EMT–Basic skills.

Introductory Paragraph
A brief chapter introduction sets the stage for the chapter's topics and provides background information as the context for the overall meaning of the chapter.

Text
The text of each chapter is broken into small sections of information to allow you to proceed through your reading and learning in a flexible but organized manner.

Information Boxes and Tables
Information boxes and tables are placed throughout the text to highlight special information, making it easier to learn and review. These special displays include

"Alerts" that call attention to critical information or safety warnings.

Principle Boxes
Many of the skills EMTs perform necessitate specific kinds of equipment that vary among EMS services. Because of these potential differences, this text strives whenever possible to focus on universal principles for how skills are performed, regardless of the specific equipment used. Principle boxes are used to emphasize the universal aspects of such skills.

Technique Boxes
The skills described in technique boxes illustrate one acceptable way to perform a skill using specific equipment. We do, however, recognize that students may be learning on slightly different equipment. Whenever there can be significant differences in the way a technique is performed because of differences in equipment, both a Principle and a Technique are included; the first emphasizing the universal steps for this skill regardless of equipment used, and the second pictorially showing the skill performed with a common type of equipment.

Review Questions
At the end of each major section of the chapter are review questions to test your comprehension of the material thus far. If you have difficulty answering any of these questions, go back and review the material before proceeding to the next section.

Illustrations
The textbook is heavily illustrated with full-color photographs and drawings. The important aspects of all essential skills are illustrated to help you see the correct steps laid out before you begin practicing them.

Chapter Summary
At the end of each chapter is a summary organized around the key topics in the chapter. This allows the student to integrate all of the key information in the chapter, as well as to return to the chapter later for a quick content review.

United States Department of Transportation National Highway Traffic Safety Administration EMT–Basic Objectives
The objectives found at the end of each chapter parallel those of the National Standard Curriculum. Cognitive objectives include what you should *know* after reading

and studying the chapter; affective objectives focus on *attitude:* what you should understand and feel about patients and family members in relation to the chapter content; and psychomotor objectives list what you should be able to *do* after studying the chapter and practicing the skills in your course.

Glossary

At the end of the text is a glossary that defines the medical and EMT terms used throughout the book. It includes all the key terms as well so that you do not need to hunt through individual chapters for definitions.

AUTHOR ACKNOWLEDGMENTS

The authors would like to thank the following individuals and organizations for their contributions to this book:

David Culverwell, David Dusthimer, Claire Merrick, and Julie Scardiglia of Mosby Lifeline for their desire to see this project through to completion. Their tremendous commitment of time and resources made this project possible. Special thanks to Lisa Esposito of Mosby Lifeline for giving us all the motivation we needed to keep us on track.

Tom Lochhaas for his work as developmental editor. His patience, sense of humor, and painstaking attention to detail made the revision process easier for all of us.

Vincent Knaus and William Hrovoski for their excellent photography.

Kimberly Battista and Stacy Lund for their beautiful illustrations.

The University of Pittsburgh Medical Center, Pittsburgh EMS, Dravosburg Volunteer Fire Department #1, and STAT MedEvac for their contributions to the artwork and development of the rescue photographs.

Parr Emergency Product Sales and Laerdal for their generous contribution of medical equipment and supplies for the illustrations.

The staff and students of the Center for Emergency Medicine for being available at a moment's notice to offer advice, opinions, or participate in a number of ways too numerous to mention.

All of our families and loved ones for their support and encouragement.

PUBLISHER ACKNOWLEDGMENTS

Mosby's EMT—Basic Textbook is the culmination of the efforts of many dedicated and gifted individuals in the field of EMS and its related medical fields. In addition to our developmental editor, Tom Lochhaas, who managed and coordinated our reviews and draft revisions, we would like to acknowledge the following individuals who contributed their time and talent to this textbook:

Barbara Aehlert, RN, for her knowledge, expertise, and the benefit of her prior writing experience, without which a project of this magnitude would not have been possible in the time alloted. Her understanding of the subject matter and her resulting contribution to the art program for this book were invaluable. We are forever in her debt.

Mick J. Sanders, for his unfailing support and author experience, not only in his role as a reviewer, but in his extensive involvement in the art program, researching and locating many of the photographs in this book.

Nancy L. Bryan, for her continued dedication not only in her special reviews but in her diligent search for much of the artwork in this text. Without her research and development in this area, coordinating the text and the artwork would have been an impossible task.

Thanks also to Maureen Anderson and Moore Medical Corporation, Inc. for supplying much of the equipment that appears in this text; Kathy Haddix and Rockingham Memorial Hospital, Harrisonburg, Virginia; for their generous contributions of time and staff to make our photo shoots a success.

Special thanks to Philip Neff, NREMT-P, Harrisonburg Rescue Squad, Harrisonburg, Virginia, for providing coordination and technical support on the photo shoots. Thanks also to the Harrisonburg Rescue Squad and Harrisonburg Fire Department for their assistance.

The editors also wish to acknowledge and thank the many reviewers of this book who devoted countless hours to intensive review. Their comments were invaluable in developing and fine tuning this manuscript.

Individuals who took part in the extensive review of this project are:

Barbara Aehlert, RN
Director, EMS Education and Research
Samaritan Health System
Phoenix, Arizona

Paul Auerbach, MD, MS, FACEP
Division of Emergency Medicine
Stanford University Hospital
Stanford, California

Jane W. Ball, RN, DrPH
Project Director, EMSC National Resource Center
Children's National Medical Center
Washington, D.C.

Anne Beauchamp, RN, BSN, CCRN, CFRN
Manager of Education
Samaritan Health Systems
Phoenix, Arizona

Ann Bellows, RN, REMT-P
Coordinator, EMS/Paramedic Program
Dona Ana Branch, Community College
Las Cruces, New Mexico

Armando Bevelacqua, EMT-P
Lieutenant, Orlando Fire Department
Training Coordinator, EMS and HAZMAT
Orlando, Florida

Russell Bieniek, MD, FACEP
Medical Director, Emergency Department
Saint Vincent Health Center
Erie, Pennsylvania

John E. Blue, II
Director, Emergency Medical Services Program
Gadsdon State Community College
Anniston, Alabama

Chip Boehm, RN, EMT-P
Falmouth, Maine

James F. Bothwell, BS, NREMT-P
Director of Operations, Stat MedEvac
Pittsburgh, Pennsylvania

Nancy L. Bryan, former BLS Training Director
Wisconsin EMS Section
Madison, Wisconsin

James A. Christopher
EMS Coordinator, EMS Department
St. Francis Hospital and Health Centers
Beech Grove, Indiana

John Clapin, BA
Director of Training
New York City EMS
New York, New York

Peter E. Connick, NREMT-P
Captain, Chatham Fire Department
Chatham, Massachusetts

Phil Currance, EMT-P, RHSP
President, Emedia Inc., Adjunct Clinical Instructor
Emergency Response Coordinator Hazardous Materials
    Program
Front Ravoe Community College
Denver, Colorado

Peter Dillman, EdD, EMT-P
Director, Wishard Ambulance Service
Wishard Memorial Hospital
Indianapolis, Indiana

John Doyle
Victor Valley College, Allied Health Department
Victorville, California

Franklin Foster, JD
Missouri Bureau of EMS
Legal Specialist
Jefferson City, Missouri

Susan Fuchs, MD, FAAP
Associate Professor of Pediatrics
University of Pittsburgh School of Medicine
Pittsburgh, Pennsylvania

Joseph J. Gadoury, BA, MICP
EMS Educator
Memorial Hospital of Burlington County
Mt. Holly, New Jersey

Charles "Punky" Garoni, BA, EMT-P
Associate Professor
UTHSC-SA EMT Department
San Antonio, Texas

Jeffrey R. Grunow, MSN, NREMT-P
Assistant Professor
Eastern Kentucky University
College of Allied Health and Nursing
Richmond, Kentucky

David J. Gurchiek, BS, NREMT-P
Education Coordinator
Big Sky EMS Education
Billings, Montana

Michael J. Hartley, REMT-P
EMS Instructor
University of Iowa Hospitals and Clinics, EMSLRC
Iowa City, Iowa

Tanas Theodore Hayda
Warren, Michigan

Karla Holmes, RN, MPA
Salt Lake City Fire Department
Training Division
Magna, Utah

Neil R. Jones, MEd, EMT-P
Director, Outreach Education
Children's Hospital of Pittsburgh
Pittsburgh, Pennsylvania

Edward J. Kalinowski, BSN, MEd
Chairman, Department of Emergency Medical Services
Kapiolani Community College
Honolulu, Hawaii

Jim Kern, EMT-P
EMS Operations Supervisor
Bromenn Regional Medical Center
EMS Training Program
Virginia at Franklin
Normal, Illinois

Randy C. Krantz, RN, EMT-P, JD
Attorney at Law
Bedford, Virginia

Perry B. Lamb, MPH
State of Idaho EMS
Boise, Idaho

Gail M. Madsen, NREMT-P
Oregon EMS Training Coordinator
Portland, Oregon

Thomas G. Martin, MD, DABMT
Director, Toxicology Treatment Program
University of Pittsburgh Medical Center
Assistant Professor of Medicine
University of Pittsburgh
Pittsburgh, Pennsylvania

Ronald G. Pirrallo, MD, MHSA
Assistant Professor, Department of Emergency Medicine
Medical College of Wisconsin
Medical Director, Milwaukee County EMS
Milwaukee, Wisconsin

David Reeves
Guilford Technical Community College
Jamestown, North Carolina

Laurie A. Romig, MD, FACEP
President, Emergency Solutions Institute
St. Petersburg, Florida

Lou E. Romig MD, FAAP
Pediatric Emergency Medicine Attending Physician
EMS Liaison
Miami Children's Hospital
Miami, Florida

Norman W. Rooker, EMT-P
Department of Public Health
City of San Francisco
San Francisco, California

Patricia Hicks Ryder, BS, EMT-P
EMS Educational Services, Inc.
Williamsport, Maryland

José Salazar
Associate, Health and Safety Services
American Red Cross National Headquarters
Health and Safety Services
Falls Church, Virginia

Mick J. Sanders, EMT-P, MSA
St. Charles, Missouri

DeeDee Sewell, NREMT-P
Acadian Ambulance Service, Inc.
Lafayette, Louisiana

Charlene M. Skaff, MS, BA, NREMT-P
Fargo, North Dakota

Gerard Sikorski
Nassau County Fire/Police/EMS Academy
Nassau County Medical Center
East Meadow, New York

Lois M. Souder, LPN, EMT-P
Apollo Career Center
Public Safety Coordinator
Lima, Ohio

Doug Stutz, PhD
GDS Communications
Miramar, Florida

Katherine H. West
Infection Control/Emerging Concepts
Springfield, Virginia

Justin W. Witt, EMT-C
James City County Fire Department
Williamsburg, Virginia

In addition, the publisher would like to thank the following professionals whose pictures and statements appear in the Division Openers:

Division 1:
Ricky Kue, NREMT-B
Ridgewood Volunteer Ambulance Corp.
Ridgewood, New York

Division 2:
Edward F. Rzepka, NREMT-D
Hartford Emergency Squad
Hartford, Wisconsin

Division 3:
James W. Hansen, NREMT-P
Firefighter/Paramedic and EMS Coordinator
Salt Lake City Fire Department
Salt Lake City, Utah

Division 4:
Paul M. Paris, MD, FACEP
Professor and Chief, Division of Emergency Medicine
University of Pittsburgh School of Medicine
Pittsburgh, Pennsylvania

Division 5:
Martin Butler, EMT-I
Leading Petty Officer
Emergency Medical Department
Naval Hospital, Roosevelt Roads
Puerto Rico

Division 6 (on left):
Lou Romig, MD, FAAP
Pediatric Emergency Medicine Attending Physician
EMS Liason
Miami Children's Hospital
Miami, Florida

Division 6 (on right):
Laurie Romig, MD, FACEP
President, The Emergency Solutions Institute, Inc.
St. Petersburg, Florida

Division 7:
Captain Eugene V. McCarthy, EMT-I
Paramedic Coordinator
Los Angeles County Fire Department
Los Angeles, California

Division 8:
Mark E. Polakoff, RN, NREMT-B
Red Lodge Volunteer Ambulance Service
Red Lodge, Montana

Finally, we gratefully acknowledge the important contributions of those who posed as models in this text:

CONTENTS

DIVISION FOUR MEDICAL/BEHAVIORAL EMERGENCIES AND OBSTETRICS AND GYNECOLOGY 232

CHAPTER 16 General Pharmacology 234

CHAPTER 17 Respiratory Emergencies 244

CHAPTER 18 Cardiovascular Emergencies 258

CHAPTER 19 Diabetes and Altered Mental Status 282

CHAPTER 20 Allergic Reactions 292

CHAPTER 21 Poisoning and Overdose 302

CHAPTER 22 Environmental Emergencies 314

As prehospital care providers, we are expected to maintain a high standard of care. Ideally, this care should be available to everyone at any given time. The importance of our duty is second to none. As the first medical professionals at the scene of an emergency, it's crucial to provide quality medical attention to the patient. To render the best possible care under any circumstance is the foundation which we as emergency medical technicians must strive to achieve.

Ricky Kue, NREMT-B
Ridgewood Volunteer
Ambulance Corp.
Ridgewood, New York

IN THIS DIVISION

DIVISION ONE

1 INTRODUCTION TO EMERGENCY MEDICAL

CARE

IN THE FIELD

It was the annual career day at the local high school. EMTs Anna and Roy had cleaned the ambulance both inside and out. They arrived at the school 15 minutes before their presentation was scheduled to begin, because they knew being punctual was important.

This was Roy's first opportunity to talk about his career with students. Anna had been to this school before, taking care of injured students, standing by at sporting events, and sharing her passion for her job with high school juniors and seniors. When it was time to begin, Roy turned down his radio so as not to disrupt the presentation, and he walked up to the microphone. He had prepared a speech discussing his career and its effect on the lives of many people.

He began his lecture by detailing a brief history of the Emergency Medical Services system. He explained what the job involved, the characteristics of his co-workers, and the personal satisfaction he felt in a job well done. He described his working relationship with doctors, nurses, and other healthcare professionals, and explained that many of these people had begun their careers as EMTs.

Anna then told the students about her experiences and thoughts about her career as an EMT–Basic. They finished the discussion with a tour of the ambulance. On the way back to the station, they felt proud of the EMS system and their involvement in providing quality care to the citizens of the town.

This chapter marks the beginning of your educational process for becoming an **Emergency Medical Technician (EMT)**. EMT–Basics who care for ill or injured patients before the patients reach the hospital require a solid foundation—a road map for learning. This chapter outlines the job roles and responsibilities to help you learn what you need to become an EMT–Basic.

This chapter also describes the **Emergency Medical Services (EMS)** system and the role of EMT–Basics within this system. This is a system of professionals who provide emergency medical care, beginning when someone initially realizes an injured or ill person requires emergency care, through the patient's admission to the hospital (Fig. 1-1).

THE EMERGENCY MEDICAL SERVICES SYSTEM

You are about to embark on a great journey that will affect not only your life but also the lives of many others. You will learn to help patients who are strangers, neighbors, friends, and even loved ones. The average person requires the assistance of emergency personnel every 7 years. Clearly, this is an important job.

Working or volunteering as an EMT–Basic is both a demanding and rewarding career. Few other professions have such an impact on people's lives on a daily basis.

Everyone has a different reason for becoming involved in the EMS system. Some students have experienced the loss of a friend or family member after a medical emergency and want to prevent others from experiencing the same loss. Others become involved because television dramas such as "Rescue 911" and "Code 3" show emergency medical care as an exciting, challenging, and fulfilling profession. Some people take the EMT–Basic program without planning to work as an EMT–Basic, but instead use the education to move toward a career as a nurse or physician. Whatever your reason, welcome to the ranks of one of the most rewarding professions in the world.

Everyday, people's lives are touched by EMTs. From an elderly patient who must reach the doctor's office for an appointment, to a child with a life-threatening airway emergency, all of the patients you will encounter have one thing in common—they need help. They require the assistance of a competent, qualified, caring individual. They need you, the EMT–Basic.

The following sections will help you better un-

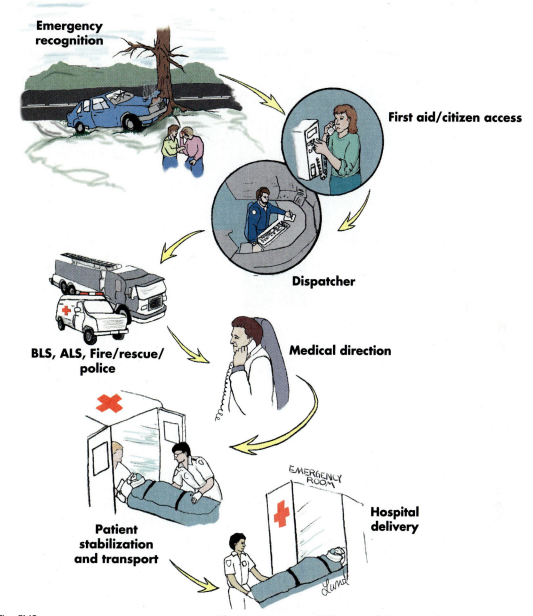

Fig. 1-1 The EMS system encompasses emergency recognition, system access, EMS personnel dispatch and response, care provided to the patient at the scene, medical direction when necessary, and patient stabilization, transportation, and delivery to the hospital.

derstand the role of EMTs in the EMS system, beginning with the national agency that sets standards for the education of EMTs.

THE NATIONAL HIGHWAY TRAFFIC SAFETY ADMINISTRATION TECHNICAL ASSISTANCE PROGRAM

The goal of the Department of Transportation (DOT) and the National Highway Traffic Safety Administration (NHTSA) is to reduce the number of deaths and disabilities caused by motor vehicle collisions on the nation's highways. NHTSA has therefore developed National Standard Curricula and Technical Assistance Programs for the states to ensure the EMS system is effective everywhere.

NHTSA has developed standards in 10 areas to guarantee high-quality EMS systems (Fig. 1-2):
• Regulation and policy
• Resource management
• Human resources and training
• Transportation

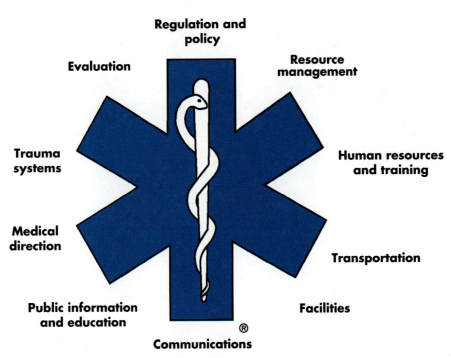

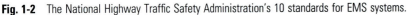

Fig. 1-2 The National Highway Traffic Safety Administration's 10 standards for EMS systems.

- Facilities
- Communications
- Public information and education
- Medical direction
- Trauma systems
- Evaluation

These aspects of the system are described below to help you better understand the overall system in which you will be working as an EMT–Basic.

Regulation and policy standards ensure that all states have a lead EMS agency, funding, regulations, and operational policies and procedures. State legislatures must pass laws that promote quality EMS care and provide adequate funding. States finance their EMS systems in various ways, but all have funds to provide high-quality, effective EMS care. As you train for your profession and begin working as an EMT–Basic, you will become familiar with state and local rules and regulations, policies, and procedures.

Resource management standards coordinate resources throughout the state. These standards allow everyone access to basic emergency medical care, including treatment by personnel trained primarily at the EMT–Basic level, and allow all patients to be transported in a well-equipped vehicle to a staffed, equipped, and prepared facility.

Human resources and training standards require all states to have good educational programs for EMT–Basics and other EMS personnel.

Transportation standards guarantee safe and effective transportation for all patients. Ambulances and air medical units must meet minimum criteria and be inspected periodically. All aspects of the state EMS system must be in a constant mode of readiness.

The facilities standard ensures that patients are transported to the closest appropriate facility. Prehospital care providers such as EMTs must understand the different hospitals' capabilities and local policies for specific emergency situations. This includes specialty facilities, such as trauma and burn centers, and children's hospitals.

Communications standards make certain that patients can call for emergency care and that emergency personnel communicate effectively with the receiving hospital and other EMS personnel.

Public information and education guidelines promote the public's involvement in the EMS system and injury prevention programs. EMTs often provide the public with information about system procedures and injury prevention. This education improves the system and helps patients receive quality care.

In the EMS system, direct patient care is delegated to four levels of providers: First Responders and three levels of EMTs—EMT–Basics, EMT–Intermediates, and EMT–Paramedics. Medical direction standards ensure that physicians stay involved in the patient care system by developing protocols or patient care guidelines, by providing medical direction and consultation, and by evaluating patient care activities and quality improvement.

Trauma is a severe wound or injury. A trauma patient requires specialized medical trauma care, provided through the state's trauma system. Across the United States, there are many state-wide trauma care systems, including designated trauma centers, trauma triage guidelines, data collection, trauma registry definitions, system management, and quality assurance.

The final standard involves evaluation of the effectiveness of patient care, including the care provided by EMT–Basics. In this way, the EMS system can continue to improve the quality of patient care delivered.

ACCESS TO THE EMERGENCY MEDICAL SERVICES SYSTEM

The manner in which the public contacts the EMS system is extremely important. In many areas of the United States, 911 is the universal access number to police, fire, and EMS (Fig. 1-3). However, some areas of the country do not have this capability and must dial a seven-digit number to access the EMS system.

Regardless of the phone number used, EMTs should educate the public on proper access to the system. Public information campaigns, such as "Make the Right Call," teach the public the proper local access number and when to call for an ambulance. EMTs at all levels should be active in these public service campaigns.

LEVELS OF EDUCATION

The **National EMS Education and Practice Blueprint** sets the standards for the education of prehospital emergency care providers. As mentioned earlier, the four established levels are:
- **First Responder**
- **EMT–Basic**
- **EMT–Intermediate**
- **EMT–Paramedic**

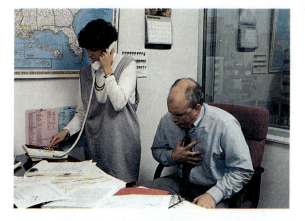

Fig. 1-3 In many areas of the United States, "911" is the universal number for access to police, fire, and EMS.

The EMS system currently lists these four levels for certification or licensure, although not all states use every level. States can also augment the levels with additional care levels. Each recognized level has its own scope of practice.

The First Responder course is for those persons who, similar to law enforcement personnel or firefighters, are likely to encounter an ill or injured person but are not trained for ambulance service. The focus at this level is to provide initial stabilization until additional EMS resources arrive.

The EMT–Basic course prepares personnel to provide primary medical care before the patient reaches the hospital. Most states require the EMT-Basic as the minimum accepted education level for ambulance staff. The EMT–Intermediate level is an advanced EMT level that includes skills such as manual defibrillation and administration of intravenous fluids and some medications. The EMT–Paramedic, currently the highest skill level, includes more advanced techniques such as tracheal intubation and administration of additional medications. The National Registry of EMTs prepares and conducts examinations designed to test the competency at these three EMT levels (Fig. 1-4). State regulations and local medical directors determine the specific procedures at all levels.

THE HEALTHCARE SYSTEM

The EMS system is a part of the overall healthcare system in the United States. This healthcare system has many components. Most important to EMT–Basics are the prehospital setting and the hospital, although many other aspects are involved.

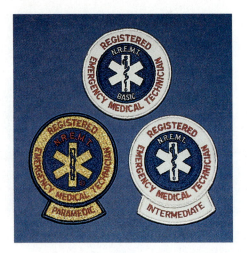

Fig. 1-4 National Registry of EMTs patches for the three EMT levels.

First Responders, EMT–Basics, EMT–Intermediates, and EMT–Paramedics are the primary emergency medical care providers outside of the hospital. The process begins when someone notices the patient's illness or injury and calls the EMS system through the local number. First Responders such as firefighters or lifeguards may already be at the scene and provide some initial care until more qualified EMTs arrive. Also involved are professional dispatchers who not only forward the emergency call to the EMS unit, but who may also give care instructions prior to arrival of the EMS unit. In many systems, **emergency medical dispatchers** have received education for dispensing medical care instructions over the phone before the EMTs arrive.

The next step in the healthcare system is the hospital. This typically begins with the arrival to the emergency department, although some states permit EMTs to transport a patient directly to a physician's office or clinic. Healthcare workers in the emergency department include physicians, nurses, nursing assistants, nurse practitioners, and physician assistants. Many people perform support services, lab work, electrocardiograms, X-rays, and other services including clerical, communications, and housekeeping support.

Some patients may require the attention of a specialty care center. EMTs transport these patients to centers such as trauma facilities, burn centers, pediatric or children's hospitals, and poison centers. These specialty centers vary in different regions. Knowledge of the specialty centers in your area is important, including the local protocol for transporting patients to one of these facilities. Your service area may have additional specialty centers.

LIAISON WITH OTHER PUBLIC SAFETY WORKERS

Most of the EMT–Basic's responsibilities involve patient care. EMTs also interact with other public safety workers including local, state, and possibly federal law enforcement. A strong working relationship with law enforcement personnel ensures the safety of EMTs, patients, and bystanders (Fig. 1-5). Depending on the system and local policies, some EMTs may interact with law enforcement on every prehospital call, whereas others work with law enforcement only at automobile crashes, crime scenes, and hazardous materials scenes. In some systems, law enforcement officers are trained to the First Responder skill level or higher and routinely arrive on the scene to provide care until other emergency personnel arrive.

EMT–Basics may also work with the local fire department. Many communities organize EMS activities as a branch of the fire department, using firefighters or EMT–Basics to work on both fire apparatus and ambulances. In some areas, EMT–Basics may also interact with the fire department by using their resources for first response to medical emergencies and traumatic injuries, vehicle rescue, special rescue situations, and hazardous materials situations.

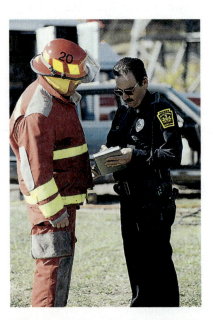

Fig. 1-5 EMTs often interact with other public safety workers, including law enforcement officials.

A strong professional relationship between EMTs and other public safety agencies is important, because this guarantees smooth operation and successful delivery of quality public safety. As an EMT–Basic, you may interact with other agencies regularly.

REVIEW QUESTIONS

THE EMERGENCY MEDICAL SERVICES SYSTEM

1. How many levels of prehospital care providers are established by the National EMS Education and Practice Blueprint?
   A. 3
   B. 4
   C. 5
   D. Not defined

2. Mark an "A" for *advanced* life support provider and a "B" for a *basic* life support provider for each of the following certification levels.
   First Responder _____
   EMT–Intermediate _____
   EMT–Paramedic _____
   EMT–Basic _____

3. The guidelines for the EMS curriculum are established by which agency?
   A. The National Registry of EMTs
   B. The National Association of EMTs
   C. The Department of Transportation/National Highway Traffic Safety Administration
   D. The National Association of EMS Physicians

4. In many communities, 911 is the phone number used to contact EMS, police, and firefighters. This number is considered:
   A. Community access
   B. National access
   C. Worldwide access
   D. Universal access

1. B
2. First Responder: B   EMT–Intermediate: A   EMT–Paramedic: A   EMT–Basic: B
3. C
4. D

THE EMERGENCY MEDICAL TECHNICIAN–BASIC

ROLES AND RESPONSIBILITIES

The roles and responsibilities of EMT–Basics are continually evolving. Job descriptions established by the service define specific requirements. EMT–Basics must understand these roles and responsibilities to be competent, professional members of the healthcare team (*see* Box 1-1).

PERSONAL SAFETY

As an EMT–Basic, you have a responsibility for your own safety. This role is discussed in depth in Chapter 2, "The Well-Being of the EMT–Basic." Ensuring personal safety includes maintaining a healthy body, remaining physically fit, and using body substance isolation precautions appropriately. Personal safety also includes surveying the emergency scene for hazards or potential hazards before entering. Chapter 8, "Scene Size-Up," describes the appropriate measures to be taken in this important procedure.

SAFETY OF THE CREW, PATIENT, AND BYSTANDERS

EMTs are also responsible for the safety of fellow crew members, patients, and bystanders. Looking out for the well-being of your partners is extremely

BOX 1-1

Roles and Responsibilities of the EMT–Basic

- Personal safety
- Safety of the crew, patient, and bystanders
- Patient assessment
- Patient care based on assessment findings
- Lifting and moving patients safely
- Transport and transfer of care
- Record keeping and data collection
- Patient advocacy (patient rights)

important. This includes maintaining scene safety and coping with stress, as you will learn in the next chapter. You also must ensure the safety of patients. You are responsible for providing the best possible care for patients, while carrying out safety precautions that will prevent further injury to patients from hazards at the scene. You must also consider the safety of bystanders. By securing a safe scene and communicating effectively with bystanders, you protect everyone's safety.

PATIENT ASSESSMENT AND CARE

Patient assessment is a primary responsibility (Fig. 1-6). EMTs assess the patient's needs and provide basic medical care established by that assessment. Chapters 9 through 13 describe how to assess a patient. As an EMT, you should practice and master these skills. The emergency care you provide is based on assessment findings. This approach allows for rapid management of life-threatening injuries and illnesses and relieves the patient's discomfort quickly.

LIFTING AND MOVING PATIENTS

When the patient has been evaluated and treated, EMTs then prepare the patient for transport. Therefore, you must be able to lift and move patients safely. You must be sure the environment is safe for lifting, for example, by moving debris off of a sidewalk before moving a patient over it. You also must use safe lifting and moving techniques as described in Chapter 6, "Lifting and Moving Patients."

TRANSPORT AND TRANSFER OF CARE

When en route to the receiving facility, or when awaiting a transport unit, EMTs continue to provide care based on ongoing patient assessment. An orderly transfer of patient care should be maintained, whether transporting to the receiving facility or another unit. This involves medical/legal issues such as preserving patient confidentiality and preventing abandonment (*see* Chapter 3, "Medical/Legal and Ethical Issues").

Chapter 14, "Communications," and Chapter 15, "Documentation," describe issues involved in the transfer of care and information. Record keeping and data collection are an important role of EMT–Basics (Fig. 1-7).

PATIENT ADVOCACY

Another role of EMTs is that of the patient advocate. You must support the patient's legal rights, privacy, and human dignity as an individual. Chapter 3, "Medical/Legal and Ethical Issues," describes the patient's legal rights. All patients should be treated with respect and dignity, regardless of their social and economic backgrounds. Always treat patients as you wish to be treated yourself.

PROFESSIONAL ATTRIBUTES

In addition to these roles and responsibilities, EMTs must behave professionally. Professional attributes include physical appearance, a positive attitude, up-to-date knowledge and skills, making

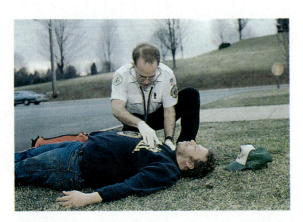

Fig. 1-6 EMTs assess patients to determine and provide adequate, appropriate care.

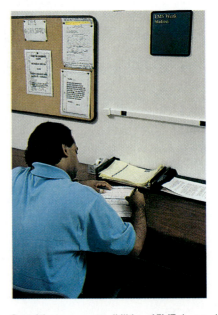

Fig. 1-7 One of the many responsibilities of EMTs is record keeping and data collection.

the patient's needs a top priority without endangering yourself or others, and expanding current knowledge of local, state, and national issues affecting EMS and healthcare.

EMTs are healthcare professionals and an important part of the healthcare team. Therefore, you should strive to project a professional appearance. Overall grooming, hair, and clothing should be neat and clean at all times. Shoes or boots should be clean and polished. Many services have a uniform policy for appropriate attire (Fig. 1-8). Some services may have duty uniforms and dress uniforms to be worn at the appropriate times.

The patient's and family's first impression of healthcare personnel can come from their initial contact with you. An unkempt EMT may imply sloppy patient care. Dressing in a crisp, clean uniform may reduce the patient's and family's anxiety.

As you enter this facet of the world of healthcare, you are choosing a profession that demands life-long continuing education and skills. Medical care will continue to evolve, and technology will provide EMS with new options for patient care. Federal, state, and regional laws and regulations will also change the way in which care is provided. EMTs have an obligation to be knowledgeable and provide technically proficient care. As a professional, you must keep abreast of changes and advances in medical care.

Continuing education is therefore an important aspect of your career. EMT–Basics should attend continuing education courses whenever possible and practice skills that are not often used (Fig. 1-9). Continuing education should not be postponed until you conclude your initial education program. You should begin to attend these programs immediately. Ask your instructor which programs can be taken before completing your initial education, and which can be taken afterward. Consider attending courses providing vehicle operation and rescue education programs. Many states require continuing education as a part of the recertification process or license renewal.

EMS–related journals can keep EMTs informed about trends in prehospital care. Several journals offer excellent information, such as *JEMS* (Journal of EMS), *Emergency, Rescue, Prehospital and Disaster Medicine*, and *Emergency Medical Services*. Check with your instructor or service to see which journal is best suited to your needs.

Another way to stay informed is to join a professional organization. Several are of benefit to EMTs, including the National Association of EMTs (NAEMT) and the National Association of EMS Physicians (NAEMSP). Both organizations keep their members abreast of changes in EMS through newsletters, journals, and conferences. In addition to these national organizations, many states and local areas have professional associations for EMS providers. This is an ideal opportunity to learn more about issues that affect EMS and to participate in decisions affecting EMT–Basics.

As described earlier, EMTs should be patient advocates. With the exception of their own safety and

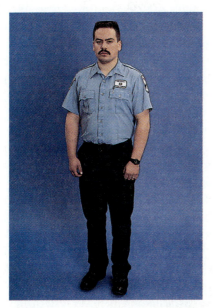

Fig. 1-8 As professionals, EMTs should maintain a neat, professional appearance.

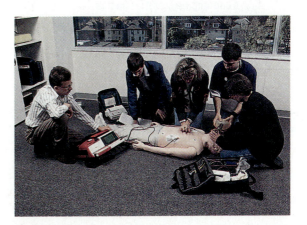

Fig. 1-9 Continuing education provides opportunities for EMTs to practice skills that are not often used.

that of the crew, EMTs must put the needs of the patient first. Serving as a patient advocate requires good judgment, which will develop further with clinical experience.

REVIEW QUESTIONS

THE EMERGENCY MEDICAL TECHNICIAN – BASIC

1. Which of the following is a role or responsibility of the EMT – Basic?
   A. Vehicle extrication
   B. Fire suppression
   C. Patient assessment
   D. Crime prevention

2. An EMT's appropriate professional appearance and confidence help to reduce a patient's _____?
   A. Blood pressure
   B. Length of stay
   C. Level of consciousness
   D. Anxiety

3. Continuing education classes help to maintain the EMT – Basic's _____?
   A. Knowledge and skills
   B. Professionalism
   C. Certification or registration
   D. All of the above

4. After ensuring safety of the EMT – Basic, the crew, the patient, and bystanders, which of the following is most important?
   A. Obtaining insurance information
   B. Being a patient advocate
   C. Teaching new EMT – Basics
   D. Vehicle maintenance

4. B
3. D
2. D
1. C

QUALITY CARE

QUALITY IMPROVEMENT

Quality improvement (QI) is a system for continually evaluating and improving the care provided within an EMS system. You may also hear terms such as *quality assurance* and *quality management*, which have similar goals of evaluating patient care to make improvements. Most EMS systems have a quality improvement system that identifies a program's strengths and weaknesses and guarantees the public receives the highest caliber of prehospital care.

The current trend in quality improvement is an approach that gives field providers such as EMT-Basics the resources, motivation, and education to detect problems, create solutions, and develop methods for maintaining quality care. The goal is to evaluate the system to determine which methods are successful and which must be further developed to improve the overall delivery of care.

As healthcare professionals, EMTs must ensure that patients receive the best possible care. This necessitates an active role in quality management —participating in patient care reviews and giving constructive criticism to both co-workers and management for methods of system improvement.

MEDICAL DIRECTION

Medical direction is the process by which physicians monitor the care given by EMT–Basics to ill or injured patients. In the past, some states required medical direction only at an advanced level and not for EMT–Basics. The nationwide curriculum change in 1994 called for a physician medical director to authorize certain skills performed by EMT–Basics.

These skills can be monitored through the two components of medical direction called **direct medical direction** and **indirect medical direction**.

Direct medical direction, also referred to as *on-line medical control*, means direct communication between the physician and the provider in the field (Fig. 1-10A and B). This communication may occur via a cellular telephone, radio, or telephone (landline). In some cases, the physician may be present at the scene of the illness or injury, allowing prehospital providers to speak directly with the attending physician. The role of a physician at the emergency scene may vary. Local protocol dictates the proper procedure for following the orders and advice of a physician at the emergency scene.

Indirect medical direction, or *off-line medical control*, consists of other ways physicians influence care, such as designing the EMS system, developing protocols and standing orders, providing initial and continuing education, and participating in quality improvement. Indirect medical direction

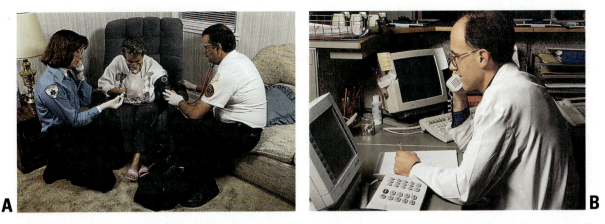

Fig. 1-10 Direct medical direction allows the EMT on the scene to consult directly with emergency medical staff at the medical treatment facility by radio or telephone to determine proper care for the patient.

encompasses all components of physician involvement beyond direct medical direction (Fig. 1-11).

The relationship of EMT–Basics and the medical director depends on the specific system. Rural and frontier providers tend to use the indirect approach because of distance factors. Urban and suburban providers often interact with medical directors more frequently. Ideally, the relationship begins when the medical director becomes involved in the education of EMT–Basics. This relationship continues as students complete courses and begin to provide patient care. The medical director participates in quality improvement of the service and aids in the development of protocols.

EMT–Basics have a responsibility to interact with the medical director in a professional manner and to abide by the decisions of the medical director. The medical director is a resource for problem solving before, during, and after patient interactions.

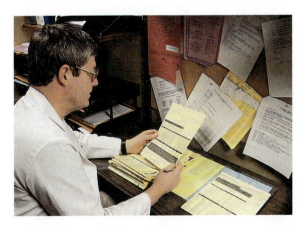

Fig. 1-11 Indirect medical direction, such as routine physician review of prehospital care reports, contributes to quality improvement and influences care to all patients.

REVIEW QUESTIONS

QUALITY CARE

Indicate whether the following activities are direct (D) or indirect (I) medical direction.

1. _____ The medical director meets with a crew to perform case reviews.

2. _____ The medical director rewrites the "Chest Pain Protocol."

3. _____ The medical director advises the EMT–Basic over the radio to administer sublingual nitroglycerin.

4. _____ The medical director advises the EMT–Basic to complete a trauma education program.

5. _____ The medical director orders the patient to be transported to a burn center.

6. Quality improvement is best described as _____?
   A. Sorting out the bad apples
   B. System audits
   C. A continuous cycle of evaluation
   D. Improving the patient care delivery system

6. C
5. D
4. I
3. D
2. I
1. I

Try to become acquainted with your EMS system of medical direction. A strong working relationship with the medical director will enhance the quality and appropriateness of the medical care you provide.

CHAPTER SUMMARY

THE EMERGENCY MEDICAL SERVICES SYSTEM

The EMS system is one of many agencies, personnel, and institutions involved in planning, providing, and monitoring emergency medical care. The National Highway Safety Traffic Administration helps states to develop EMS systems through established technical standards and assessments of EMS delivery in each state. These standards include: Regulation and policy; Resource management; Human resources and training; Transportation; Facilities; Communications; Public information and education; Medical direction; Trauma systems; and Evaluation. Each area addresses specific concerns for the quality delivery of EMS.

The four recognized levels of prehospital care providers as defined by the National EMS Education and Practice Blueprint are: First Responder, EMT–Basic, EMT–Intermediate, and EMT–Paramedic. All EMS personnel interact with other healthcare system professionals. EMT–Basics also interact with law enforcement officials and firefighters. EMT–Basics should establish a strong working relationship with these other personnel.

THE EMERGENCY MEDICAL TECHNICIAN–BASIC

The EMT–Basic has many roles and responsibilities, including personal safety; the safety of crew, patient, and bystanders; patient assessment; patient care based on assessment findings; lifting and moving patients safely; transportation of patients and transfer of care; record keeping and data collection; and patient advocacy. The individual ambulance service provides the EMT–Basic with a job description outlining specific roles and responsibilities.

The EMT–Basic is a healthcare professional with certain professional attributes: attending continuing education programs, projecting a professional appearance, maintaining knowledge and skills at a competent level, participating in issues that affect EMS on a local, state, and national level, and serving as a patient advocate.

QUALITY CARE

Quality improvement and medical direction go hand in hand. They are an important aspect of quality prehospital care. Quality improvement includes comprehensive planning, reviews of patient care delivery, and development of methods to improve the delivery system.

Medical direction establishes that all care given a patient is medically appropriate. Direct medical direction involves direct contact between the physician and providers in the field. Indirect medical direction includes other activities such as system planning, protocol development, education, and quality management.

UNITED STATES DEPARTMENT OF TRANSPORTATION NATIONAL HIGHWAY TRAFFIC SAFETY ADMINISTRATION EMT–BASIC OBJECTIVES

Check your knowledge. The National Registry of EMTs and many state EMS agencies use the objectives below to develop EMT–Basic certification examinations. Can you meet them?

COGNITIVE

1. Define Emergency Medical Services (EMS) systems.
2. Differentiate the roles and responsibilities of the EMT–Basic from those of other prehospital care providers.
3. Describe the roles and responsibilities related to personal safety.
4. Discuss the roles and responsibilities of the EMT–Basic toward the safety of the crew, the patient, and bystanders.
5. Define quality improvement and discuss the EMT–Basic's role in the process.
6. Define medical direction and discuss the EMT–Basic's role in the process.
7. State the specific statutes and regulations in your state regarding the EMS system.

AFFECTIVE

1. Assess areas of personal attitude and conduct of the EMT–Basic.
2. Characterize the various methods used to access the EMS system in your community.

THE WELL-BEING OF THE EMT–BASIC

KEY TERMS

Body substance isolation (BSI) precautions: Measures taken to prevent EMTs from coming in contact with body fluid.

Critical incident: Any situation that causes an emergency worker to experience unusually strong emotional reactions and that interferes with their ability to function immediately or at some time in the future.

Critical incident stress debriefing (CISD): A debriefing process conducted by a team of peer counselors and mental health professionals to help emergency workers deal with their emotions and feelings after a critical incident.

Hazardous materials: Materials that pose a threat or unreasonable risk to life, health, or property if not properly controlled during manufacture, processing, packaging, handling, storage, transportation, use, and disposal.

Stress: Bodily or mental tension caused by a physical, chemical, emotional, or other factor.

IN THE FIELD

A week after the fatal plane crash, John again woke from a nightmare of the crash scene. He still couldn't accept that a crash with no survivors had happened in his town. He remembered the radio call to implement the airport disaster response, his hurried drive to the ambulance station, and the drive to the incident command post. Dozens of ambulances responded within minutes, but there were no survivors for whom to give medical care. All of the EMTs had strong feelings of helplessness.

John had been thinking about the crash every day. He had lost his appetite and was having trouble concentrating at work. Everyone involved in the response was supposed to talk to the Critical Incident Stress Debriefing (CISD) team, but John didn't feel that talking would help.

When John arrived at work that day, his supervisor, Mary, and his partner, Lisa, met him at the door. "I think we need to talk," Mary said. Lisa had noticed his change in attitude and had tried to approach him, but he hadn't wanted to talk. She discussed the problem with Mary, and together they asked John to see the CISD team.

After talking to the team and the other EMTs at the crash, John still thinks about the crash, but without the negative emotions and tension of several weeks ago. The team was able to help John work through his frustration of being unable to care for the victims of the crash, and helped him remember the value of the work he does everyday.

EMS is a stressful profession. EMTs and other healthcare professionals are regularly called upon to help the sick, injured, and dying. EMTs must deal not only with physical illnesses and injuries but also with the emotions of the patient and the family, as well as their own emotions (Fig. 2-1). EMTs who are prepared to deal with these stresses may be better able to cope with the consequences.

EMTs also face personal risk in the form of scene hazards, exposure to disease, and stress. Knowing the warning signs of stress and how to deal with personal protection can help you to have a long and healthy career in EMS.

EMOTIONAL ASPECTS OF EMERGENCY CARE

DEATH AND DYING

Death is the natural end to all living things. At some time in our lives, we will all face death—the death of a friend or family member, our own, or that of a patient. Different people have different ways of coping with death, but there are some similarities in their general coping mechanisms.

Dr. Elisabeth Kubler-Ross observed that people facing death are likely to go through a series of stages as they discover their death is imminent and begin to deal with that fact. Understanding these stages will help you understand the patients', their family members', and your own reactions to death.

1. *Denial: "Not me."* This is a defense mechanism that allows people to feel that there must be a mistake when they learn they are dying: the medical tests were wrong, the results were misinterpreted, or something else went wrong. People often deny the facts even in the face of overwhelming evidence. As an EMT, do not agree with patients who are denying their illness. Be straightforward and honest if the patient and family question you about your knowledge of their illness or condition.

2. *Anger: "Why me?"* Once patients begin to accept the fact that they are dying, a common response is anger. Patients may become angry at those nearby who are in good health, the doctor who informs them of their condition, their family, or EMTs who respond to their home to try to help. Remember that the patient is not actually angry with you, and do not take any insults or anger

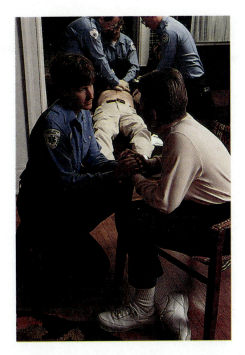

Fig. 2-1 EMTs must handle the emotions of patients and their family members as well as their own emotions.

personally. Be tolerant and patient, and do not become defensive. Listen to what the patient has to say, and answer all questions truthfully. Do not make false reassurances, such as saying, "Of course you will be all right," or "Don't worry, everything is fine."

3. *Bargaining: "OK, but first let me . . ."* Once patients begin to accept their imminent death, they may try to postpone the inevitable event by bargaining. "OK, I know I'm going to die, but let me live a while longer to see my first grandchild." Patients may try to bargain with doctors, themselves, or God.

4. *Depression: "OK, but I haven't. . ."* Once patients realize that bargaining won't work, sadness and despair may set in. They think of all of the happy things in their lives they will miss, and all of the things they will never get to do. These patients are often silent and retreat into their own world. They are preparing and grieving for their own death.

5. *Acceptance: "OK, I'm not afraid."* At this stage, people have made peace with themselves and are willing to accept that they are dying. Acceptance does not imply that the patient will be happy about dying, only that they realize their fate. Some family members still may not accept death at this stage and may require more emotional support than the patient. Be supportive of family members and the patient's wishes.

Not everyone moves through these stages in the same way or in the same time frame. Some patients may experience the stages in a different order or skip stages. Some people never make it through all of the stages, or they may return to a previous stage. The response to death is as varied as people are. The patient's progression through these stages is influenced by age, duration of illness, and family support.

Dealing with a dying patient and family members is not an easy task. Kindness, compassion, and understanding may help the patient or family members cope with their emotions.

Patients should always be treated with respect, and their privacy should be protected. Patients may feel the need to have some control over their treatment, and their wishes should be honored when possible. Always explain your actions to the patient and family members, and treat the patient with dignity, even when they are unresponsive. Often a gentle touch, such as holding the patient's hand on the ride to the hospital, will be remembered more than expert medical care.

Family members may feel rage and helplessness. Listen to their concerns in a way that shows you understand their concerns, but do not falsely reassure them that their loved one will get better. Let the family and patient know that everything possible is being done to help. Unless it interferes with care, allow family members to remain with the patient. It is important that they be allowed to express their love and sorrow to their family member. Allow family members to express their feelings. People grieve in different ways: some may cry, some may scream in anger, and others may show little reaction. Support the family and provide any comfort measures that you can.

STRESSFUL SITUATIONS

Stress and a career in EMS go hand in hand. EMTs feel stress in many different situations. Although different people find different situations stressful, some situations cause almost all EMS workers to feel stress (Box 2-1).

EMTs not only have their own stress to deal with, but often also have to manage bystanders or other patients who are experiencing stressful reactions.

Stressful situations may lead to stress long after the incident. After caring for an injured child, EMTs

BOX 2-1

Situations That Cause Stress

- Mass casualty incident
- Infant and child trauma
- Traumatic amputation
- Infant or child abuse, elder abuse, or spouse abuse
- Death or injury of a co-worker or other public safety personnel
- Emergency response to the illness or injury of a friend or family member

BOX 2-2

Stress Warning Signs

- Irritability with co-workers, family, friends, or patients
- Inability to concentrate
- Physical exhaustion
- Difficulty sleeping or nightmares
- Anxiety
- Indecisiveness
- Guilt
- Loss of appetite
- Loss of interest in sexual activities
- Isolation
- Loss of interest in work
- Increased substance use or abuse (alcohol, medications, illegal drugs)
- Depression

may be more protective of their children in the days and weeks to follow. Stress can also be caused by a slow buildup of smaller stressful situations. You must know the warning signs of severe stress and be able to recognize them in yourself or co-workers.

STRESS MANAGEMENT

Stress is a bodily or mental tension caused by physical, chemical, or emotional factors. Stress also involves the person's response to events that are threatening or challenging. Not all stress is negative. If we didn't feel the stress of knowing there is an exam at the end of the course, we might not read the book for class. If not for the stress of being late for work, we might never get out of bed. Stress becomes a problem when it is felt so strongly that it begins to hinder our ability to function. Emergency workers are not immune to the stress of an emergency situation. You must be aware of the signs of stress in yourself and in co-workers so that you know when to take steps to manage stress. Signs of stress are exhibited in different ways by different people (Box 2-2).

As different as people's reactions to stress, so are the ways stress is dealt with. Too much stress can unquestionably affect your health. Following are some proven guidelines that can help many people deal with their stress and avoid burnout (Fig. 2-2).

1. *Change your diet.* A healthy diet keeps your body in good condition and prepared to respond to an emergency. Consume only small amounts of sugar, caffeine, and alcohol. Avoid fatty foods, but increase carbohydrates. Also avoid excessive salt, which may increase your blood pressure. It is easy to miss meals during a busy day; don't forget to take care of yourself, and eat meals regularly.

2. *Stop smoking.* Cigarette smoking has been shown to double your chances of a fatal heart attack. Cigarettes contain hundreds of toxins that increase your chances of lung disease and cancer and contribute to thousands of deaths every year. Although it is difficult to quit smoking, most people can do it once they are committed to their decision. The benefits of quitting smoking are unquestionable. Cigarette smoking is the number one changeable risk factor for heart disease, which is the number one cause of death in the United States.

3. *Get regular exercise.* Regular exercise leads to improved cardiovascular fitness, strength, and flexibility and lowers your chances of becoming ill or injured. Exercise contributes to psychological and physical well-being.

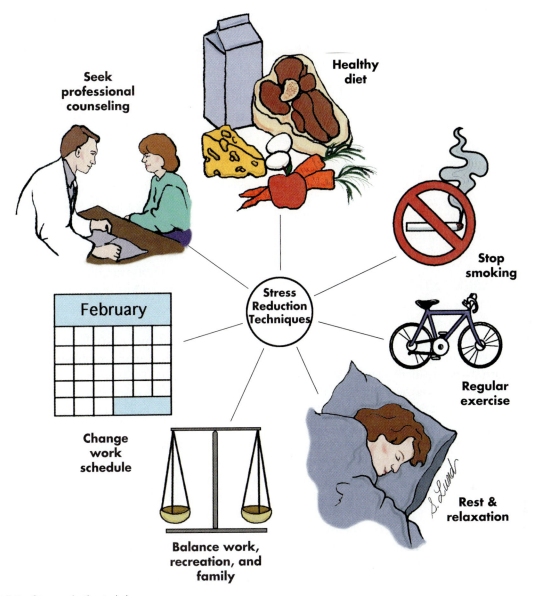

Seek professional counseling

Healthy diet

Stop smoking

Stress Reduction Techniques

February

Regular exercise

Change work schedule

Rest & relaxation

Balance work, recreation, and family

Fig. 2-2 Stress reduction techniques.

4. *Learn to relax.* Many people have learned to manage their stress by practicing relaxation techniques, meditation, visual imagery, and other methods.

5. *Balance work, recreation, and family.* Many EMTs and other emergency workers become heavily involved in their jobs. They may begin to define themselves based on their work, and may have trouble separating their professional and personal lives. Plan time away from EMS, and don't lose interest in your outside activities.

6. *Change work schedule.* If you find that you are feeling severe effects of stress, request a change of shift or duty assignment to a less busy area. No one expects emergency workers to be immune to stress, and it is not a weakness to need time to recover from stressful situations.

7. *Seek professional help.* You can benefit from professional help if the symptoms of stress are severe and you feel you can't deal with them on your own.

EMTs and other emergency workers are not the only ones who experience stress on the job. Family and friends of emergency workers also experience stress. Spouses of EMTs often want to share the burden of stressful situations on the job but may not understand the situations their spouse faces. At other times, family and friends may not want to hear about the emergency situations that their loved ones face when the EMT needs to talk. On-call shifts, rotating shifts, and late ambulance calls also make it hard to plan family activities. Families of emergency workers also have to deal with the fears of injury or death on the job. Talk with your family about these concerns and work out the best solution for you. Share your concerns with your family. Balancing work, family, rest, and social activities can help to alleviate the stress both you and your family may experience.

CRITICAL INCIDENT STRESS DEBRIEFING

Although EMTs deal with stressful situations every day, some situations cause reactions that are more severe than usual. For EMTs with children, the death or serious injury of a child may trigger great stress. For others, a patient who dies after a long rescue attempt may cause severe stress. Although the type of incident that causes severe stress varies from person to person, the result is often the same. A **critical incident** is a specific situation that causes an emergency worker to experience unusually strong emotional reactions and interferes with their ability to function immediately or in the future.

EMTs may also place undue stress on themselves if they have unrealistic expectations about their abilities to help. It is important to realize that there are limitations to your ability to help patients, and not every patient situation will turn out for the best.

One way to deal with a critical incident is through a process called **critical incident stress debriefing (CISD).** The debriefing process is conducted by a team of peer counselors and mental health professionals who help emergency care workers deal with critical incident stress. The meeting is held within 24 to 72 hours after a critical incident. During the discussion, emergency care workers are encouraged to discuss their fears, feelings, and reactions openly and honestly. The discussion is not an investigation into the causes of the stress, how the event was handled, or any technical matters. It is a chance to discuss the events and feelings with people who will listen and provide understanding and support, not judgement or criticism. All information is kept confidential so that everyone

involved can feel free to discuss anything. The debriefing team then offers suggestions for dealing with and overcoming the stress.

Everyone who was involved in the incident should become involved in the debriefing, including fire, police, EMS, dispatch, and emergency department personnel.

CISD helps people work through their emotional responses more quickly than they may be able to on their own. CISD accelerates the normal recovery process after experiencing a critical incident. Emergency workers get the opportunity to let out their feelings quickly after the incident. The nonthreatening, nonjudgmental environment encourages all workers to discuss their feelings. Often during CISD, general stresses related to the job but not related to the critical incident are discussed also.

Dozens of books have been written on stress, stress management, and CISD. Stress has become recognized as a real-world problem that affects emergency workers. EMTs are encouraged to expand their knowledge of job stress and become involved in helping themselves and their co-workers deal with stress.

Find out how to access your local CISD team, and remember that the service is there for you to use when you need it. Emergency workers shouldn't feel embarrassed or uncomfortable seeking help. We are all human, and we will need help dealing with our response to emergency situations.

COMPREHENSIVE CRITICAL INCIDENT STRESS MANAGEMENT

In addition to dealing with the stress after the occurrence of a critical incident, systems have been developed to help emergency workers, their families, and the community in general deal with stress in a more comprehensive manner.

Preincident stress education helps emergency workers understand how to deal with the stresses they will be facing as part of their job. By knowing the signs of stress and how to find the help you need, you may be able to avoid critical stress. In addition to preincident stress education, other health and wellness programs are in place to help you stay in good physical and psychological shape. On-scene and one-on-one support provides a network of other emergency workers to rely upon during times of stress. This support is focused not only on disasters and critical incidents, but also on the daily stresses that emergency workers face.

In times of disaster, support services are provided to emergency workers, their families, and the community. CISDs are a part of the support provided. Families of emergency workers also learn how to deal with the stress their loved ones are facing, as well as the stress they face themselves as families of emergency workers. In times of disaster, the community as a whole may need to have a place to turn to discuss their feelings of loss and sorrow. An earthquake, for example, not only affects those working to help victims of the disaster, but everyone involved in the earthquake. Community outreach programs are designed to provide a way for the entire community to become involved in the healing process of dealing with their feelings.

Follow-up is provided so that emergency workers are able to deal with their feelings after critical incidents. Some workers may not feel the effects of their stress for weeks or even months.

These comprehensive programs are a way of dealing with the effects of stress before stressful events occur, during times of great stress, and after the events are over. Remember these situations do not have to be something as big as a natural disaster to cause stress, but any situation that involves stress reactions.

SCENE SAFETY

Every EMT who responds to an emergency call is responsible for the safety of that scene. As an EMT, you are responsible for your own personal safety, the safety of other crew members, the patient, and bystanders, in that order. It is in the caring nature of emergency workers to begin treating an ill or injured patient as soon as possible. However, to be able to help anyone, you must first take precautions so that you are not harmed. EMTs who become injured cannot provide care or help to anyone else and must be cared for themselves by other EMTs, taking away from the care that can be provided to the patient.

You also must work as a team and watch out for the safety of your partners. As a team you can perform more efficiently and safely than as separate individuals. You must also take responsibility for the safety of the patients and do your best to allow no further injuries. With the help of law

REVIEW QUESTIONS
EMOTIONAL ASPECTS OF EMERGENCY CARE

1. Number the stages of death and dying according to Elisabeth Kubler-Ross in order, and match them with the phrase on the right that corresponds to the stage.

Order Matching

____	____	Anger	A.	"Not me."
____	____	Denial	B.	"OK, I'm not afraid."
____	____	Acceptance	C.	"OK, but I haven't . . ."
____	____	Bargaining	D.	"Why me?"
____	____	Depression	E.	"OK, but first let me . . ."

2. Everyone moves through all of these stages in the same order. True or False?

3. List at least three warning signs of stress.

_____, _____, _____

4. Critical incident stress debriefing should:
   A. Take place at least two weeks after the incident.
   B. Not include the person in charge of the call.
   C. Be an open and honest discussion of feelings and emotions.
   D. Involve criticism and judgement about actions taken on the call.

4. C
3. Fatigue; irritability; change in appetite; or symptoms listed in Box 2-1
2. False
   Matching: D, A, B, E, C
1. Order: 2, 1, 5, 3, 4;

enforcement personnel, you also protect bystanders by restricting them to areas out of the path of danger. Once the scene is safe, you should take further steps to ensure your personal safety by following body substance isolation precautions.

BODY SUBSTANCE ISOLATION PRECAUTIONS

One of the first steps in personal protection is to prevent the spread of communicable diseases from patients to you. Although some patients clearly present a disease exposure risk, it is impossible to evaluate any patient as safe. Patients infected with diseases such as hepatitis or HIV do not have a certain appearance, dress, or particular socioeconomic class. Contact with the blood or other body fluid of any patient should be considered a risk, and you should follow steps to avoid such contamination.

Body substance isolation (BSI) precautions are designed to prevent you from coming in contact with body fluid. Preventive measures to avoid exposure to a communicable disease are also a part of good patient care. EMTs could transfer a disease to other patients, healthcare workers, or family members if they are careless. To prevent the spread of infection, take the measures described in the following sections.

HAND WASHING

Hand washing is the single most important procedure for preventing the spread of disease. Effective hand washing involves vigorously rubbing the hands together with lathered soap, and then rinsing under a stream of water (Fig. 2-3). Hand washing should last for at least 10 to 15 seconds. Dry hands thoroughly with a clean cloth or disposable towel. Be sure to wash hands thoroughly after every patient contact, even if you were wearing gloves. There are also waterless hand-washing substitutes available for use when you do not have access to a sink and water but need to wash your hands. These solutions are usually alcohol based. The rubbing action causes friction, and the alcohol kills surface organisms. You must thoroughly wash your hands when you have access to a sink, even if you use waterless hand-washing substitutes.

EYE PROTECTION

Eye protection is available in a variety of forms and should be worn when there is the possibility of blood or body fluid splashing into the face or eyes. Any type of eye protection that stops fluids from reaching the eyes is sufficient; high-quality, expensive goggles are not required. Remember, the splashing of body fluids can occur in many situations, not only in trauma situations. Assisting in childbirth, for example, will likely place you at risk for contact with splashing fluids. If you wear

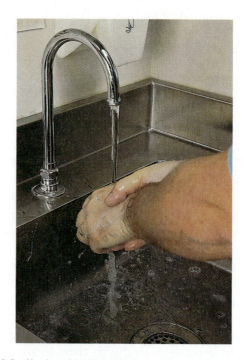

Fig. 2-3 Hand washing is the single most important procedure for preventing the spread of disease.

prescription glasses, you can apply removable side shields to them.

GLOVES

Wear disposable vinyl or latex gloves any time you are in contact with blood or body fluids, when there is a high chance that there will be blood or body fluids present, or that you will come in contact with mucous membranes or broken skin. Gloves should also be worn if you will be dealing with equipment that has been in contact with blood or other body fluids or mucous membranes. If a patient complains of nausea but has not vomited, you face a high likelihood of contact with vomit during the call, and it is too late to put on gloves once the patient begins to vomit. Prepare ahead and wear gloves if it seems possible that the situation could include contact with blood or other body fluids. Many EMTs find it convenient to don gloves before leaving the ambulance (Fig. 2-4).

Change gloves between contact with different patients to prevent cross-contamination. To remove gloves, turn them inside out using the cuff to pull them off so you do not touch the outside of the gloves with your hands.

You may not need gloves for all patient contacts. If a patient twisted an ankle while playing softball and has no open injuries, gloves may not be required. It is not always possible, however, to know

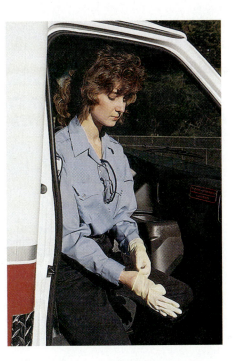

Fig. 2-4 EMTs should put on vinyl or latex gloves if it seems likely that the situation could include blood or other body fluids.

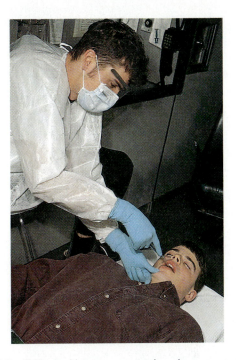

Fig. 2-5 EMTs should wear eye protection, gloves, gown, and a mask to protect against splattering during some procedures, such as suctioning.

when gloves will be needed at the beginning of a call. Therefore, many EMS providers are in the habit of wearing gloves for every patient contact. Consult your department's exposure control plan for your policy.

Utility gloves are required for cleaning vehicles and maintaining equipment.

GOWNS

Gowns are used for calls when large amounts of blood or bodily fluids are expected, such as in assisting childbirth. Regular EMS uniforms are also part of the protective barrier against body fluid contamination. Wearing a gown over your uniform keeps you from soiling your uniform. A change of uniform should always be readily available.

MASKS

Masks can be worn by emergency workers to prevent body fluids from spattering into the EMT's mouth or nose. If it is likely that body fluids will come in contact with your nose and mouth, it is likely these fluids will also contact your eyes; therefore, eye protection should also be worn (Fig. 2-5). Masks can be worn by a patient who has an airborne disease. If the patient is unwilling to wear a mask, you should wear one. For a patient

diagnosed with tuberculosis, specialty masks known as *high-efficiency particulate air (HEPA)* respirators are required (Fig. 2-6). Some models of these masks must be fitted to each individual EMT. Table 2-1 provides examples of BSI precautions used in certain circumstances.

REPORTING AN EXPOSURE

The Occupational Safety and Health Administration (OSHA), states, regions, and individual

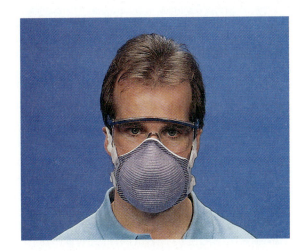

Fig. 2-6 EMTs should wear a high-efficiency particulate air (HEPA) respirator when transporting a patient with tuberculosis.

TABLE 2-1	Recommended Personal Protection Against Blood-Borne Pathogens in Prehospital Settings			
	PROTECTIVE EQUIPMENT			
TASK OR ACTIVITY	**DISPOSABLE GLOVES**	**GOWN**	**MASK**	**PROTECTIVE EYEWEAR**
Bleeding control with spurting blood	Yes	Yes	Yes	Yes
Bleeding control with minimal bleeding	Yes	No	No	No
Emergency childbirth	Yes	Yes	Yes, if splashing is likely	Yes, if splashing is likely
Endotracheal intubation	Yes	No	No, unless splashing is likely	No, unless splashing is likely
Oral/nasal suctioning, manually clearing airway	Yes*	No	No, unless splashing is likely	No, unless splashing is likely
Handling and cleaning instruments with microbial contamination	Yes	No unless soiling is likely	No	No
Measuring blood pressure	No	No	No	No
Measuring temperature	No	No	No	No
Giving an injection	No	No	No	No

Note: The examples provided in this table are based on the application of universal precautions. Universal precautions are intended to supplement rather than replace recommendations for routine infection control, such as hand washing and using gloves to prevent gross microbial contamination of hands (eg, contact with urine or feces).
* Although not clearly necessary to prevent HIV or hepatitis B virus transmission unless blood is present, gloves are recommended to prevent transmission of other agents (eg, Herpes simplex).
(From Centers for Disease Control Guidelines for Prevention of Transmission of Human Immunodeficiency Virus and Hepatitis B Virus to Healthcare and Public Safety Workers. MMWR 1989; 38 [NOS-6:35])
Note: BSI precautions may differ from universal precautions.

ambulance services are required to have policies and regulations for BSI precautions. The requirements for notification and testing after an exposure incident depend on the region. It is vitally important that all healthcare workers understand their rights and responsibilities under these laws and fulfill their obligations for reporting exposures. Each EMS service will review its exposure control plan with the crew members.

ADVANCE SAFETY PRECAUTIONS

Before new healthcare workers become EMTs or begin patient contact, steps are taken to help ensure their physical well-being. Your immune status to commonly transmitted contagious diseases such as rubella, measles, mumps, and polio is verified, and you may also be vaccinated against hepatitis B. In addition, you should receive a tetanus booster. Tuberculin-purified protein derivative (Mantoux) testing should be conducted in accordance with local or regional policies.

PERSONAL PROTECTION

Although every emergency response involves risk to the safety of the EMT, some particular scenes carry a greater risk. Three potentially dangerous situations are: hazardous materials spills, rescues, and violent scenes.

HAZARDOUS MATERIALS

A **hazardous material** is a substance that poses a threat or unreasonable risk to life, health, or property if not properly controlled during manufacture, processing, packaging, handling, storage, transportation, use, and disposal. Hazardous materials incidents should be handled by specialized hazardous materials teams. In general, specialty equipment and knowledge are needed, and crews not educated or equipped to handle the situation should let the hazardous materials team handle the situation. Call for the assistance of the specialty team as soon as a hazardous materials incident has been identified, and protect yourself and bystanders from harm.

Use binoculars to identify hazards at the scene. This allows you to identify any placards or marking symbols without coming close to the hazardous material. For hazardous materials incidents involving motor vehicles carrying hazardous materials, a placard will be displayed on the vehicle. A placard is a diamond-shaped sign displayed on hazardous materials containers (Fig. 2-7). If the placard can be identified from a safe distance, information from that placard should be provided to the responding hazardous materials team so it is prepared for the type of incident. The *Hazardous Materials Emergency Response Guidebook*, a publication of the United States Department of Transportation, contains concise reference information about hazardous materials and their identification numbers. This book allows you to identify the materials on the scene. For hazardous materials incidents at farms

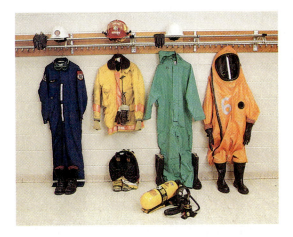

Fig. 2-8   There are four levels of protective clothing required to be worn for hazardous materials exposure. The self-contained breathing apparatus on the floor is worn with the two highest protection levels at right. An air purifying respirator is worn with the next highest level.

or industries, placards may not be displayed. In these situations, employees should know what chemicals are involved and can provide you with valuable information about them. Regardless of the type of hazardous material, do not attempt to enter the scene; wait for the hazardous materials team. For an overview of hazardous materials, please refer to Chapter 32, "Overviews: Special Response Situations."

The protective clothing required to deal with hazardous materials depends on the hazardous material involved. Different levels of hazardous materials suits and self-contained breathing apparatus may be required (Fig. 2-8). The type of suit varies according to local protocol and the type of incident. The suit protects the wearer from liquid and dry chemicals, and the breathing apparatus protects from inhaled contaminants.

EMTs provide emergency care to patients only after the scene is safe. It is not safe to enter a scene to remove a contaminated patient until the patient has been decontaminated and the hazardous materials specialists have informed you it is safe to do so. Premature entry could pose a risk to the patient, bystanders, and you.

If you are interested in receiving additional education for hazardous materials incidents, contact your local hazardous materials team or emergency management agency to find out about such education programs.

RESCUE

In a variety of situations, the patient must be rescued from places that are difficult to access. For

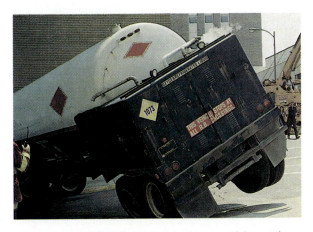

Fig. 2-7   A placard displayed on hazardous materials containers provides information about the materials inside.

heavy rescue or specialty situations such as water rescue or entrapment in a heavily damaged car, special rescue teams are required.

Most accident scenes involve a variety of threats to life. Most EMTs respond to car accidents, and the hazards at these scenes can be numerous. Along many highways are electrical wires and poles that can become obstacles when struck by a vehicle. High-voltage electricity could be conducted through those wires, and they should never be touched until the utility company has turned off the power. Fire and explosions are also possible risks, and you must carefully evaluate the situation before entering the scene. Broken glass, sharp jagged metal, and unstable surfaces are only a few of the concerns at most auto crashes.

Protective clothing is a must for all rescue situations, including the following (Fig. 2-9):

1. Turnout gear that prevents or resists puncturing.
2. Puncture-proof gloves.
3. Helmet with ear protection and a chin strap to keep the helmet on your head. Many helmets are equipped with face shields as well.
4. Eye protection, such as heavy goggles made specifically for working with power equipment. Face shields and prescription glasses are not sufficient eye protection.
5. Boots with steel toes and insoles are recommended.

If you are interested in participating in rescue operations, you must attend continuing education courses to prepare yourself for these incidents. Such courses cover safety issues, equipment, and rescue techniques.

VIOLENCE

Violent scenes should always be controlled by law enforcement personnel before you enter to provide patient care. Consider your own safety first. Allow law enforcement officials to determine that the scene is safe, and then provide care to the patient. Information about dealing with violent patients is covered in Chapter 23, "Behavioral Emergencies."

> **ALERT**
> EMTs should not enter violent scenes. Patient care can begin after law enforcement officials have determined that the scene is safe for EMS personnel to enter.

At a crime scene, disturb as little evidence as possible. Evidence you protect at the scene may solve a crime case. Do not disturb anything unless you must to provide medical care. If you must disturb something, make note of what you see, where it was, how and where it was moved, by whom, and why. This topic is discussed further in Chapter 3, "Medical/Legal and Ethical Issues."

CHAPTER SUMMARY

EMOTIONAL ASPECTS OF EMERGENCY CARE

EMTs face many emotional situations, including patients and their family members who are dealing with death and dying. Patients respond differently to injury, illness, and death. People pass through a series of stages when encountering their own

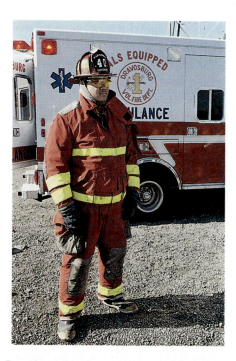

Fig. 2-9 Protective clothing is essential for all rescue situations. This equipment should include turnout gear, puncture-proof gloves, helmet with ear protection and a chin strap, eye protection (heavy goggles made specifically for working with power equipment), and boots.

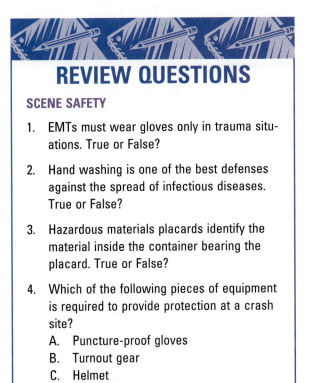

REVIEW QUESTIONS

SCENE SAFETY

1. EMTs must wear gloves only in trauma situations. True or False?

2. Hand washing is one of the best defenses against the spread of infectious diseases. True or False?

3. Hazardous materials placards identify the material inside the container bearing the placard. True or False?

4. Which of the following pieces of equipment is required to provide protection at a crash site?
   A. Puncture-proof gloves
   B. Turnout gear
   C. Helmet
   D. All of the above

5. EMTs should wait for law enforcement at all scenes of crime or violence, even if the patient states the violent individual has left the scene. True or False?

5. True
4. D
3. True
2. True
1. False

death: Denial ("Not me."); Anger ("Why me?"); Bargaining ("OK, but first let me . . ."); Depression ("OK, but I haven't . . ."); and Acceptance ("OK, I'm not afraid.").

Treat dying patients and their families with respect and dignity. Explain all your actions and honor the patient's wishes when possible. Patients may need to feel they have some control over the situation. Family members' responses to the impending death of a loved one may be stronger than the patient's, who may have already accepted their own death.

Almost all emergency workers experience severe stress when responding to situations such as: mass casualty incidents, infant and child trauma, amputations, abuse, death of a co-worker, or the injury or illness of a family member or friend. EMTs may feel the effects of stress immediately after a call, or the reaction may be delayed or cumulative.

Stress can be detected by a variety of warning signs including irritability with co-workers, family, friends, or patients; inability to concentrate; physical exhaustion; difficulty sleeping or nightmares; anxiety; indecisiveness; guilt; loss of appetite; and loss of interest in sexual activities.

Stress can be managed in many ways, not all of which work for all people. Some options for stress management include eating a balanced diet, not smoking, exercise, relaxation techniques, and balancing work, family, and recreation. Find professional help if stress is severe and you can't manage it alone. Families of EMS providers also feel the effects of stress. CISD allows emergency workers to discuss their emotions while counselors help them work through their problems.

SCENE SAFETY

As an EMT, you are responsible for your own safety and the safety of your partners, the patient, and bystanders.

BSI precautions include hand washing, masks, gloves, gowns, and eye protection. These precautions should be followed any time there is a chance you will encounter body fluids. It is not always possible to determine at the beginning of a call if body fluids will be involved. It is often impossible to apply gloves once a patient begins to vomit or bleed, so evaluate the need for precautions early.

Healthcare workers who come in contact with patients should be vaccinated against common communicable diseases and tested for others on a regular basis.

EMTs should not enter scenes that are unsafe or that require special knowledge and equipment. Specialty crews should be called to deal with hazardous materials and rescues. Law enforcement personnel should be called upon to control scenes of crime or violence. You may be able to identify hazardous materials by the placards on the container.

UNITED STATES DEPARTMENT OF TRANSPORTATION NATIONAL HIGHWAY TRAFFIC SAFETY ADMINISTRATION EMT–BASIC OBJECTIVES

Check your knowledge. The National Registry of EMTs and many state EMS agencies use the objectives below to develop EMT–Basic certification examinations. Can you meet them?

COGNITIVE

1. List possible emotional reactions that the EMT–Basic may experience when faced with trauma, illness, death, and dying.
2. Discuss the possible reactions that a family member may exhibit when confronted with death and dying.
3. State the steps in the EMT–Basic's approach to the family confronted with death and dying.
4. State the possible reactions that the family of the EMT–Basic may exhibit due to their outside involvement in EMS.
5. Recognize the signs and symptoms of critical incident stress.
6. State possible steps that the EMT–Basic may take to help reduce/alleviate stress.
7. Explain the need to determine scene safety.
8. Discuss the importance of body substance isolation.
9. Describe the steps the EMT–Basic should take for personal protection from airborne and blood-borne pathogens.
10. List the personal protective equipment necessary for each of the following situations: hazardous materials; rescue operations; violent scenes; crime scenes; exposure to blood-borne pathogens; exposure to airborne pathogens.

AFFECTIVE

1. Explain the rationale for serving as an advocate for the use of appropriate protective equipment.

PSYCHOMOTOR

1. Given a scenario with potential infectious exposure, the EMT will use appropriate personal protective equipment. At the completion of the scenario, the EMT–Basic will properly remove and discard the protective garments.
2. Given the above scenario, the EMT–Basic will complete disinfection/cleaning and all reporting documentation.

MEDICAL/LEGAL AND ETHICAL ISSUES

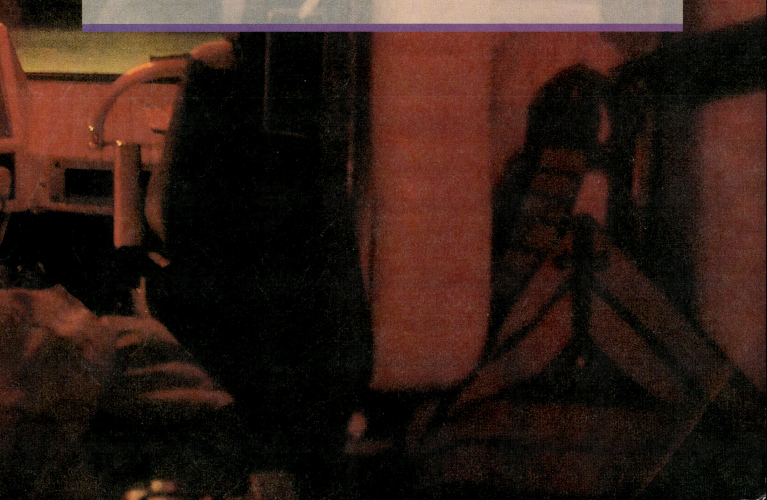

KEY TERMS

Abandonment: Termination of care without the patient's consent and without making any provisions for continuing care at the same or a higher level.

Advance directives: Orders from patients and their physicians regarding what care should be provided or withheld in certain emergency situations.

Assault: Threatening or attempting to inflict offensive physical contact.

Battery: Offensive touching of a person without the person's consent.

Duty to act: Legal obligation that certain personnel, either by statute or function, have a responsibility to provide patient care when the opportunity presents itself.

Expressed consent: Condition in which the patient agrees to the treatment plan and gives the EMT permission to proceed, while understanding any risks associated with the treatment.

Implied consent: Condition in which EMTs have legal permission to provide treatment to a person who is mentally, physically, or emotionally unable to provide expressed consent or otherwise unable to agree to treatment when treatment is needed due to a serious or life-threatening injury or illness. Care is given on the assumption that the patient would ask for and agree to treatment if able to.

Negligence: Failure to act as a reasonable, prudent EMT would under similar circumstances.

Scope of practice: The range of duties and skills EMTs are allowed to and supposed to perform when necessary.

Standard of care: The minimum acceptable level of care readily provided within a general area.

IN THE FIELD

On a warm summer morning, 7-year-old Tory and her mother were at the playground where she was learning to ride her bicycle without training wheels for the first time. Suddenly, Tory lost her balance and crashed to the ground. Almost immediately she cried in an anguished voice, "Mommy, my arm! My arm!"

The child's crying drew a small crowd of onlookers. Tory's mother asked one of them to call 911 for an ambulance, while she tried to comfort her crying child. Tory was sitting on the ground supporting her right arm across her chest with her left hand. Her right forearm was obviously deformed, and it was already beginning to swell. The bystander returned and reported that the 911 operator said an ambulance would be sent right away.

A few minutes later, two EMTs arrived in the ambulance. They quickly reassured Tory's mother and calmed the child while assessing her for any injuries beyond the obvious one. Her mother answered their questions about Tory's allergies and past medical problems while they splinted the injured arm. Tory was wearing her bicycle helmet, and although there were no indications of head, neck, or back injuries, the EMTs decided to use spinal immobilization procedures as a precaution. Throughout the process they took time to explain each procedure and why they were important to both Tory and her mother.

After moving to the ambulance, one crew member showed the child's mother where to sit and helped her fasten her seat belt. She asked that they be taken to the local Children's Hospital.

While en route, Tory complained that her arm still hurt, and her mother asked why the trip was taking so long. The EMT riding with them in the patient compartment explained that there was a lot of traffic at this time of day. He said that using their siren and emergency lights would make little difference in the transport time because of the heavy traffic, and would increase their risk of being involved in a traffic accident—a risk not warranted by Tory's condition. A few minutes later, they arrived safely at the hospital, and Tory's care was transferred over to the emergency department staff.

Most of the time, when a call for help goes out, EMTs find a patient who is in some degree of medical distress and who truly wants and expects to be helped by care on the scene and be transported to a hospital or other advanced-care facility. That is how things went in the opening scenario, but situations are not always that simple.

In addition to your essential medical knowledge, you must also understand the legal issues involved in EMS service. For example, in the opening story, what would the legal ramifications be if Tory had been alone and no parent or guardian could be found? What if her injury had occurred at home and Tory wouldn't say what happened but the story from her mother was inconsistent with her injury? How would the situation be different if the patient was a 260-pound person who, besides being obviously injured, was intoxicated, belligerent, and refusing treatment?

These are situations you can face on any call. How you medically, ethically, and legally handle such cases could mean the difference between a long and rewarding career in EMS and a long and painful journey through the legal system.

SCOPE OF PRACTICE

EMTs must function within both maximum and minimum performance guidelines called the *scope of practice*. **Scope of practice** identifies the range of duties and skills EMTs are allowed and are supposed to perform when necessary.

For example, driving an ambulance to the scene

of a motor vehicle accident and taking a patient's blood pressure are within the scope of practice for EMTs. Writing prescriptions and performing surgery are appropriate for physicians, but are beyond EMTs' scope of practice. Ignoring an accident victim's plea for help or failing to treat an obvious life-threatening injury would also be serious violations of the EMT's scope of practice because these actions are below the expected level of performance.

LEGAL DUTIES TO THE PATIENT, MEDICAL DIRECTOR, AND PUBLIC

EMTs have legal duties to their patients, medical director, and the public in general. Each state has legislation that defines the scope of practice for EMTs. Most states base their regulations on the United States Department of Transportation National Highway Safety Administration's National Standard Curriculum for the EMT–Basic (Fig. 3-1). Consult with an attorney, the state Attorney General's office or its equivalent, the attorney for the ambulance service, or local, regional, or statewide agencies with oversight authority if you have any questions about how state laws apply to your EMS activities.

EMTs have the duty to provide necessary care for the well-being of the patient as outlined by this scope of practice. However, the scope of practice does not automatically grant EMTs the authority to perform every identified skill. The **standard of care** is the minimum acceptable level of care normally provided in the area. EMTs may not be permitted to perform certain skills by their medical director if the local medical community or state regulations deem it inappropriate for EMTs to provide that particular care in their area.

The scope of practice may be broadened through protocols and standing orders. These are written policies that allow EMTs in the particular EMS system to carry out some treatments or procedures— in whole or in part—before consulting with the medical director. However, these are also at the discretion of the local, regional, or statewide medical director and must be approved by the agency with oversight authority.

As an EMT, your legal right to provide certain care depends on the availability of medical direction. EMTs can perform certain procedures only after consulting with a medical direction physician, such as assisting with patient medications or advanced airway control procedures. Whether permission is required depends on the nature of the skill, your own level of experience, the condition of the patient, and the physician's comfort level with your abilities.

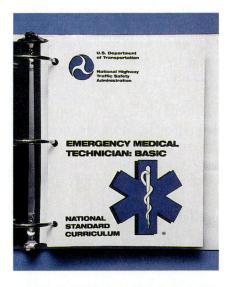

Fig. 3-1 In each state, legislation defines the scope of practice for EMTs. Most states base their regulations on the United States Department of Transportation National Highway Traffic Safety Administration's National Standard Curriculum for the EMT–Basic.

ALERT
Laws pertaining to patient care delivery vary from state to state. You should know how you are affected by your state's Medical Practice Act and other regulations. The information in this chapter is general and is not a complete guide to any state's legislative system, EMS laws, or regulations.

The way in which you obtain permission to give certain care also depends on various factors. You may be required to consult directly with a physician by radio or telephone, or face to face if there is a physician at the scene. In some cases, permission to carry out certain procedures is granted in advance by written protocols or standing orders. These enable you to carry out specified skills before speaking to a physician when the patient has specific signs and symptoms.

Standing orders may also be used in circumstances when direct consultation is not possible. This may occur with a patient who has a life-threatening problem requiring immediate attention or during multiple casualty incidents where there isn't time to speak to a physician about every patient. This may also occur if there is a failure of the communications system, such as when a severe storm knocks out telephone and power lines or in a disaster situation where radio and telephone communications are already overburdened with other emergency transmissions.

Because EMTs function as an extension of the physician within the defined scope of practice, the medical director has responsibility for the treatment rendered in the field. For this reason, the physician has the right to evaluate the performance of all the EMTs he or she has responsibility for and to withhold medical direction privileges from anyone who fails to comply with the established standard of care.

ETHICAL RESPONSIBILITIES

As an EMT you also have ethical responsibilities, including carrying out duties in a professional manner. A professional manner includes your attitude toward the care you give, regardless of whether you receive a salary for that service. In other words, there's more to being an EMT than just driving around in an ambulance with lights and sirens. You must address your responsibilities to the patient, the medical director, and the general public *on every call*.

Think back to the story at the opening of this chapter and try to view the events through Tory's eyes: It's not bad enough that you've wrecked your bicycle, but the pain in your arm won't stop. Your mother, who always knows what to do and makes you feel better when you get hurt, looks frightened and hasn't done anything to make the pain go away. There are several total strangers standing over you with frightened looks on their faces. And now, two strangers dressed like policemen are trying to tie some white thing onto your injured arm, which only hurts worse because they're touching it.

For Tory, this is a terribly painful ordeal both physically and emotionally. For the EMTs, it is a routine call in which they have a medical responsibility to treat Tory's obvious injury as well as other potential injuries. They have a moral responsibility to try to make what may be the most frightening experience of her life a little less traumatic. That means they need to help her mother calm down so she can try to help Tory be less frightened. They must be courteous to the onlookers who, although they are not doing much, would like to help but do not know how. They have a responsibility to drive carefully and safely to the hospital. They have a responsibility to use their emergency warning devices only when necessary (which means not in this case, since Tory's condition doesn't warrant it). In other words, even the most routine call demands that you perform at nothing less than your very best, with all of your concerns relating back, either directly or indirectly, to the welfare of the patient.

Your responsibilities do not end when the call is over. You have a responsibility to practice and maintain all of your skills. Because one can never know when, where, or which skill will be needed next, you must practice all to the point of mastery. You also have a responsibility to maintain and upgrade your knowledge by participating in continuing education programs to remain current in patient care trends and treatments. All oral and written reports must be honest and accurate because of the associated medical/legal and educational issues. You must examine your own performance (driving ability, treatment, response times, communications skills, patient outcomes, etc.) in an effort to improve upon any areas of weakness and to advance to the currently available standard of care.

DUTY TO ACT

In the simplest of terms, **duty to act** means that you as an EMT have a legal responsibility to provide emergency medical care when called upon or presented with the opportunity to do so.

LEGAL CONSIDERATIONS

Duty to act is complex because it can involve either a legal or contractual obligation, which may be either formal or implied.

A formal obligation exists, for example, when an ambulance service has a written contract with a municipality to provide service. Specific clauses in the contract identify when and to what degree service will be provided, and when service can be refused.

An informal contract is not likely to be written, but is just as binding. For example, in the opening story of this chapter, an informal contract was established when the bystander called 911 on behalf of Tory's mother. The caller gave the 911 dispatcher the information about Tory's accident, and the dispatcher told the caller that an ambulance would be sent. In other words, a call for help was accepted and help was promised as soon as possible; a contract had been made, even if it was only implied.

In some states you will be "licensed," while in others you will be "certified." In either case, the implication is that you have been educated to provide appropriate care and will do so when the need arises. In other words, regardless of the term that a state uses to indicate that EMTs have met some minimum educational requirement, you may always have an implied duty to act merely by being "licensed" or "certified." However, the laws pertaining to duty to act vary widely from state to state. Check with your ambulance service and local, regional, or state EMS agencies to determine when you have a duty to act.

Negligence. In any of the previous examples, if a formal or implied contract existed and if the service or EMT failed to follow through on it, then there was a failure to act. This could lead to charges of negligence.

Negligence occurs when a patient suffers damage or injury because an EMT fails to perform at the accepted standard of care. The judgment of the EMT's performance will be based on what any other EMT with similar education and experience would have done under similar circumstances.

Before negligence can be proven, four criteria must be met:

1. *There was a duty to act.* That is, as an EMT you had the responsibility to provide services.
2. *There was a breach of duty.* You failed to act, or failed to provide the level of service that another EMT of equal education and experience would have provided in a similar situation.
3. *Damage occurred.* That is, the patient suffered some physical or psychological injury.
4. *There was proximate cause.* This means that the physical or psychological injury that the patient suffered was caused by your actions or inactions.

Again, all four of these criteria must be met. In other words: if you did not have a duty to act, there was no negligence; if you did act and you acted appropriately, there was no negligence; if the patient did not suffer an injury (either physical or psychological), there was no negligence; and finally, even if the patient did suffer a physical or psychological injury, if it was not as a result of your actions or inactions, there was no negligence.

Abandonment. An **abandonment** situation occurs when care is discontinued without the patient's consent and without ensuring that care is being continued at the same or a higher level. Once you begin care, you must not stop until a person of equal or greater training assumes responsibility for the patient. For example, you cannot turn patient care over to a First Responder, nor can you leave the scene of an accident once you start to provide patient care except in these situations:

- You relinquish care to someone with equal or greater qualifications;
- You transport the patient(s) to a higher care facility;
- Your personal safety is threatened by uncontrolled hazards at the scene.
- The patient no longer needs or wants your services.

ALERT

Once you accept responsibility for taking action (beginning care, stopping at a scene, or even taking the call from the dispatch center), an implied contract to provide service has been established between you and the patient. Failure to provide or continue service could cause the patient harm and may potentially lead to a lawsuit for negligence against you.

ETHICAL CONSIDERATIONS

Some situations may not involve a legal duty to act but may still involve moral and ethical considerations. For example, in some states, EMTs have no legal duty to act when they are off duty. While riding in an ambulance with the purpose of rendering care to persons in need, there is clearly a duty to act. However, after your shift ends and you are driving home in your own personal vehicle (even if still in a work uniform), you may have no legal obligation to take action if you come upon a medical emergency by chance.

In a situation where a crew of EMTs are in their ambulance and proceeding through a municipality that is not part of their service area, they may not have to stop to render care at an accident scene that they come upon if they have no legal obligation to provide service to that community and therefore have no duty to act.

Although the EMTs may not have a legal duty to act in the situations above, is there a moral or ethical duty to act? What action is appropriate with respect to the profession of emergency medicine? How would the public feel if a patient was not given care in such a situation? How would you feel if you were the patient, lying injured on the street, to watch an ambulance drive by without stopping to help? How would you feel if you drove by and did nothing? On the other hand, how would you feel if you watched a loved one die of a heart attack, and found out later that your community's only ambulance had stopped to bandage the hand of the "town drunk" in a neighboring community while traveling back from a local hospital, although they had no legal obligation to do so?

If you have no legal duty to act, then you must answer such questions for yourself within the guidelines of your ambulance service, and within your own personal beliefs. Moral and ethical issues are inherent in EMS and cannot be ignored.

Even if you cannot decide purely on the basis of ethical responsibility, it may be wise to render aid as necessary even when there is no duty to act, because the benefit of doing so exceeds the risk. In other words, if you choose to provide care even though you have no clear legal obligation to do so, your care probably will benefit the patient and you will eliminate the possibility of being accused of being negligent for failing to act. In any case, you must thoroughly document the facts surrounding such an event and clearly identify what was done or not done and provide justification for your actions.

Remember, the laws pertaining to duty to act vary widely from state to state. Check with your own service and local, regional, and state EMS agencies to determine exactly when you have a duty to act.

REVIEW QUESTIONS

SCOPE OF PRACTICE

1. List the four criteria that must be present for an EMT to be guilty of negligence.

2. _____ refers to the range of duties and skills the EMT is allowed to and supposed to perform when necessary.

3. Abandonment occurs when an EMT ends _____ without transferring the patient to a healthcare provider at an equal or higher level.

1. The EMT had a duty to act; there was a breach of duty; damages occurred to the patient; the damages were caused by the EMT's action or inactions.
2. Scope of practice
3. Care

CONSENT FOR TREATMENT AND TRANSPORT

Consent means that one gives approval for what another does or proposes to do. In general, consent means the patient must give you permission to carry out any treatments and procedures, including transportation to a medical facility, before those treatments and procedures can be carried out. Laws concerning the specifics of consent vary from state to state. Therefore, you must be familiar with the statutes in your area and how they affect the scope of your practice.

EXPRESSED CONSENT

A patient may give expressed or implied consent for care. **Expressed consent** means the patient directly agrees to accept your treatment and gives permission to proceed with it. In short, the patient expresses a desire for treatment.

Expressed consent depends on two criteria:

1. The patient must be of legal age and able to make a rational decision. *Legal age* means an adult, but, this term is defined differently in each state. You must know what is considered legal age in your own jurisdiction. *Able to make a rational decision* means that the patient is responsive and of sound mind, and has a full understanding of the ramifications of his or her actions (or inactions).

2. You must explain to the patient all the steps of the procedure(s) and any associated risks. In other words, the patient has the right to know what to expect during a procedure, what can go wrong, and what the outcome could be if it does. This allows the patient to make an informed decision to let you perform the entire procedure, part of the procedure, or none of it at all. Remember, expressed consent must be obtained from all responsive, mentally competent adults before you can legally begin to treat them.

IMPLIED CONSENT

Implied consent assumes that all responsive and rational patients suffering from an immediately life-threatening or disabling injury or illness would want to receive treatment and would provide expressed consent if they could. Therefore, implied consent applies in cases where the person requiring treatment is mentally, physically, or emotionally unable to provide expressed consent (Fig. 3-2). Life-saving measures should never be withheld because doing so would likely be considered as negligence.

CHILDREN AND MENTALLY INCOMPETENT ADULTS

When a child requires medical care, consent for treatment must be obtained from a parent or legal guardian. Consent from an adult relative usually is enough if a parent is unavailable. If the parent gives consent, you have the legal right and obligation to treat the child, even if the child does not want to be treated.

On the other hand, a parent or legal guardian also has the right to refuse treatment on behalf of a child. This is a fairly rare event unless the child's injury or illness is very minor. However, you have little recourse in this situation unless the child's welfare is clearly in danger.

Attempting to physically take a child from a parent or guardian may be appropriate in very rare critical circumstances, but this action would almost

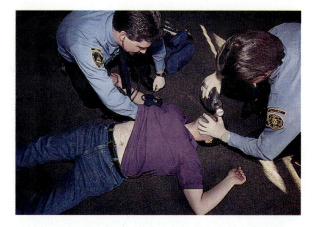

Fig. 3-2 Implied consent applies in cases where the person requiring treatment is unresponsive and therefore unable to provide expressed consent.

certainly lead to a physical confrontation and possibly injuries (or worse) to all concerned. That would probably do little to immediately help the child and could eventually lead to charges being filed against you.

In a case of a parent refusing care for a child in a life-threatening situation, your best option may be to quickly ask for the police to respond to the scene so that the child could be taken into protective custody. The child then becomes a ward of the state, and treatment can be rendered under implied consent. Consult with the medical director as quickly as possible in this situation for other options or suggestions.

Implied consent also applies in situations involving children when no parent, guardian, or other adult relative is available to give expressed consent. The presumption is that they would want the child to be treated if they were present to give their consent.

The one exception occurs when a child is an emancipated minor. *Emancipation*, in this case, means the child is free from parental care and responsibility. Emancipated minors have control over their own lives and are free to make their own decisions. In short, they are legally considered adults. Emancipated minors have the right to consent to treatment or refuse care for themselves. In most states, minors are considered emancipated if they are married, pregnant, or out on their own and able to provide for themselves. The specific statutes pertaining to emancipation vary from state to state. Therefore, you must consult with local authorities to determine the legal definition of emancipation in your area.

For a mentally incompetent adult, you must obtain consent the same way as for a child. Expressed consent from the patient's legal guardian is required before care can be given. Patients who cannot make or communicate decisions concerning themselves are considered to be incompetent. Persons who are mentally, emotionally, or developmentally unable to make rational decisions typically fit this definition. Also, as with children, if a life-threatening condition exists and no competent relative or guardian is available, life-saving measures should be carried out under implied consent.

Patients who are under the influence of drugs or alcohol and those who have a diminished level of consciousness because of their injury or illness may also be unable to make rational decisions. If no family member is available to give expressed consent on the patient's behalf, care should be given based on implied consent.

REFUSAL OF TREATMENT AND TRANSPORT

Adult patients who are of sound mind and who understand the consequences of their actions, even though injured or ill, have the legal right to refuse treatment. Treating patients against their will may lead to charges of assault or battery being filed against you. Transporting patients against their will may even be interpreted as kidnapping.

The patient also has the right to terminate treatment at any time after it has begun. For example: two EMTs respond in their ambulance to a private residence. Upon arrival they find an adult male who has experienced a sudden and unexpected loss of consciousness. They begin to treat the patient under the conditions of implied consent. After a few moments, the patient regains consciousness and then refuses further treatment and transportation to the hospital. He is an adult, and the only thing that has changed is that he is now responsive. As long as he is of sound mind (ie, he understands what has happened and can make rational decisions about his current situation), he has the right to refuse any further care.

However, to avoid liability for negligence, the EMTs in this situation should not simply pack up and leave at the patient's first refusal of treatment. They should first try to persuade the patient to at least go to the hospital for further evaluation of the injury or illness, even if he doesn't want to be treated by them immediately.

The EMTs also must inform the patient of the potential risks and consequences of refusing further treatment or transport. In other words, refusal of treatment and transport must also be informed and expressed, just the same as consent to treatment and transport. In this situation, the EMTs must explain the potential seriousness of a sudden loss of consciousness and explain to the patient why medical evaluation is needed to find the underlying cause. Because the unconsciousness in the above example happened without warning once, it could happen again, and the consequences could be life-threatening to the patient and to others.

The EMTs must be sure that the patient is not suffering from a mental impairment, either temporary (induced by drugs, alcohol, or the current injury or illness) or permanent (such as a mental illness), that prevents making a rational, informed decision. An impaired patient can be treated under implied consent, but unimpaired patients have the right to refuse their treatment efforts.

If the patient is mentally competent and still refuses treatment and transport even though it is clearly needed, the EMTs should consult with their medical director. This physician may be able to suggest alternatives or may talk directly with the patient to try to gain cooperation. It may also be appropriate to call for law enforcement personnel. However, police also have little recourse unless it can be determined that the patient intends to do harm to self or another or that the patient truly does have some type of mental impairment after all. In any case, the decision not to transport a patient should be made in consultation with other EMS officials.

At this point, if the patient has sound judgment and still refuses treatment or transport, you must thoroughly document all assessment findings, any care that you gave, and the facts related to the patient's refusal of treatment or transport. Then have the patient sign a "release from liability" form (Fig. 3-3). The form should explain that, after being evaluated for a potential medical emergency, the patient was offered treatment or transport to a medical facility and against the better judgment of the EMT refuses one, the other, or both. Also document that the potential consequences of refusal of care were explained, that the patient clearly and willfully expressed refusal of treatment or transport, and that treatment or transport would be provided if the patient called back at a later date (Fig. 3-4).

Try to have at least one witness sign the refusal form to attest to the fact that care was offered and

---

REFUSAL OF SERVICES

I hereby refuse the emergency medical services and/or transportation offered and advised by the above named service provider and its emergency personnel, _____ hospital, and the emergency medical and nursing personnel from said hospital giving directions to the service provider. I understand that my refusal may jeopardize the health of the patient, and hereby release the above named parties from any and all claims of liability in connection with my refusal.

_____
Signature of Patient or Legally Authorized Representative

_____
Signature of EMT/Field RN

_____   _____
Witness   Date

Fig. 3-3 A sample "release from liability" form.

refused. Preferably, the witness should be someone not affiliated with your ambulance service or the patient, such as a police officer, neighbor, or bystander. Documenting the witness's address, phone number, and reason for being there is important also in case later questions arise.

Just as the patient has the right to refuse care, the patient also cannot be made to sign the refusal form. Having a witness sign the form attesting to that fact is even more important in this situation.

Finally, if the patient has a life-threatening condition and you have any doubt about the patient's ability to understand the risks of the refusal or about the soundness of the patient's judgment, you should provide care. It is worse to be sued for wrongful death resulting from gross negligence than for giving care without expressed consent.

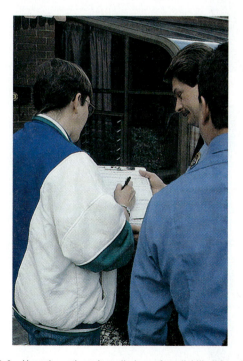

Fig. 3-4 Have the patient sign a "release from liability" form if the patient meets the criteria for sound judgment but still refuses treatment or transport.

ALERT

Merely having a patient's signature on a refusal of treatment form does not relieve you from liability. Thorough supporting documentation is crucial. Your documentation in such cases may be the deciding factor as to whether you get into, or keep out of, court.

ASSAULT AND BATTERY

The specific definitions and degrees of assault or battery vary from state to state. In general, **assault** occurs when someone threatens or attempts offensive physical contact with another person, or makes another person fear such contact. **Battery** occurs when a person is touched offensively without consent.

Consent means all people have a legal right to determine what happens to their body. Assault and battery go against this right. That is why adults who are of sound mind and have a full understanding of the consequences of their actions, even though injured or ill, have the legal right to refuse treatment.

If you defy the patient's wishes in such circumstances and try to give treatment (even by simply laying a hand on the patient, as in taking a pulse), you may be found guilty of battery. Even if you only cause the patient fear at the thought of being touched or treated after refusing care, you may be found guilty of assault. For example, saying something like, "If you don't let us splint your broken arm, we'll call the police and they'll come and hold you down so that we can," could certainly make a patient apprehensive about being treated and could therefore be considered assault.

ADVANCE DIRECTIVES

An **advance directive** is a written document some patients use to state what care they want to receive, or refuse, should they become unable to express their wishes in the future.

LIVING WILLS

A living will is a type of advance directive that is becoming more common. It is a written document that describes the kind of life-sustaining treatment that a patient wants (or does not want) if the patient later becomes unable to request, consent to, or refuse that treatment. The patient identifies how long and how extensive any resuscitative effort should be. This could be only compassionate care (accepting only nourishment, water, and possibly pain relief), only basic life support, or every possible advanced procedure that's available. The directive might also request several resuscitative attempts, one attempt only, or no attempts at all.

Life-sustaining treatment is an important phrase. It

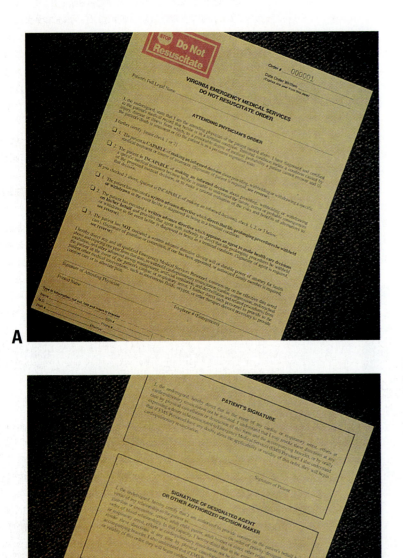

Fig. 3-5 Example of a Do Not Resuscitate (DNR) order. **A,** Front of form. **B,** Back of form.

means that the living will applies only in life-threatening circumstances. In all other cases where injuries or illnesses are less severe, appropriate care must be given when there is expressed or implied consent. For example, a patient's statement requesting no extraordinary life-saving efforts if diagnosed with terminal cancer doesn't mean a refusal of treatment for a broken arm.

DURABLE POWER OF ATTORNEY

Durable Power of Attorney is another type of advanced directive. In this chapter, the discussion will deal only with Durable Power of Attorney for Healthcare, although Durable Power of Attorney may exist for other matters as well.

Durable Power of Attorney is a written document identifying a guardian (one individual or possibly a group) to make medical decisions for the patient (eg, a parent being responsible for providing expressed consent or refusal of care on behalf of a child, as discussed earlier) when the patient no longer can make these decisions.

You are most likely to encounter this situation when responding to a terminally ill patient being cared for at home. Someone, often but not necessarily a family member, produces a document indicating Durable Power of Attorney for Healthcare for the patient. The document should bear the patient's and witnesses' signatures and be notarized. If the patient is no longer able to make rational decisions about care, the person(s) identified in the document has (have) the authority to make those decisions.

DO NOT RESUSCITATE ORDERS

Do Not Resuscitate (DNR) orders are another type of advance directive. They are written by the patient's physician, usually at the patient's request, stating that no (or very few) life-saving measures are to be taken if the patient experiences cardiac arrest (Fig. 3-5A and B).

These orders are also most commonly found in situations involving terminally ill patients being cared for at home or at long-term care facilities such as hospices or nursing homes. Because of issues concerning prolonged suffering, quality of life, and the cost of providing care for a loved one in a terminal and irreversible state, many patients are requesting that limited or no resuscitative efforts be performed.

An important consideration is that, although a written DNR order may exist, it may not be present at the scene. It may be kept on file at the patient's hospital or at the physician's office. Some patients and physicians provide copies of their orders to the local ambulance service so that responding crews can be given this information when they are dispatched. However, if you face a situation where you are informed of a DNR request but the physician's order cannot be produced, then there is little choice but to begin CPR or other life-saving measures. Consult with your medical direction physician if you encounter a situation such as this.

Also, you must not withhold care from patients with a living will who change their mind about life-sustaining care at the last minute, or if the person(s) having Durable Power of Attorney for Healthcare changes their mind.

Some states do not regulate EMS personnel in regard to DNR orders, living wills, or advanced directives. In fact, in some states DNR orders are considered beyond the EMT's scope of practice, leaving no choice but to start resuscitative efforts in these

REVIEW QUESTIONS

CONSENT FOR TREATMENT AND TRANSPORT

1. When a patient agrees to the treatment plan of an EMT and understands the associated risks, _____ consent has been obtained.

2. Implied consent can be used in the case of a patient who is _____, but is seriously injured and needs immediate care.

3. Emancipated children have control over their own lives and make their own decisions. True or False?

4. _____ occurs when someone threatens or attempts to inflict offensive physical contact. _____ occurs when someone actually touches another person without consent.

5. EMTs can honor DNR orders even if they do not see them. True or False?

1. Expressed
2. Unresponsive
3. True
4. Assault; Battery
5. False

situations. You must therefore learn about any state and local laws or protocols that govern your actions regarding DNR orders, living wills, and advanced directives.

PATIENT CONFIDENTIALITY

Confidentiality comes from the word *confide*. To confide in someone means to entrust that person with something. When receiving treatment, patients entrust EMTs with their lives, possessions, personal information, and privacy.

CONFIDENTIAL INFORMATION

You learn much personal information from patients in the course of assessing them and providing care. The patient's age, past and recent medical history, and personal information coming from the physical examination are all confidential. Treatments given also become confidential information.

Like everyone else, the patient has a right to privacy. All this information is considered the property of the patient. No one but the patient has the right to share this information with others.

The patient usually must sign a written release form before any personal information can be given out. You must not speak to friends, family, the media, or anyone else about the details of a call, including the patient's name, the injury or illness, what the patient said or did, what care was provided or refused, or where the patient was transported.

RELEASING CONFIDENTIAL INFORMATION

In certain situations, a signed release form is not required for you to share patient information with others. Some examples are:
1. When patients are delivered to other healthcare providers, you must relay information about them and their conditions and treatments to provide a complete transfer of care (such as reporting to a nurse when a patient is delivered to the emergency department).
2. Certain incidents require notifying law enforcement, and you must provide appropriate information in those situations. A police report may be required for industrial accidents, animal bites, rape, suspected child abuse, or gunshot wounds. Because reporting regulations vary from state to state, check with your local law enforcement agency to find out what incidents must be reported.
3. Third-party payment for services is fairly common for EMS providers. A third-party payer is an insurance company that covers the patient's expenses. EMTs or others in the service submit patient and insurance information so that the third-party reimbursement process can be started.
4. EMTs can be subpoenaed for information. A *subpoena* is a legal document from a court requiring information or an action. In such a case you must honor the subpoena or face the consequences for refusing to follow a court order.

SITUATIONS REQUIRING SPECIAL REPORTING

You may encounter other unusual situations that require additional reports or notifications. Suspected child, elderly, or spouse abuse commonly requires additional reporting. Crimes of violence such as a shooting, suicide, stabbing, or rape may also require additional reporting (Box 3-1). These reports may be required by service policy or local or state law. In some states, EMTs can be found negligent for failing to notify law enforcement when there is suspicion of abuse.

Other situations that may require special reporting include:
1. Exposure to an infectious disease. This type of reporting enables tracking of both the patient and you for follow-up evaluations or treatments to ensure the health and welfare of both as well as that of the general public.
2. Restraining a patient. Usually EMTs do not have the authority to restrain or transport patients against their will, and law enforcement should be called to handle this task. However, if this is the only way to protect the patient or others, it may be appropriate to restrain the patient, such as if the patient is attacking your partner. In this case, a special report documenting what happened is usually required. (Specific information pertaining to restraining a patient is presented in Chapter 23, ''Behavioral Emergencies.'')
3. Treating a patient without consent. This situation might occur, for instance, if you treat an intoxicated patient with an obvious serious in-

BOX 3-1

Cases Reportable Under Law in Most States

- Neglect or abuse of children
- Neglect or abuse of older adults
- Rape
- Gunshot wounds
- Stab wounds
- Animal bites
- Certain communicable diseases

jury who refuses care. A report may be necessary to document the facts that led to your decision that the patient was mentally incompetent and that treatment was necessary under implied consent.

Because the requirements vary from service to service and state to state, you must check with your service and local law enforcement agency to determine exactly what situations require special reporting measures.

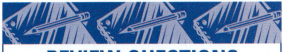

REVIEW QUESTIONS

PATIENT CONFIDENTIALITY

1. EMTs can usually restrain patients against their wishes without the aid of law enforcement personnel. True or False?

2. List at least three situations when EMTs may have to divulge confidential information about a patient.

1. False
2. Child abuse, spouse or elder abuse, rape, gunshot or stab wounds, animal bites, communicable diseases, infectious disease exposure, restraining a patient, treating patients against their will.

SPECIAL SITUATIONS

POTENTIAL ORGAN DONORS

Your greatest accomplishment as an EMT may be to save a patient's life. Unfortunately, even after the most dedicated efforts, that does not always happen with all patients.

Organ donation is sometimes described as the gift of life. If a patient has decided to donate their organs after death, you may have an opportunity to help save the life of another by acting on the patient's wish. However, legal issues are involved.

A situation may occur where the patient's survival is questionable and you learn that the patient is a potential donor. The law requires that there be a legal document, signed by the person, making known the intent to be an organ donor at death. This may be an organ donor sticker on the person's driver's license or a separate donor card (Fig. 3-6).

In this situation, you must not treat the prospective organ donor differently from any other patient. Such patients do not sign away their right to treatment. The card simply means that upon their death, the patient is offering his or her organs for possible life-saving transplantation into another human being. As with any patient, if you fail to give life-saving care to an organ donor you may be liable for negligence.

In any case, saving the patient's life is always the first priority. Saving the patient's organs is a secondary concern.

MEDICAL CONDITION IDENTIFICATION INSIGNIA

When assessing a patient or giving care, you may come across a medical condition identification insignia on a necklace, bracelet, or even ankle brace-

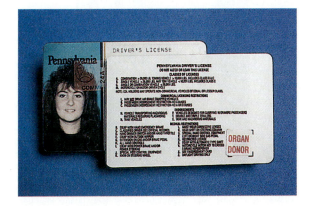

Fig. 3-6 A person may make known the intent to be an organ donor upon his or her death with an organ donor sticker on a driver's liscense or a separate donor card.

let. Its purpose is to inform healthcare providers of the wearer's medical condition in case the person is unresponsive or cannot communicate directly (Fig. 3-7). Patients wear such devices because they have a potentially serious medical condition such as diabetes, severe allergies, epilepsy, or asthma that requires rapid intervention. A caduceus is sometimes engraved on one side and the patient's medical problem on the other. There may also be an identification number or telephone number for obtaining more information about the patient's medical condition.

Some patients carry a wallet card identifying their medical condition(s). Most patients carrying a wallet card also wear an insignia necklace or bracelet. If the insignia device suggests checking the wearer's wallet for additional information, then you should do so if you can retrieve the wallet without causing unnecessary movement or worsening of the patient's medical condition.

CONSIDERATIONS AT POSSIBLE CRIME SCENES

You may know that you are going to a crime scene when you are dispatched. In this case, police are probably already on the scene or being dispatched. Your first concern should be for your own safety. Stand by at a safe location near the scene and wait for the police to arrive. After the police have secured the scene, you can enter and begin to treat the patient.

If the police are already on the scene, check with them first to see if the scene has been secured. If

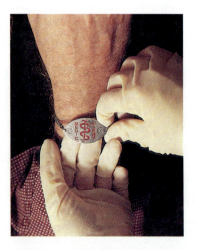

Fig. 3-7 The Medic-Alert® tag informs healthcare providers of the wearer's medical condition if the person is unresponsive or cannot communicate directly.

your personal safety is relatively assured, you may enter the scene and treat the patient.

In a different situation, you may not be aware that a violent crime has taken place until after you are already on the scene. If violence is still occurring or seems possible, call for police assistance immediately and take measures to ensure your own safety, even if that means leaving without providing care. If you find it necessary to leave the scene without the patient, go to a safe location from which you can quickly return to the scene. Remain at this location of safety until police arrive to secure the scene, and then return to provide patient care when needed or called upon.

You may arrive at a scene that appears to be safe if the perpetrator of the violence has already left. Police may not yet be present or en route because the crime has not yet been reported. In this case, you should request police assistance if there is reason to believe a crime has been committed.

In any event, your primary concern once the scene is safe and personal safety is assured, is to provide emergency medical care to the patient. Any time care is delayed in any of these situations —while awaiting police arrival or leaving the scene for safety reasons—be sure to document the reason for the delay and the event(s) that caused it.

If possible, try not to disturb anything at the scene unless absolutely necessary to provide patient care. Blood trails, the position of furniture, small items on the floor, and the location and position of the victim are all evidence and may provide clues about the crime. If something must be moved, try to remember its exact location, and tell the police.

If the victim has been shot or stabbed, try to avoid cutting, tearing, or otherwise damaging or destroying knife or bullet holes in the clothing. The clothing is an important piece of evidence, and the police can learn much about the crime and the perpetrator from the size, shape, and location of holes that are still intact.

Finally, pay close attention to what you see and hear in a possible crime scene, especially anything out of the ordinary. Include any observations in the prehospital care report. If you observe things that you do not include in the prehospital care report form because they do not involve patient care (for example, the patient's state of dress or the presence of money strewn about the scene), make additional documentation listing this other information. Most services have generic special or supplemental report forms for documentation of nonpatient care issues and events. All this information is extremely important, particularly if the patient must be transported before the police arrive on scene. Your observations may be crucial pieces of information.

REVIEW QUESTIONS

SPECIAL SITUATIONS

1. Name at least 3 conditions for which patients commonly wear medical condition identification insignia.

2. EMTs should not treat patients who have been the victim of violent crimes because they may destroy evidence while treating them. True or False?

1. Diabetes; allergies; epilepsy; asthma; contact lenses
2. False

CHAPTER SUMMARY

SCOPE OF PRACTICE

EMTs have legal responsibilities to patients, the medical director, and the public at large. These responsibilities are identified by the EMT's scope of practice and the standard of care in the area.

EMTs provide care measures as outlined by the state's EMS legislation. That legislation identifies the scope of practice, (ie, the maximum and minimum performance guidelines for functioning). Any legal questions about an EMT's actions are based on how those specific activities compare with the actions of any other EMT with the same education and experience under similar conditions.

Duty to act refers to the legal responsibility that requires EMTs to take action by rendering care when needed. In some cases, there may actually be no legal responsibility to take action. However, EMTs should also consider the moral and ethical consequences of not taking action when facing such a dilemma.

Failure to provide care, or providing care incorrectly or inappropriately, may make EMTs liable for negligence. Starting but failing to follow through with care or to transfer care to another provider with equal or greater education may make an EMT liable for abandonment.

CONSENT FOR TREATMENT AND TRANSPORT

Adult patients who are of sound mind and understand the consequences of their actions have the legal right to refuse treatment or transport to a care facility, even when obviously ill or injured. The legal basis for this is the right of people to determine what happens to their own body. Therefore EMTs must have the patient's permission to provide any and all treatment or transport. If the patient is an adult of sound mind who is asking for help or agrees to be helped, and fully understands the risks associated with the procedures, then the patient gives expressed consent. With an unresponsive patient, EMTs can provide care under the guidelines of implied consent. Under implied consent, the presumption is that any rational adult, if able to, would provide expressed consent to have life-threatening or severely disabling injuries treated.

Children and adults who are mentally incompetent cannot be expected to make rational judgments about the care they receive or deny, and therefore a parent or legal guardian has the responsibility for giving or withholding expressed consent. If there is a severe or life-threatening injury or illness, EMTs may initiate care within the guidelines of implied consent, until expressed consent can be obtained.

Adults who are of sound mind have the right to accept or refuse treatment, even if obviously sick or injured. EMTs who treat the patient without consent may be found guilty of battery for touching the patient against his or her will. Even if the EMT only suggests that treatment will be provided and thereby instills some fear in the patient, assault could be charged. Thorough documentation of the events is extremely important.

A living will is an advance directive. It is a written document that describes the kind of life-sustaining treatment that a patient wants (or does not want) if the patient later becomes unable to request, consent to, or refuse that treatment.

Do Not Resuscitate (DNR) orders, another type

of advance directive, are written standing orders from a physician that identify what treatments should and should not be rendered to the patient in the event of cardiac arrest. They are most frequently encountered when dealing with terminally ill patients being cared for at home or in a long-term care facility. The purpose of DNR orders is to allow patients to die with dignity by not prolonging their suffering. An EMT facing a cardiac arrest patient has little choice but to start resuscitative efforts if written DNR orders cannot be produced. Also, some states consider acceptance of DNR orders to be outside the EMT's scope of practice.

PATIENT CONFIDENTIALITY

EMTs learn a significant amount of personal information about a patient. All of that information is considered private and therefore cannot be released without the patient's written permission. There are a few instances when EMTs either may or must release confidential patient information; these are all related to line of duty events (transferal of the patient's care to another, for third-party billing purposes, or when subpoenaed to do so).

Other unusual situations may also require EMTs to release confidential patient information. These situations depend on the nature or circumstances of the incident (child, elderly, spouse abuse; rape; shootings or stabbings; treating or transporting a patient without consent; exposure to infectious disease; etc.).

SPECIAL SITUATIONS

EMTs should treat a patient who is a prospective organ donor the same as any other patient. Any legal document that patients signed to become an organ donor does not sign away their right to treatment. EMTs who become aware that the patient is a prospective donor, if the patient's survivability is in question, should consult with the medical direction physician. Continued resuscitation efforts are likely to be ordered, even if the patient will not survive.

EMTs may also encounter patients wearing medical condition identification insignia, usually in the form of a necklace, bracelet, or ankle bracelet. The item is designed to alert healthcare providers that the patient has a serious medical condition. They are usually readily visible and easily seen during the physical examination. Other patients may carry a wallet card with medical information listed on it in place of but usually in addition to a necklace or bracelet.

When dispatched to treat a patient who was injured as a result of a crime, an EMT's first concern is for personal safety. If the scene is not secure and there are indications of personal danger, EMTs should take whatever measures are necessary to ensure their safety, even if that means leaving the scene without providing care. The EMT can provide patient care after returning to the scene once it is secure.

After personal safety is relatively assured at a scene of crime or violence, the EMT should provide life-saving care to the patient, and touch or move as few things as possible so that the crime scene may be preserved. Make a mental note of where things are and other observations, as this information may provide valuable evidence for the police investigation.

If the patient was shot or stabbed, EMTs should attempt to avoid cutting or tearing any knife or bullet holes in the clothing. Clothing is also evidence, and the size, shape, number, and location of bullet or knife holes may be very valuable in helping to solve the crime.

Check your knowledge. The National Registry of EMTs and many state EMS agencies use the objectives below to develop EMT–Basic certification examinations. Can you meet them?

COGNITIVE

1. Define the EMT–Basic scope of practice.
2. Discuss the importance of Do Not Resuscitate (DNR) [advance directives] and local or state provisions regarding EMS application.
3. Define consent and discuss the methods of obtaining consent.
4. Differentiate between expressed and implied consent.
5. Explain the role of consent of minors in providing care.
6. Discuss the implications for the EMT–Basic in patient refusal of transport.
7. Discuss the issues of abandonment, negligence, and battery and their implications to the EMT–Basic.
8. State the conditions necessary for the EMT–Basic to have a duty to act.
9. Explain the importance, necessity, and legality of patient confidentiality.
10. Discuss the considerations of the EMT–Basic in issues of organ retrieval.
11. Differentiate the actions that an EMT–Basic should take to assist in the preservation of a crime scene.
12. State the conditions that require an EMT–Basic to notify local law enforcement officials.

AFFECTIVE

1. Explain the rationale for the needs, benefits, and usage of advance directives.
2. Explain the rationale for the concept of varying degrees of DNR.
3. Explain the role of EMS and the EMT–Basic regarding patients with DNR orders.

THE HUMAN BODY

KEY TERMS

Accessory breathing muscles: The additional muscles used by patients in respiratory distress to draw more air into the chest.

Adrenaline: A hormone that helps prepare the body for emergencies.

Anatomic position: The position in which the patient is standing upright and facing forward, with palms facing forward.

Bilateral: A directional term describing the right and left sides of the body relative to each other.

Blood pressure: A measure of the pressure exerted against the walls of the arteries.

Breath sounds: The sound of air moving in and out of the lungs.

Central pulse: A pulse point in or near the trunk.

Heart rate: The number of times the heart beats per minute.

Hemoglobin: The chemical that carries oxygen in the blood and releases it when it reaches the tissues.

Hormones: Body chemicals secreted by glands in the endocrine system that regulate body activities and functions in many body systems.

Insulin: A hormone that is crucial for the body's use of sugars.

Intercostal muscles: The muscles located between each rib that move with breathing.

Midaxillary line: An imaginary line that extends vertically from the armpits to the ankles, dividing the body into anterior (front) and posterior (back) halves.

Midclavicular line: Each of two imaginary lines that divide the clavicles (collar bones) in two and extend down the trunk through each nipple.

Midline: An imaginary line through the middle of the body that starts at the top of the head and goes through the nose and the umbilicus.

Perfusion: The process of circulating blood to the organs, delivering oxygen, and removing wastes.

Peripheral pulse: A pulse point in an extremity.

Platelets: The blood component that plays an important role in blood clotting.

Red blood cells: The blood cells that contain hemoglobin.

Sutures: The joints between the skull bones.

Thorax: The bone structure composed of twelve pairs of ribs and the sternum.

Tidal volume: The volume of air per breath.

White blood cells: The blood cells that are a main part of the body's defense against infection.

IN THE FIELD

EMTs Scott and Stacy were dispatched to a scene in which a young girl had fallen off her bike. Dispatch reported that her arm was bleeding and her mother thought her leg might be broken. When they arrived they found that a small crowd had gathered around a little blonde girl who was being comforted by her mother. After checking scene safety and taking body substance isolation precautions, Stacy approached the little girl. "Hi, my name is Stacy. I'm an EMT, and I'm here to help you. What's your name?" The tearful, scared child squeaked out a meek answer, "Tahnee."

"I see you fell off of your bike. Where do you hurt?" Stacy asked in a reassuring, sympathetic voice as she noticed the blood oozing from Tahnee's hand and elbow.

The 8-year-old girl couldn't hold back the tears as she cried, "My knee really hurts and I skinned my hand."

After establishing rapport with Tahnee and her mother, Stacy and Scott stabilized Tahnee's cervical spine, bandaged her wounds, splinted her knee, and placed her on a long backboard. En route to the hospital, Scott called the emergency department. After the preliminary information, he described Tahnee's injuries over the radio: "She has an abrasion on the ventral surface of her right hand, and a 4-cm laceration just distal to her right elbow. The right patella is deformed medially, and there is some tenderness just proximal to the knee."

The doctor responded, "Thanks. We'll be ready for her when you get here."

As the opening example shows, the patient, the parent, and the EMT all described the same injury in different ways. They each spoke with different needs and from different levels of experience. You already know the common names of most body parts, and this is important when you speak with patients. However, this everyday vocabulary is not precise enough for medical purposes. As a medical professional you need to describe to other clinicians your physical examination findings and the location of injuries. This ability requires a familiarity with human anatomy and medical terminology.

ANATOMIC TERMS

THE ANATOMIC POSITION

To communicate effectively, healthcare professionals follow medical conventions of language. The most basic concept is the **anatomic position.** All directional and anatomic terms for the human body assume that the patient is standing upright and facing forward, with palms facing forward (Fig. 4-1). Obviously, patients are rarely found in the anatomical position, but agreement on what is "normal" enables us to accurately describe parts of the body in relation to this fixed standard. For example, an injury "above the elbow" is still referred to as "above" even if the hand and arm are pointing up and the injury would, in nonmedical language, seem at that moment "below" the elbow. Using the anatomical position removes any doubt about what directional terms mean.

The body can be divided by a number of imaginary lines. These lines are very useful when you are describing the specific location of injuries on the torso (trunk). The **midline** is an imaginary line through the middle of the body that starts at the top of the head and goes through the nose and the umbilicus (belly button). The midline divides the body into right and left halves. Whenever you refer to the sides of the body, you always refer to the patient's right or left. For example, the heart lies immediately to the left of the midline.

The term **bilateral** is used when describing the right and left sides relative to each other. For example, the right side of the chest rising at the same time and to the same degree as the left side is called *equal chest rise, bilaterally*. An injury or finding on one side of the body is called *unilateral*.

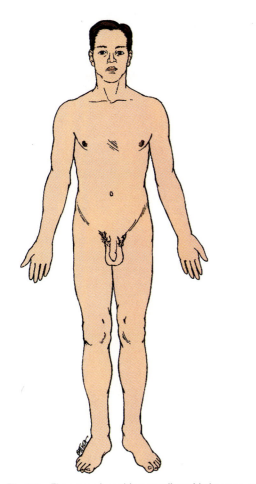

Fig. 4-1 The anatomic position: standing with the arms at the sides and the palms, head, and feet facing forward.

The left and right **midclavicular lines** are imaginary lines that divide the clavicles (collar bones) in two and extend down the trunk through the nipples. The **midaxillary line** extends vertically from the armpits to the ankles. The midaxillary line divides the body into anterior (front) and posterior (back) halves (Fig. 4-2).

DESCRIPTIVE ANATOMIC TERMS

The directional terms in Table 4-1 are important for communicating with fellow EMTs and other healthcare professionals. This terminology can be used to accurately describe physical examination findings and the location of pain or injuries. Notice how these terms work in pairs of opposites. It is important that you integrate these words into your vocabulary so that they become second nature when talking with other health professionals.

Many terms are used to describe the position of the whole body. As an EMT you must be familiar with at least the five positions described in

Table 4-2. These terms are useful as you explain how patients are positioned when you find them or how you position them for transportation.

BODY SYSTEMS

The human body is the envy of modern engineering. Never has an engineer even come close to creating anything as well designed and constructed. The complexity of the human body can be better understood by considering its separate parts, although no body system functions independently. A body system is a group of organs that work together to perform a function. Although each body system is described in the following sections as an independent component, they are all interconnected.

THE RESPIRATORY SYSTEM

The respiratory system plays a crucial role in the delicate balance of life. The body is composed of trillions of cells that convert sugar to energy in the presence of oxygen. This process gives off carbon dioxide as a waste product. The respiratory system takes oxygen from the air and makes it available for the blood to transport to every cell and rids the body of excess carbon dioxide.

THE AIRWAY

Air enters and exits the respiratory system through the mouth and the nose (Fig. 4-12). These two structures play an important role in warming, cleaning, and humidifying inhaled air. The pharynx is a muscular tube commonly referred to as the *throat*.

The pharynx is divided into two areas: the nasopharynx and the oropharynx. The nasopharynx lies directly behind the nose. The oropharynx is just behind the mouth and extends to the level of the epiglottis. The epiglottis is a leaflike flap that prevents food and liquid from entering the trachea (windpipe) during swallowing. The pharynx is a common pathway for both food and air. Because air and food pass through the pharynx, it is often the location of airway obstructions by foreign bodies.

Just inferior to the epiglottis is the opening to the trachea. The larynx, or voice box, is just below this opening. The vocal cords are bands of cartilage that vibrate when we speak. The most prominent structure of the larynx is the thyroid cartilage, which

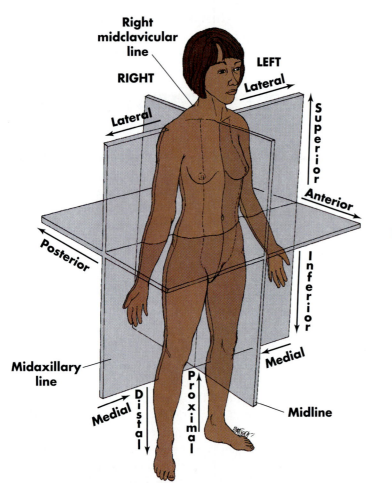

Fig. 4-2 Directions and planes of the body.

TABLE 4-1	Directional Terminology	
Term	**Definition**	**Example**
Medial	Toward the midline	The eyes are medial to the ears
Lateral	Away from the midline	The ears are lateral to the eyes
Proximal	Toward the trunk	The elbow is proximal to the forearm
Distal	Away from the trunk	The ankle is distal to the knee
Superior	Toward the top of the body	The shoulder is superior to the hips
Inferior	Toward the bottom of the body	The stomach is inferior to the heart
Right	To the patient's right	The appendix is on the right side of the body
Left	To the patient's left	The stomach is to the left of the liver
Posterior (dorsal)	Toward the back	The shoulder blades are on the posterior (dorsal) of the torso
Anterior (ventral)	Toward the front	The belly button is on the ventral surface
Plantar	The bottom of the foot	The sole of the foot is the plantar surface
Palmar	The palm of the hand	In the anatomic position, the palmar surface of the hand faces forward

TABLE 4-2   Positional Terminology

Term	Definition	
Prone	The patient lying flat on the stomach (Fig. 4-3).	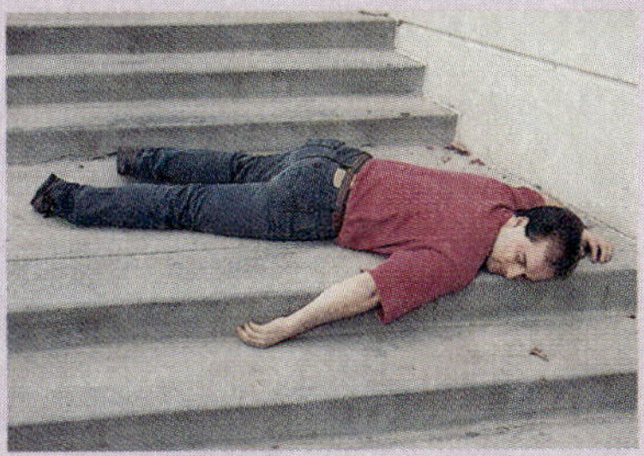 **Fig. 4-3** This patient is lying prone.
Supine	The patient lying flat on the back (Fig. 4-4).	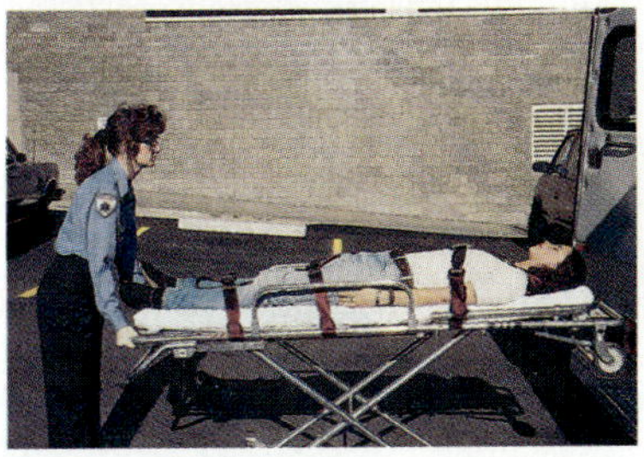 **Fig. 4-4** Patient in supine position.
Fowler's	The patient lying on the back with an approximately 45° bend at the hips (Fig. 4-5).	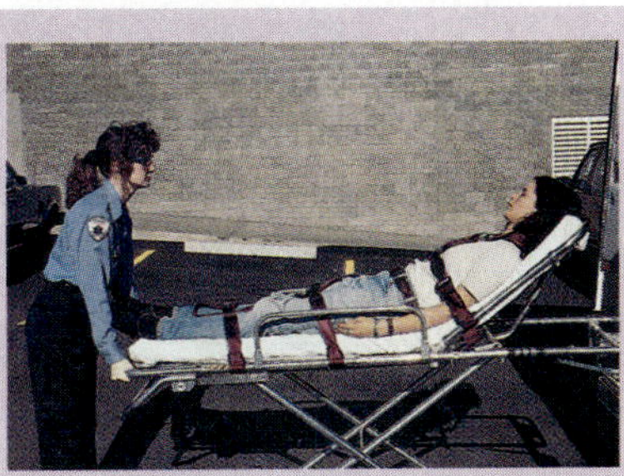 **Fig. 4-5** Patient in Fowler's position.
Trendelenburg's	The patient lying flat on the back, on an incline, and with feet elevated approximately 12 inches above the head (Fig. 4-6).	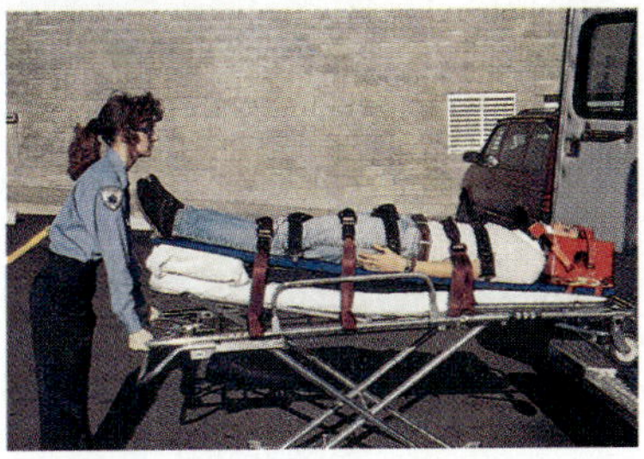 **Fig. 4-6** Patient in Trendelenburg's position.
Shock position	The patient lying flat on the back, bent at the hips with feet lifted approximately 12 inches off of the ground (Fig. 4-7).	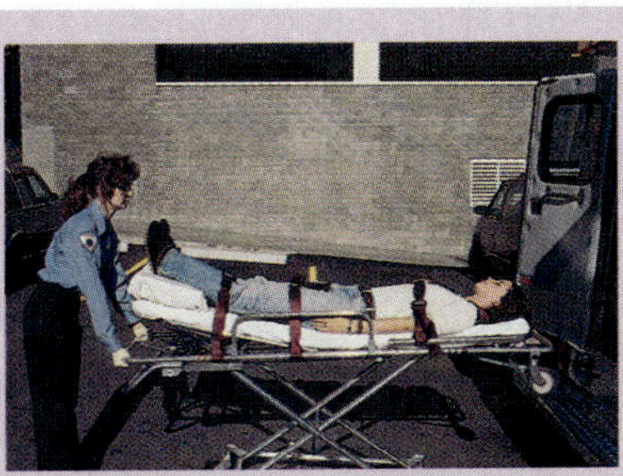 **Fig. 4-7** Patient in shock position.

REVIEW QUESTIONS

ANATOMIC TERMS

Using descriptive anatomic terms and referencing body planes (when appropriate), describe the location of the following injuries:

1. Fig. 4-8

2. Fig. 4-9

3. Fig. 4-10

4. Fig. 4-11

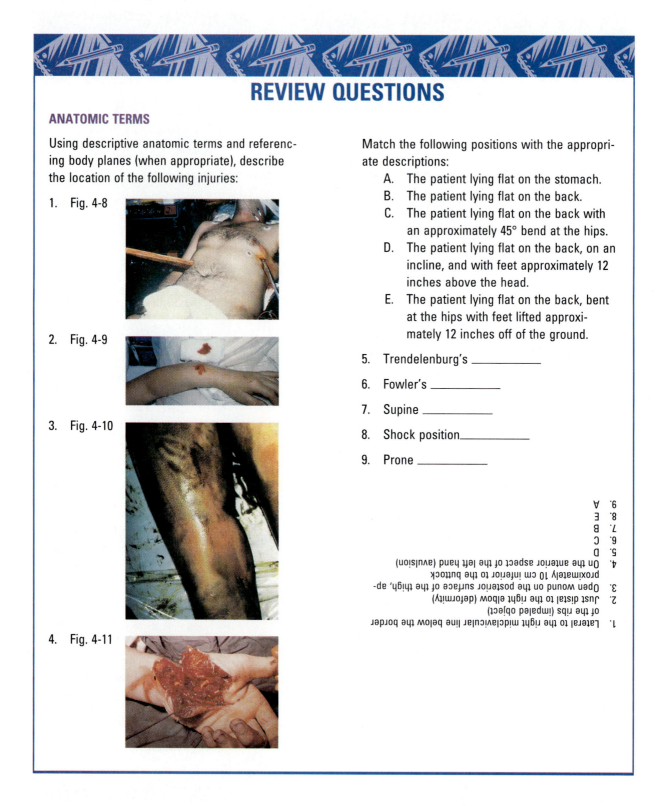

Match the following positions with the appropriate descriptions:

   A. The patient lying flat on the stomach.

   B. The patient lying flat on the back.

   C. The patient lying flat on the back with an approximately 45° bend at the hips.

   D. The patient lying flat on the back, on an incline, and with feet approximately 12 inches above the head.

   E. The patient lying flat on the back, bent at the hips with feet lifted approximately 12 inches off of the ground.

5. Trendelenburg's _____

6. Fowler's _____

7. Supine _____

8. Shock position_____

9. Prone _____

9. A
8. E
7. B
6. C
5. D
4. On the anterior aspect of the left hand (avulsion)
3. Open wound on the posterior surface of the thigh, approximately 10 cm inferior to the buttock
2. Just distal to the right elbow (deformity)
1. Lateral to the right midclavicular line below the border of the ribs (impaled object)

forms the Adam's apple. The cricoid cartilage is a firm cartilage ring just inferior to the lower portion of the larynx.

THE LUNGS

The trachea extends inferiorly from the cricoid cartilage and is the common pathway for the air that enters the lungs. The trachea splits into two main-stem bronchi, which are the major branches into each lung. The bronchi subdivide into smaller and smaller air passages until they end at the alveoli, which are the microscopic air sacs of the lungs.

Gas exchange occurs in the alveoli. These air sacs

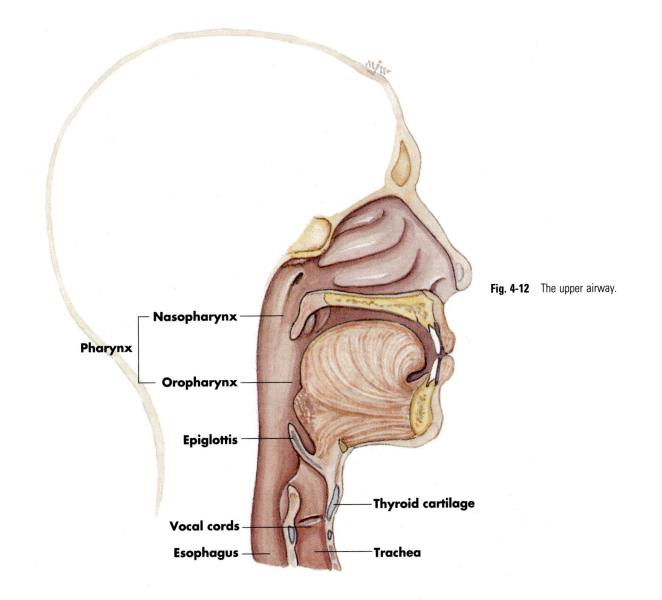

Fig. 4-12 The upper airway.

Nasopharynx

Pharynx

Oropharynx

Epiglottis

Thyroid cartilage

Vocal cords

Esophagus

Trachea

are only one cell thick and are surrounded by capillaries. The alveoli increase the surface area of the lungs so that respiration is adequate to deliver enough oxygen to the body (Fig. 4-13). The average adult human lungs have a total inside surface area equivalent to the size of a tennis court!

The process of ventilating the lungs with a constant supply of fresh air uses two main sets of muscles: the diaphragm and the intercostal muscles. The diaphragm is the large, dome-shaped muscle separating the thoracic and abdominal cavities. When muscle fibers in the diaphragm contract, the dome of the diaphragm flattens and lowers.

The intercostal muscles are located between each rib. Because of the way that they are attached to the ribs, contraction of the intercostal muscles moves the ribs upward and outward. Inhalation begins with the contraction of the diaphragm and

the intercostal muscles. This contraction increases the size of the thoracic cavity, and air is pulled into the lungs through the mouth and nose, much like pulling the plunger back on a syringe. Inhalation is an active process resulting from muscle contraction, and therefore the muscles must act for inhalation to occur (Fig. 4-14A).

Exhalation begins with the relaxation of the intercostal muscles and diaphragm. As these muscles relax and return to their resting position, the size of the thoracic cavity is decreased and air rushes out through the mouth and nose. Normally, exhalation is a passive process and therefore muscle action is not needed for exhalation to occur (Fig. 4-14B). In some cases of disease or obstructions, exhalation becomes an active process. A cough is one example of a forced exhalation.

Gas Exchange. There are two sites for the ex-

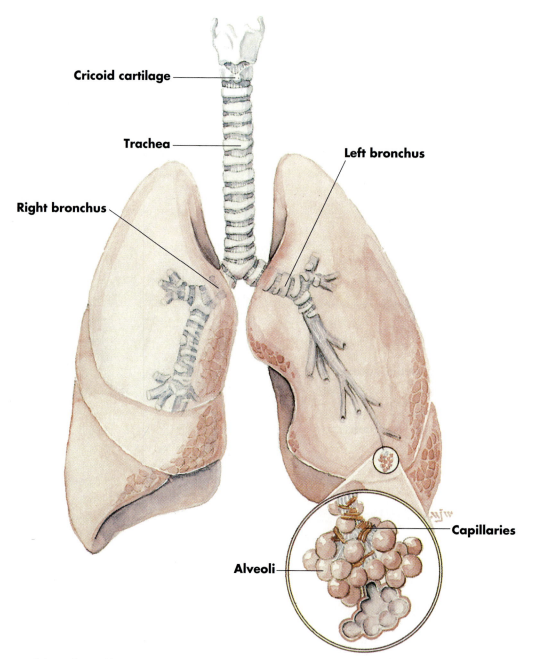

Cricoid cartilage

Trachea

Left bronchus

Right bronchus

Capillaries

Alveoli

Fig. 4-13 Anatomy of the trachea and lungs.

exchange of oxygen and carbon dioxide: the alveolar/capillary interface and the capillary/cellular interface. During inhalation, air is drawn into the lungs. Normally, air contains 21% oxygen and almost no carbon dioxide. As this oxygen-rich air enters the alveoli, blood with low levels of oxygen and high levels of carbon dioxide is flowing through the capillaries surrounding the alveoli. Gases move from areas of greater concentration to areas of lesser concentration, and therefore oxygen enters the blood and carbon dioxide is removed (Fig. 4-15).

The oxygenated blood is then pumped by the heart to the rest of the body. As this oxygen-rich blood approaches its destination, the blood vessels decrease in size until they branch into thin-walled capillaries. At the tissue level, the blood is highly oxygenated and low in carbon dioxide. However, the cells are low in oxygen and high in carbon dioxide. The capillaries give up oxygen to the cells, and the cells give carbon dioxide to the blood in the capillaries (Fig. 4-16). The blood is then collected in the veins and returned to the lungs for reoxygenation.

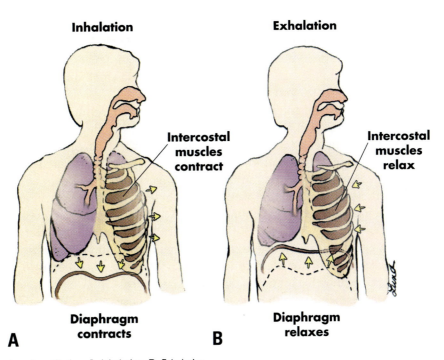

Inhalation   **Exhalation**

Intercostal muscles contract   **Intercostal muscles relax**

Diaphragm contracts   **Diaphragm relaxes**

A   **B**

Fig. 4-14   The mechanics of ventilation. **A,** Inhalation. **B,** Exhalation.

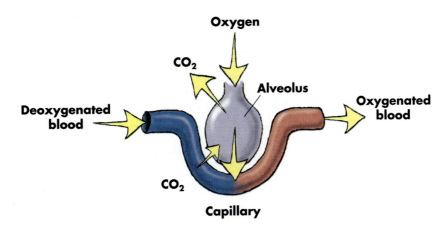

Oxygen

CO₂   **Alveolus**

Deoxygenated blood   **Oxygenated blood**

CO₂

Capillary

Fig. 4-15   Pulmonary gas exchange.

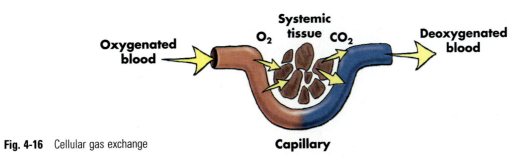

Systemic tissue

Oxygenated blood   **O₂**   **CO₂**   **Deoxygenated blood**

Fig. 4-16   Cellular gas exchange   **Capillary**

NORMAL BREATHING

A healthy adult breathes between 12 and 20 times a minute when at rest. The oxygen needs of infants and children are greater than the adult, and therefore they must breathe faster. Table 4-3 lists the normal ranges of respiration.

Under normal conditions, the respiratory cycle occurs at regular intervals. Irregularities in the rhythm of breathing may be a sign of an abnormality.

Normally, when a person takes a breath, both lungs inflate equally. The movement of air in and out of the lungs creates **breath sounds** that can be heard by placing a stethoscope on the chest wall. These sounds should be bilaterally equal in volume and pitch.

If breath sounds on either side of the chest are diminished or absent, some condition is affecting the amount of air that is reaching that lung. Absent or diminished breath sounds in one or both lungs is an important sign of inadequate breathing.

Equal expansion of both lungs can also be assessed by watching the chest rise. Both sides of the chest should rise and fall equally with each breathing cycle. Breathing should not require excessive effort. When breathing becomes labored, additional muscles, **accessory breathing muscles,** are used to draw more air into the chest. The use of abdominal or neck muscles is regarded as a sign of respiratory distress.

Finally, an adequate amount of air must be exchanged with each breath. This volume of air per breath is the **tidal volume,** which is a measure of how deep the patient is breathing. With experience you will be able to easily assess the depth of a patient's breathing.

THE RESPIRATORY SYSTEM OF INFANTS AND CHILDREN

Infants and children are not just small adults. There are considerable anatomic and physiologic differences between pediatric and adult patients.

The most obvious difference is that the airway structures are smaller. The smaller diameter of the airway makes obstructions much more common in young patients. Airway obstructions can occur when foreign bodies are lodged in the trachea or with even a small amount of swelling of airway tissues.

Two factors combine to make infant's and children's airways more easily obstructed. First, the tongue is much larger in proportion to the size of the mouth in infants and children. Second, the younger the patient, the softer the trachea. Because of these factors, the airway can be more easily obstructed if the pediatric patient is placed on the back. The chest wall is softer and more pliable in infants and children. Pediatric patients tend to rely heavily on the diaphragm for breathing and are often referred to as belly breathers, because their abdomen rises and falls even during normal respirations. The use of chest or neck muscles is regarded as a sign of respiratory distress in infants and children.

THE CIRCULATORY SYSTEM

In the growing fetus, the heart begins to pump in the 4th week of development and on the average will keep beating continuously for the next 75 years! Contracting over 100,000 times a day, the heart is a marvel of endurance and reliability. The heart pumps blood to the body organs through the cardiovascular system. This process is so vital to life that any interruption for more than a few minutes can mean death to the individual.

THE HEART

The heart is a pump consisting of four chambers. Two of the chambers are the atria, which function to receive blood and pump it to the ventricles. The two ventricles pump blood out of the heart. Because of one-way valves between the chambers, heart contraction propels blood in only one direction.

The left ventricle pumps blood rich in oxygen to the body to be used by the cells. After the oxygen is used, blood is returned to the heart into the right atrium, which pumps it to the right ventricle. The right ventricle pumps this oxygen-poor blood to the lungs for oxygenation. The oxygen-rich blood is returned into the left atrium. The left atrium pumps blood to the left ventricle, and the circuit starts all over again (Fig. 4-17).

The heart has specialized cells that generate electrical impulses and serve as the heart's pacemaker. Electrical signals are carried through the

TABLE 4-3	Normal Respiratory Rates
Adult	12–20 breaths/min
Child	15–30 breaths/min
Infant	25–50 breaths/min

Normal blood flow

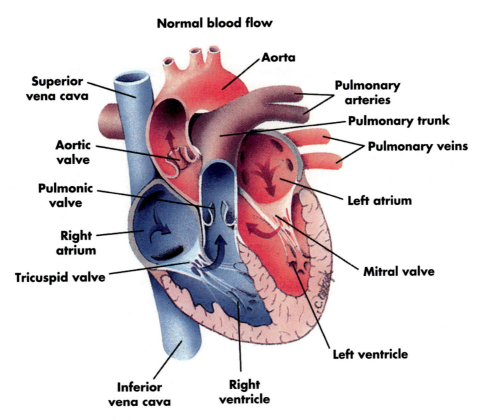

Fig. 4-17 Normal blood flow through the heart.

heart by conductive tissue. These signals give the heart the amazing ability to beat on its own. The number of times the heart beats per minute is the **heart rate,** which varies with age, physical condition, situation, and a number of other factors.

BLOOD VESSELS

Blood vessels are the ''pipes'' of the body. These vessels carry blood to every organ. Arteries carry blood away from the heart. The major artery of the body is the aorta, which is a vessel about the diameter of your thumb. It originates from the base of the heart and arches in front of the spine, then descends through the thoracic and abdominal cavities. Figure 4-18 shows the location of the major arteries in the body.

Pulsations in the carotid arteries can be felt on either side of the trachea in the neck. The femoral arteries can be palpated in the groin area, at the crease between the abdomen and the thigh. In the arm, the brachial artery is used to take a pulse or the blood pressure in an infant. The radial artery is very useful for taking the patient's pulse and can be felt along the thumb side of the wrist. Pulsations in the posterior tibial artery and the dorsalis pedis artery are important for assessing lower extremity circulation.

Arteries branch as they get further away from the heart. The smallest branch of an artery is an arteriole. The arterioles contain smooth muscle, which can change the internal diameter of the blood vessel. The arterioles play an important role in regulating blood flow and blood pressure. Other smooth muscles are described later in this chapter.

The arterioles lead to capillaries, which are the smallest blood vessels in the body. The exchange of oxygen and nutrients for carbon dioxide and other wastes occurs in the thin-walled capillaries (Fig. 4-19). The capillaries are microscopic structures, only about one twenty-fifth of an inch in length and just one cell thick, but they are present in astronomical numbers. If all of the capillaries in your body were placed end to end, they would extend for 62,000 miles!

Many capillaries join together to form a venule, which is the smallest branch of a vein. The venules in turn form veins. Most veins carry oxygen-poor blood back to the heart. Figure 4-20 shows the location of the major veins.

THE BLOOD

An average-sized adult man has about 5 to 6 L of blood circulating in the body. This complex fluid

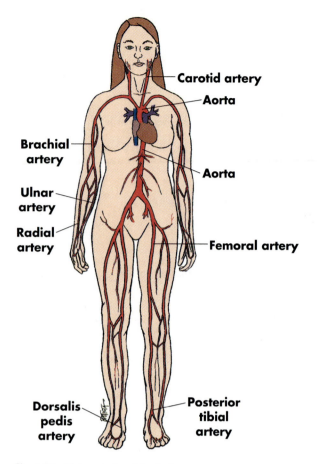

Fig. 4-18 Major arteries of the body.

serves many functions and contains many components. The **red blood cells** give blood its characteristic color. They contain **hemoglobin,** which is the chemical that carries oxygen in the blood and releases it when it reaches the tissues.

Platelets play an important role in blood clotting. The **white blood cells** are a main part of the body's defense against infection. White blood cells increase in number when the body is fighting invasion from microorganisms.

Plasma is the fluid component of blood, providing a fluid medium for the red and white blood cells and platelets. Plasma also carries nutrients to the

tissues and plays an important role in the elimination of the waste products of metabolism.

THE CIRCULATION OF BLOOD

As the left ventricle contracts, pumping blood to the body, a wave of pressure is sent through the arteries. This pressure wave can be felt anywhere an artery passes close to the skin and over a bone. These locations are called *pulse points* and occur both in the extremities and near the trunk. When the pulse point is in an extremity, it is a **peripheral pulse;** when it is in or near the trunk, it is a **central pulse.**

Blood pressure is a measure of the pressure exerted against the walls of the arteries. Blood pressure is generally measured in millimeters of mercury (mm Hg), which is a standard method of measuring blood pressure in terms of the force required to support a column of mercury in the tube of the device used to measure blood pressure.

Because a rise in this pressure occurs during each ventricular contraction, there are two pressures. The systolic pressure, which is the first number reported in a blood pressure, is the pressure in the arteries when the heart contracts, causing blood to flow through the artery. The diastolic pressure, which is the second number, is the pressure in the arteries when the heart is at rest.

A blood pressure reported as 138/86 means that a pressure equivalent to the weight of 138 mm Hg is pushing on the arteries during heart contraction and that the equivalent of 86 mm Hg is pushing on the arteries when the heart is relaxed. Blood pressure varies depending on age and various individual factors. The procedure for taking a blood pressure is described in Chapter 5, "Baseline Vital Signs and SAMPLE History."

For the body's cells to function properly, they must have a continuous supply of oxygenated blood. This supply requires adequate pressure to circulate the blood to all parts of the body. The

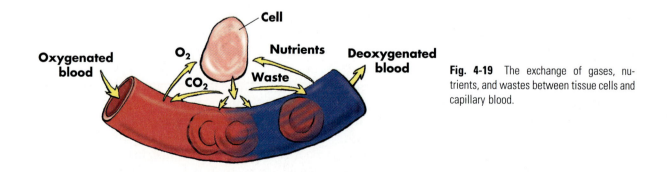

Fig. 4-19 The exchange of gases, nutrients, and wastes between tissue cells and capillary blood.

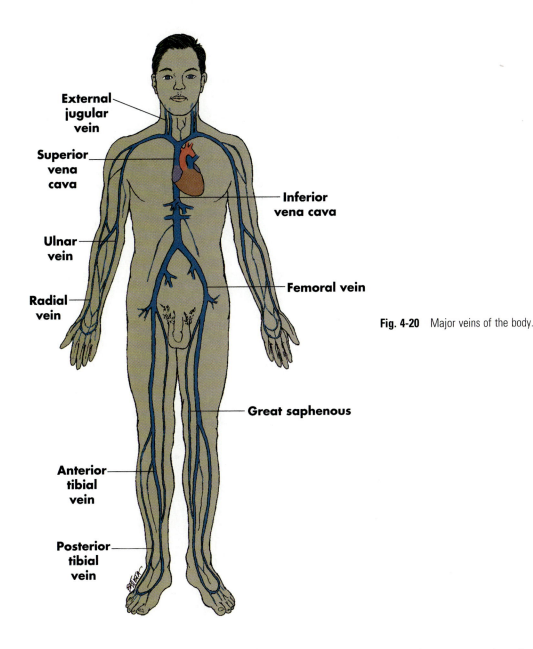

Fig. 4-20 Major veins of the body.

(Labels on figure, top to bottom left:) External jugular vein; Superior vena cava; Ulnar vein; Radial vein; Anterior tibial vein; Posterior tibial vein.

(Labels on figure, right:) Inferior vena cava; Femoral vein; Great saphenous.

process of circulating blood to the organs, delivering oxygen, and removing wastes is **perfusion.** When perfusion is inadequate, a state known as *shock* develops. Shock is a widespread depression of perfusion and is also known as *hypoperfusion.*

THE MUSCULOSKELETAL SYSTEM

THE SKELETON

The skeletal system is the scaffolding of the body. Not only do bones give the body shape and rigidity, but they also protect the vital internal organs. For example, the skull completely surrounds the delicate brain and protects it from everyday bumps and bruises. The ribs, sternum, and vertebrae also play important roles in protecting the heart and other important organs from damage.

Along with the muscles, the bones also serve as attachment points to enable the body to move. The skeleton creates levers and fulcrums through the body. The contracting of muscles moves these levers with incredible precision. Figure 4-21 shows the major bones of the body.

The Skull. This structure consists of the cranium and the bones of the face. The brain is the most important organ in the human body and is housed completely within the rigid bony box called the *cranium.* The cranium consists of eight bones. These flat bones fit together with very tight joints, very much like a jigsaw puzzle. These joints, which are called **sutures,** enable the bones to move slightly

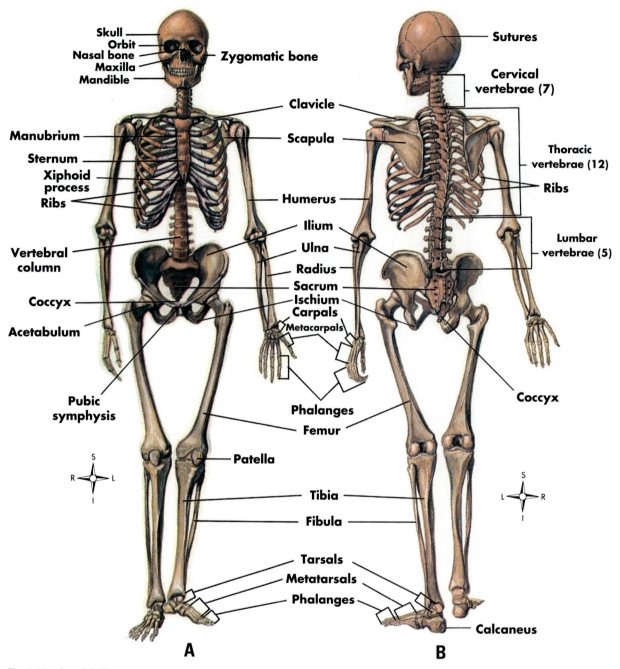

Fig. 4-21   A and B, The skeletal system.

without breaking. This feature provides the brain with excellent protection from external forces.

The face is formed by fourteen bones fitting together in a tremendously intricate three-dimensional puzzle. Some of these bones are very thin and are easily damaged in traumatic injuries. The following are the major bones of the face:

1. The orbits form the eye sockets.
2. The nasal bones are a collection of bones that create the nose.
3. The zygomatic bones form the cheek bones.

4. The maxilla is the main bone of the upper jaw.
5. The mandible is commonly referred to as the *jaw*.

The Spinal Column and Rib Cage   The spinal column serves four main functions:

1. Supporting the weight of the head and trunk.
2. Protecting the spinal cord.
3. Allowing spinal nerves to branch off the spinal cord.
4. Allowing for movement of the head and trunk.

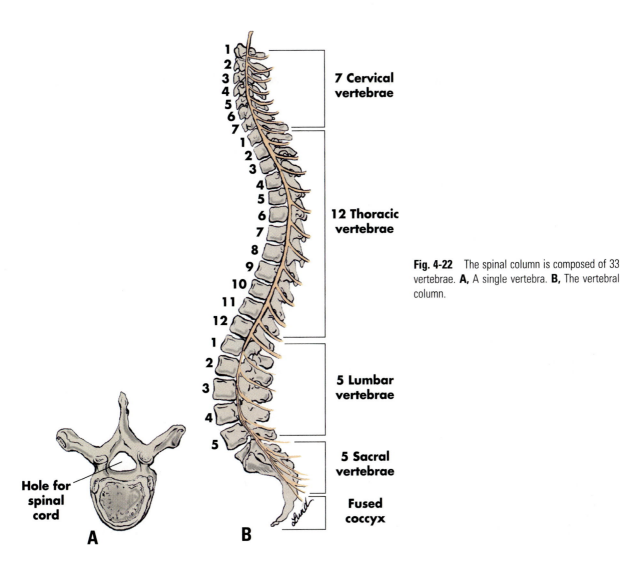

Hole for spinal cord

A

B

1
2
3
4
5
6
7

7 Cervical vertebrae

1
2
3
4
5
6
7
8
9
10
11
12

12 Thoracic vertebrae

1
2
3
4
5

5 Lumbar vertebrae

5 Sacral vertebrae

Fused coccyx

Fig. 4-22 The spinal column is composed of 33 vertebrae. **A,** A single vertebra. **B,** The vertebral column.

The bones of the spinal column are the vertebrae (Fig. 4-22). The vertebrae of the neck and back each have a vertical hole in them. These vertebrae stack on top of each other, and the holes line up to create a tube for the spinal cord. If one of these bones becomes misaligned or damaged, it can cause damage to the spinal cord.

The 33 vertebrae of the spinal column are divided into five regions: seven small cervical vertebrae in the neck; twelve thoracic vertebrae, which attach to the ribs in the upper back; five heavy lumbar vertebrae, which support the weight of the head and trunk in the lower back; five sacral vertebrae, which fuse and form the back of the pelvis; and four coccyx, which fuse together to form the tailbone.

The **thorax** contains 12 pairs of ribs. Each rib is attached posteriorly to one of the thoracic vertebrae. The first through the 10th ribs are attached anteriorly to the sternum. The 11th and 12th ribs are the floating ribs because they simply extend laterally from the vertebrae. The floating ribs help protect the kidneys. The attached ribs provide protection to all of the organs in the thorax and assist in breathing.

The sternum, commonly called the *breastbone*, protects the heart and gives rigidity to the thoracic cage. The superior one third of the sternum is the manubrium. The body of the sternum comprises the remaining two thirds of the sternum. The xiphoid process extends from the posterior end of the sternum. This bony point is sharp and delicate and can be broken and can damage important organs (such as the liver) during cardiopulmonary resuscitation.

The Pelvis and Lower Extremities. The sacral vertebrae form the back of the pelvis. Six fused bones create the pelvic girdle. The iliac crests are the wings of the pelvis. The pubis bones join anteriorly at the pubic symphysis. The ischium bones are

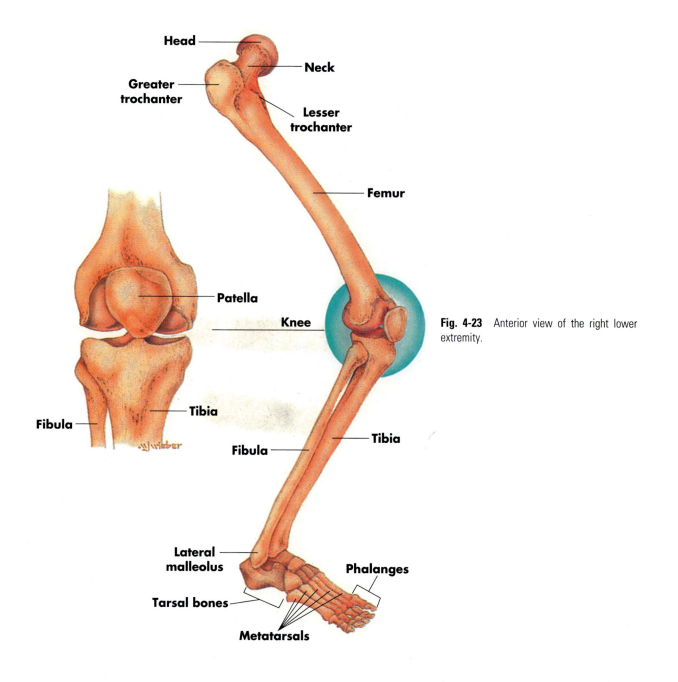

Fig. 4-23   Anterior view of the right lower extremity.

the posterior portion of the pelvis and are the two looped bones on which we sit. The acetabulum is the socket of the hip joint.

The head of the femur, the long bone of the thigh, is spherical and fits into the acetabulum to form the hip joint. The neck of the femur joins the body at the greater trochanter, which can be felt over your hip. The patella (kneecap) protects the knee from damage if you fall directly onto your knee.

The lower leg has two bones. The tibia (shin) is the main weight-bearing bone of the lower leg and forms the rounded medial malleolus of the ankle joint. The fibula does not bear weight but assists in the movement of the ankle. The distal portion of the fibula forms the lateral malleolus.

The tarsal and metatarsal bones provide structure to the foot, and the calcaneus is the bony prominence at the heel. The phalanges are the skeletal support for the toes (Fig. 4-23).

The Upper Extremities.   The arms join the trunk at the shoulder girdle. The shoulder girdle consists of two bones: the scapula posteriorly and the clavicle, or collarbone, anteriorly. The acromion process can be felt at the tip of the shoulder. The humerus is the bone of the upper arm.

The olecranon process of the ulna, which is the medial bone of the forearm, along with the distal

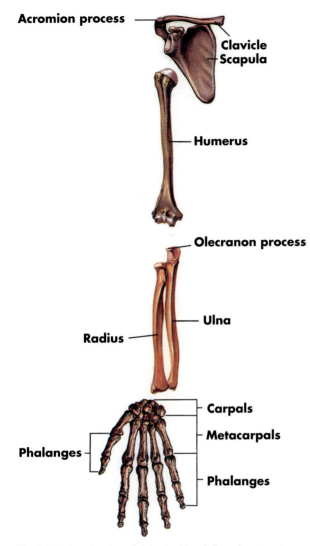

Acromion process

Clavicle
Scapula

Humerus

Olecranon process

Ulna

Radius

Carpals

Metacarpals

Phalanges

Phalanges

Fig. 4-24 Anterior view of right shoulder girdle and upper extremity.

end of the humerus, make up the elbow. The radius is the lateral bone in the forearm. The carpals are tiny bones in the wrist that enable the hand to move in many intricate positions. The metacarpals and the phalanges form the hand and fingers (Fig. 4-24).

JOINTS

A joint is a place where bones come together. Joints serve many functions, but most importantly, they provide a system of fulcrums and levers that makes movement of the body possible. There are many types of joints, but the two most common and most important for EMTs are the hinge and the ball-and-socket joints.

Hinge joints consist of a cylinder that fits into a cradle (Fig. 4-25A). Hinge joints allow movement only in one plane and are found in the elbow, knee, and all of the fingers and toes. Ball-and-socket joints exist when the head of one bone fits into a socket of another bone (or combination of bones) (Fig. 4-25B). This type of joint allows for movement in many directions and is found in the shoulder and the hip.

MUSCLES

No movement in the body could occur without muscles. Every physical activity, from riding a bike to turning the pages of this book, occurs with the contraction of muscles. Additionally, muscles protect vital organs and help give the body shape.

There are three types of muscles found in the human body: skeletal, smooth, and cardiac. All three types of muscle have the unique ability to contract (shorten) (Fig. 4-26).

Skeletal Muscles. As the name implies, these muscles are attached to bones. When these muscles shorten, they provide the force to move the levers of the skeletal system (Fig. 4-27). Skeletal muscles make up the major muscle mass of the body. Weight lifters and athletes exercise to strengthen and develop skeletal muscles.

Tap your right foot three times. To accomplish this task, your brain sent a signal to the muscles in your calf to shorten, and your foot extended. Then your brain told your calf to relax and the muscles in the front of your lower leg to contract, and this process was repeated twice more. Although you did not have to consciously think about each step, it was voluntary because you chose to do it. Therefore, skeletal muscles are called *voluntary muscles*.

Smooth Muscles. These muscles are found in the walls of tubular structures in the gastrointestinal tract, the urinary system, the blood vessels, and the bronchi. Because they are circular, contraction changes the inside diameter of the tube (Fig. 4-28). This contraction is very important for controlling flow through the tubes of the body.

For instance, when you are cold, the body decreases blood flow to the arms and legs because significant body heat can be lost from the blood through the skin in these areas. The blood flow to the extremities is reduced by contracting the smooth muscles in the arteries that lead to the arms and legs.

You have no control over this process. Smooth muscles carry out many of the automatic muscular functions such as digestion, blood vessel control, and modifying the diameter of your airway. Be-

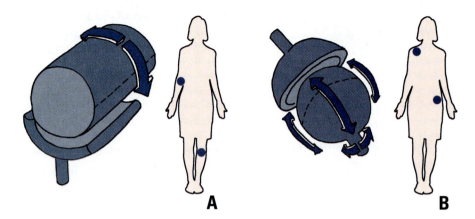

Fig. 4-25   Two common types of joints. **A,** A hinge joint. **B,** A ball-and-socket joint.

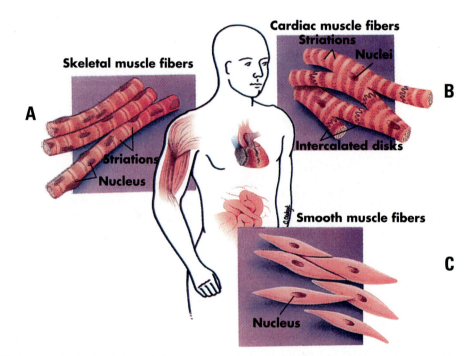

Fig. 4-26   **A,** Skeletal muscle attaches to bone. **B,** Cardiac muscle is located in the heart. **C,** Smooth muscle is located in organs such as the stomach and intestine.

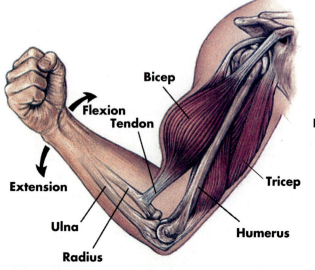

Fig. 4-27   Skeletal muscles provide the force to move the body.

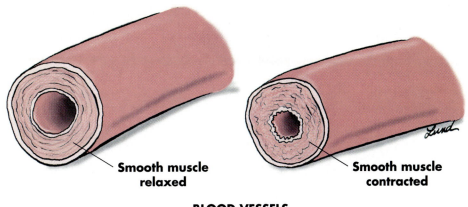

Smooth muscle
relaxed

Smooth muscle
contracted

BLOOD VESSELS

Fig. 4-28 Smooth muscles are found in the walls of some tubular structures and can contract to change the diameter of the tube and thus affect flow through it.

cause no conscious thought is required for these activities, the smooth muscles are called *involuntary*.

Cardiac Muscle.   The heart is the most important muscle in the body. The heart muscle has tremendous stamina. Imagine squeezing a tennis ball 60 times per minute. How long do you think that you could keep up with that pace? Certainly not 60 times per minute, 24 hours a day like the heart.

To accomplish this amazing feat of stamina, the heart must have a continuous supply of blood. The coronary arteries deliver oxygen and nutrients to the heart muscle. Cholesterol in the bloodstream is deposited in plaques on the inside walls of the coronary arteries. When these plaques rupture, a clot forms and blood flow to a portion of the heart is decreased. If this flow of blood is interrupted for more than a few minutes, part of the heart will be damaged. The damaged muscle causes the most common sign of a heart attack—chest pain.

Because your heartbeat is not under conscious control, cardiac muscle is also involuntary, but cardiac muscle has the unique property of being able to contract on its own. This phenomenon, known as *automaticity*, helps to ensure that the heart will continue to deliver blood to the body even if other body systems are damaged.

THE NERVOUS SYSTEM

The human nervous system is incredibly well developed and complex. It is the root of all thought, memory, and emotion. It also controls the voluntary and involuntary activities of the body. Anatomically, the nervous system has two components: the central nervous system and the peripheral nervous system (Fig. 4-29).

The central nervous system consists of the brain, which is located within the cranium, and the spinal cord, which is located within the spinal column from the base of the skull to the lumbar vertebrae. The central nervous system is responsible for all higher mental functions, such as thought, decision making, and communication, and also has an important role in the regulation of body functions.

The peripheral nervous system consists of sensory and motor nerves that lie outside the skull or spinal cord. These nerves serve as wires, carrying information between the central nervous system and every organ and muscle in the body.

Sensory nerves carry information from the body to the central nervous system. They provide information about the environment, pain, pressure, and body position to the brain for decision making. Motor nerves carry information from the central nervous system to the body. Signals from the motor nerves cause contraction of skeletal muscles, which are responsible for all body movement (Fig. 4-30).

THE SKIN

Most people think of the skin as just a covering for the body. In reality it is a very important organ that performs many functions. The skin protects the body from the environment. Not only does it keep us from drying out, it also serves as a barrier to prevent invasion of the body by bacteria and other organisms.

The skin also plays a crucial role in temperature regulation. When you are too hot, the blood vessels dilate and the skin secretes sweat, which evaporates and cools the body. When you are cold, the blood vessels to the skin contract to decrease the heat loss to the environment.

Skin is also an important sensory organ. Special

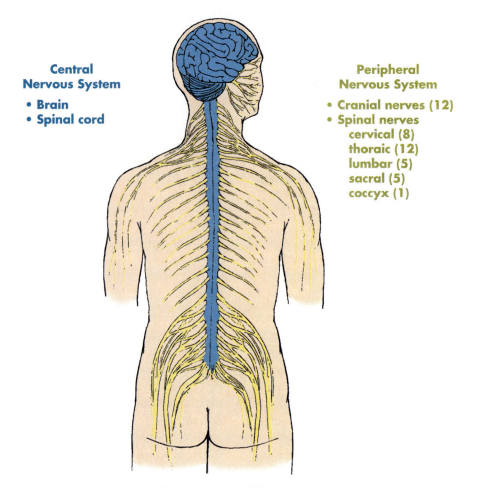

Central Nervous System

• **Brain**
• **Spinal cord**

Peripheral Nervous System

• **Cranial nerves (12)**
• **Spinal nerves**
   cervical (8)
   thoraic (12)
   lumbar (5)
   sacral (5)
   coccyx (1)

Fig. 4-29 The central nervous system consists of the brain and spinal cord. The peripheral nervous system consists of nerves that lie outside the skull and spinal cord.

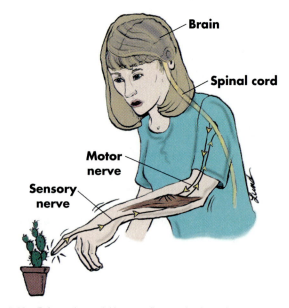

Brain

Spinal cord

Motor nerve

Sensory nerve

Fig. 4-30 Pain, such as pricking your finger, stimulates the sensory nerves, which carry the information to the brain. The brain then signals the motor nerves to withdraw your finger.

receptors in the skin can detect heat, cold, touch, pressure, and pain. Information from these receptors is transmitted to the central nervous system by sensory nerves.

The skin has three layers (Fig. 4-31). The epidermis is the outermost layer. The dermis is the deeper layer, containing the sweat glands, hair follicles, blood vessels, and nerve endings. The subcutaneous layer lies just below the dermis and connects the skin to the underlying tissue. The subcutaneous layer also stores fat, which serves an important function in insulation and storing energy.

THE DIGESTIVE SYSTEM

Food provides our bodies with substances that cells need to produce energy and build new tissue. The digestive system breaks down food so that it can be absorbed into the blood and delivered to the cells as nutrients, vitamins, and minerals (Fig. 4-32).

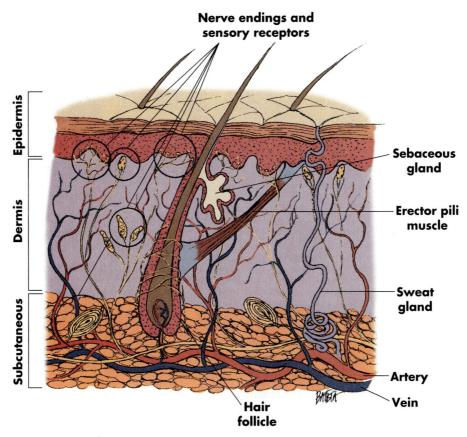

Nerve endings and sensory receptors

Epidermis

Dermis

Subcutaneous

Sebaceous gland

Erector pili muscle

Sweat gland

Artery

Vein

Hair follicle

Fig. 4-31   The epidermis, dermis, and subcutaneous layers of the skin.

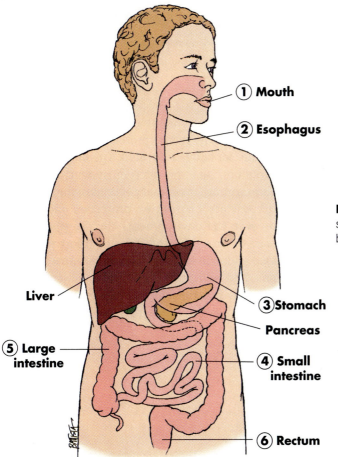

① **Mouth**

② **Esophagus**

Liver

⑤ **Large intestine**

③ **Stomach**

Pancreas

④ **Small intestine**

⑥ **Rectum**

Fig. 4-32   The pathway food follows through the digestive system. The liver and pancreas add chemicals to aid in the breakdown of food.

Food passes through the hollow organs of the digestive system from the mouth to the anus. The breakdown of food begins in the mouth as the food is chewed and mixes with saliva. This breakdown continues in the stomach where the food is churned and combined with stomach acids. Chemicals from the liver and pancreas further break down food into its component parts.

Once food has been broken down, the nutrients are absorbed into the blood as the food passes through the small intestine. Liquid is removed from the food as it passes through the large intestine, which is also called the *colon*. Undigestible material is eliminated from the body as feces.

THE ENDOCRINE SYSTEM

The endocrine system is a very complicated system, consisting of a number of glands inside the body (Fig. 4-33) that produce chemicals called **hormones.** These chemicals, when secreted into the bloodstream, regulate body activities and functions in many body systems. Two examples of such hormones are **adrenaline,** which helps prepare the body for emergencies, and **insulin,** which is crucial for the body's use of sugars.

CHAPTER SUMMARY

ANATOMIC TERMS

As a healthcare professional, you need to know the vocabulary and language used for the human body. This common medical terminology and descriptive anatomical terminology allows you to explain the exact location of injuries in both verbal and written communications. All terms and planes of the body refer to the body in the anatomical position. Positional terminology is used to describe the position in which you find or transport patients.

BODY SYSTEMS

The human body can be divided into systems to make the study of function easier. The respiratory system makes oxygen available to the blood and rids the body of carbon dioxide. The circulatory

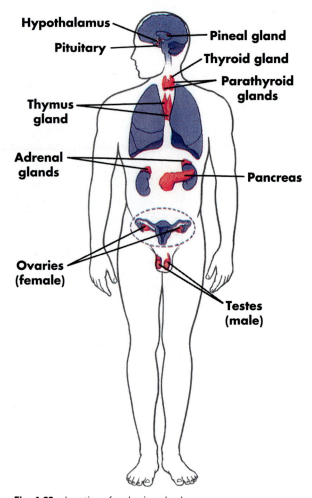

Fig. 4-33 Location of endocrine glands.

system delivers the oxygen to and removes waste products from the organs of the body. The skeleton gives the body shape, protects vital organs, and provides for body movement. The muscles provide movement, and the nervous system controls all voluntary and involuntary actions of the body. The skin provides a barrier for protection and interaction with the environment. The digestive system breaks down food so that it can be absorbed into the blood and delivered to the cells as nutrients, vitamins, and minerals. The endocrine system regulates body function through the release of chemicals called *hormones* into the bloodstream.

REVIEW QUESTIONS

BODY SYSTEMS

1. _____ blood pressure is the pressure exerted on the arteries during ventricular contraction, and _____ blood pressure is the pressure on the arteries during relaxation of the heart.

2. List the three functions of the skeletal system:

    _____

    _____

    _____

3. Match the following by location and number of vertebrae:
    1. Cervical   ___ ___
    2. Thoracic   ___ ___
    3. Lumbar   ___ ___
    4. Sacral   ___ ___
    5. Coccyx   ___ ___
       A. Lower back   i.   12
       B. Pelvis   ii. 7
       C. Upper back   iii. 5
       D. Tail bone   iv. 4 fused
       E. Neck   v.   5 fused

4. Which muscle type has the unique property of automaticity?
    A. Skeletal
    B. Smooth
    C. Voluntary
    D. Cardiac

5. The peripheral nervous system consists of _____ nerves, which carry information to the central nervous system, and _____ nerves, which carry information from the central nervous system.

6. List the three layers of the skin, from superficial to deep.

    _____

    _____

    _____

7. The chemicals released by the endocrine system are called _____.

1. Systolic; diastolic
2. Gives the body shape and rigidity, provides protection for the internal organs, serves as the attachment point for muscles
3. 1-E-ii
   2-C-i
   3-A-iii
   4-B-v
   5-D-iv
4. D
5. Sensory; motor
6. Epidermis; dermis; subcutaneous
7. Hormones

UNITED STATES DEPARTMENT OF TRANSPORTATION NATIONAL HIGHWAY TRAFFIC SAFETY ADMINISTRATION EMT–BASIC OBJECTIVES

Check your knowledge. The National Registry of EMTs and many state EMS agencies use the objectives below to develop EMT–Basic certification examinations. Can you meet them?

COGNITIVE

1. Identify the following topographic terms: medial, lateral, proximal, distal, superior, inferior, anterior, posterior, midline, right and left, midclavicular, bilateral, and midaxillary.

2. Describe the anatomy and function of the following major body systems: respiratory, circulatory, musculoskeletal, nervous, and endocrine.

KEY TERMS

Accessory muscles: The additional muscles used to facilitate breathing in a person in respiratory distress.

Capillary refill: The amount of time required to refill the capillary bed after applying and releasing pressure on a fingernail.

Crowing: A long, high-pitched sound when breathing in; indicates a respiratory problem.

Diastolic blood pressure: The measurement of the pressure exerted against the walls of the arteries while the heart is at rest.

Grunting: Respirations that sound like the patient is grunting when attempting to breathe. The sound comes from the airway and is unintentional; indicates a respiratory problem.

Gurgling: A liquid sound during breathing; indicates a respiratory problem.

History: A concise and inclusive set of information that EMTs gather about the patient.

Labored respirations: An increase in the effort expended to breathe.

Noisy respirations: Any noise coming from the patient's airway; indicates a respiratory problem.

Normal respirations: Respirations occurring without airway noise or effort from the patient, usually occurring at a rate of between 12 to 20 breaths per minute.

Reactive to light: A term referring to pupil constriction when exposed to a penlight.

Shallow respirations: Respirations that have low volumes of air in inspiration and expiration.

Sign: Any medical or trauma condition that can be observed and identified in the patient.

Snoring: A sound that indicates the patient is unable to keep the airway open; the tongue is falling back into and partially obstructing the upper airway.

Stridor: A loud, high-pitched airway noise that indicates a respiratory problem.

Symptom: Any nonobservable condition described by the patient.

Systolic blood pressure: The measurement of the pressure against the walls of the arteries during contraction of the heart.

Trending: The process of comparing sets of vital signs or other assessment information over time.

Wheezing: A high-pitched whistling sound that is usually caused by constriction of the smaller airways or bronchioles; indicates a respiratory problem.

IN THE FIELD

EMTs Joe and Heather were called to respond with a second ambulance crew to a car crash at the intersection of Route 51 and Coal Valley Road. They arrived at the scene within 5 minutes and began to assess the driver of one car, while the other ambulance crew assessed the driver of the other car. Their patient was a 27-year-old white man named Mark who said he had pain in his abdomen and his neck. Mark was able to talk with them and did not initially appear to be seriously injured.

They immobilized him with a cervical spine immobilization device, a short backboard, and then a long backboard. After they quickly assessed him from head to toe, they moved Mark into the ambulance, and Heather took a set of baseline vital signs. Mark's pulse was 100, his respiratory rate was 18, and his blood pressure was 118/76. His skin was warm and dry, and his pupils were equal and reactive to light.

Joe drove the ambulance while Heather remained in the patient compartment with Mark. Although Mark was still responsive and answering questions, he was becoming confused. Heather repeated her initial assessment and reassessed the vital signs. Mark's pulse had increased to 116, his respiratory rate was now 22, and his blood pressure had decreased to 110/70. The change in vital signs and mental status alerted Heather that Mark might have serious internal injuries. Heather informed Joe of the changes in Mark's condition. Heather's repeated assessment and her detection of the change in Mark's vital signs allowed her to recognize a change in Mark's condition quickly and provide appropriate care.

Some information about the patient is obvious when you first begin interacting with the patient. The patient's approximate age, gender, and race can be determined quickly and easily. Although this information may not change your treatment, it is beneficial in your documentation and communication with medical direction. This information may give the medical direction physician insight to direct changes in your treatment plan.

In addition, patients can provide you with other valuable information about themselves and their medical history. It is important to determine quickly the patient's chief complaint—the reason why EMS was called. After introducing yourself, ask the patient to describe the signs and symptoms related to the chief complaint at this time. If the patient begins a long description of ailments dating back several years, try to focus the patient on the immediate problem that prompted the call for assistance today.

After gathering this general information, as part of the assessment process, you assess the vital signs and gather additional information about the patient.

Vital signs are an important part of every patient assessment. Except in the most extreme cases, you always assess vital signs. In cases in which the patient's condition is immediately life threatening, you may not have the time to assess vital signs. For example, with a trauma patient who is unable to maintain an open airway, you may need to constantly maintain the airway by positioning and suctioning fluids from the mouth; in this case you should not stop care to assess the vital signs. Except in such extreme cases, you should assess vital signs of every patient.

BASELINE VITAL SIGNS

The vital signs are breathing; pulse; skin color, temperature, and condition; pupil size and reactivity; and blood pressure. They are called *vital signs* because they can reveal much about the patient's condition and the body's life-sustaining functions. The baseline vital signs are those vital signs you measure or assess when you first encounter the patient; these baseline vital signs can then be used for comparison with other measurements as the patient's condition changes. **Trending** is the process of comparing sets of vital signs or other assessment information over time. A single set of vital signs does not provide as much information as does a trend in the patient's vital signs.

Take care to record vital signs accurately. Record these assessment specifics as you take each vital sign, rather than trying to remember all the numbers and recording them later. Some EMTs prefer to record the vital signs on an available piece of paper during the assessment, and then copy them later into the prehospital care report.

BREATHING

Breathing is assessed by observing the patient's chest rise and fall. One breath is one complete cycle of breathing in and out. You assess the patient's breathing rate and quality. Breathing is also called *respiration*.

RATE

You can determine the patient's respiratory rate by counting the number of breaths in 30 seconds and multiplying by two. If the patient's breathing rate is irregular, count the respirations for 1 full minute to obtain a more accurate rate. Because patients may subconsciously change their rate of breathing if they know you are monitoring their respirations, do not tell the patient that you are assessing the breathing rate. A good way to avoid telling the patient is to count respirations immediately after you assess the pulse. Keep your hand in contact with the patient's wrist, and the patient generally thinks you are still taking the pulse and

will not think about breathing or subconsciously alter respirations.

A patient's respiratory rate is affected by the patient's age, size, and emotional state at the time. Patients often breathe faster than normal when they are ill or injured. The average range of respiratory rates for adults is 12 to 20 breaths per minute. Average ranges by age are listed in Table 5-1.

QUALITY

The quality of breathing is the second part of the respiratory assessment. There are four basic categories for the quality of breathing: normal, shallow, labored, and noisy.

Normal respirations are characterized by average chest wall motion, ie, the chest moves outward and downward in a smooth regular manner. The rhythm of normal breathing is regular and even. Normal breathing is effortless. As the work of breathing increases, accessory muscles are used. To determine if a patient is using accessory muscles, watch the abdominal, shoulder, and neck muscles for excessive movement. Also look at the muscles between the ribs. If the patient is working hard to breathe, these accessory muscles may be used.

Shallow respirations have slight chest or abdominal wall motion and usually indicate that the patient is moving only small volumes of air into the lungs. Even when the breathing rate is within the average range, patients with shallow respirations may not be receiving enough oxygen with each respiration to support the needs of their bodies.

TABLE 5-1	Average Vital Sign Ranges by Age		
AGE	**PULSE**	**RESPIRATIONS**	**BLOOD PRESSURE**
Newborn	120–160	40–60	80/40
1 year	80–140	30–40	82/44
3 years	80–120	25–30	86/50
5 years	70–115	20–25	90/52
7 years	70–115	20–25	94/54
10 years	70–115	15–20	100/60
15 years	70–90	15–20	110/64
Adult	60–80	12–20	120/80

Labored respirations indicate a dramatic increase in the patient's effort to breathe. **Grunting** and **stridor** are often present. Grunting is the sound created when the patient forcefully exhales against a closed glottic opening which traps air and keeps the alveoli open. This sound often indicates respiratory distress. Stridor is a loud, high-pitched sound usually heard during inspiration. Stridor typically indicates an upper airway obstruction. **Accessory muscles** are used predominantly when the patient has difficulty breathing (Fig. 5-1). Patients may also seem to be gasping for air. Nasal flaring (the widening of the nostrils during inhalation) and supraclavicular and intercostal retractions also indicate labored respirations, especially in infants and children (Fig. 5-2). Because children and infants normally rely heavily on their diaphragm for breathing, do not assume that the abdominal motion of their breathing automatically indicates labored breathing.

Noisy respirations are abnormal respiratory sounds. Any time you hear noisy breathing, something is obstructing the flow of air. Noisy breathing includes **snoring**, **wheezing**, **gurgling**, and **crowing**. Snoring is a sign that the patient cannot keep the airway fully open. The tongue is falling back into and partially obstructing the upper airway. Wheezing is a high-pitched whistling sound that is usually caused by constriction of smaller airways or bronchioles. Gurgling indicates liquid in the airway. Crowing is a long, high-pitched sound when breathing in.

A noisy airway always indicates a respiratory problem. Any abnormal breathing quality is always an emergency, and you need to intervene to manage the patient's airway and/or breathing. Chapter 7, "The Airway," discusses the techniques to maintain an open airway and administer oxygen.

PULSE

The pulse is the wave of pressure in the blood generated by the pumping of the heart. You can feel the pulse wherever an artery passes over a bone near the surface of the skin. Figure 5-3 shows the location of key pulse points in the body. The pulse should be assessed for both rate and quality.

RATE

The pulse rate is the number of beats in 1 minute. The pulse is assessed by counting the number

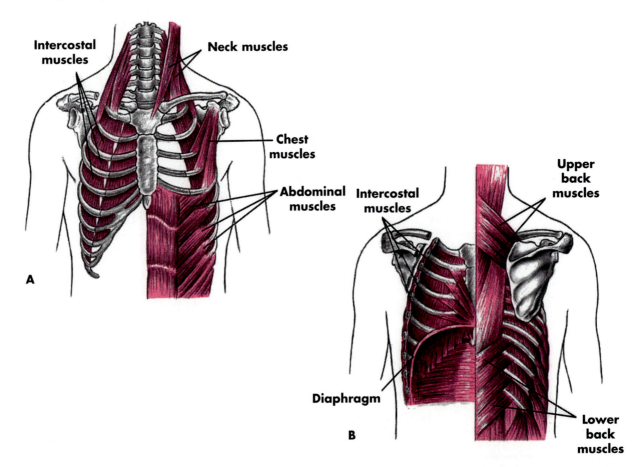

Fig. 5-1 When breathing becomes labored, accessory muscles are used to draw more air into the chest. **A,** Anterior view. **B,** Posterior view.

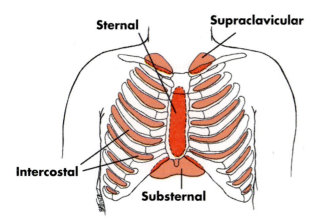

Fig. 5-2 Retractions indicate labored respirations, especially in infants and children.

of beats you feel in 30 seconds and multiplying by two. The pulse rate is affected by factors such as the patient's age, physical condition, blood loss, and anxiety. The average range for a resting pulse in adults is 60 to 80. An individual's normal pulse may not fall within this average range, however. For instance, a well-conditioned athlete may have

a resting pulse of 50; although this pulse is outside the average range, it is normal for this patient. When you measure the pulse and obtain low or high rates outside the average range, ask patients if they know their normal resting pulse.

QUALITY

The quality of the pulse is defined as its strength and regularity. The strength of the pulse can be strong or weak. The rhythm can be regular or irregular.

The pulse should feel strong as you palpate with your fingertips. If the heart is not pumping effectively, or if there is a low volume of blood, the pulse may feel weak. A weak pulse is an early sign of shock (hypoperfusion), which may help you prioritize the patient.

The pulse should also feel regular. A regular pulse does not speed up or slow down but has a constant time between beats. If there is not a constant time between beats, the pulse is irregular. An irregular pulse rate may indicate cardiovascular compromise.

Initially, assess the radial pulse in all responsive patients 1 year of age or older (Fig. 5-4). The radial pulse is the pulse in the wrist on the thumb side of the forearm. Using two fingers, slide your fingertips from the center of the patient's forearm just proximal to the point where the wrist bends, toward the thumb side of the arm. By applying moderate pressure, you should be able to feel the beats of the pulse. If the pulse is weak, applying more pressure may help you feel a pulse. Too much pressure, however, may occlude the artery, and you will not be able to feel the pulse. If you cannot feel a radial pulse in one arm, try the other arm.

If you are unable to feel a radial pulse in either arm, use the carotid pulse (Fig. 5-5). The carotid

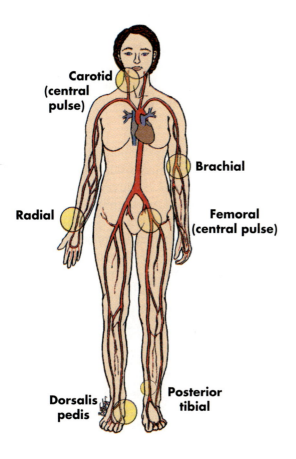

Fig. 5-3 Key pulse points in the body.

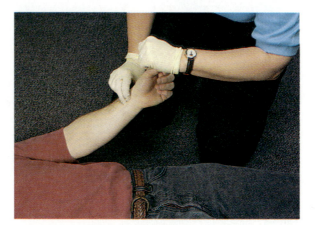

Fig. 5-4 Locating the radial pulse.

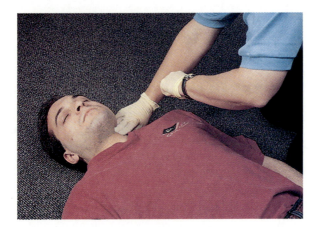

Fig. 5-5 Locating the carotid pulse.

pulse is felt in the neck along the carotid artery. Locate the Adam's apple in the center of the patient's neck, and slide two fingers toward one side of the neck. Never exert excessive pressure on the neck when feeling for a carotid pulse, especially with geriatric patients. Excessive pressure may dislodge a clot, with serious effects in the body. You should never assess the carotid pulse on both sides of the neck at the same time because this could cause a drop in the patient's heart rate.

For patients less than 1 year of age, assess the brachial pulse (Fig. 5-6). The carotid pulse is normally difficult to locate due to the small size of the infant's neck.

To assess the pulse, follow these steps:
1. Locate the radial pulse for patients 1 year of age or older, and locate the brachial pulse for those less than 1 year of age.
2. Count the number of beats in 30 seconds and multiply this number by two to determine the pulse rate.

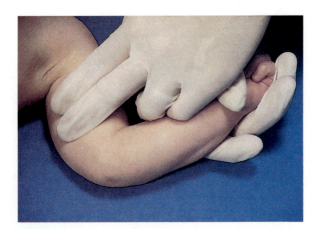

Fig. 5-6 Palpate the brachial pulse in an infant.

3. Characterize the quality of the pulse as strong or weak and as regular or irregular.

SKIN

The patient's skin color, temperature, and condition are assessed because they are good indicators of the patient's **perfusion**. Capillary refill is also assessed in infants and children less than 6 years of age.

COLOR

Assess skin color in the nail beds, oral mucosa (inside the mouth), and conjunctiva (inside the lower eyelid). These places accurately reflect the level of oxygen in the blood and are easy to assess because the capillary beds run close to the surface of the skin. The normal skin color in these areas is pink for patients with light or dark skin. For infants and children, assess the soles of the feet or the palms of the hands.

Abnormal skin colors include pale, cyanotic (blue-gray), flushed (red), or jaundiced (yellow). Pale skin color indicates poor perfusion, which is caused by a lack of effective blood flow reaching all body tissues. Cyanosis (blue-gray color) indicates inadequate oxygenation (lack of oxygen reaching the cells) or poor perfusion. Flushed skin indicates exposure to heat or carbon monoxide poisoning. Finally, a jaundiced or yellow skin color indicates the patient's liver may not be functioning properly.

TEMPERATURE

Assess skin temperature by placing the back of your hand against the patient's skin (Fig. 5-7). The back of your hand is more sensitive to temperature changes than the palm. Assess the skin temperature in more than one location and compare findings. The patient's extremities are more susceptible to environmental changes in temperature than the trunk. Normally the skin is warm. Hot skin indicates a fever or exposure to heat. Cool skin indicates poor perfusion or exposure to cold. If the skin is cold, the patient has been exposed to extreme cold.

CONDITION

The condition of the skin is normally dry—but not so dry that it appears cracked. Wet, moist, or extremely dry skin conditions are abnormal. Extremely dry skin may be a sign of dehydration. When the skin is cool and moist, the skin is termed *clammy*. Clammy skin is a sign of shock

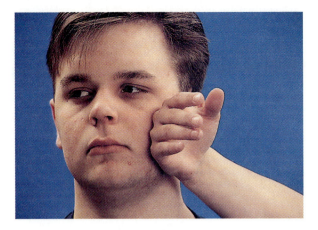

Fig. 5-7 Assess skin temperature with the back of your hand.

(hypoperfusion). For more information on shock (hypoperfusion), see Chapter 25, ''Bleeding and Shock''.

CAPILLARY REFILL

Capillary refill is the time it takes for the capillary beds to fill after being blanched (Fig. 5-8). Capillary refill is checked only in patients less than 6 years of age because it is not reliable as an indicator of the signs and symptoms of shock (hypoperfusion) in older patients.

To assess capillary refill, press on the nail beds, release the pressure, and determine the time it takes for the nail bed to return to its initial color. If the capillary refill time is less than 2 seconds, then the capillary refill is normal. Any capillary refill time longer than 2 seconds is abnormal and indicates poor perfusion.

PUPILS

The pupils are the dark centers of the eye, which react to changes in the amount of light reaching the eye by constricting (getting smaller) or dilating (getting bigger). The pupils should constrict when exposed to light and dilate when covered from light. Normally both eyes react in the same manner. Sometimes, head injuries or neurological problems can cause the pupils not to be **reactive to light** (termed *nonreactive*) or cause one pupil to react as expected and the other to be nonreactive (termed *unequally reactive*). The pupils are normally midsize, which is neither constricted nor dilated.

To assess the pupils, follow these steps:
1. Look at the patient's pupils and determine how the pupils look in the ambient light. Note if the pupils are dilated, constricted, or normal.
2. Using a penlight, pass the light across each pupil and note the response. Each pupil should constrict to the same extent (Fig. 5-9).

If the area is brightly lighted, such as in bright sunlight, a penlight may not cause the pupils to react. In this case, cover each eye from the light for a few seconds and then uncover it. Note the reaction of the pupils. Head injuries, eye injuries, or

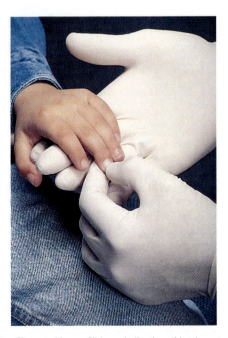

Fig. 5-8 Slow capillary refill is an indication of inadequate perfusion in children less than 6 years of age.

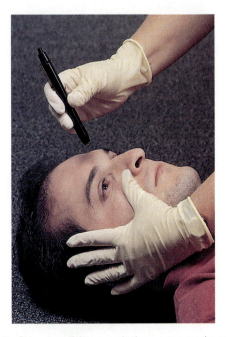

Fig. 5-9 Shine a penlight across both eyes to note the pupillary reaction.

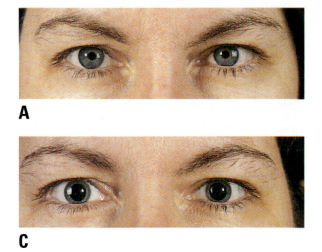

A

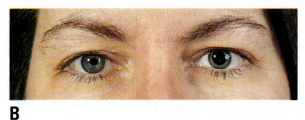

B

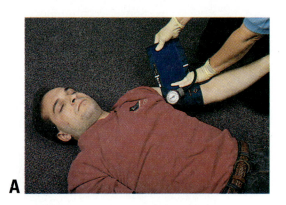

C

Fig. 5-10 The assessment of pupils. Normal pupils are equal and reactive, neither dilated nor constricted. **A,** Constricted pupils. **B,** Uneven pupils. **C,** Dilated pupils.

TECHNIQUE 5-1
Measuring Blood Pressure by Auscultation

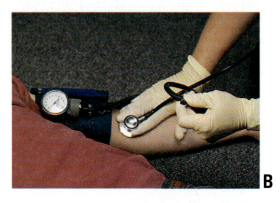

A

B

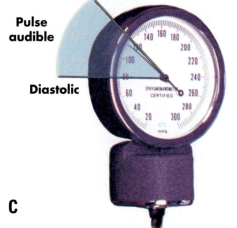

Systolic

Pulse
audible

Diastolic

C

Fig. 5-11 Choose a cuff of the appropriate size. Palpate the brachial pulse. **A, Place the blood pressure cuff around the patient's upper arm.** The lower edge of the cuff should be about 2.5 cm above the point where the brachial pulse was palpated. **B, Place the head of the stethoscope over the pulse location of the brachial artery distal to the blood pressure cuff.** Close the valve on the blood pressure cuff and inflate it to 200 mm Hg. Slowly release the pressure in the cuff while listening with the stethoscope. **C, Note the number when you hear the first beat. This is the systolic pressure. Note the number when you hear the beat disappear or become muffled. This number is the diastolic pressure.** Record both pressures.

drugs can all influence the size and reactivity of the pupils. Note all assessment findings.

Figure 5-10A through C shows constricted pupils, uneven pupils, and dilated pupils.

BLOOD PRESSURE

Blood pressure is a measurement of the force the blood exerts against the walls of blood vessels during the heart's contraction and relaxation phases. The **systolic blood pressure** is a measurement of the pressure exerted against the walls of the arteries as the wave of blood produced by the contraction of the heart passes that point in the artery. During each contraction of the heart, the pressure rises momentarily as blood is pumped through the arteries.

The **diastolic pressure** is the force exerted against the walls of the blood vessels as the heart relaxes. It represents the pressure exerted against the walls of the arteries between the waves of blood passing through the arteries.

It is important to understand that one blood pressure reading is not valuable, unless it is extremely high or low. Changes in successive blood pressure readings, however, may provide valuable clues about the patient's condition. This information must be documented on the prehospital care report. Any values outside the average range or significant changes should be included in your verbal and written report.

There are two methods for obtaining a patient's blood pressure. Auscultation is the preferred method for assessing blood pressure. This method uses a blood pressure cuff and stethoscope (*see* Technique 5-1).

Palpation is an alternate method to measure blood pressure. You measure the systolic blood pressure by feeling for return of the pulse with deflation of the cuff. You can use the palpation method in situations when you can not hear stethoscope sounds well because the patient's pulse is too weak or because the environment is too noisy. Technique 5-2 describes how to perform this method.

Blood pressure should be measured in all patients more than 3 years of age. The average ranges of blood pressures for adults and children are listed in Table 5-1. Remember that these are only average ranges and that a blood pressure outside of these ranges can still be normal for that individual. Ask patients if they know the usual range of their blood pressure.

VITAL SIGN REASSESSMENT

With stable patients, reassess the vital signs every 15 minutes. Stable patients are alert and ori-

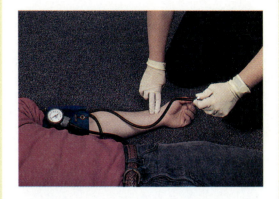

TECHNIQUE 5-2
Palpation of Blood Pressure

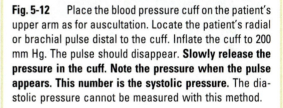

Fig. 5-12   Place the blood pressure cuff on the patient's upper arm as for auscultation. Locate the patient's radial or brachial pulse distal to the cuff. Inflate the cuff to 200 mm Hg. The pulse should disappear. **Slowly release the pressure in the cuff. Note the pressure when the pulse appears. This number is the systolic pressure.** The diastolic pressure cannot be measured with this method.

ented, with vital signs within the normal limits and with no signs that their condition is worsening. Vital signs in unstable patients should be reassessed every 5 minutes as you monitor their condition constantly (Fig. 5-13). Patients are unstable when they have mental status changes, poor vital signs outside average limits, or a worsening condition. Also assess patients' vital signs before and after every intervention. If the transport time is less than 15 minutes, at least obtain a baseline set of vital signs and one more set before arrival at the hospital.

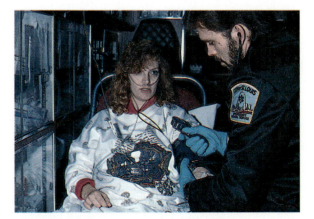

Fig. 5-13   Repeat the vital sign assessment every 5 minutes for an unstable patient.

Remember that your general assessment of the patient, especially in infants or children, is more important than the vital signs. Notice if the patient appears sick, is in respiratory distress, or is unresponsive. These are better assessments of status than vital signs.

It is important to remember that the vital sign numbers provided in this chapter are only average ranges. For any individual person, a blood pressure, pulse, or respiratory rate not within the average limits can still be appropriate for them. Trends in vital signs allow us to track changes in the patient's condition.

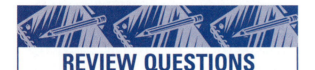

REVIEW QUESTIONS

BASELINE VITAL SIGNS

1. Two methods to measure blood pressure are _____ and _____ .

2. Baseline vital signs should be assessed soon after determining the patient's chief complaint. True or False?

3. Skin temperature and appearance are not good indicators of the patient's perfusion. True or False?

1. Auscultation; palpation
2. True
3. False

SAMPLE HISTORY

A patient **history** is a concise and inclusive set of information you gather about patients and their medical problems. The acronym SAMPLE stands for the six elements of the history:

- **S**igns and symptoms
- **A**llergies
- **M**edications
- **P**ertinent past medical history
- **L**ast oral intake (solid or liquid)
- **E**vents leading to injury or illness

Signs and symptoms are different kinds of indications of a possible problem. A **sign** is any medical or trauma condition EMTs can observe in the patient and identify. For example, signs include skin color and temperature, blood pressure, pulse, respirations, lacerations, bleeding, or a rigid abdomen. A **symptom** is any nonobservable condition described by the patient. For example, patients may state that they feel nauseous, have a headache, or just feel sick. You cannot see these symptoms and can only ask the patient about them. Sometimes patients state symptoms that are unclear or not specific, or they may have reported several symptoms that seem equally important. Encourage them to state clearly the problem that caused them to call the ambulance. Signs and symptoms are important because these form the basis for how you care for the patient.

Ask the patient about any *allergies* to medications, foods, or environmental factors, and always look for a medical alert tag. Some people are allergic to certain medications such as penicillin or sulfa drugs. Other people may be allergic to shellfish or other foods such as milk. Try to obtain specific information from the patient about allergies. This information may lead you to suspect that an allergic reaction has occurred and to guide appropriate treatment. In addition, if the patient's mental status changes en route to the hospital, you can provide the receiving facility staff with this valuable information.

Identify any *medications* the patient is taking. Ask the patient if the medications are current or recent and if they have been prescribed. Again, look for a medical identification tag. The medical direction physician may authorize you to assist with certain prescribed medications. Determining that the patient is taking a medication and investigating this information may enable you to provide additional care.

Ask for *pertinent past medical history* including recent or past medical problems, surgeries, and injuries. Keep the patient focused on recent or pertinent medical history. Surgery on a patient's ankle 20 years ago, for example, usually is not relevant to the patient's chief complaint. However, heart surgery 5 years ago might be important to the patient's current problem. This information may guide you to look for subtle signs and symptoms that may not be obvious at first. In addition, give this information to the medical direction physician, who may request that additional care be provided to the patient.

Last oral intake includes the time and quantity of both solid and liquid food. Get specific information about any recent change in eating habits or lack of eating. Some patients may intentionally not eat or overeat. Also consider alcohol intake or ingestion of other nonfood substances. The time of last oral intake is relevant in case emergency surgery is required. Any solids or liquids in the patient's stomach have the potential to cause airway compromise if the patient is unable to protect their own airway.

Events leading to the injury or illness should be identified. Chest pain with exertion or at rest should be noted. Other symptoms such as dizziness or confusion may also provide the receiving facility with important information. Sometimes the order in which the symptoms occurred is important. For example, dizziness may be the chief complaint, but the patient may state that it occurred after chest pain began. When assessing ill patients, remember the OPQRST questions, although not all signs and symptoms fit into this acronym. O is for onset—the original onset of the patient's illness or condition, such as the original diagnosis of heart disease, not necessarily the specific episode the patient is now experiencing. P is for provocation—what makes the sign or symptom better or worse. Q represents quality—the patient's subjective description of the sign or symptom. R is for radiation—question the patient to determine if the pain radiates to any other location. S is severity—it is helpful to ask the patient to rate the severity of the sign or symptom. A 1-to-10 scale with 1 meaning no symptoms and 10 meaning the worst the patient can imagine will help you judge the symptoms. T represents time—the length of time that the signs or symptoms have been present.

The information you gather in the SAMPLE history can help you provide care to the patient. Knowing information about past medical problems, allergies, and medications can help the medical direction physician give you guidance. Should a patient become unresponsive after the initial contact with EMS, you will have gained valuable information to help the receiving facility make decisions in the care provided to the patient.

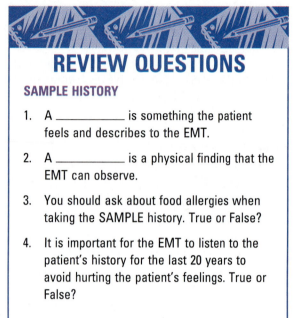

REVIEW QUESTIONS

SAMPLE HISTORY

1. A _____ is something the patient feels and describes to the EMT.

2. A _____ is a physical finding that the EMT can observe.

3. You should ask about food allergies when taking the SAMPLE history. True or False?

4. It is important for the EMT to listen to the patient's history for the last 20 years to avoid hurting the patient's feelings. True or False?

1. Symptom
2. Sign
3. True
4. False

CHAPTER SUMMARY

BASELINE VITAL SIGNS

A patient's vital signs include breathing; pulse; skin color, temperature, and condition; pupils; and blood pressure. Breathing and pulse are both evaluated for rate and quality. Skin colors include pink (normal), pale, cyanotic, flushed, and jaundiced. Skin should be warm and dry. Abnormal skin temperatures include hot, cool, and cold; abnormal skin conditions include wet, moist, and excessively dry. Pupils should be equal in size and reactive to light. Blood pressure measurements are taken for patients more than 3 years of age. Trends in vital signs can reveal changes in the patient's condition. Vital signs should be evaluated every 5 minutes for unstable patients and every 15 minutes for stable patients.

SAMPLE HISTORY

The SAMPLE history is a systematic approach for EMTs to assess the patient's history. The acronym SAMPLE stands for:

- Signs and symptoms
- Allergies
- Medications
- Pertinent past medical history
- Last oral intake
- Events leading to the injury or illness

UNITED STATES DEPARTMENT OF TRANSPORTATION NATIONAL HIGHWAY TRAFFIC SAFETY ADMINISTRATION EMT–BASIC OBJECTIVES

Check your knowledge. The National Registry of EMTs and many state EMS agencies use the objectives below to develop EMT–Basic certification examinations. Can you meet them?

COGNITIVE

1. Identify the components of vital signs.
2. Describe the methods to obtain a breathing rate.
3. Identify the attributes that should be obtained when assessing breathing.
4. Differentiate between shallow, labored, and noisy breathing.
5. Describe the methods to obtain a pulse rate.
6. Identify the information obtained when assessing a patient's pulse.
7. Differentiate between a strong, weak, regular, and irregular pulse.
8. Describe the methods to assess the skin color, temperature, condition (capillary refill in infants and children).
9. Identify the normal and abnormal skin colors.
10. Differentiate between pale, blue, red, and yellow skin colors.
11. Identify the normal and abnormal skin temperature.
12. Differentiate between hot, cool, and cold skin temperatures.
13. Identify normal and abnormal skin conditions.
14. Identify normal and abnormal capillary refill in infants and children.
15. Describe the methods to assess the pupils.
16. Identify normal and abnormal pupil size.
17. Differentiate between dilated (big) and constricted (small) pupil size.
18. Differentiate between reactive and nonreactive pupils and equal and unequal pupils.
19. Describe the methods to assess blood pressure.
20. Define systolic pressure.
21. Define diastolic pressure.
22. Explain the difference between auscultation and palpation for obtaining a blood pressure.
23. Identify the components of the SAMPLE history.
24. Differentiate between a sign and a symptom.
25. State the importance of accurately reporting and recording the baseline vital signs.
26. Discuss the need to search for additional medical identification.

AFFECTIVE

1. Explain the value of performing the baseline vital signs.
2. Recognize and respond to the feelings patients experience during assessment.
3. Defend the need for obtaining and recording an accurate set of vital signs.
4. Explain the rationale of recording additional sets of vital signs.
5. Explain the importance of obtaining a SAMPLE history.

PSYCHOMOTOR

1. Demonstrate the skills involved in assessment of breathing.
2. Demonstrate the skills associated in obtaining a pulse.
3. Demonstrate the skills associated with assessing skin color, temperature, condition, and capillary refill in infants and children.
4. Demonstrate the skills associated with assessing the pupils.
5. Demonstrate the skills associated with obtaining a blood pressure.
6. Demonstrate the skills that should be used to obtain information from the patient, family, or bystanders at the scene.

6 LIFTING AND MOVING PATIENTS

KEY TERMS

Body mechanics: The principles of effective movement used in lifting and moving patients.

Emergency move: A patient move used when there is an immediate danger to the patient or crew members if the patient is not moved, or when life-saving care cannot be given because of the patient's location or position.

Nonurgent move: A patient move used when there is no present or anticipated threat to the patient's life and care can be adequately and safely administered.

Power grip: A hand position that provides maximum force to the object being lifted, using a maximum surface area of the hands; the fingers and palm come into complete contact with the object.

Recovery position: The left lateral recumbent position for a patient to maintain an open airway by allowing secretions to drain by gravity and prevent the tongue from occluding the posterior aspect of the mouth.

Urgent move: A patient move used when the patient's condition may become life-threatening.

IN THE FIELD

The EMTs Joe and Jeff responded to the emergency call of an 82-year-old woman complaining of shortness of breath. It was the middle of summer, and the temperature outside was 98° F (37° C). When Joe and Jeff arrived at the scene, they reached the third floor by narrow, steep stairs. In the third floor apartment, they began care for the patient and realized that using the ambulance stretcher would place the patient and crew at risk. The stairway was too narrow and steep to maneuver a stretcher.

While Joe assessed the patient and provided additional care, Jeff retrieved the stair chair from the ambulance. The crew safely moved the patient in the stair chair from the apartment to the street level. Then they transferred the patient to the wheeled ambulance stretcher and began transport to the hospital.

In this situation, the wheeled stretcher would have been dangerous for both the crew and patient. The crew could have been stuck in the narrow and steep hallway with no option but to back up the stairs to the third floor. Knowing how to use their available equipment helped them make the correct decision.

Lifting and moving patients is an important area of EMT education and practice. As an EMT, you will care for patients in many difficult situations and positions. When you arrive on scene, the patient is not always in an accessible location or a position that is easy to load for transport. You may have to extricate a patient from a vehicle, carry a patient down from a third floor apartment through a narrow, dark stairwell, or move the patient from a bedroom that is inaccessible to your ambulance stretcher. Your patient may be in remote, rugged terrain. You may find your patients in many situations. Using the principles of proper patient lifting and moving and the tools available to you, you can safely and quickly transport patients to the emergency vehicle and the hospital.

EMTs frequently sustain disabling injuries when performing their duties. Most of these injuries can be prevented by using proper lifting and moving techniques.

BODY MECHANICS

Of the many ways to injure yourself as an EMT, one of the most common is through poor body mechanics. **Body mechanics** are the principles of effective movement used in lifting and moving patients. Use of proper body mechanics is essential in performing your duties and greatly reduces your chances of being injured.

LIFTING

Lifting patients poses one of the greatest dangers for healthcare providers. The risk of lower-back injury is high. EMTs can damage their backs over long periods of time by lifting with poor body mechanics. Chronic back pain may not be disabling but can limit lifestyle and work capabilities. A sudden traumatic back injury can also occur, such as a ruptured disk. This injury causes immediate and crippling pain that could end your career.

Take safety precautions when lifting a patient. Keep your back straight and use your legs, not your back, to lift the patient. The closer you hold the patient's weight to your body, the less strain is placed on you. Figure 6-1A illustrates an improper lifting technique with the back bent.

When preparing to lift a patient, consider the patient's weight and if your crew requires additional help to safely lift the patient. Every crew member has different lifting capabilities, and it is your responsibility not to surpass your own limit.

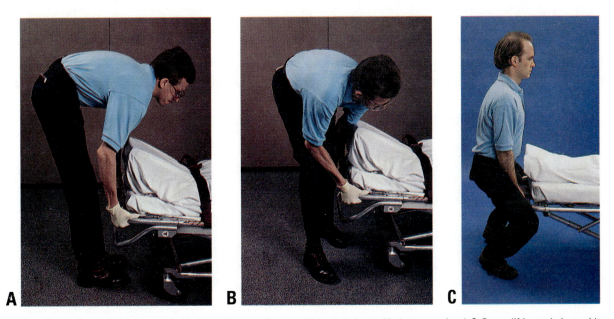

Fig. 6-1. **A,** Improper lifting technique with the back bent. **B,** Improper lifting technique with the torso twisted. **C,** Proper lifting technique with knees bent.

When lifting, do not twist your torso. This increases the strain on your lower spine and may cause injury; this is also the main cause of ruptured disks. Figure 6-1B illustrates an improper lifting technique with the torso twisted.

Position your feet about shoulder width apart, making sure you have good traction under your feet and that you are positioned close to the patient you are lifting (Fig. 6-1C). Always communicate with your crew. Don't be afraid to let your crew know if you need help carrying a patient. Don't try to be a hero; you may injure yourself and place the patient and your crew at risk.

Proper lifting depends on understanding several key principles (eg, the weight of the patient). Again, be sure you and the crew can handle the lift. At the very minimum, two people are required for a successful lift. Call for more help if necessary. The more help available, the easier and safer the lift will be. Use an even number of people to maintain the balance of the patient and the lifting and moving device.

The crew must also know the weight limitations of any equipment being used. Most lifting and moving equipment has a warning label similar to that shown in Figure 6-2. Check the manufacturer's guidelines for equipment weight limits. You may have to improvise if the patient's weight exceeds the capacity of the equipment. There is no set rule other than to use skillful common sense in moving the patient. If the situation appears unsafe

to you, do not move the patient until you are comfortable with the method to be used.

When lifting from the ground, use the squat lift, also called the *power-lift,* position. This position keeps your back locked during the lift. The squat lift (*see* Technique 6-1) is the ideal method for lifting from the ground, particularly for crew members with weak knees or thighs. If only two crew members are present, maintain balance by standing opposite each other at the sides or ends of the stretcher when lifting the patient.

CARRYING

Sometimes EMTs must carry patients from the scene to the ambulance. As a general rule, always

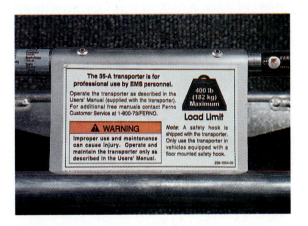

Fig. 6-2. Warning labels on lifting equipment specify weight limits.

TECHNIQUE 6-1
The Squat Lift for Lifting a Stretcher

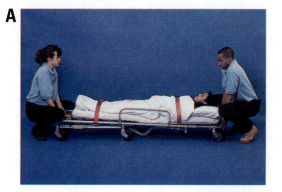

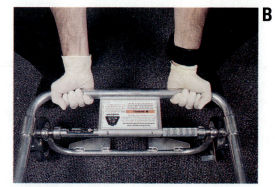

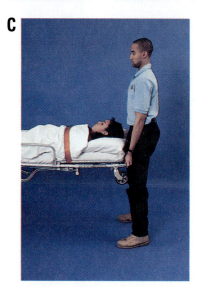

Fig. 6-3 **A,** Stand facing the stretcher with your feet shoulder width apart. (This can be done at either the ends or the side of the stretcher.) **Squat down to the stretcher, bending at the knees. Keep your back tight, with the abdominal muscles locking your back in a normal slight inward curve. B, Always use the power grip to get the maximum force from your hands. The palm and fingers should come into complete contact with the object and all fingers should bend at the same angles. Your hands should be at least 25 cm (10 in) apart. C, Keep your feet flat and distribute your weight to the balls of your feet, or just behind them. Stand up, making sure that your back is locked and your upper body comes up before your hips.** When lowering the stretcher, reverse the above steps.

try to wheel patients to the ambulance rather than carry them. Let the stretcher wheels do the work for you. However, in some situations, the crew has to physically carry a patient and device to the ambulance. In this case, the safety precautions and guidelines are the same as for lifting a patient.

Ideally, EMTs would work with partners of similar height to maintain better balance when lifting and carrying. This is usually impossible, so crew members should try to adapt to height differences. Be careful not to hyperextend your back or lean to either side to compensate for any imbalance when carrying a patient. When carrying a stretcher or backboard with only two crew members, face each other in opposing positions from the sides or ends (Fig. 6-4). The more crew members available to

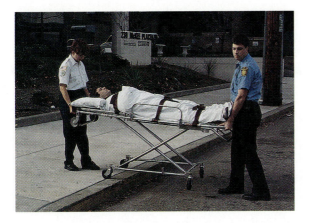

Fig. 6-4. When carrying the stretcher with only two crew members, face each other in opposing positions from either the sides or ends of the stretcher.

help, the easier it is to carry the patient. The stretcher or backboard can be carried using the one-handed technique with multiple rescuers (Fig. 6-5). This is much safer than a two-person carry, because the stretcher or backboard is balanced and the weight is evenly distributed, and there is less weight for each person to carry.

When you must carry a patient down stairs, a stair chair should be used (Fig. 6-6). Stair chairs allow the crew more flexibility for handling and transporting the patient. The patient is strapped to the stair chair, and the smaller size of the stair chair makes it easier to maneuver in tight, steep areas. Although a stair chair is the best method for steep stairs, it should not be used for a patient with a possible spinal injury. In this case, the patient can be transported down stairs, immobilized on the long spine board.

REACHING

Reaching for patients can also lead to injury. Reaching may simply be reaching across the stretcher to fasten a buckle or straining to pull the patient onto a backboard. Try to keep your back in a locked position, avoid leaning back over your hips, and avoid twisting your back. All of these actions place strain on the spine and increase the chance of injury. Generally, try not to reach more than 0.5 m (20 in) in front of you, and avoid situations where you must reach for longer than 1 minute to perform a task. Reaching for longer than 1 minute may fatigue body muscles, increasing the chance of injury. When performing a log roll with the patient on the ground, keep your back straight when leaning over the patient, lean from the hips, and use your shoulder muscles to help with the roll. Figure 6-7 demonstrates proper technique when preparing for a log roll.

PUSHING AND PULLING

Whenever possible, it is preferable to push rather than pull a patient into position, although in some situations pulling may be the only option. Again, keep your back locked in. The back is simply not strong enough to bear the weight of your body along with the added stress of the patient's weight. Keep the weight close to your body. When pulling the patient, keep the line of pull through the center of your body by bending your knees. The line of pull is the path from the patient directly to you. Push the patient with your arms between your waist and shoulder.

Be careful whenever the weight load is below your waist level. In this case, kneel down to meet

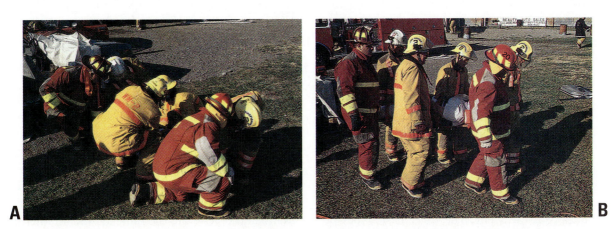

A **B**

Fig. 6-5. **A,** Multiple rescuers preparing to lift a backboard using the one-handed technique. **B,** Multiple rescuers lifting and carrying a patient.

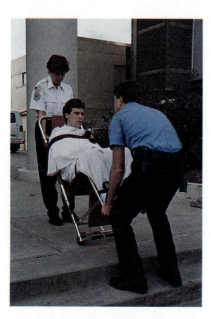

Fig. 6-6. A stair chair provides more flexibility for handling and transporting the patient in narrow or steep areas.

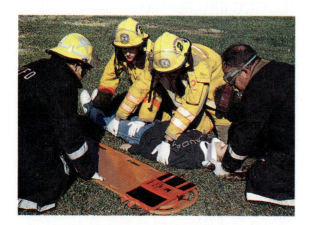

Fig. 6-7. When performing a log roll with the patient on the ground, keep your back straight while leaning over the patient, lean from the hips, and use your shoulder muscles to help with the roll.

the patient to prevent back injury. Avoid pushing or pulling from above if possible, and keep your elbows bent with arms close to the sides.

PRINCIPLES OF MOVING PATIENTS

Movement of any patient depends on two major considerations: the seriousness of the patient's condition and the presence of any life-threatening conditions at the scene. The three basic types of

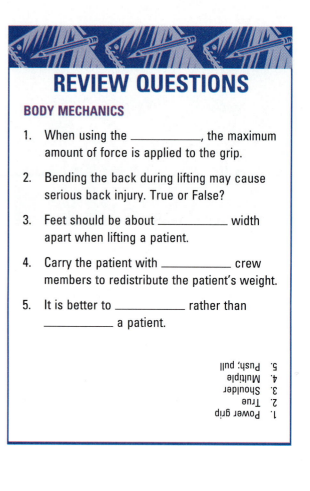

REVIEW QUESTIONS

BODY MECHANICS

1. When using the _____, the maximum amount of force is applied to the grip.

2. Bending the back during lifting may cause serious back injury. True or False?

3. Feet should be about _____ width apart when lifting a patient.

4. Carry the patient with _____ crew members to redistribute the patient's weight.

5. It is better to _____ rather than _____ a patient.

1. Power grip
2. True
3. Shoulder
4. Multiple
5. Push; pull

patient moves are: emergency moves, urgent moves, and nonurgent moves.

An **emergency move** is required when there is an immediate danger to the patient or to you if the patient is not moved, or when life-saving care cannot be given because of the patient's location or position. An **urgent move** is used when the patient's condition may become life-threatening. A **nonurgent move** is appropriate when there is no threat to life, and care can be adequately and safely administered.

EMERGENCY MOVES

Once you have determined an emergency move is necessary (*see* Principle 6-1), take caution not to aggravate a possible spinal injury. However, there is no time to properly immobilize the spine in an emergency move. Attempt to protect the spine by pulling the patient in the direction of the long axis of the body while keeping the patient's body in a straight line. It is impossible to remove a patient from a vehicle quickly and simultaneously provide as much protection to the spine as with an interim

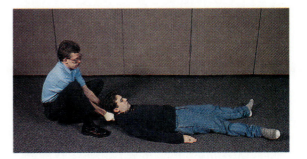

Fig. 6-8. The clothing pull technique for moving a patient.

immobilization device. A patient who is lying on the floor or ground can be moved by pulling on the patient's clothing in the neck and shoulder area, putting the patient on a blanket and dragging the blanket, dragging the patient with your hands under the patient's armpits from the back, or by grasping the patient's forearms. Again, the general principle is to maintain as much in-line spine con-

trol as possible. The clothing pull uses the patient's clothing as the point for balance. Your arms cradle the patient's head and the pulling comes from the patient's clothing. The blanket drag has the same principle, except the patient is placed onto a blanket. If a patient is difficult to handle because of size or lack of cooperation, then securing your arms under the patient's arms will help to maintain bal-

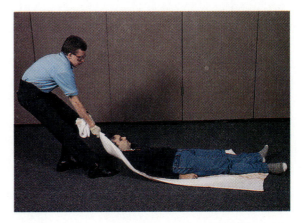

Fig. 6-9. The blanket drag technique for moving a patient.

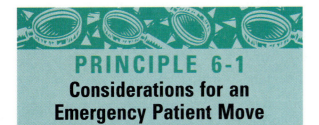

PRINCIPLE 6-1
Considerations for an Emergency Patient Move

There is an immediate danger to the patient or crew members if the patient is not moved in these situations:

1). Fire or danger of fire.

2). Explosives or other hazardous materials.

3). Inability to protect the patient from other hazards at the scene.

4). Inability to gain access to other patients in a vehicle who need life-saving care.

5). Any other situation that has the potential for causing injury.

6). Life-saving care cannot be given because of patient location or position: for example, a cardiac arrest patient sitting in a chair.

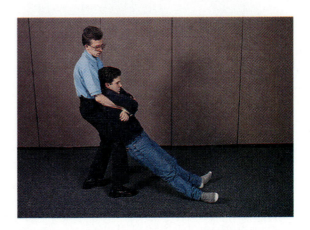

Fig. 6-10. Pulling the patient under the arms is also a technique used for moving or lifting a patient.

ance and control. Figures 6-8 through 6-10 show three common methods for emergency moves.

URGENT MOVES

In an urgent move, the patient's condition can become life threatening at any moment, requiring rapid movement of the patient for treatment (*see* Principle 6-2). If the patient does not have a suspected spine injury, then the patient may be moved to the ambulance as soon as possible using the safest method available. However, if a patient is in a vehicle, the principle for rapid extrication should be followed, with consideration for a potential spinal injury (Technique 6-2).

NONURGENT MOVES

For a nonurgent move, there are two major techniques to move the patient from the ground to a stretcher: the direct ground lift (Technique 6-3) and the extremity lift (Technique 6-4).

Transfer of a supine patient from a stretcher to a bed may be accomplished by the direct carry (Technique 6-5) or the draw sheet method (Technique 6-6).

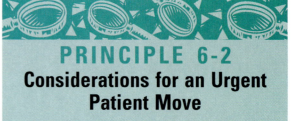

PRINCIPLE 6-2
Considerations for an Urgent Patient Move

1). Unresponsive or incoherent patient
2). Inadequate breathing
3). Signs and symptoms of shock

TECHNIQUE 6-2
Rapid Extrication of a Patient from a Vehicle

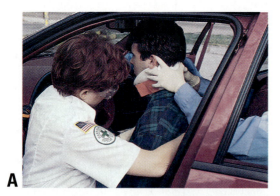 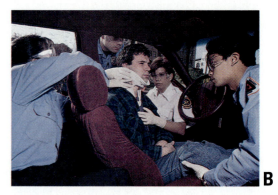

Fig. 6-11   **A,** An EMT steps into the vehicle behind the patient and carefully maneuvers the cervical spine into neutral in-line position and provides manual stabilization. The airway is then quickly assessed and opened by using a jaw thrust if necessary. **Another EMT approaches the patient from the side, quickly examines the neck, applies the cervical immobilization device, and supports the torso. B,** A third EMT places a long backboard near the door and **moves to the opposite side of the car to free the patient's legs. At the direction of the EMT at the patient's head, the patient is rotated in several short, coordinated moves until the patient's back is in the open doorway with feet on the passenger seat.** The patient's back is quickly examined.

Continued

TECHNIQUE 6-2
Rapid Extrication of a Patient from a Vehicle

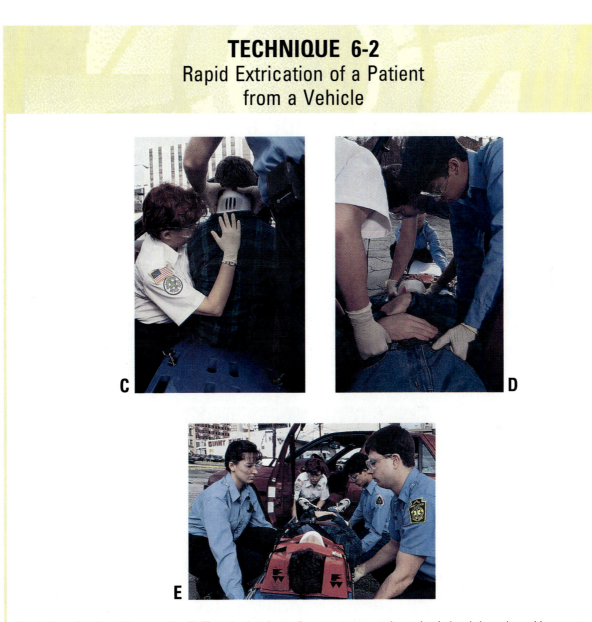

Fig. 6-11 *Continued* Because the EMT at the head usually cannot support the patient's head throughout this process, another EMT must step in and support the patient's head and neck. **C, The end of the long backboard is placed on the seat, under the patient's buttocks. [Other public safety officials support the other end of the board as the patient is lowered onto the board.]** The neck and back are moved as one unit. **D, The EMTs then slide the patient into proper position on the board in short, coordinated moves, as directed by the EMT at the patient's head. E, The patient should then be quickly moved to the ambulance for further evaluation and treatment and secured to the long backboard as soon as possible.** Several variations of this technique are possible. This technique must be accomplished without compromise to the spine.

TECHNIQUE 6-3
Direct Ground Lift (No Suspected Spine Injury)

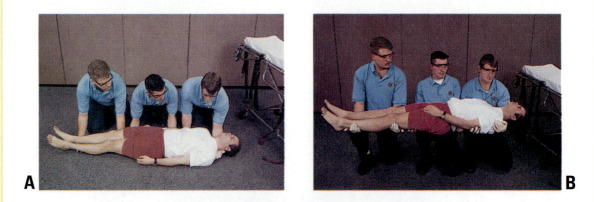

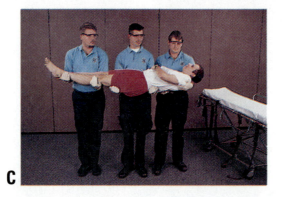

Fig. 6-12   A, Three EMTs line up on one side of the patient and kneel for lifting power. The patient's arms are placed on the chest if possible. **EMT 1 at the patient's head places one arm under the patient's neck and shoulder, cradles the patient's head, and places the other arm under the patient's upper back. EMT 2 places one arm under the patient's waist and one arm below the patient's buttocks. EMT 3 should place both arms under the patient's waist and EMT's 1 and 2 should slide their arms either up to the midback or down to the buttocks, depending on the weight distribution. B, On signal from EMT 1, all three EMTs lift the patient onto their knees and roll the patient in toward their chests. C, Again on signal, the EMTs stand and move the patient to the cot or stretcher.** To lower the patient, the steps are reversed.

TECHNIQUE 6-4
Extremity Lift (No Suspected Spine Injury)

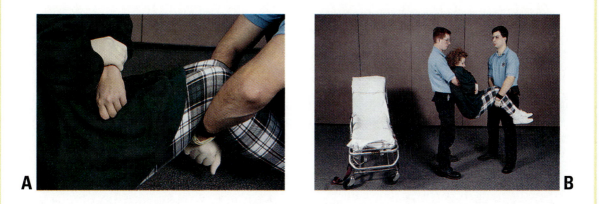

Fig. 6-13   **A, EMT 1 kneels at the patient's head and EMT 2 kneels at the patient's side by the knees. EMT 1 places one hand under each of the patient's arms and grasps the wrists. EMT 2 reaches under and grasps the patient's knees, reaching as closely under the patient's hips as possible to redistribute the weight.** (Otherwise, EMT 1 lifting the patient's chest area will have to bear the major portion of the patient's weight.) Both EMTs then move up to a crouching position. **B, The EMTs stand up simultaneously and move with the patient to a stretcher.**

TECHNIQUE 6-5
Transfer of Supine Patient from the Stretcher to the Bed by the Direct Carry Method

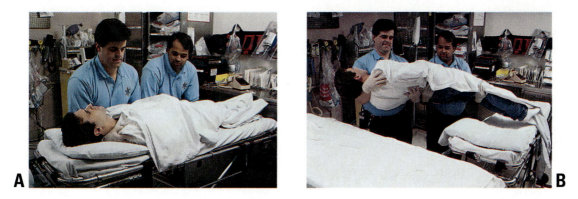

Fig. 6-14   **A,** Position the stretcher perpendicular to the bed with the head end of the stretcher at the foot of the bed. Prepare the bed to receive the patient. **EMTs 1 and 2 stand between the bed and stretcher, facing the patient. EMT 1 slides one arm under the patient's neck and cradles the patient's shoulders, while EMT 2 slides one hand under the patient's hip and lifts slightly. EMT 1 then slides the other arm under the patient's back. EMT 2 places arms underneath the hips and calves of the patient.** Both EMTs together slide the patient to the edge of the stretcher. **B, The patient is then lifted and curled in toward the EMT's chests.**
Continued

TECHNIQUE 6-5
Transfer of Supine Patient from the Stretcher to the Bed by the Direct Carry Method

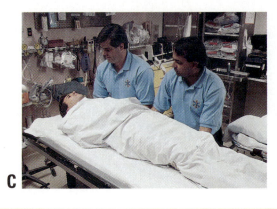

C

Fig. 6-14 *Continued* **C,** Rotating as one unit, the EMTs turn and place the patient gently onto the bed.

TECHNIQUE 6-6
Transfer of a Supine Patient from the Stretcher to the Bed by the Draw Sheet Method

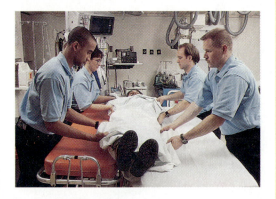

Fig. 6-15 Loosen the bottom sheet of the stretcher and position the stretcher next to the bed. Prepare the stretcher by adjusting the height to that of the bed, lowering the rails, and unbuckling the straps. Reach across the stretcher and grasp the sheet firmly at the patient's head, chest, hips, and knees. Pull the sheet to slide the patient gently onto the bed.

REVIEW QUESTIONS

PRINCIPLES OF MOVING PATIENTS

Mark each statement True or False.

1. An emergency move is considered for a patient in a vehicle on fire.

2. A cardiac arrest patient should be moved immediately if you cannot provide CPR because of the patient's position.

3. An urgent move is used for a patient with the signs and symptoms of shock.

4. An emergency move is used for a patient with a swollen, painful left ankle as long as no danger is present to the patient or crew members.

5. A nonurgent move means there is no threat to the patient's or your life.

1. True
2. True
3. True
4. False
5. True

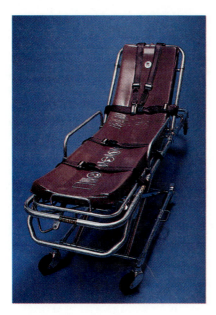

Fig. 6-16. The wheeled stretcher.

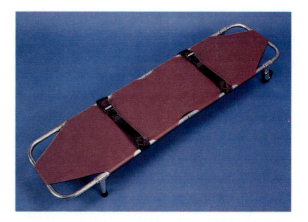

Fig. 6-17. A portable stretcher.

EQUIPMENT

Once you decide how to move the patient, choose and prepare the right equipment to do the job.

STRETCHERS AND COTS

When using stretchers and cots, use common sense in securing the patient to the device. There are numerous techniques and materials available for this purpose. The principle objective is to secure the patient to prevent the patient from moving or falling off the stretcher or cot. Depending on the weather, a blanket or waterproof cover may be required.

WHEELED STRETCHER

The most common device used for patient movement is the wheeled stretcher (Fig. 6-16). Whenever possible, move patients by rolling them on a wheeled stretcher. This saves the crew from injury or exhaustion caused by carrying a patient. However, a wheeled stretcher can be used only on smooth terrain. Direct the stretcher by guiding the foot end, while another crew member at the head of the patient pushes the stretcher. This prevents the patient from becoming dizzy or disoriented.

Lifting the stretcher is preferable in narrow, steep spaces, but this technique requires more crew strength. It is difficult to roll wheels over steep

steps. With two EMTs, one should be positioned at the patient's head and the other at the feet. This allows for greatest control and balance. A four-person carry is better because it provides more stability and places less strain on the rescuers. Each crew member carries a corner. The four-person carry is considered much safer over rough terrain.

The primary concern for loading the patient into a ambulance is safety. Follow the equipment manufacturer's directions, and ensure all stretchers and patients are secured before the ambulance moves. Be careful of traffic around the ambulance. If passing traffic is not aware of the crew's location, then crew members may be struck by passing traffic.

PORTABLE STRETCHER

A portable stretcher (Fig. 6-17) is used to transport a second patient to the same ambulance or for extrication from areas where a wheeled stretcher does not fit. The portable stretcher is commonly folded in half to allow for easy storage. There are usually brackets on the bench seat in the patient compartment of the ambulance for securing the stretcher to the bench seat before moving the ambulance. The principles are the same for securing the patient as for the wheeled stretcher.

SCOOP STRETCHER

A scoop stretcher (Fig. 6-18) is used to lift a patient from a supine position onto the stretcher for transport. The scoop stretcher is hinged and opens at the head and feet to "scoop" around and under the patient. Once the scoop stretcher is fastened, the patient can be lifted onto the transport stretcher. Because there is controversy regarding the use of a scoop stretcher for individuals with a suspected spine injury, follow local protocol. If you

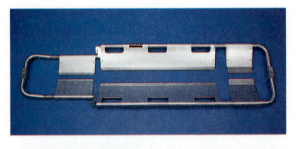

Fig. 6-18. A scoop stretcher.

do use a scoop stretcher in this case, use it to transfer a patient to a long spine board.

FLEXIBLE STRETCHER

A flexible stretcher (Fig. 6-19) can be used when there is no suspected spine injury. The flexible stretcher is made of material strong enough to hold the patient's weight, with handles at each corner to assist in moving the patient. The flexible stretcher is excellent for cases where the crew must carry the patient from an upper floor to the ground floor. The flexible stretcher provides great flexibility in patient handling.

BASKET STRETCHER

A basket stretcher is used primarily in rescue situations. The basket stretcher is constructed as a secure, rigid device that can withstand a great deal of strain (Fig. 6-20). Patients are secure when strapped down inside the stretcher. A long backboard can be placed into the stretcher when spinal immobilization is required. Ropes and other lifting devices can be attached to the basket stretcher to raise or move the stretcher over rough terrain or to evacuate the patient. The basket stretcher is the preferred device for removing patients from wilderness or rough terrain.

STAIR CHAIR

The stair chair (Fig. 6-21) is the preferred method for transporting the patient down stairs or

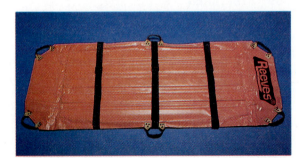

Fig. 6-19. A flexible stretcher.

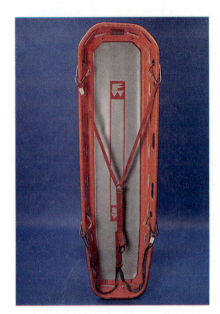

Fig. 6-20. A basket stretcher.

through narrow hallways to a stretcher. After securing the patient to this device, two EMTs can safely carry the chair. Most stair chairs have wheels at the rear, which can be used to roll the patient to the stretcher.

BACKBOARDS

Backboards come in both long and short forms. The long backboard (Fig. 6-22) is used to immobilize the entire patient. Straps must be secured across the patient's torso, waist, and legs along with a cervical immobilization device for the patient to be properly immobilized. Several varieties of long

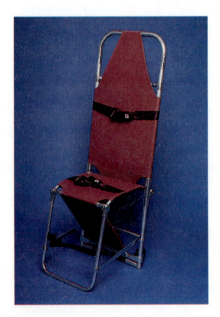

Fig. 6-21. A stair chair.

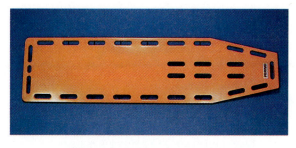

Fig. 6-22. The long backboard.

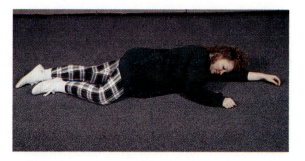

Fig. 6-24. The recovery position.

boards are in use. Chapter 28, "Injuries to the Head and Spine," describes the use of backboards in detail.

Short boards are available in two types: the traditional wooden device and commercially available vest types (Fig. 6-23). These are used to immobilize the patient's spine during extrication and must be used in conjunction with the long spine board after extrication to provide full spinal immobilization.

For each device, follow the manufacturer's directions for use and maintenance.

PATIENT POSITIONING

The patient's condition determines how you position the patient for transport. An unresponsive patient without a suspected spine injury should be placed in the **recovery position** to allow secretions to drain from the patient's airway. To place the patient in the recovery position, roll the patient onto the left side, place the left arm under the head, and bend the left knee to balance the patient (Fig. 6-24).

A patient with chest pain, discomfort, or difficulty in breathing should be allowed to sit in a position of comfort. Usually, the patient breathes easier sitting on the stretcher rather than lying down.

Remember, any patient with a suspected spine injury should be transported immobilized on a long

backboard. Place a patient with the signs and symptoms of shock (hypoperfusion) lying flat on the back, bent at the hips with feet lifted 20 to 30 cm (8 to 12 in) (shock position). If a pregnant patient has hypotension, position her on her left side. The fetus may be pressing on the vessel that returns blood to the mother's heart from the lower part of her body (the vena cava), impeding the return of blood to the heart. Positioning the patient on her left side alleviates the pressure on the vena cava (Fig. 6-25). Patients who complain of nausea or who are vomiting should be allowed to remain in a position of comfort.

Stay in a position to maintain the patient's airway or suction the airway if required. For trauma patients who are fully immobilized, special care must be taken for airway control. Suction must be available, and you may have to log roll a patient strapped to a long backboard onto their side to prevent aspiration.

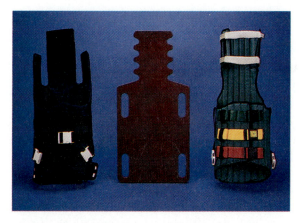

Fig. 6-23. The XP1 (*left*), short wooden backboard (*center*), and KED (*right*).

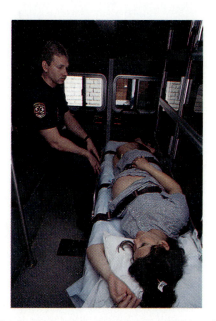

Fig. 6-25. Positioning a pregnant patient in the left lateral recumbent position alleviates the pressure on the vena cava.

Pediatric patients present a unique situation. Often children struggle against being immobilized. Pediatric immobilizers can be used that secure the patient by wrapping the infant or child completely with restraints. This prevents any movement of the infant or child and protects the spine from further damage. Figure 6-26 illustrates transportation of a child in a specially designed safety seat. Sometimes a young child is more relaxed when transported in the arms of a parent. In this case, secure both the parent and child. Situations may vary considerably, and there is no one method that works best in all cases. Use common sense to transport the parent and child safely.

When a patient is responsive and does not have a suspected spine injury, you may ask the patient for assistance in moving to the stretcher or cot. Not all patients are unresponsive or unable to assist you.

Geriatric patients often require special care as well. Older patients may move slowly and deliberately, requiring extra time for patient positioning. Be patient with elderly patients because they may be slower in following your requests. Decreased hearing and vision may also impair an elderly patient's ability to follow your directions and may also hinder the patient in moving. Certain diseases such as osteoporosis (a common disease of the elderly that causes bone thinning) may precipitate further injury. Depending on the patient's positioning, there may be difficulty in breathing. Elderly pa-

tients may startle more easily as well. Remember the special needs of the elderly when administering care to them.

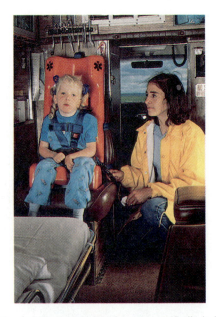

Fig. 6-26. A child secured in a safety seat specifically designed for ambulance transport.

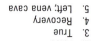

REVIEW QUESTIONS

EQUIPMENT

1. The _____ is used to fully immobilize the spine of a patient.

2. A short spine board is adequate to immobilize a patient complaining of back pain after a fall. True or False?

3. When using multiple rescuers to lift or carry a stretcher, the carry will be much safer than when only two rescuers carry the stretcher. True or False?

4. An unresponsive patient without a suspected spine injury is placed in the _____ position.

5. A pregnant patient should be placed on her _____ side because the fetus may be occluding the _____.

1. Long spine board
2. False
3. True
4. Recovery
5. Left; vena cava

CHAPTER SUMMARY

BODY MECHANICS

Use your legs, not your back, to lift a patient. Either the squat lift or the power-lift method is acceptable. Do not attempt to lift a weight beyond your physical limitations. Carrying the patient requires excellent balance and more work by the crew than rolling the patient on a wheeled stretcher. Preferably, the patient should be wheeled. A stair chair is used on tight or narrow passages and for moving up or down steps. Reaching for the patient puts much stress on the back.

Never try to reach overhead or hyperextend the back, as these lead to possible injury. It is preferable to push a patient or stretcher into position rather than pull.

PRINCIPLES OF MOVING PATIENTS

An emergency move is for patients who are in immediate danger or when life-saving care cannot be given because of the patient's location or condition. An urgent move is used when the patient has an altered mental status, inadequate breathing, or signs and symptoms of shock. A patient who has no life-threatening conditions may be moved when the patient is ready for transportation.

EQUIPMENT

Wheeled stretchers, portable stretchers, scoop stretchers, flexible stretchers, basket stretchers, stair chairs, and backboards are tools used to move the patient from the scene to the ambulance for transport. Patients should be positioned based on their condition and comfort.

UNITED STATES DEPARTMENT OF TRANSPORTATION NATIONAL HIGHWAY TRAFFIC SAFETY ADMINISTRATION EMT–BASIC OBJECTIVES

Check your knowledge. The National Registry of EMTs and many state EMS agencies use the objectives below to develop EMT–Basic certification examinations. Can you meet them?

COGNITIVE

1. Define body mechanics.
2. Discuss the guidelines and safety precautions that need to be followed when lifting a patient.
3. Describe the safe lifting of cots and stretchers.
4. Describe the guidelines and safety precautions for carrying patients and/or equipment.
5. Discuss one-handed carrying techniques.
6. Describe correct and safe carrying procedures on stairs.
7. State the guidelines for reaching and their application.
8. Describe correct reaching for log rolls.
9. State the guidelines for pushing and pulling.
10. Discuss the general considerations of moving patients.
11. State three situations that may require the use of an emergency move.
12. Identify the following patient-carrying devices:
    Wheeled ambulance stretcher
    Portable ambulance stretcher
    Scoop stretcher
    Flexible stretcher
    Basket stretcher
    Stair chair
    Long spine board

AFFECTIVE

1. Explain the rationale for properly lifting and moving patients.

PSYCHOMOTOR

1. Working with a partner, prepare each of the following devices for use, transfer a patient to the device, properly position the patient on the device, move the device to the ambulance, and load the patient into the ambulance:
    Wheeled ambulance stretcher
    Portable ambulance stretcher
    Scoop stretcher
    Flexible stretcher
    Basket stretcher
    Stair chair
    Long spine board
2. Working with a partner, the EMT–Basic will demonstrate the techniques for the transfer of a patient from an ambulance stretcher to a hospital stretcher.

AIRWAY

When we talk about the airway, we get back to the basics we learned in our first CPR course—the ABCs. We learned that the first step in providing good care is to make sure the patient's airway is clear. As EMS providers, we've come a long way in the handling and maintenance of patient airways. Whether it's maintaining the airway of a child or an adult, the importance of having good airway skills cannot be overemphasized. And maintaining these skills is just as important.

Edward F. Rzepka, NREMT-D
Hartford Emergency Squad
Hartford, Wisconsin

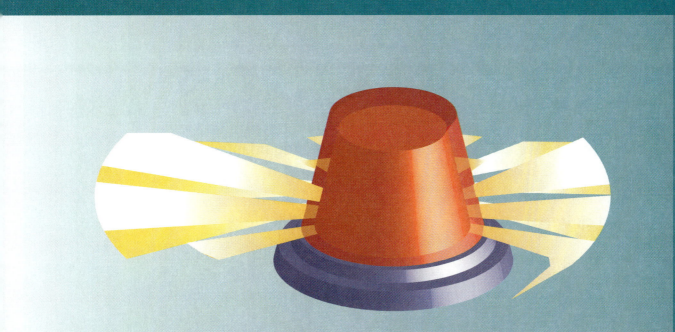

DIVISION TWO

7 THE AIRWAY

KEY TERMS

Airway: The respiratory system structures through which air passes.

Alveoli: The air sacs in the lungs where gas exchange takes place.

Bag-valve-mask (BVM): A common ventilation device consisting of a self-inflating bag, a one-way valve, a mask, and an oxygen reservoir.

Bronchi: The two major branches of the trachea into each lung.

Cricoid ring: A firm cartilage ring just inferior to the lower portion of the larynx.

Cyanotic: Bluish discoloration of mucous membranes and skin caused by hypoperfusion of tissues.

Diaphragm: The large, dome-shaped muscle that separates the thoracic from the abdominal cavities; used in breathing.

Epiglottis: The flaplike structure that prevents food and liquid from entering the trachea during swallowing.

Gag reflex: A reflex that causes the patient to retch when the back of the throat is stimulated; this reflex helps unresponsive patients protect their airways.

Glottis: The passageway into the trachea from the pharynx.

Intercostal muscles: Muscles located between the ribs that move with breathing.

Jaw thrust: A method of opening the airway by displacing the jaw forward; used instead of the head-tilt chin-lift in patients with suspected spinal injury.

Laryngectomy: A surgical procedure in which the larynx is removed.

Larynx: The voice box, or vocal cords, consisting of bands of cartilage that vibrate when we speak.

Nasal cannula: A device for delivering oxygen from tubing that has holes that blow oxygen directly into the patient's nostrils.

Nasopharyngeal airway: A flexible tube of rubber or plastic that is inserted into the patient's nostril to provide an air passage.

Nasopharynx: The part of the pharynx behind the nose.

Nonrebreather mask: A high-flow device for delivering oxygen to the patient.

Oropharyngeal airway: A curved piece of plastic that goes into the patient's mouth and lifts the tongue out of the oropharynx.

Oropharynx: The part of the pharynx behind the mouth.

Pharynx: The part of the airway behind the nose and mouth, divided into two regions: the nasopharynx and the oropharynx.

Suction devices: Devices used to suction secretions and fluids from the mouth and oropharynx of unresponsive patients.

Trachea: The windpipe.

Tracheal stoma: A permanent artificial opening in the trachea.

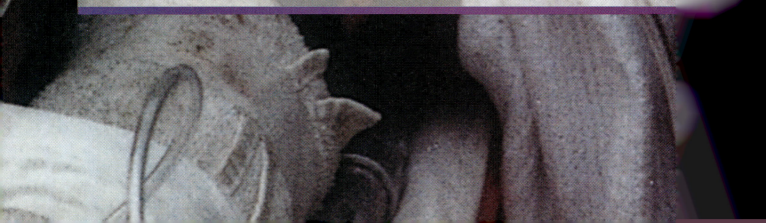

THE RESPIRATORY SYSTEM

The respiratory system includes all the body structures through which air passes. These tubes and passageways make up what is known as the **airway**. Because the body requires a continual supply of fresh air, anything that blocks or obstructs the airway is a serious life threat. As an EMT, you use your most critical skills to ensure that the patient's airway remains clear and open.

RESPIRATORY ANATOMY

Familiarity with the anatomy of the airway helps you understand airway management (Fig. 7-1). The airway begins with the mouth and nose and continues into the **pharynx**. The pharynx is divided into two regions: the **nasopharynx** and the **oropharynx**. The area just behind the nose is the nasopharynx, and the oropharynx lies just inferior to the nasopharynx and is commonly called the *back of the throat*.

The passageway into the **trachea,** or windpipe, is called the **glottis**. The **epiglottis** is a flaplike structure that prevents food and liquid from entering the trachea during swallowing.

The **larynx**, or *voice box*, lies just inferior to the glottic opening. The larynx forms the prominence commonly called the *Adam's apple*. Inferior to the larynx is the **cricoid ring**. The cricoid ring is a important landmark because it is the only airway structure that is a complete ring of firm cartilage.

As the trachea descends from the cricoid ring, it divides into two **bronchi**. Each bronchi subdivides into smaller and smaller branches, ending at the **alveoli**, where gas exchange takes place (Fig. 7-2).

The main muscles of respiration are the **diaphragm** and the **intercostal muscles**. The diaphragm is the large, dome-shaped muscle that separates the thoracic from the abdominal cavities. The intercostal muscles between the ribs cause the ribs to flare outward and upward when they contract.

When the diaphragm contracts, it flattens. Contraction of the diaphragm and the intercostal muscles increases the size of the chest, and air is pulled into the lungs through the mouth and nose. Inhalation is therefore an active process controlled by muscle contraction. During exhalation, the diaphragm and intercostal muscles relax. The diaphragm moves upward, and the ribs move downward and inward. This movement decreases the size of the chest, moving air out through the mouth and nose. Ordinarily, exhalation is a passive process that occurs when the muscles relax. In cases of respiratory distress, the abdominal and intercostal muscles are used to force exhalation.

RESPIRATORY PHYSIOLOGY

The process of exchanging oxygen and carbon dioxide is essential for life. Any interruption of respiration can be fatal within minutes. This gas ex-

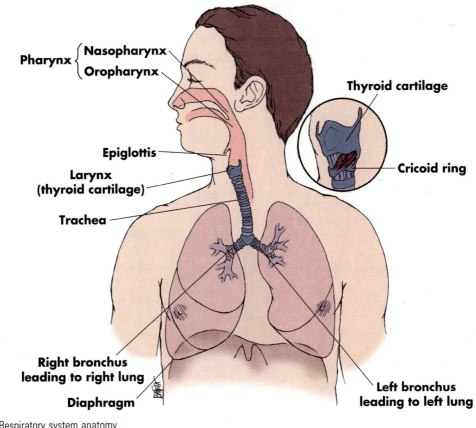

Fig. 7-1 Respiratory system anatomy.

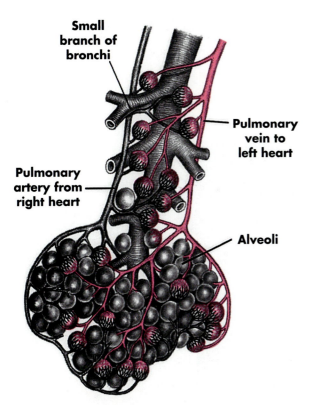

Fig. 7-2 In the lungs, capillaries surround the alveoli.

change occurs at two sites: the alveolar/capillary exchange and the capillary/cellular exchange.

Air entering the lungs is rich in oxygen and low in carbon dioxide. The blood pumped to the lungs from the right side of the heart is low in oxygen and high in carbon dioxide. At the alveolar/capillary interface in the lungs, oxygen enters the bloodstream, and carbon dioxide moves out of the blood into the alveoli, where it will be exhaled from the lungs.

The process is reversed at the capillary/cellular level. Blood in the arteries entering the capillaries is high in oxygen and low in carbon dioxide. The cells give up their carbon dioxide to the blood in the capillaries, and the blood in the capillaries releases oxygen to the cells.

ADEQUATE BREATHING

To support the oxygen demands of the body, a person must breathe at an adequate rate and depth. The number of breaths in 1 minute is called the *respiratory rate*. Box 7-1 lists the normal ranges of respiratory rates. The amount of air that a person exchanges in one breath is called the *tidal volume*.

BOX 7-1

Normal Respiratory Rates

- Adult   12–20
- Children   15–30
- Infants   25–50

The tidal volume for an average-sized adult man is approximately 800 mL.

Normal breathing is regular and relaxed. Patients feel they are getting enough air, and the chest expands equally on both sides. Breath sounds are present and equal bilaterally. There is no visible effort associated with breathing.

INADEQUATE BREATHING

In almost all cases, respiratory difficulty is a true emergency. Quickly recognizing inadequate breathing is one of the most important skills to master as an EMT. The most important sign of inadequate breathing is that the patient's rate is either too fast or too slow. It is possible, however, for the patient's respiratory rate to be normal while the volume of each breath (tidal volume) is below normal. This results in inadequate breathing. The easi-

est way to be sure that a patient has an adequate tidal volume is to be sure that the chest rises and falls with each ventilation. If the chest is only moving slightly, the tidal volume is inadequate.

Patients who are breathing inadequately often complain of being "starved for air." Any time patients state that they are having difficulty breathing or are short of breath is a symptom of respiratory distress. Box 7-2 lists the major signs and symptoms of inadequate breathing.

CONSIDERATIONS FOR INFANTS AND CHILDREN

Because the airway structures in infants and children are smaller than in adults, the airway is more easily obstructed. The tongue takes up proportionally more space in infants' and children's mouths (Fig. 7-3). The large tongue can easily fall against the back of the throat and block the airway if the patient is in the supine position.

Because the trachea in infants and children is very narrow, it can become easily obstructed by even a small amount of fluid or swelling. The infant's trachea is so soft and flexible that it can be kinked by positioning the head incorrectly, especially by tilting the head back too far. The cricoid ring is pliable and less developed than in adults.

The chest wall of infants and children is also very pliable. Because the intercostal muscles are weaker, children use the diaphragm more than the rib cage for inspiration. An important sign of inadequate respiration in infants and children is the visi-

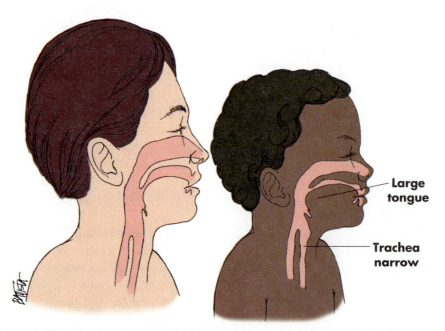

Large tongue

Trachea narrow

Fig. 7-3 In infants and children the airway is more easily obstructed, and the tongue takes up proportionally more space in the mouth.

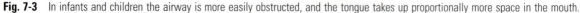

BOX 7-2

Signs and Symptoms of Inadequate Breathing

- Difficulty breathing, shortness of breath
- A rate that is too fast or too slow
- A rhythm that is irregular
- Diminished or absent breath sounds
- Unequal or inadequate chest expansion
- Increased effort of breathing
- Inadequate tidal volume, shallow breathing
- Cyanotic, pale, or cool and clammy skin
- Use of accessory muscles, retractions above the clavicles and between the ribs, nasal flaring, and see-saw breathing in infants and children

ble use of the muscles in the chest and neck to assist breathing.

OXYGEN

Oxygen is the element of life. A constant supply of oxygen is required by every cell in the body. Normally the body gets enough oxygen from the air breathed during adequate respiration. In illness or injury, however, the amount of oxygen in the blood may decrease as a result of respiratory difficulty, cardiac failure, or airway obstruction. In these situations, the patient requires oxygen to decrease the possibility of permanent damage.

OXYGEN SOURCES

The oxygen used in most EMS systems is stored in high-pressure tanks. Tanks come in several common sizes (Fig. 7-4; Table 7-1). Oxygen tanks are usually filled to about 2000 pounds of pressure per square inch. Because this great pressure could be explosive if a tank were damaged, always handle oxygen tanks carefully. The most delicate parts of the tanks are the valves and the gauges. Secure oxygen tanks during transport to prevent them from falling or rolling around.

Some EMS systems use liquid oxygen systems. Some patients receiving oxygen at home have a

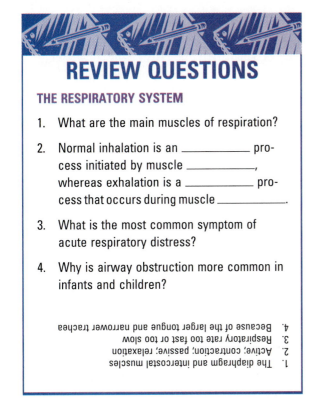

REVIEW QUESTIONS

THE RESPIRATORY SYSTEM

1. What are the main muscles of respiration?
2. Normal inhalation is an _____ process initiated by muscle _____, whereas exhalation is a _____ process that occurs during muscle _____.
3. What is the most common symptom of acute respiratory distress?
4. Why is airway obstruction more common in infants and children?

1. The diaphragm and intercostal muscles
2. Active, contraction; passive; relaxation
3. Respiratory rate too fast or too slow
4. Because of the larger tongue and narrower trachea

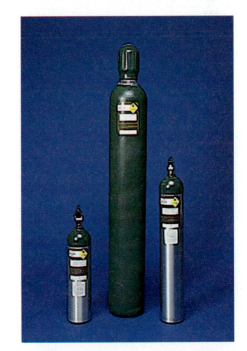

Fig. 7-4 Common sizes of oxygen tanks. The D tank is small, the E tank medium, and the M tank large.

TABLE 7-1	Sizes of Oxygen Cylinders	
CYLINDER	**CAPACITY (L)**
D	350
E	625
M	3000
G	5300
H	6900

similar system. Large amounts of liquid oxygen can be stored in a small container, but these systems are more expensive and not as widely used as standard high-pressure oxygen tanks.

EQUIPMENT FOR OXYGEN DELIVERY

OXYGEN REGULATORS

To deliver the oxygen to the patient at the correct pressure and flow rate, a regulator is used (Fig. 7-5). The regulator attaches to the valve of the tank to control the flow of oxygen. Just as with a water faucet, you control the flow rate by adjusting the regulator. Technique 7-1 describes how to attach the regulator to the tank.

Some regulators have humidifiers that moisten the oxygen before it reaches the patient. Humidified oxygen is used more often in long-term oxygen therapy and usually is not used by EMTs.

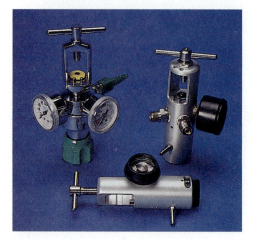

Fig. 7-5 Three different kinds of oxygen flow regulators.

MASKS

Once the flow of oxygen is regulated to the desired rate, it is delivered to the patient by a mask. Many types of oxygen masks are available, but only two are generally used by EMTs in prehospital care: nonrebreather masks and nasal cannulas. If you work in a setting where another type of mask is used, be sure to learn about it (Fig. 7-7).

Nonrebreather masks. This mask is the preferred prehospital method of delivering oxygen to the patient. This is a high-flow device that can deliver up to 90% oxygen when the flow rate is set at a rate of 15 L/min. The nonrebreather mask stores oxygen in a reservoir bag. Inflate this bag with oxygen before you place the mask on the patient, and be sure that it does not collapse completely while the patient is breathing (Fig. 7-8).

Nonrebreather masks come in a variety of sizes. The proper mask should fit from the bridge of the patient's nose to just below the bottom lip. Regardless of the mask size, the flow rate should be set at a rate of 15 L/min.

> ## ALERT
> **Any patient who complains of difficulty breathing (or shortness of breath) or who is cyanotic and whose skin is cool or clammy should receive oxygen by nonrebreather mask.**

In the past, EMTs were instructed to withhold high-flow oxygen administration in certain patients. The standard has changed, however, for prehospital settings. Any adult, child, or infant who is in respiratory distress should receive high-concentration oxygen.

Some patients become very apprehensive when a mask is placed on their face. Usually, if you explain that they are receiving high concentrations of oxygen and that this will help them breathe easier, they will calm down. Some patients are more comfortable if they hold the mask on their face, instead of having the strap around their head. Having a parent hold the mask close to a child's mouth and nose may help calm a child. If the patient will not tolerate an oxygen mask, you may need to use a nasal cannula.

TECHNIQUE 7-1
Attaching the Regulator to the Oxygen Tank

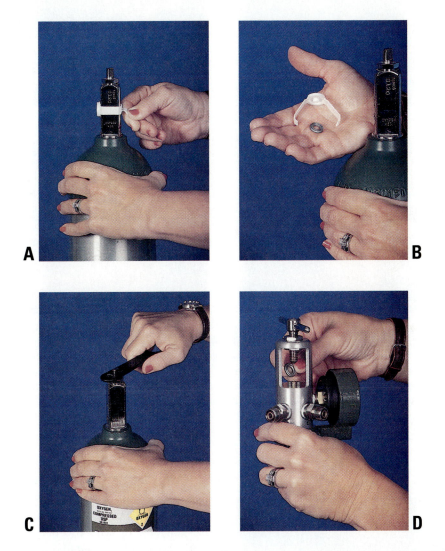

Fig. 7-6   A, Remove the protective seal from the valve on the tank. B, Attached to the seal is a washer that provides an air-tight seal between the regulator and the tank. Be sure not to lose it. C, Quickly open and close the valve to blow any dirt or contamination out of the tank opening. Be sure that the valve is facing away from you or anyone else. **D, Place the washer over the inlet port on the regulator.**

Continued

TECHNIQUE 7-1
Attaching the Regulator to the Oxygen Tank

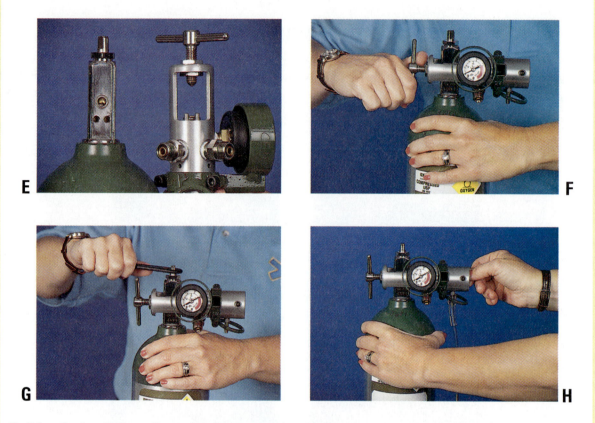

Fig. 7-6 *Continued* **E, Line up the regulator inlet port and pins with the tank opening and holes in the tank valve.** The pins are designed so that only the correct regulator fits the tank. Be sure that the flow meter is turned off. **F, Tighten the screw by hand. G, Open the tank valve to test that you have an air-tight seal.** If oxygen is leaking, tighten the screw until the leak stops. **H, Adjust the flow meter to the desired setting.** When finished, turn off the flow meter and close the tank valve. Release the pressure from the regulator by momentarily opening the flow meter.

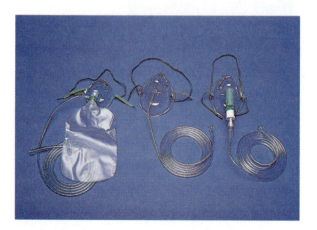

Fig. 7-7 Nonrebreather, simple, and venturi oxygen masks.

Nasal cannulas. These devices are an alternative to delivering oxygen by mask (Fig. 7-9). They are simply a piece of tubing that has holes that blow oxygen directly into the patient's nostrils. Nasal cannulas are often used for long-term oxygen therapy in a medical facility or at home. With a nasal cannula, you should set the flow rate up to 6 L/min.

In prehospital settings, nasal cannulas should be used only for patients who are still uncomfortable with the mask after you have reassured them that they are getting plenty of oxygen. The nasal cannula is a low-flow device and is a poor alternative to the nonrebreather mask. It is, however, better than nothing if the patient absolutely will not tolerate the mask.

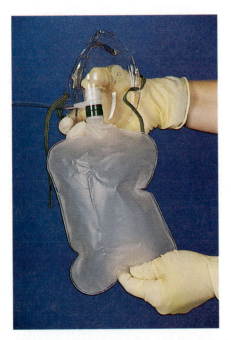

Fig. 7-8 Inflate the nonrebreather bag with oxygen before you place the mask on the patient.

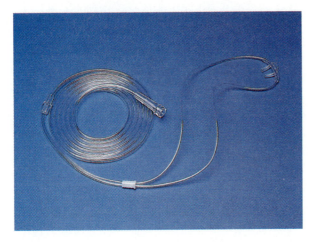
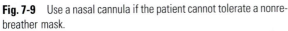

Fig. 7-9 Use a nasal cannula if the patient cannot tolerate a nonrebreather mask.

OPENING THE AIRWAY

ALERT
Anything that compromises the continuous flow of air in and out of the lungs is an immediate life threat. Ensuring that the patient's airway is open is the most important job of the EMT.

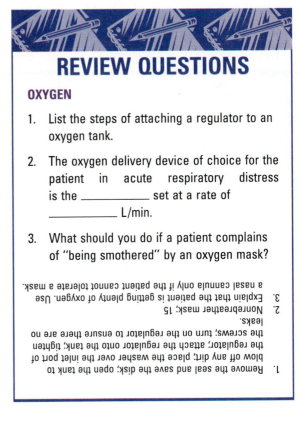

REVIEW QUESTIONS

OXYGEN

1. List the steps of attaching a regulator to an oxygen tank.

2. The oxygen delivery device of choice for the patient in acute respiratory distress is the _____ set at a rate of _____ L/min.

3. What should you do if a patient complains of "being smothered" by an oxygen mask?

1. Remove the seal and save the disk; open the tank to blow off any dirt; place the washer over the inlet port of the regulator; attach the regulator onto the tank; tighten the screws; turn on the regulator to ensure there are no leaks.
2. Nonrebreather mask; 15
3. Explain that the patient is getting plenty of oxygen. Use a nasal cannula only if the patient cannot tolerate a mask.

MANUAL POSITIONING

Unresponsive patients lose muscular control of the jaw. If the patient is in the supine position, the jaw falls posteriorly and the base of the tongue contacts the back of the throat, and the epiglottis blocks the glottic opening (Fig. 7-10). These three actions close the airway and make it impossible to move air from the mouth and nose to the lungs.

In your CPR course you learned that there are different ways to manually open the airway. The most common method of opening the airway is the head-tilt chin-lift technique. Tilting the head back and lifting the chin pulls the base of the tongue out of the oropharynx and lifts the epiglottis away from the glottis (Fig. 7-11). This simple technique requires no equipment and should be performed immediately whenever you are treating an unresponsive nontrauma patient.

When using this technique with infants and children, avoid tilting the head past the point where the nose is perpendicular to the surface upon which the patient is lying. If an elderly patient has a curvature of the upper back that places the head in a hyperextended position, you should use padding under the head to maintain the correct position.

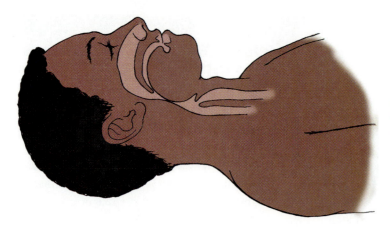

Fig. 7-10   Unresponsive patients lose muscular control of the jaw. This may cause the tongue to contact the back of the throat, obstructing the airway.

If trauma is suspected, moving the neck could damage the patient's spinal cord. In this case, perform a **jaw thrust** by simply displacing the jaw forward which opens the airway. This technique is generally accomplished by placing your index fingers at the angles of the jaw and the meaty parts of your thumbs on the maxilla. Use your thumb tips to keep the mouth open (Fig. 7-12). This procedure enables you to quickly open the airway of unresponsive trauma patients while keeping the head in the neutral position.

AIRWAY ADJUNCTS

Oropharyngeal airways and **nasopharyngeal airways** are devices that help open and maintain the airway. One of these two devices should be used when patients are unable to control their airway.

OROPHARYNGEAL AIRWAY

The oropharyngeal airway (Fig. 7-13) is a curved piece of plastic that goes into the patient's mouth and lifts the tongue out of the oropharynx (Fig. 7-14). It is also called an *oral airway* or an *OP airway*.

The **gag reflex** causes the patient to retch when the back of the throat is stimulated. This reflex helps unresponsive patients protect their airways. Unresponsive patients who lose the gag reflex are at very high risk for airway obstructions and aspiration of material into the lungs. The oral airway should be used any time the patient is unresponsive and has no gag reflex. If the oral airway is used in a patient who has a gag reflex, the patient may gag or vomit. This can seriously threaten the airway. Technique 7-2 describes the steps for inserting an oral airway in an adult. Technique 7-3 describes the steps for inserting an oral airway in a child or infant.

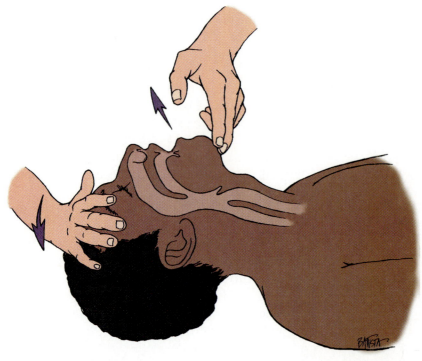

Fig. 7-11   When you tilt the head back and lift the chin, the base of the tongue and the epiglottis are lifted out of the airway.

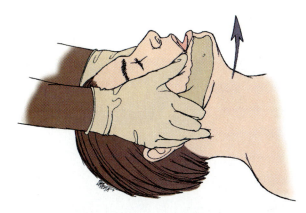

Fig. 7-12 Use the jaw thrust to open the airway in a patient with suspected spinal trauma.

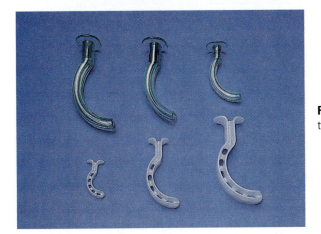

Fig. 7-13 Oropharyngeal airways are available in several sizes and types.

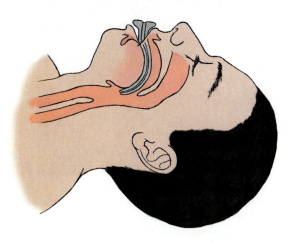

Fig. 7-14 The oropharyngeal airway displaces the tongue from the oropharynx.

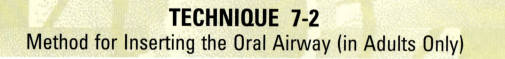

TECHNIQUE 7-2
Method for Inserting the Oral Airway (in Adults Only)

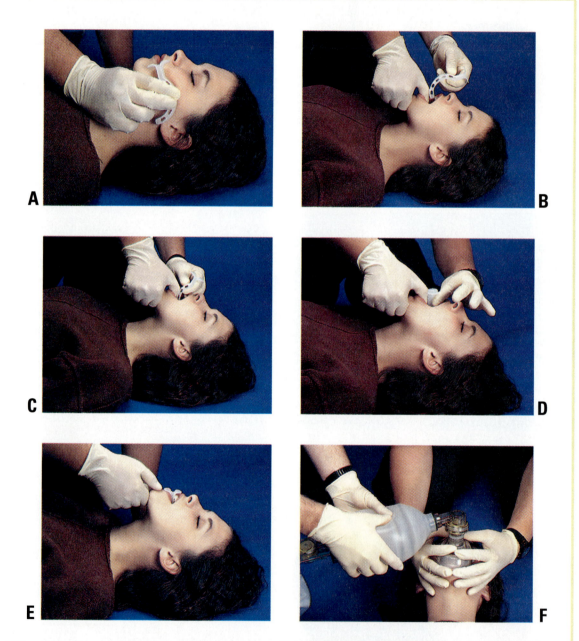

Fig. 7-15   Put on gloves. **A, Select the properly sized airway, which should measure from the corner of the patient's mouth to the earlobe or angle of the jaw.** Position yourself at the patient's side. **B, Open the patient's mouth by lifting the jaw and tongue. Insert the airway upside down (with the tip facing toward the roof of the patient's mouth). C, Advance the airway gently until you feel resistance. D, Turn the airway 180° so that it E, comes to rest with the flange on the patient's teeth. F, Ventilate the patient as needed.**

TECHNIQUE 7-3
Method for Inserting the Oral Airway (Preferred Method for Infants and Children)

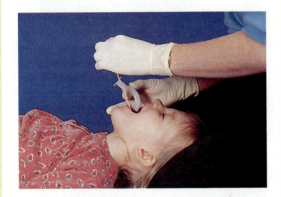

Fig. 7-16 Put on gloves. Select the properly sized airway, which should measure from the corner of the patient's mouth to the earlobe or angle of the jaw. Position yourself at the top of the patient's head. Open the patient's mouth and use a tongue depressor to press the tongue forward and out of the airway. **Insert the airway right side up (with the tip facing toward the floor of the patient's mouth).** Advance the airway gently until the flange comes to rest on the patient's lips or teeth. Ventilate the patient as needed.

NASOPHARYNGEAL AIRWAY

The nasopharyngeal airway is a flexible tube of rubber or plastic (Fig. 7-17). It is inserted into the patient's nostril to provide an air passage (Fig. 7-18). The nasopharyngeal airway is commonly

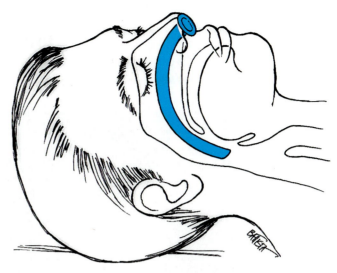

Fig. 7-18 Nasopharyngeal airways can be used in responsive and semiresponsive patients to maintain an open airway.

called a *nasal airway* or *NP airway*. The nasopharyngeal airway is less likely to stimulate vomiting and is a valuable adjunct in patients who are responsive but need assistance in maintaining their airway. They are well tolerated in patients of all ages and are the easiest airway adjunct to use if the patient is actively seizing. Technique 7-4 describes the steps for inserting a nasopharyngeal airway in a patient of any age.

If you meet resistance, do not force the airway. Remove it from that nostril, lubricate it, and try the other side. Even a well-lubricated nasopharyngeal airway may be uncomfortable for the patient and may elicit a painful response. Keep in mind that the nasal airway may become clogged by mucous, blood, or vomit. If this occurs, you should suction the airway to restore patency.

SUCTION

Fluid such as blood, vomit, mucous, or saliva in the airway can obstruct the free passage of air into the lungs. This fluid can also be inhaled into the lungs with resulting damage to lung tissue. Any

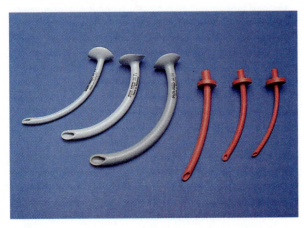

Fig. 7-17 Different types and sizes of nasopharyngeal airways.

ALERT
Gurgling is the most common sign of liquid in the airway! Any time that you hear gurgling:
1. Open the airway immediately.
2. Suction the airway immediately.

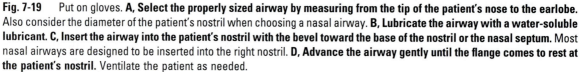

TECHNIQUE 7-4
Inserting a Nasopharyngeal Airway (All Ages)

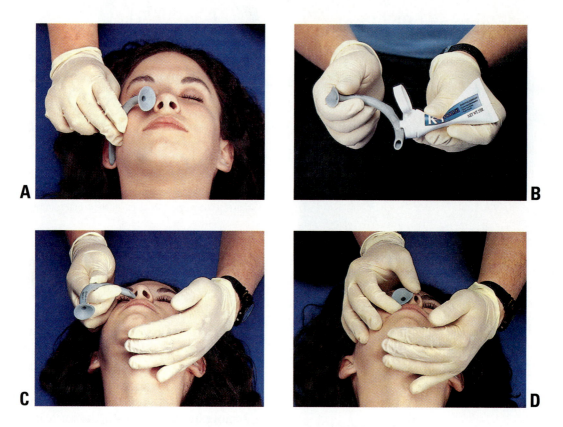

Fig. 7-19 Put on gloves. **A, Select the properly sized airway by measuring from the tip of the patient's nose to the earlobe.** Also consider the diameter of the patient's nostril when choosing a nasal airway. **B, Lubricate the airway with a water-soluble lubricant. C, Insert the airway into the patient's nostril with the bevel toward the base of the nostril or the nasal septum.** Most nasal airways are designed to be inserted into the right nostril. **D, Advance the airway gently until the flange comes to rest at the patient's nostril.** Ventilate the patient as needed.

time liquid is in the airway, it must be immediately removed using suction. Some suction units are capable of removing small solid objects (eg, broken teeth, gum, or pieces of food) from the airway.

Suction devices are important emergency equipment. Almost all ambulances have a built-in suction unit, usually mounted near the patient's head. This suction unit is generally powered by the ambulance's battery (Fig. 7-20).

Because it is important to have suction immediately available whenever you are treating a patient, you should have a portable suction device within reach. Your portable suction unit is one of your most important pieces of equipment and should always be close at hand. Most portable suction de-

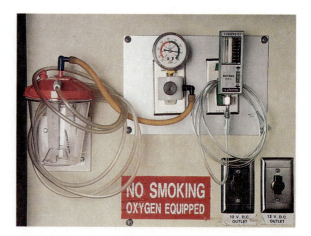

Fig. 7-20 Almost all ambulances have a built-in suction unit.

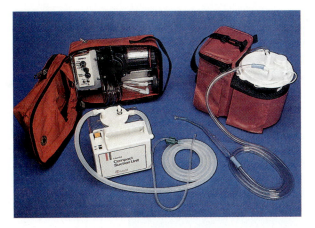

Fig. 7-21 Examples of portable suction units.

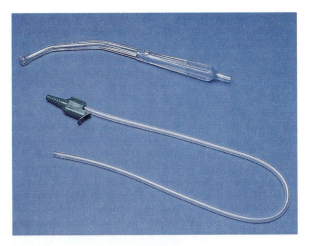

Fig. 7-23 Rigid (top) and soft (bottom) suction catheters.

vices have rechargeable battery systems (Fig. 7-21). Some hand-operated suction units have become very popular because of their lightweight, compact design and their reliability, low cost, and size (Fig. 7-22).

Most suction units generate negative pressure using a vacuum pump. A length of tubing empties into a collection canister. With most devices you attach a suction catheter to the end of this tubing before you place it into the patient's mouth. Most suction catheters have a hole you must cover with your finger during suctioning. If the material that you are suctioning is so thick that it clogs the suction catheter, use the tubing without a catheter attached. If there is a large volume of material that needs to be cleared from the airway, roll the patient on the side and continue to suction.

Suction catheters are either rigid or soft (Fig. 7-23). The rigid catheters are also called ''hard,'' ''tonsil tip,'' and ''tonsil sucker'' catheters. These

hard plastic catheters are easy to control while suctioning. They are used to suction the mouth and oropharynx of unresponsive patients. The tip of the rigid catheter should always remain visible when you insert it into the mouth. Never insert the catheter so far that you lose sight of the tip.

The rigid catheter can be used in infants and children. In younger patients, however, stimulation of the back of the throat can cause changes in the heart rate. If you use a rigid suction catheter, avoid touching the back of the airway to decrease the chances of slowing the heart rhythm.

Soft suction catheters are also commonly called ''French'' catheters because of the way they are sized. These long, flexible pieces of plastic are used to suction the nasal passages or in other situations where the rigid catheter cannot be used. Soft catheters often become clogged because of the small diameter of the tubing. Just as with the rigid catheter, these catheters should not be inserted further than the base of the tongue.

A bulb syringe is used to suction infants. This simple device is effective for suctioning the nose and mouth of a newborn and can be used to suction an infant up to approximately 3 to 4 months of age. This device is useful to clear obstructions from the nasal passages because newborns and infants are not able to voluntarily breathe through their mouths. The bulb syringe is compressed before placing it in the baby's mouth or nose. Once the bulb syringe is in the mouth or nose, release the bulb and allow the fluids to fill the syringe. Withdraw the syringe and release the contents of the syringe onto a towel. Do not place the syringe far enough into the mouth to touch the back of the throat.

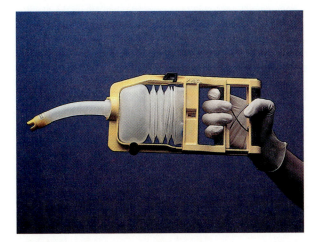

Fig. 7-22 A hand-operated portable suction unit.

TECHNIQUE 7-5
Suctioning

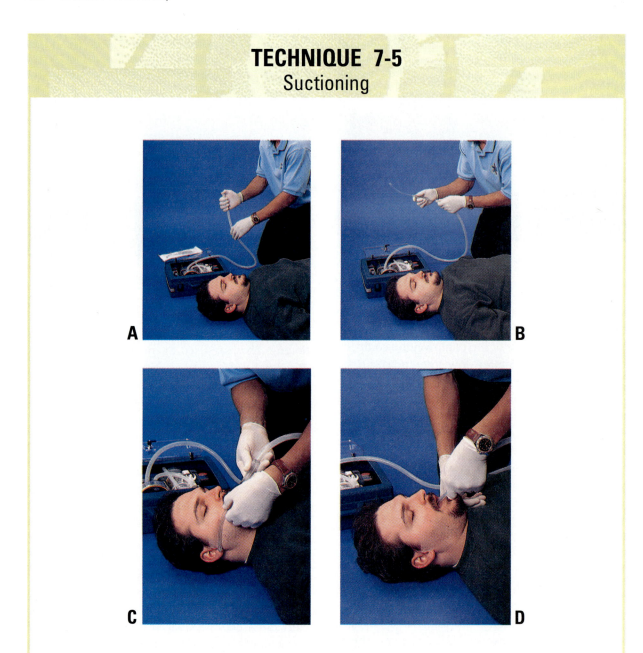

Fig. 7-24 Inspect the portable and on-board suction units at the beginning of each shift to ensure that they are working and cleaned properly. If the unit has a pressure gauge, check the pump to be sure that it can generate a 300 mm Hg vacuum. Battery-operated units should be fully charged at all times and ready for use. Put on gloves, mask, and eye protection. Turn on the power. **A, You will hear the motor start and you should check to be sure that the suction is working by placing your thumb over the end of the suction tubing. B, Select and attach a catheter to the end of the suction tubing. C, Measure the distance from the corner of the patient's mouth to the earlobe and place your fingers at this mark on the catheter.** Insert the catheter into the mouth without suction. This makes it easier to control the tip of the catheter during insertion. You can either keep your finger off of the hole in the catheter or turn the unit off until after you place the catheter into the patient's mouth. If there are copious amounts of fluid in the mouth, suction immediately upon placing the catheter into the patient's mouth. **D, Insert the catheter until your fingertips reach the patient's lips. This prevents inserting the catheter too far.** Continued

TECHNIQUE 7-5
Suctioning

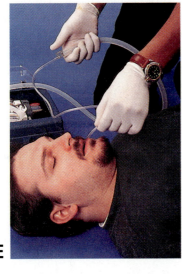

E

Fig. 7-24 *Continued.* **E, Once you have placed the catheter into the patient's mouth, apply suction by turning the unit on or occluding the hole in the catheter.** Never suction for more than 15 seconds at a time to prevent the patient from becoming deprived of oxygen. Infants and children should be suctioned for less time. If you cannot clear the patient's mouth in 15 seconds, log roll the patient on the side immediately. This position enables the fluid to drain from the mouth and clears the oropharynx. To prevent the suction catheter or tubing from becoming clogged, you can intermittently suction water to clear the lines.

Principle 7-1 lists the key principles for suctioning all patients. Technique 7-5 describes one technique for suctioning an adult.

In some patients blood, vomit, or secretions may enter the airway as rapidly as you can suction. In this case, do not continuously suction without oxygenating the patient. Suction for 15 seconds and then stop to ventilate. Provide artificial ventilation for 2 minutes and suction in 15-second intervals. This is a difficult situation, and you should contact medical direction for advice.

ARTIFICIAL VENTILATION

Previous sections in this chapter have described how to maintain the patient's airway by positioning the head, neck, and jaw and how to keep it clear of obstructions by suctioning. These airway management skills help keep the passageways open but do not deliver oxygen to the lungs. Patients who are breathing inadequately, or not at all, must be artificially ventilated in order to stay alive.

There are four preferred ways that you can assist patients who are not breathing on their own. Not all are equally effective. These four techniques of artificial ventilation are listed in decreasing order of preference:

1. Mouth-to-mask
2. Two-person bag-valve-mask
3. Flow-restricted, oxygen-powered ventilation device
4. One-person bag-valve-mask

Mouth-to-mouth ventilation is not included in

PRINCIPLE 7-1
Principles of Suctioning

1. Make sure that the suction unit is working before you use it.
2. Follow body substance isolation precautions.
3. Use a catheter that is appropriate for the situation.
4. Do not insert the catheter further than the base of the tongue.
5. Ensure that the patient does not become deprived of oxygen.
6. Keep the catheter and the tubing clean.

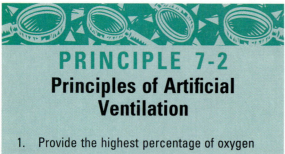

PRINCIPLE 7-2
Principles of Artificial Ventilation

1. Provide the highest percentage of oxygen possible.
2. Maintain an open airway.
3. Ensure an airtight seal between the mask and the patient's face.
4. Prevent air from going into the stomach.
5. Ventilate the patient with an adequate volume and rate.
6. Allow complete, passive exhalation.

this list of preferred methods, even though you learned this skill in your basic life-support course. Because of the direct physical contact with the patient and lack of body substance isolation precaution with this procedure, mouth-to-mouth ventilation is not a preferred EMT skill. You should stay skilled with the mouth-to-mouth technique in case you need to ventilate a family member or friend when you are not working as an EMT and do not have a mask available.

The first step in performing mouth-to-mouth ventilation is to open the airway. This is usually accomplished by the head-tilt chin-lift method. Then take a deep breath, pinch the patient's nostrils closed, and make an airtight seal with your mouth on the patient's lips. Exhale enough breath to make the patient's chest rise, delivering it over 1.5 to 2 seconds. Continue ventilations at a rate of one breath every 5 seconds for an adult or every 3 seconds for a child. Ventilate infants by sealing your mouth over both the infant's mouth and nose, giving one breath every 3 seconds. Principle 7-2 lists the key principles of artificial ventilation.

MOUTH-TO-MASK WITH SUPPLEMENTAL OXYGEN TECHNIQUE

You learned about the mouth-to-mask technique of ventilation in your CPR class. Mouth-to-mask ventilation is the preferred method of ventilating a nonbreathing patient. It is a simple technique, and because of the two-handed mask seal it provides excellent ventilatory volumes. It is described in Technique 7-6.

TECHNIQUE 7-6
Mouth-to-Mask Ventilation With Supplemental Oxygen

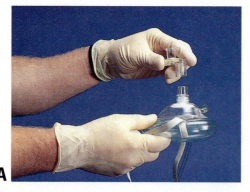
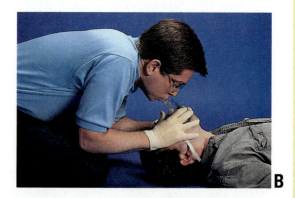

A   **B**

Fig. 7-25   Follow body substance isolation precautions. **A, Connect the one-way valve to the mask, if it is not already attached.** Attach oxygen tubing to the mask and set the flow rate at 15 to 30 L/min. Open the airway by tilting the head back (if no trauma is suspected) and lifting the jaw, and inserting a oral or nasal airway. From a position at the top of the patient's head, place the mask on the patient. **B, Seal the mask to the patient's face with your thumbs and index fingers. Take a normal breath, seal your lips over the ventilation port, and exhale slowly and constantly for 1.5 to 2 seconds. Stop ventilating when the patient's chest rises.** Allow the patient to passively exhale between breaths. Ventilate the adult patient once every 5 seconds and infants and children once every 3 seconds.

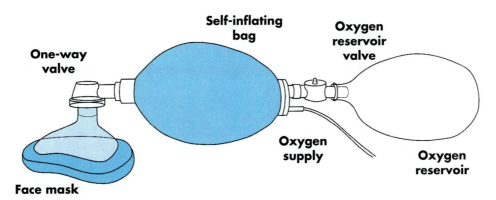

Fig. 7-26   The bag-valve-mask device consists of a self-inflating bag, a one-way valve, a mask, and an oxygen reservoir.

TWO-PERSON BAG-VALVE-MASK TECHNIQUE

The **bag-valve-mask (BVM)** is a ventilation device commonly used in medicine. The BVM consists of a self-inflating bag, a one-way valve, a mask, and an oxygen reservoir (Fig. 7-26). The adult bag has a volume of approximately 1600 mL, which is squeezed to ventilate the patient. The BVM typically delivers less volume than mouth-to-mask technique.

The BVM is most effective when used with two EMTs. When properly performed, two-person BVM ventilation can deliver 90% to 100% oxygen to a nonbreathing patient when attached to an oxygen source. The procedure is described in Technique 7-7.

A few years ago, a number of BVMs were manufactured with pressure pop-off valves designed to prevent overinflation during ventilating. Research showed that these pop-off valves sometimes

TECHNIQUE 7-7
Two-Person Bag-Valve-Mask Procedure

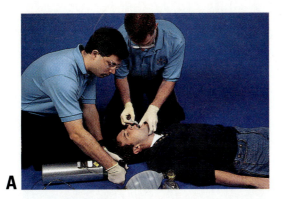

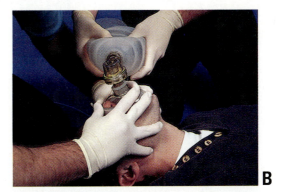

Fig. 7-27   A, The first EMT manually opens the patient's airway from the patient's side. The second EMT assembles and prepares the BVM (including attaching to oxygen) from a position at the top of the patient's head. The first EMT then inserts the properly sized oral or nasal airway (if tolerated). B, The first EMT holds the bag portion of the BVM with both hands. The second EMT seals the mask by placing the apex of the mask over the bridge of the patient's nose and then lowers the mask over the patient's mouth and upper chin. The second EMT's thumbs are positioned over the top half of the mask and the index and middle fingers over the bottom half. If the mask has a large round cuff surrounding a ventilation port, the port is centered over the mouth. The first EMT squeezes the bag slowly and steadily to deliver the breath over 1.5 to 2 seconds until the chest rises. The second EMT maintains the airway by using the ring and little fingers to bring the jaw up to the mask and evaluates the chest rise. The first EMT continues to ventilate the patient at least once every 5 seconds for adults or every 3 seconds for infants and children. The second EMT maintains the mask seal and open airway and continually monitors the chest rise.

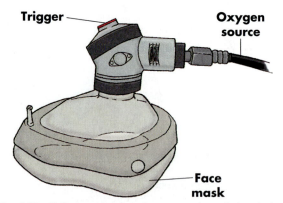

Fig. 7-28 A flow-restricted, oxygen-powered ventilation device may be used in place of a BVM.

BOX 7-3

Features of Bag-Valve-Masks

- A self-refilling bag that is either disposable or easily cleaned and sterilized
- A valve that allows a maximum oxygen inlet flow rate of 15 L/min
- Standardized 15/22 mm fittings
- An oxygen inlet and reservoir to allow for a high concentration of oxygen
- A one-way valve that prevents the rebreathing of exhaled air
- Constructed of materials that work in all environmental conditions and temperatures
- Available in infant, child, and adult sizes

FLOW-RESTRICTED, OXYGEN-POWERED VENTILATION DEVICE

The flow-restricted, oxygen-powered ventilation device (Fig. 7-28) is an alternative to bag-valve-mask ventilation. This device provides 100% oxygen at a peak flow rate of 40 L/min. The valve is designed to prevent overpressurization of the lungs by an inspiratory pressure relief valve that opens when the pressure exceeds 60 cm of water. Most valves have an audible alarm that sounds when the relief valve is activated. The flow-restricted, oxygen-powered ventilation device should never be used on infants or children because it may cause lung tissue damage and cause air to enter the stomach.

resulted in inadequate ventilation. Bag-valve-masks used in emergency situations should not have pop-off valves. Box 7-3 lists the features of BVMs.

TECHNIQUE 7-8
Flow-Restricted, Oxygen-Powered Ventilation Procedure

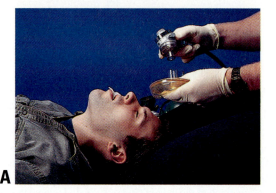 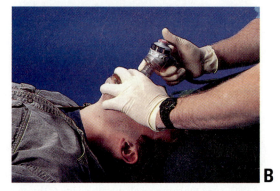

Fig. 7-29 Manually open the patient's airway from the top of the patient's head. Insert the properly sized oral or nasal airway. **A,** Attach the mask to the flow-restricted, oxygen-powered ventilation device. **B,** Seal the mask by placing the apex of the mask over the bridge of the patient's nose, and then lower the mask over the mouth and upper chin. Position your thumb over the top half of the mask, and the index and middle fingers over the bottom half. Maintain the airway by using the ring and little fingers to bring the jaw up to the mask. Trigger the flow-restricted, oxygen-powered ventilation device until the chest rises. Release the trigger and allow for passive exhalation. Continue to ventilate the patient at least once every 5 seconds (for adults).

The flow-restricted, oxygen-powered ventilation devices used by EMTs operate in all environmental conditions. The trigger is positioned so that you can maintain the mask seal and airway while ventilating the patient. The main advantage of this technique is that it can be used by one EMT. The flow-restricted, oxygen-powered ventilation device is preferred over the BVM if only one EMT is available to ventilate the patient. The procedure is described in Technique 7-8.

ONE-PERSON BAG-VALVE-MASK TECHNIQUE

Ventilation with a BVM appears to be a simple skill when practiced on manikins, but on real patients it is very difficult for one EMT to maintain an open airway, seal the mask, and squeeze the bag. One person BVM ventilation should be used only as a last resort when none of the other techniques of ventilation is possible. The procedure is described in Technique 7-9.

ALERT
One person bag-valve-mask ventilation requires a tremendous amount of practice and experience to do properly.

CONSIDERATIONS FOR TRAUMA PATIENTS

Unresponsive trauma patients present a considerable challenge in airway management. In addition to bleeding into the airway and the possibility of facial trauma, spinal injuries require special care. All of the techniques of ventilation have to be modified so that the head is not tilted. These modifications are described in Technique 7-10.

TECHNIQUE 7-9
One-Person Bag-Valve-Mask Ventilation Procedure

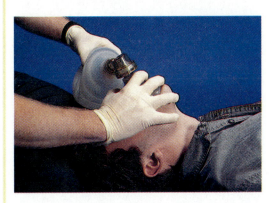

Fig. 7-30 Manually open the patient's airway from a position at the top of the patient's head. Insert the properly sized oral or nasal airway. Attach oxygen tubing to the oxygen port, and attach the mask to the BVM. **Seal the mask by placing the apex of the mask over the bridge of the patient's nose, and then lower the mask over the mouth and upper chin. Make a "C" with your index finger and thumb around the ventilation port. Maintain the airway by using the middle, ring, and little fingers under the jaw to maintain the chin lift. Squeeze the bag with your other hand slowly and steadily to deliver the breath in 1.5 to 2 seconds until the chest rises.** Allow the patient to passively exhale. Evaluate the chest rise and continue to ventilate the patient at least once every 5 seconds for adults or once every 3 seconds for infants and children.

TECHNIQUE 7-10
Modifying Ventilation Techniques for Trauma Patients

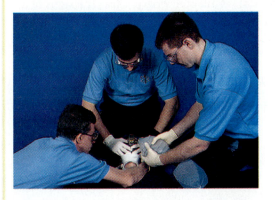

Fig. 7-31 Position yourself at the top of the patient's head. **A second EMT can stabilize the patient's head and neck, or you can use your knees to prevent head movement. Maintain a mask seal with the thumbs and index fingers on top of the mask, and the middle, ring, and little fingers under the chin. This allows for a jaw thrust to be performed at the same time, helping to maintain an open airway. Do not push down on the chin, because this may occlude the airway. Another EMT should ventilate the patient with the bag-valve-mask, as a much better seal with the mask can be achieved by using two hands rather than one. Ventilate once every 5 seconds for adults or once every 3 seconds for infants and children without tilting the head back.** Allow for passive exhalation after each breath. Evaluate the chest rise and fall on every breath.

BOX 7-4

Signs of Adequate Ventilation

- The chest rises and falls with each artificial ventilation
- The patient is being ventilated at least 12 times per minute for adults, or 20 times per minute for children and infants
- The heart rate returns to normal
- The skin color improves

ASSESSING THE ADEQUACY OF ARTIFICIAL VENTILATION

Whenever you ventilate a patient, it is very important to assess the adequacy of the artificial breathing. Regardless of the technique, you must continually evaluate the effectiveness of the ventilation. Everybody on the crew, not only the EMT ventilating the patient, should continually evaluate artificial ventilation. Box 7-4 lists the signs of adequate ventilation. Box 7-5 lists the signs of inadequate ventilation.

BOX 7-5

Signs of Inadequate Ventilation

- The chest fails to rise and fall with each ventilation
- The rate is either too fast or too slow
- There is gastric distention
- The heart rate does not return to normal
- Cyanosis is present or worsens

Chest rise is the best indicator that ventilations are being delivered effectively. There are a number of causes of inadequate chest rise. Use the four-step approach described in Box 7-6 for correcting poor chest rise while ventilating a patient.

BOX 7-6

Correcting Poor Chest Rise During Ventilation

Step	Rationale
• Reposition the jaw	• An improperly opened airway is the most common cause of poor chest rise
• Check the mask seal	• Poor mask seal is the next most common cause of poor chest rise; you can generally hear air leaking through the sides of the mask
• Use an alternative technique	• Some patients are ventilated more effectively with one technique than another
• Check for an obstruction	• Foreign body airway obstructions may cause poor ventilation. You may need to perform the Heimlich maneuver or suction the patient.

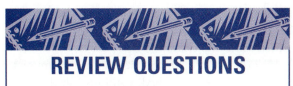

REVIEW QUESTIONS

ARTIFICIAL VENTILATION

1. Place the following ventilation techniques in decreasing order of preference.
   A. One-person bag-valve-mask
   B. Flow-restricted, oxygen-powered ventilation device
   C. Mouth-to-mask
   D. Two-person bag-valve-mask

2. List at least four of the desirable features of the bag-valve-mask.

3. In two-person bag-valve-mask technique the EMT at the top of the head is responsible for _____ and _____.

4. The flow-restricted, oxygen-powered breathing device provides _____ % oxygen at a rate of _____ L/min with a pop-off valve set at _____ cm of water.

5. For all artificial ventilations, the inspiratory time should be _____ to _____ seconds.

6. List three signs of inadequate ventilations.

7. Describe the four steps that you take when you ventilate a patient and the chest does not rise.

(answers, printed upside down)

7. Reposition the jaw; check the mask seal; use an alternative technique; check for an obstruction

6. The chest does not rise and fall; rate is either too fast or too slow; heart rate is not returning to normal; cyanosis is present or worse

5. 1.5 to 2

4. 100; 40; 60.

3. Holding the mask seal; maintaining an open airway

2. Self inflating bag; easily cleaned and sterilized; 15/22 mm fittings/oxygen inlet and reservoir; a valve that prevents rebreathing; works in all environments; available in adult, child, and infant sizes

1. C; D; B; A

SPECIAL SITUATIONS IN AIRWAY MANAGEMENT

PATIENTS WITH LARYNGECTOMIES

A **laryngectomy** is a surgical procedure in which the voice box is removed, usually because of throat cancer. After a laryngectomy the patient may have a **tracheal stoma,** which is a permanent artificial opening into the trachea (Fig. 7-32). In some cases, the patient has a tube that fits into the stoma. If this tube becomes obstructed, use suction to remove the occlusion.

If a patient with a tracheal stoma must be ventilated, you can usually ventilate with a mask directly through the stoma. Use a small mask to get a seal on the neck. Because you are inflating below the level of the tongue and epiglottis, the head and neck do not need to be positioned.

In some cases, patients have a partial laryngectomy, in which there is still an air passage from the trachea to the mouth and nose. If air escapes from the mouth and nose when you ventilate a patient with a stoma, close the patient's mouth and pinch the nose shut. If ventilating through the tracheal

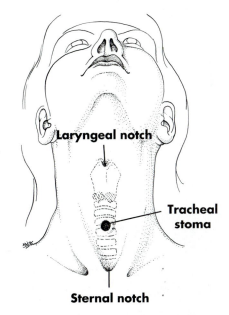

Fig. 7-32 A tracheal stoma is a permanent artificial opening into the trachea.

stoma proves to be difficult, try to suction the hole. If ventilation is still difficult, you should seal the tracheal stoma with a gloved hand, provide proper head tilt, and ventilate through the mouth and nose.

VENTILATING INFANTS AND CHILDREN

Respiratory emergencies are quite common in children, and you need to be able to artificially ventilate pediatric patients. Because the airway is more pliable, you must pay particular attention to head position. Infants should be ventilated with the head in the neutral position. Children may need to have their head slightly extended. Avoid hyperextension or flexion of the head in any child or infant. Ventilate infants and children once every 3 seconds and be prepared to suction to help clear the small airways.

Ventilate the patient every 3 seconds with just enough oxygen to make the chest rise. Excessive pressure will cause gastric distention, which severely compromises the effectiveness of ventilation and increases the possibility of vomiting. Do not use pop-off valves because they can lead to unrecognized hypoventilation. Use an oral or nasal airway if other methods fail to provide an adequate airway.

FACIAL INJURIES

Facial trauma can pose considerable difficulty for managing the airway and ventilating trauma patients (Fig. 7-33). The head and face have a rich blood supply, and blunt injuries to the face cause significant bleeding and swelling.

Be prepared to use suction and positioning (jaw thrust without head tilt) to keep the airway clear of blood and vomit. Use an oral or nasal airway to help maximize the airway without tilting the head. Be cautious when using a nasal airway in patients with

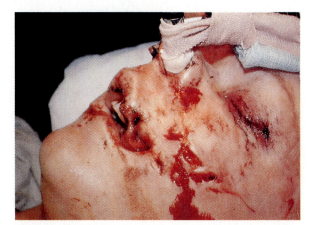

Fig. 7-33 Facial trauma can pose considerable difficulty for managing the airway and ventilating trauma patients.

facial trauma. If there is significant injury to the bones of the skull, it is possible to insert the airway directly into the cranial cavity.

If you cannot open the airway in a trauma patient and all else has failed, you must tilt the head back to ventilate the patient. Although moving the neck may cause spinal cord injury, if you do not open the airway, the patient will die.

OBSTRUCTIONS

In your CPR class you learned the American Heart Association or the American Red Cross procedures for dealing with a foreign body airway obstruction, including abdominal thrusts, finger sweeps, and ventilation attempts. A combination of back blows and chest thrusts are used in infants. If three cycles of attempts to clear a foreign body airway obstruction fail to open the airway, you should transport the patient immediately, while continuing the cycle en route to the hospital.

DENTAL APPLIANCES

Dentures and partial dentures can create a problem for managing the airway. If at all possible, at-

---

REVIEW QUESTIONS

SPECIAL SITUATIONS IN AIRWAY MANAGEMENT

1. A patient with a laryngectomy may have an artificial opening in the trachea called a
   _____.
   A. Laryngectomy
   B. Tracheostomy
   C. Stoma
   D. Trachea

2. What should you do if you cannot get the chest to rise when you ventilate a spine-injured patient with massive facial injures?

3. Dental appliances should be left in place while ventilating a patient unless they
   _____.

1. C
2. Tilt the head to provide an adequate airway if no other techniques are successful
3. Become dislodged

tempt to keep dentures in place when ventilating a patient. They add form and structure to the mouth and make it easier to get a mask seal.

If dentures become dislodged, they can create an airway obstruction. If this happens, you should remove them immediately.

CHAPTER SUMMARY

THE RESPIRATORY SYSTEM

The respiratory system maintains the delicate balance of oxygen and carbon dioxide in the body. The airway consists of the passageways from the lips and nostrils to the lungs. Airway structures include the nose, nasopharynx, mouth, oropharynx, epiglottis, glottis, larynx, cricoid ring, trachea, bronchi, and alveoli. Air is moved in and out of the lungs by the contraction and relaxation of the diaphragm and intercostal muscles. Normal breathing is relaxed and regular. The airway of the pediatric patient is easily obstructed. Great care must be taken to maintain this vital passageway of life in all patients.

OXYGEN

High-concentration oxygen should be given to all patients with signs or symptoms of inadequate breathing. Oxygen is stored in high-pressure tanks and controlled by regulators. In prehospital care, oxygen is delivered to the patient using either a nonrebreather mask or a nasal cannula. The mask is the preferred method of providing oxygen because it delivers much higher concentrations of oxygen. The nasal cannula should be used only if the patient will not tolerate the mask.

OPENING THE AIRWAY

Ensuring an open airway is the most important job of an EMT. Many circumstances can prevent the free passage of air from the mouth to the lungs. In an unresponsive patient the base of the tongue can create an airway obstruction. Foreign bodies, such as teeth, gum, and dentures, can also create airway problems. Fluid (blood, saliva, vomit, etc.) should be suctioned from the airway immediately. The head-tilt chin-lift technique is the simplest airway skill and should be performed immediately on any unresponsive, nontrauma patient. Nasal and oral airway devices are very useful in helping maintain the airway.

ARTIFICIAL VENTILATION

Once the airway has been opened, the next priority in patient management is ventilation. EMT–Basics use four methods for providing artificial ventilation. Mouth-to-mask ventilations are the preferred method of ventilating a patient. In this technique, one EMT seals the mask to the patient's face with both hands and exhales into the mask until the chest rises. The next option is the two-person bag-valve-mask technique where one EMT uses both hands to seal the mask to the patient's face and open the airway while a second EMT squeezes the bag with both hands. The next option for ventilation uses the flow-restricted, oxygen-powered ventilation device. One EMT uses both hands to seal the mask and open the airway, and ventilation is given until the chest rises. The last option for ventilating a patient is the one-person bag-valve-mask technique. Because one EMT must seal the mask, open the airway, and squeeze the bag, this technique is the least preferred method of artificial ventilation.

When ventilating a trauma patient, take care to open the airway using the jaw thrust and ventilate the patient without moving the head or neck. Everyone on the crew is responsible for continuously assessing the adequacy of ventilations. The four-step procedure to use when the chest does not rise is to reposition the airway, check the mask seal, use an alternative technique, and check for obstruction.

SPECIAL SITUATIONS IN AIRWAY MANAGEMENT

Special situations present challenges when managing the airway and ventilating certain patients. Patients with stomas can generally be ventilated directly through the stoma. The airways of infants and children are easily compromised by head position, swelling, or fluid. Facial injuries can cause considerable bleeding and swelling. Foreign body airway obstructions should be managed by abdominal thrusts, finger sweeps, and ventilation attempts. If they remain in place, dental appliances should be kept in place during artificial ventilation.

UNITED STATES DEPARTMENT OF TRANSPORTATION NATIONAL HIGHWAY TRAFFIC SAFETY ADMINISTRATION EMT–BASIC OBJECTIVES

Check your knowledge. The National Registry of EMTs and many state EMS agencies use the objectives below to develop EMT–Basic certification examinations. Can you meet them?

COGNITIVE

1. Name and label the major structures of the respiratory system on a diagram.
2. List the signs of adequate breathing.
3. List the signs of inadequate breathing.
4. Describe the steps in performing the head-tilt chin-lift.
5. Relate mechanism of injury to opening the airway.
6. Describe the steps in performing a jaw thrust.
7. State the importance of having a suction unit ready for immediate use when providing emergency care.
8. Describe the techniques of suctioning.
9. Describe how to artificially ventilate a patient with a pocket mask.
10. Describe the steps in performing the skills of artificially ventilating a patient with a bag-valve-mask while using the jaw thrust.
11. List the parts of a bag-valve-mask system.
12. Describe the steps in performing the skill of artificially ventilating a patient with a bag-valve-mask for one and two rescuers.
13. Describe the signs of adequate artificial ventilation using the bag-valve-mask.
14. Describe the signs of inadequate artificial ventilation using the bag-valve-mask.
15. Describe the steps for artificially ventilating a patient with a flow-restricted, oxygen-powered ventilation device.
16. List the steps in performing the actions taken when providing mouth-to-mouth and mouth-to-stoma artificial ventilation.
17. Describe how to measure and insert an oropharyngeal (oral) airway.
18. Describe how to measure and insert a nasopharyngeal (nasal) airway.
19. Define the components of an oxygen delivery system.
20. Identify a nonrebreather face mask and state the oxygen flow requirements needed for its use.
21. Describe the indications for using a nasal cannula versus a nonrebreather face mask.
22. Identify a nasal cannula and state the flow requirements needed for its use.

AFFECTIVE

1. Explain the rationale for basic life support artificial ventilation and airway protective skills taking priority over most other basic life support skills.

2. Explain the rationale for providing adequate oxygenation through high inspired oxygen concentrations to patients who, in the past, may have received low concentrations.

PSYCHOMOTOR

1. Demonstrate the steps in performing the head-tilt chin-lift.
2. Demonstrate the steps in performing the jaw thrust.
3. Demonstrate the techniques of suctioning.
4. Demonstrate the steps in providing mouth-to-mouth artificial ventilation with body substance isolation (barrier shields).
5. Demonstrate how to use a pocket mask to artificially ventilate a patient.
6. Demonstrate the assembly of a bag-valve-mask unit.
7. Demonstrate the steps for performing the skills of artificially ventilating a patient with a bag-valve-mask for one and two rescuers.
8. Demonstrate the steps in performing the skills of artificially ventilating a patient with a bag-valve-mask while using the jaw thrust.
9. Demonstrate artificial ventilation of a patient with a flow-restricted, oxygen-powered ventilation device.
10. Demonstrate how to artificially ventilate a patient with a stoma.
11. Demonstrate how to insert an oropharyngeal (oral) airway.
12. Demonstrate how to insert a nasopharyngeal (nasal) airway.
13. Demonstrate the correct operation of oxygen tanks and regulators.
14. Demonstrate the use of a nonrebreather face mask and state the oxygen flow requirements needed for its use.
15. Demonstrate the use of a nasal cannula and state the flow requirements needed for its use.
16. Demonstrate how to artificially ventilate the infant and child patient.
17. Demonstrate oxygen administration for the infant and child patient.

PATIENT ASSESSMENT

When I told my father I was going to be a firefighter, he expressed his apprehension. His concern was that I was too impulsive—he was worried about my safety. He advised me that nothing was so urgent that I could not take the time to think about my own safety. He never used the term "scene size-up," but I know now that's what he was talking about. On one of my first medical calls I found two men down and unconscious, in the bottom of a manhole. My impulse was to rush down in there and help them. But my father's words, "stop and think," came to mind. So I did. I realized there must be a reason for the men's condition. I took the time to put on my full protective gear and completed a successful rescue, rather than becoming a victim myself. (Thanks, Dad, for 20 years of safe emergency service.)

James W. Hansen, NREMT-P
*Firefighter/Paramedic
and EMS Coordinator
Salt Lake City Fire
Department
Salt Lake City, Utah*

IN THIS DIVISION

DIVISION THREE

8 SCENE SIZE-UP

IN THE FIELD

EMTs Phil and Jamal were dispatched to the home of Mrs. Fields, who had called EMS because she was experiencing a severe headache. She met the EMTs at the front door. They entered the home and began their patient assessment. Jamal smelled natural gas as they walked in. They immediately moved the patient into the yard. Phil asked Mrs. Fields if anyone else was in the house, and Mrs. Fields answered that she lived alone. Jamal used the cellular phone in the ambulance to request additional help at the scene from the gas company and to request that a fire crew be sent to the home.

Was the scene safe for the EMT crew? Was natural gas the agent that had caused the illness? The most important thing was to move to a safe environment first and then call for additional help.

Before starting to provide care for a patient, EMTs must first ensure that the scene is safe, a process called **scene size-up**. Although scene size-up may occur along with the beginning of patient assessment, it is a separate action from patient care.

The scene size-up may affect how you position yourself to provide care. Always remember that the first step of any patient evaluation is scene size-up, followed by patient assessment.

Scene size-up depends on the knowledge,

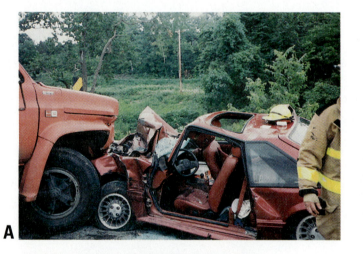

A

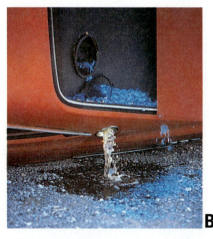

B

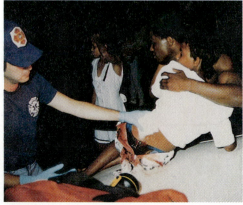

C

Fig. 8-1 A, Glass and torn metal often present safety hazards at the scene of an automobile crash. **B,** A gasoline leak can cause fire and explosion at a crash scene. **C,** Violent scenes, such as this drive-by shooting, can be especially dangerous. Be sure police have secured the scene before entering.

attitude, and skills necessary to stay alive and well as an EMT. The scene size-up includes checking scene safety, determining the mechanism of injury or nature of illness, finding out how many patients are involved, and determining whether you need additional help.

Everything you see and hear at the scene, as well as what you do not see or hear, helps to indicate whether the scene is safe. Trauma scenes with broken glass, torn metal, and spilled hazardous fluids are not the only scenes that result in injuries (Fig. 8-1A). Any of the following examples may also be a significant hazard: a patient in a car with the engine still running and the transmission in drive; a bystander smoking a cigarette down the street from the scene of an accident where gasoline is beginning to drip from a ruptured gas tank (Fig. 8-1B); a violent situation (Fig. 8-1C); an overzealous bystander attempting to help provide care and inadvertently mishandling equipment. Any factors like these, either alone or in combination with other factors, may lead to an unsafe or unstable situation.

You must take extreme caution on every call, regardless of how simple the call may seem. First and foremost, as an EMT you must take care of yourself. Rushing into a scene before evaluating it for safety may result in becoming injured or killed. EMTs who do not carefully evaluate the situation before entering the scene not only create a danger for themselves but also put their fellow healthcare professionals at risk. The goal of the first provider on the scene is to provide care for the patient. Additional responding personnel should not have to confront a situation in which they have to provide care for both the patient who initially needed EMS and an EMT who has also become a patient. Your responsibility is to ensure your own safety before addressing the safety of the patient or bystanders. Use your good judgement and experience to determine whether the scene is safe.

BODY SUBSTANCE ISOLATION PRECAUTIONS

Before beginning the scene size-up, always consider the need for body substance isolation (BSI) precautions. BSI precautions protect healthcare professionals from contact with blood and other body fluids. Healthcare professionals must be protected from both blood-borne and air-borne pathogens that may result in severe illness or death (Fig.

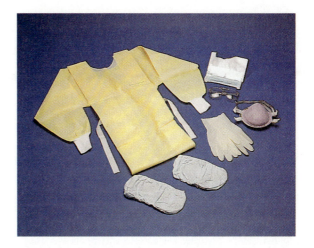

Fig. 8-2 Body substance isolation (BSI) precautions protect EMTs from contact with blood and other body fluids.

8-2). It is your responsibility to take the necessary precautions to protect yourself from contagious diseases. Chapter 2, "The Well-Being of the EMT–Basic", discusses BSI precautions and how and when to use gloves, masks, gowns, and eye protection.

SCENE SAFETY

The goal of checking scene safety is to ensure that you are not harmed while providing care. Scene size-up is the evaluation of the entire environment for any possible risks (Fig. 8-3). The scene size-up is the process by which EMTs evaluate the area before entering the scene. This size-up provides valuable information to help you stay alive and well. To protect yourself and your crew, use your senses of smell, vision, and sound to evaluate every patient situation. In time you will gain an intuitive sense for evaluating the scene.

PERSONAL PROTECTION

EMS systems use different methods of personal protection. If your roles and responsibilities as an

> **ALERT**
> The most important thing to remember as an EMT is that if the scene is not safe, and you can not make it safe, do not enter the scene.

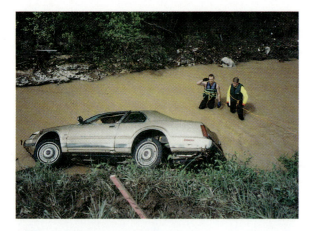

Fig. 8-3 EMTs may place themselves at risk by not checking for hazards, such as this unsecured car.

EMT involve rescue and extrication, then your service is responsible for making sure that you have the appropriate protective equipment (Fig. 8-4). You are responsible for wearing and using this protective equipment appropriately. If you provide patient care in the presence of hazardous materials, you must also be provided the proper protective equipment.

EMTs have different roles and responsibilities in different EMS systems. EMTs who work in systems that have a separate rescue division may not need added education in rescue and hazardous

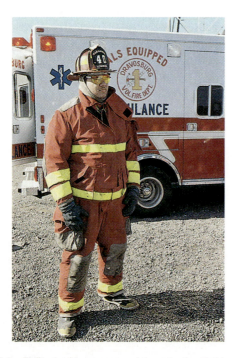

Fig. 8-4 EMTs should wear appropriate protective clothing when working at any hazardous scene.

materials. Although these courses are beneficial as continuing education, they may not be needed for day-to-day care. However, EMTs who want to work in rescue do need continuing education programs about extrication, including special equipment and skills. Because your EMS system determines your exact roles and responsibilities, you should be provided with the appropriate instruction and equipment for the situations in which you give care.

Any EMT may encounter special situations such as crash scenes, rescue situations, toxic substances, unstable surfaces, and crime scenes. These specific situations are discussed in more detail in other chapters. During the size-up of any scene, check for any special circumstances and decide how best to deal with them.

PROTECTION OF THE PATIENT

Once you have checked that the scene is safe to provide care, you also have responsibility for ensuring the safety of the patient. If you are first to arrive at a crash scene, for example, after making sure the scene is safe for you and other EMTs, your role includes protecting the patient from additional injury that may occur from traffic or other hazards. Bystanders who have inappropriately parked their cars nearby and who are close to the scene create hazards for themselves, the patient, and you. An approaching vehicle that swerves to miss hitting a bystander might end up in the patient care area. In rescue and extrication operations, the patient must be protected from metal, flying glass, or sparks created by extrication tools. Patients also require protection from the environment, such as extreme heat or cold.

PROTECTION OF BYSTANDERS

In some situations you need to ensure the safety of bystanders at the scene after protecting yourself and the patient. Usually law enforcement personnel have this role, but if you are first on the scene you may have to assume this responsibility. Bystanders are often not aware of potential hazards. They may become so engrossed in the emergency that they fail to watch out for themselves. You may need to move bystanders away from the immediate area for their safety and that of others.

In other situations, bystanders may be beneficial. In many EMS systems you may use bystanders to assist in caring for a patient. In such situations, take extra time to be certain that they adequately

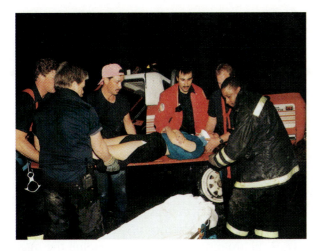

Fig. 8-5 Bystanders can assist with some tasks as long as they are well directed and are not a danger to themselves or to others at the scene.

understand their duty and role at the scene. The bystander's role may be as simple as assisting with moving the patient onto the stretcher or as complex as assisting in the removal of a patient from a vehicle onto a long backboard (Fig. 8-5). Always give bystanders enough information about their role to prevent any threat to their safety, the safety of the patient, or your own safety.

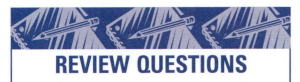

REVIEW QUESTIONS

SCENE SAFETY

1. EMTs should protect bystanders first and patients second. True or False?

2. Bystanders often can be used as assistance when extra help is needed. True or False?

3. EMTs should assess _____ before assessing the patient.

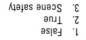

1. False
2. True
3. Scene safety

NATURE OF ILLNESS AND MECHANISM OF INJURY

After ensuring safety at the scene, you should evaluate the nature of illness or the mechanism of injury. The **nature of illness** is the patient's description of the chief complaint, or why EMS was called. The **mechanism of injury** is the event or forces that caused the patient's injury.

NATURE OF ILLNESS

Before entering the scene, assess for dangers and take appropriate BSI precautions. On entering the scene, speak with the patient to learn more about the situation (Fig. 8-6). The patient, if responsive, is usually the best source of information about the nature of illness. If the patient is unresponsive or unable to provide information, a family member or a bystander who has witnessed the situation may be able to provide information about the patient.

The appearance of the patient or the clinical signs may make the nature of illness obvious, or you may determine it shortly after your arrival as the patient describes the symptoms. The nature of illness is ultimately what the patient describes as the chief complaint.

The nature of illness for patients who are short of breath, for example, is respiratory distress. Patients who are experiencing chest pain may be having a cardiac problem. Ask patients what their chief complaint is, and provide care based on this information and your assessment findings. Ask questions such as: "Why did you call the ambulance?" and "How are you feeling?"

TRAUMA PATIENTS

For trauma patients, after ensuring scene safety and taking BSI precautions, determine the mechanism of injury. There are usually signs of the mechanism of injury, and you may be able to simply look at the surroundings and determine the mechanism of injury (Fig. 8-7A and B). If the patient is unresponsive or cannot provide information regarding the mechanism of injury, ask family, friends, or bystanders. The situation may not be what it seems at first. Ask specific questions about the situation, and do not jump to conclusions. The following are examples of questions to consider or ask others when determining the mechanism of injury:

- **For motor vehicle crashes:** How fast was the vehicle traveling? What did the vehicle hit? How

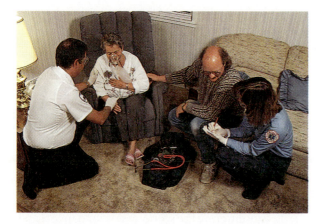

Fig. 8-6 Talk to the patient and the patient's family to gain more information about the nature of the patient's illness.

much damage was done to the vehicle? Were the occupants wearing their seat belts or helmets?
- **For falls:** How far did the patient fall? What did the patient land on? What part of the patient's body hit first?
- **For gunshot victims:** What kind of gun was used?

The patient may have sustained injuries in addition to the ones you first see. Often internal injuries are far more serious than the obvious external injuries to the patient. Evaluating the mechanism of injury helps you know when to suspect hidden injuries and guides you toward providing the most appropriate patient care.

NUMBER OF PATIENTS AND NEED FOR ADDITIONAL HELP

Calls for individuals with a medical problem usually involve only one patient. However, trauma calls such as motor vehicle crashes often involve more than one patient. When evaluating the scene, therefore, also determine whether additional patients are present. If you see a car seat in or outside the vehicle, an infant or child patient may be present somewhere in the scene. Gender-specific articles (such as a woman's purse or a man's wallet) may suggest the presence of an unseen patient. Look all around the scene to determine the total number of patients.

If more patients are present than you can adequately handle, you must request additional EMS units (Fig. 8-8). Do not delay the call for assistance; it is better to have the extra help return unneeded than to need them and not have them available. If more patients are present than your EMS system can care for, you must activate a mass casualty incident plan, as described in Chapter 32, "Overviews: Special Response Situations."

Sometimes you may require additional help for actions other than patient care. You may need help to lift a large patient. You may need law enforcement officials to deal with traffic problems, uncooperative bystanders, or with potentially violent scenes. Special assistance from fire personnel or equipment, rescue personnel or equipment, or utility companies may be needed. When possible, call for additional help before beginning the patient

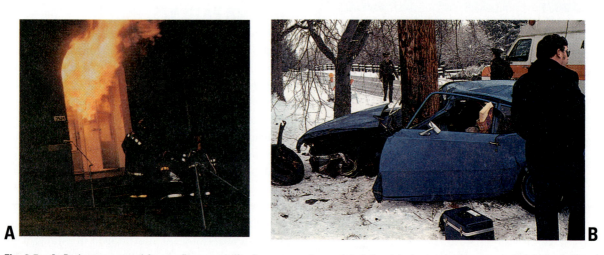

Fig. 8-7 A, Patients removed from a fire may suffer from severe burns, inhalation injuries, and other traumatic injuries inflicted during escape attempts. **B,** You should expect the driver of this car to have significant internal injuries.

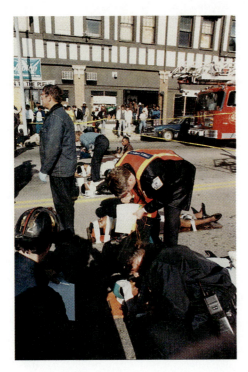

Fig. 8-8 Multiple-patient incidents often require additional EMS assistance.

care or as soon as you realize assistance is needed. Avoid getting into a situation in which you become so involved in patient care that you do not remember to or have a chance to call for additional help.

CHAPTER SUMMARY

BODY SUBSTANCE ISOLATION PRECAUTIONS

EMTs should take precautions to prevent or minimize contact with a patient's blood or other body fluids. Gloves, eye protection, gowns, and masks should be worn as necessary.

SCENE SAFETY

After taking care of themselves, EMTs should next protect the patient and then bystanders. Patients should be protected from further injury from traffic hazards, rescue operations, heat, cold, or any other danger.

NATURE OF ILLNESS AND MECHANISM OF INJURY

If the patient has a medical condition, the nature of illness is determined. If the patient has sustained a traumatic injury, the mechanism of injury is determined.

REVIEW QUESTIONS

NATURE OF ILLNESS AND MECHANISM OF INJURY/NUMBER OF PATIENTS AND NEED FOR ADDITIONAL HELP

1. Before entering the scene, what should you do to protect yourself?

2. The nature of illness described by a medical patient is also referred to as the

   _____.

3. If more patients are present than you can handle, what should you do?

1. Assess for danger and take appropriate BSI precautions
2. Chief complaint
3. Request additional help immediately

UNITED STATES DEPARTMENT OF TRANSPORTATION NATIONAL HIGHWAY TRAFFIC SAFETY ADMINISTRATION EMT–BASIC OBJECTIVES

Check your knowledge. The National Registry of EMTs and many state EMS agencies use the objectives below to develop EMT–Basic certification examinations. Can you meet them?

COGNITIVE

1. Recognize hazards/potential hazards.
2. Describe common hazards found at the scene of a trauma and a medical patient.
3. Determine if the scene is safe to enter.
4. Discuss common mechanisms of injury/nature of illness.
5. Discuss the reason for identifying the total number of patients at the scene.
6. Explain the reason for identifying the need for additional help or assistance.

AFFECTIVE

1. Explain the rationale for crew members to evaluate scene safety prior to entering.
2. Serve as a model for others explaining how patient situations affect your evaluation of mechanism of injury or illness.

PSYCHOMOTOR

1. Observe various scenarios and identify potential hazards.

9 INITIAL ASSESSMENT

IN THE FIELD

EMTs Joe and Michelle responded to Jake's home for a chest pain call. On arrival they were met at the door by his wife, Amanda, who appeared quite distressed. As they approached the patient, they were already evaluating Jake's condition. They heard him gasping for breath. He appeared to be in severe distress, was sweating profusely, and was clenching his fist against his chest. As they touched him, they felt his skin was clammy and his pulse weak, rapid, and irregular. Even after this brief patient contact, Joe and Michelle knew that Jake needed rapid treatment and transport to the hospital for his medical condition.

Later in the day, Joe and Michelle responded to a call for a patient with a cut finger. They sized up the scene and were invited into the patient's kitchen. They found him sitting at the table, holding his finger wrapped in a dish towel. As they approached the patient, they had already started the initial assessment. Their general impression of the patient was that he appeared to be calm, alert, and oriented. No life threats appeared to be present. The patient was talking clearly and calmly to them, his airway was patent, and his breathing was regular. After Joe shook hands with the patient, he felt for his pulse and noted a strong regular pulse. The initial assessment was complete, and they had determined that the patient needed evaluation only for a simple cut finger.

The first decisions about patient assessment and care are typically made within the first few seconds of seeing the patient. EMTs often can determine if the patient has a medical problem or is suffering from trauma by simply looking at the patient and the scene. During the initial assessment, you quickly evaluate the patient to:

- Form a general impression
- Assess mental status
- Assess the airway
- Assess breathing rate and quality
- Assess circulation
- Identify any life-threatening injuries and provide care based on those findings
- Make an initial transport decision

GENERAL IMPRESSION OF THE PATIENT

After completing the scene size-up and taking appropriate BSI precautions, the first thing to do when approaching a patient is to form a **general impression**. The general impression is your immediate assessment of the environment and the patient's problem. The process takes place in seconds.

The general impression usually allows you to determine the patient's priority of care and to form a plan of action for continuing to assess the patient and provide care (Fig. 9-1).

In the general impression, decide first if the patient has a medical condition or is injured. If the patient has a medical condition, determine the **nature of illness** (Fig. 9-2). The nature of illness for a person who complains of shortness of breath is

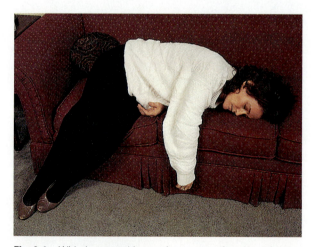

Fig. 9-1 With the general impression you can often determine the patient's priority and begin to plan care.

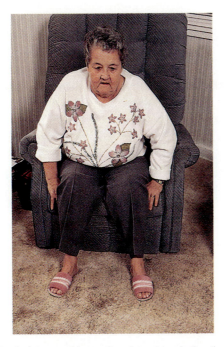

Fig. 9-2 In the general impression, determine whether the patient is injured or has a medical condition, and the nature of the illness.

respiratory distress. The nature of illness for a patient with chest pain is a potential cardiac emergency. Sometimes you cannot easily and quickly determine the nature of illness.

If the patient has been injured, identify the **mechanism of injury**. Examples of mechanisms of injury include motor vehicle crashes, falls, and stab wounds. Remember that acute medical problems may sometimes lead to trauma, such as a car driver who suffers from a heart attack and crashes the car, or a person who has a seizure and strikes the head on falling. While forming the general impression of the patient, also note the patient's age, gender, and race.

The final aspect of the general impression is to determine if the patient has any life-threatening injuries. Life-threatening injuries include major bleeding, inadequate breathing, inadequate circulation, and a variety of other conditions, which are discussed in later chapters. If a life threat is identified, it must be corrected immediately. For example, if there is blood, vomit, or teeth in the airway of a trauma patient, you must clear the airway before performing any other assessment or care. If a patient has no pulse, cardiopulmonary resuscitation (CPR) must begin immediately. By looking at, listening to, and touching the patient, you can identify threats to life.

Your general impression should be guided by the

nature of illness or the mechanism of injury as well as the patient's general appearance. For example, if a patient was in a roll-over car crash that caused severe damage to the car, the patient has potential for serious injury. Even if the patient appears to be stable or has only minor injuries, you should be suspicious that the patient may have severe internal injuries.

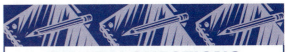

REVIEW QUESTIONS
GENERAL IMPRESSION OF THE PATIENT

1. EMTs should not interrupt the initial assessment to clear the patient's airway. True or False?

2. The general impression is used to guide the care provided to the patient. True or False?

3. During the general impression, the EMT should determine the nature of the patient's illness or _____.

1. False
2. True
3. Mechanism of injury

ASSESSING THE PATIENT'S MENTAL STATUS

After forming a general impression and before continuing the assessment, you must stabilize or immobilize the spine if the mechanism of injury suggests that a spinal injury may be present. Specific techniques for stabilizing and immobilizing the spine are discussed in Chapter 28, "Injuries to the Head and Spine." For now, remember that patients with potential spinal injuries should not be moved or be allowed to move before appropriate immobilization.

To assess the patient's mental status, begin by speaking to the patient. Introduce yourself, tell the patient that you are an EMT, and explain that you are there to help and provide care for the illness or injury. Note the patient's response.

The patient's mental status can be described in

one of four categories. Patients may be <u>A</u>lert; may not be fully alert but still respond to <u>V</u>erbal stimuli; may respond only to <u>P</u>ainful stimuli; or may be completely <u>U</u>nresponsive. The acronym *AVPU* is a reminder of these four categories, which are described in more detail below.

An alert patient is one who interacts with you without prompting. Alert patients know their name, where they are, what time it is, and the reason why EMS was called. Some patients may know their names but be unable to remember why EMS was called, or be unsure of where they are or what time it is. These patients are still alert but are considered to be disoriented. In a child, alert responses depend on the child's developmental stage. An alert child at almost any age clearly prefers being with the usual caretakers than strangers such as you. Remember that sick and injured children often regress in behavior. For example, children 3 years of age who usually can say their name may or may not be able to do so when they are hurt or scared.

Some patients appear to be sleeping but respond when you talk to them. These patients are considered to be responsive to verbal stimuli. Some patients may respond only to loud verbal stimuli. Responses in children, from oldest to youngest, may range from following a command, to actively trying to locate a parent's voice, to crying after a loud noise.

Patients who do not respond to a verbal stimulus may respond to a painful stimulus (Fig. 9-3). Pinching the patient's skin between the neck and shoulder is an adequate painful stimulus. Patients may respond to painful stimuli by making a noise, trying to remove the painful stimulus, or trying to pull away from the stimulus.

If a patient does not respond to verbal or painful stimuli, the patient is considered to be unresponsive. Relatively few patients are completely unresponsive. Most patients with altered mental status have some response to pain.

To assess the patient's level of responsiveness, first determine if the patient interacts with you without prompting. If so, the patient is alert. If not alert, will the patient respond to verbal stimuli? If not, will the patient respond to painful stimuli? A patient who does not respond to any stimulus is unresponsive.

It is important to note the mental status of the patient in your first interaction and also to note

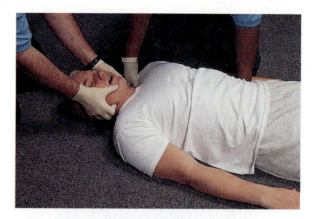

Fig. 9-3 Check the patient's response to painful stimuli if the patient does not respond to verbal stimuli.

any later changes. If the patient becomes more or less responsive, this trend is important to communicate to the receiving facility and document in the prehospital care report. Be prepared to provide airway support or to treat the patient for signs and symptoms of shock if you note that the patient's mental status is deteriorating.

REVIEW QUESTIONS

ASSESSING THE PATIENT'S MENTAL STATUS

Match the following:

1. Alert   _____   A. Responds to
    Verbal   _____   being pinched
    Painful   _____   B. Responds with-
    Unresponsive _____   out prompting
                                C. Does not
                                    respond
                                D. Responds to
                                    questions asked

2. Mental status changes can signify a changing trend in the patient's condition. True or False?

1. B; D; A; C
2. True

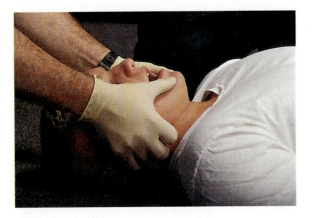

Fig. 9-4 The modified jaw thrust is performed by pushing the patient's jaw forward while stabilizing the head. This technique prevents or minimizes cervical spine movement.

ASSESSING THE PATIENT'S AIRWAY STATUS

The airway is assessed in one of two ways depending on whether the patient is alert or has an altered mental status. Alert patients may be talking or crying. If they are, the airway is open and you should move immediately to evaluating their breathing. If the patient is responsive to verbal or painful stimulus only and is not talking or crying, you may need to open the airway.

The airway is opened in one of two ways depending on whether the patient has a medical condition or an injury. For medical patients, perform the head-tilt chin-lift as described in Chapter 7, "The Airway." If the airway is not clear, it must be cleared immediately. Place the patient in the recovery position after the airway is cleared (*see* Chapter 6, "Lifting and Moving Patients").

For trauma patients or patients with an unknown nature of illness or mechanism of injury, manually stabilize the spine with your hands and perform a modified jaw thrust as described in Chapter 7, "The Airway" (Fig. 9-4). If the airway is not clear, clear it. You may need to log roll the patient onto the patient's side to clear the airway. Maintain spinal stabilization if trauma is suspected. Once the airway is open, the next step is to assess breathing.

ASSESSING THE PATIENT'S BREATHING

Assess the patient's breathing efforts as described in Chapter 5, "Baseline Vital Signs and

SAMPLE History" (Fig. 9-5). Even if an adult patient is breathing adequately at a rate between 8 and 24 breaths per minute, oxygen may be indicated. Medical direction or local protocol dictates when to administer oxygen to patients whose breathing rate is adequate and who have no obvious medical condition that indicates the use of oxygen.

Some adult patients may be breathing at a rate that is either too fast (more than 24 breaths per minute) or too slow (less than 8 breaths per minute). If these patients are responsive, they should be placed on high-flow oxygen via a nonrebreather mask at a rate of 15 L/min. If the patient will not

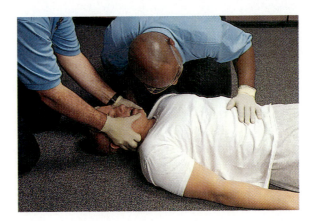

Fig. 9-5 Assess breathing by looking for chest rise, listening for air movement, and feeling the movement of exhaled air against your cheek.

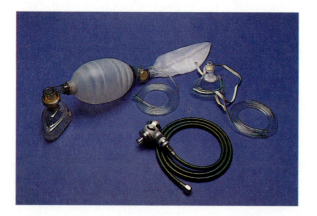

Fig. 9-6 Bag-valve-mask *(top left)*, pocket mask with oxygen port *(top right)*, and flow-restricted oxygen-powered ventilation device *(foreground)*.

tolerate a mask, you may have to use a nasal cannula. Patients who are breathing too slowly require artificial ventilation. Chapter 7, "The Airway," describes the techniques of oxygen administration. The EMT who is assessing the patient should not stop the assessment to administer oxygen, but should let another crew member perform this task.

If the patient has decreased responsiveness but is breathing adequately, the airway should be maintained in an open position and the patient placed on high-flow oxygen via a nonrebreather mask. Patients who are not breathing adequately must have their airway maintained in an open position, and oxygen provided by a ventilatory adjunct. Adjuncts for ventilation include pocket masks,

bag-valve-masks, and flow-restricted oxygen-powered ventilation devices, along with oral or nasal airways (Fig. 9-6).

Priorities for assessing breathing and providing necessary treatment are the same for infants and children as for adults. Normal breathing rates depend on the patient's age (*see* Chapter 5, "Baseline Vital Signs and SAMPLE History"). Younger children breathe more quickly. Respiratory rates slow as people grow older. A child who is breathing too slowly is much sicker than one who is breathing too fast.

ASSESSING THE PATIENT'S CIRCULATION

After evaluating the patient's level of responsiveness, airway, and breathing, and providing interventions as necessary, assess the circulation. This assessment involves checking the pulse, looking for major bleeding, and assessing perfusion.

PULSE

In adult patients, assess circulation by palpating the radial artery. If you cannot feel a radial pulse, palpate the carotid pulse. For children, palpate the radial and carotid pulses as you would in adults. For infants, use the brachial pulse (Fig. 9-7).

For patients who have a pulse, palpate both the distal and central pulses at the same time (Fig. 9-8). If the distal pulse is absent or weaker than the central pulse, the patient is showing a sign of shock.

If no pulse is present, begin CPR. For medical patients who are older than 12 years of age or weigh more than 40 kg (90 lbs.) an automated external defibrillator (AED) is also used. AEDs and their use are discussed in Chapter 18, "Cardiovascular Emergencies." For medical patients who are less than 12 years of age or less than 40 kg (90 lbs.), and for trauma patients, start CPR and transport the patient; AEDs are not used in these cases.

MAJOR BLEEDING

Next, evaluate the patient for major bleeding. In your general impression at the beginning of the initial assessment, major bleeding is one of the life threats for which you look. As part of assessing the patient's circulation, check again for major bleeding. You may need to expose injured areas by removing clothing to assess for bleeding. For patients with major trauma, all clothing should be removed

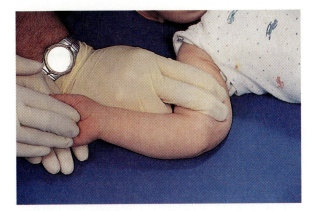

Fig. 9-7   For infants, assess the brachial pulse.

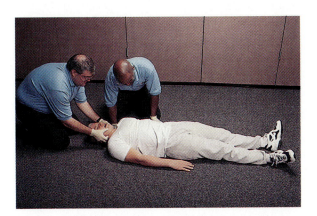

Fig. 9-8   Take radial and carotid pulses simultaneously for comparison.

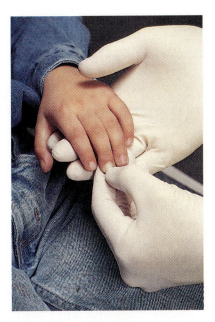

Fig. 9-9   Capillary refill is an effective technique for assessing perfusion in children less than 6 years of age.

to assess properly for injury and bleeding. If you see significant bleeding as you assess the patient, treat it as a life-threatening condition as described in Chapter 25, "Bleeding and Shock."

PERFUSION

The patient's perfusion is assessed by looking at the color of the nail beds, the inside of the lips, or the skin inside the eyelids. Normally the color of these areas is pink, regardless of race. Abnormal colorations include pale, cyanotic or blue-gray, flushed or red, and jaundiced or yellow.

In infants and children less than 6 years of age, evaluate **capillary refill** by pushing on the nail bed skin until it blanches, and then count the time it takes for the color to return to normal (Fig. 9-9). Normal capillary refill is less than 2 seconds. Delayed capillary refill is greater than 2 seconds. Delayed capillary refill indicates that there is decreased peripheral perfusion due to shock (hypoperfusion), fever, or hypothermia.

Assess skin temperature by putting the back of your hand against the patient's skin. Normal skin is warm to the touch. Abnormal skin temperatures are hot, cool, cold, or clammy (cool and moist). It is

REVIEW QUESTIONS

ASSESSING THE PATIENT'S CIRCULATION

1. AEDs should not be used for patients in cardiac arrest following traumatic injuries. True or False?

2. Major bleeding is first assessed during the _____.

3. Abnormal skin colors include _____, _____, or _____.

4. Capillary refill is assessed by pushing on the nail bed and counting as the color returns. Normal capillary refill is under _____ seconds.

1. True
2. General impression
3. Pale; cyanotic; flushed or jaundiced
4. 2

not necessary to take the patient's temperature with a thermometer in prehospital settings; the basic assessment with your hand is sufficient. If the patient's skin is cool and clammy, the patient may be in a state of hypoperfusion (shock). If the skin is hot and dry, the patient may be suffering from a medical condition or having a heat-related emergency.

The skin's condition should also be evaluated. Normally the skin is dry, but it may be moist or wet in patients with abnormal conditions.

IDENTIFYING PRIORITY PATIENTS

Patients who are seriously ill or injured need to be transported quickly to an appropriate facility where they can receive definitive treatment. The initial assessment gives you much information, and based on these findings, you may identify the patient as a priority patient. The following findings help determine if the patient is a priority patient and should be rapidly transported:

1. Poor general impression
2. Unresponsive patients with no gag reflex or cough
3. Responsive patient who is unable to follow commands
4. Patients experiencing difficulty breathing
5. Patients with the signs and symptoms of shock
6. Patients having complicated childbirth
7. Patients with chest pain and a blood pressure of less than 100 systolic
8. Patients with uncontrolled bleeding
9. Patients with severe pain anywhere

Any of these types of patients should be transported immediately. In EMS systems working with advanced life support (ALS) intercept or ALS backup, notify dispatch to send these additional crew members to the scene or to meet you en route to the hospital as designated by your EMS service. If ALS help is not available, transport rapidly to the nearest appropriate facility.

After identifying the patient priority, your initial assessment is complete. You then proceed to either the medical or trauma focused history and physical examination to continue the assessment process and to provide additional care. For patients with life-threatening illnesses or injuries, the next step in the assessment process—the focused history and physical examination—may be continued after the patient is inside the ambulance and transport has begun. For most patients, it is clear from the beginning of the assessment whether the patient has suffered from a traumatic injury or is a medical patient. For some patients, it may not be obvious until after the initial assessment. If it is unknown if an unresponsive patient is a medical patient or a trauma patient, proceed to the focused history and physical examination for trauma and take precautions to protect the spine.

With experience and practice, you will be able to perform the initial assessment for most patients in less than a minute. The initial assessment is a crucial component in the patient assessment process. A properly performed initial assessment provides valuable information about the patient's condition and allows correction of any life-threatening conditions that are found.

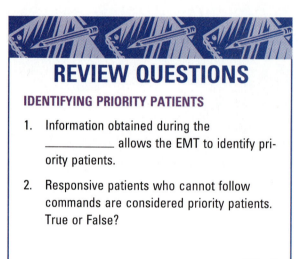

REVIEW QUESTIONS

IDENTIFYING PRIORITY PATIENTS

1. Information obtained during the _____ allows the EMT to identify priority patients.

2. Responsive patients who cannot follow commands are considered priority patients. True or False?

1. Initial assessment
2. True

CHAPTER SUMMARY

GENERAL IMPRESSION

A general impression of the patient should be formed during the first few seconds of contact with the patient. The mechanism of injury or nature of illness is identified during the general impression. Life-threatening conditions should be identified and corrected.

ASSESSING THE PATIENT'S MENTAL STATUS

Patients can be classified by the acronym *AVPU*: Alert, responsive to Verbal stimuli, responsive to Painful stimuli, or Unresponsive.

ASSESSING THE PATIENT'S AIRWAY STATUS

Patients who are alert may need oxygen or artificial ventilation. EMTs must maintain an open airway for patients who have decreased responsiveness. The head-tilt chin-lift maneuver is used for medical patients and the modified jaw thrust for trauma patients.

ASSESSING THE PATIENT'S BREATHING

Patients who are breathing too rapidly, too slowly, or inadequately need to have oxygen administered or receive artificial ventilations.

ASSESSING THE PATIENT'S CIRCULATION

EMTs assess circulation by assessing the radial, carotid, or brachial pulse, depending on the patient's age; by looking for major bleeding; and by assessing skin color temperature and condition. Assess capillary refill in children less than 6 years of age.

IDENTIFYING PRIORITY PATIENTS

Information obtained in the initial assessment helps to identify priority patients. All priority patients should be transported immediately to the nearest appropriate receiving facility. ALS intercept or back-up should be used for these patients when it is available.

UNITED STATES DEPARTMENT OF TRANSPORTATION NATIONAL HIGHWAY TRAFFIC SAFETY ADMINISTRATION EMT–BASIC OBJECTIVES

Check your knowledge. The National Registry of EMTs and many state EMS agencies use the objectives below to develop EMT–Basic certification examinations. Can you meet them?

COGNITIVE

1. Summarize the reasons for forming a general impression of the patient.
2. Discuss methods of assessing altered mental status.
3. Differentiate between assessing the altered mental status in the adult, child, and infant patient.
4. Discuss methods of assessing the airway in the adult, child, and infant patient.
5. State reasons for management of the cervical spine once the patient has been determined to be a trauma patient.
6. Describe methods used for assessing if a patient is breathing.
7. State what care should be provided to the adult, child, and infant patient with adequate breathing.
8. State what care should be provided to the adult, child, and infant patient without adequate breathing.
9. Differentiate between a patient with adequate and inadequate breathing.
10. Distinguish between methods of assessing breathing in the adult, child, and infant patient.
11. Compare the methods of providing airway care to the adult, child, and infant patient.
12. Describe the methods used to obtain a pulse.
13. Differentiate between obtaining a pulse in the adult, child, and infant patient.
14. Discuss the need for assessing the patient for external bleeding.
15. Describe normal and abnormal findings when assessing skin color.
16. Describe normal and abnormal findings when assessing skin temperature.
17. Describe normal and abnormal findings when assessing skin condition.
18. Describe normal and abnormal finding when assessing skin capillary refill in the infant and child patient.
19. Explain the reason for prioritizing a patient for care and transport.

AFFECTIVE

1. Explain the importance of forming a general impression of the patient.
2. Explain the value of performing an initial assessment.

PSYCHOMOTOR

1. Demonstrate the techniques for assessing mental status.
2. Demonstrate the techniques for assessing the airway.
3. Demonstrate the techniques for assessing if the patient is breathing.
4. Demonstrate the techniques for assessing if the patient has a pulse.
5. Demonstrate the techniques for assessing the patient for external bleeding.
6. Demonstrate the techniques for assessing the patient's skin color, temperature condition, and capillary refill (infants and children only).
7. Demonstrate the ability to prioritize patients.

FOCUSED HISTORY AND PHYSICAL

EXAMINATION FOR TRAUMA PATIENTS

KEY TERMS

Crepitation: A grating or crackling sound or sensation, such as that caused when fractured ends of bone move against each other.

DCAP–BTLS: An acronym standing for the eight components of assessment: deformities, contusions, abrasions, penetrations or punctures, burns, tenderness, lacerations, and swelling.

Distal pulse: A pulse taken away from the center of the body, such as at the wrist.

Iliac wings: The anteriosuperior tips of the pelvis.

Jugular vein distention: The abnormal enlargement of the veins on the sides of the neck.

Motor function: Testing the ability to move.

Multitiered response system: A system in which EMS responses to calls involve basic and advanced levels; may include First Responders, EMTs, paramedics, and other healthcare professionals. Various levels of healthcare professionals may arrive at the scene or meet en route to facilities to provide patient care.

Paradoxical motion: An abnormal movement of the chest wall during inspiration and exhalation in which the affected portion moves opposite the unaffected portion.

Sensation: The ability to feel a touch against the skin.

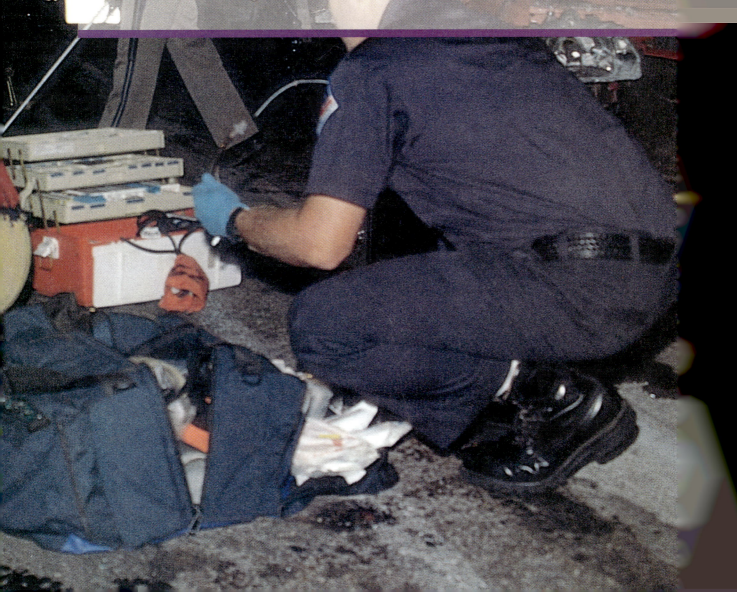

IN THE FIELD

EMTs Jake and Amanda responded to a vehicle crash. The patient was sitting on the ground outside the vehicle talking to bystanders. Their scene size-up revealed no dangers to the EMTs. The mechanism of injury was obvious as they looked around the scene: the patient's car had struck a utility pole, causing moderate damage to the car. The patient had been helped from the car by bystanders, and no other patients were involved. The initial assessment revealed that the patient was alert, had a patent airway, was breathing at a normal depth and rate, and had a strong and regular pulse.

Jake then moved on to the next step—the focused history and physical examination for trauma patients. The mechanism of injury was a front-end collision of a car into a utility pole. The inside of the vehicle seemed intact, but because of the amount of damage to the exterior, Amanda realized that they must quickly evaluate the patient from head to toe to look for any unseen life threats not detected in the initial assessment. The mechanism of injury suggested that there may be serious hidden life-threatening injuries even though the patient seemed to be stable.

Jake quickly evaluated the patient from head to toe, inspecting, palpating, and auscultating to assess for injuries. This rapid assessment was completed in about 90 seconds. Jake and Amanda determined that no life threats were present. The patient continued to appear stable. They moved him onto a long backboard and into the ambulance and began transport to the appropriate facility.

While en route to the hospital, Jake obtained the baseline vital signs SAMPLE history.

As explained in the preceding chapter, all patients receive an initial assessment. The focused history and physical examination that follows the initial assessment may differ somewhat depending on whether the patient has a medical or trauma condition. Most patients clearly fit into one of these categories. For a patient with a medical condition, use the focused history and physical examination for medical patients (described in Chapter 11, "Focused History and Physical Examination for Medical Patients"). If you are not immediately sure whether the patient has a trauma or medical condition, treat the situation as trauma and perform the rapid trauma assessment. This chapter describes the assessment process used for trauma patients.

The focused history and physical examination may differ for particular trauma patients depending on whether they have a serious injury (or a serious mechanism of injury) or a simple injury with no serious mechanism of injury. Both categories of trauma patients receive a focused history and physical examination. Patients with injuries to multiple body systems, unresponsive patients, and patients with serious mechanisms of injury should also receive a rapid head-to-toe trauma assessment

(Fig. 10-1). Patients with an isolated, specific injury, such as a painful, swollen, deformed extremity or a cut finger with no significant mechanism of injury, should receive a focused history and physical examination directed toward that injury site.

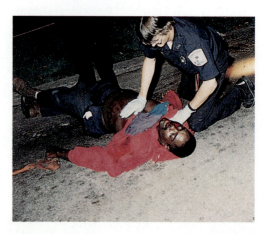

Fig. 10-1 Use the rapid head-to-toe trauma assessment for patients with injuries to multiple body systems, unresponsive patients, and patients with serious mechanisms of injury.

MECHANISM OF INJURY

As you begin the focused history and physical examination for trauma patients, reconsider the mechanism of injury. Patients with mechanisms of injury such as those listed in Box 10-1 are at greater risk for hidden injuries, which you may not find unless you look for them. These are only a few of the situations that place patients in the category to receive a rapid head-to-toe trauma assessment.

In vehicle collisions, there may be hidden injuries caused by seat belts, air bags, or other devices. Although seat belts unquestionably save lives, they can also cause injuries, especially when used inappropriately. Ask patients if they were wearing their seat belt, and check for any related injuries, such as bruises to the chest or waist. Bruising caused by seat belts may indicate hidden internal injuries.

Air bags are becoming increasingly standard equipment in automobiles. Air bags are deployed when a force is applied to the front of the vehicle. Air bags cushion the vehicle's occupant from hitting the steering wheel or dashboard. Air bags are less effective if seat belts are not used, and they do not prevent patients from hitting the steering wheel or dashboard after the air bag has deflated. Air bags are designed to deflate automatically within a few seconds after they are deployed. In all cases, lift a deployed air bag and check the steering wheel for deformity, which could indicate that the occupant struck the steering wheel, making an internal injury more likely.

With infants and children, falls greater than 3 m (10 ft) or twice their height, bicycle collisions, and vehicle collisions at medium speed can cause serious injury. Less force is required to seriously injure an infant or child than to injure an adult. Inquire whether infant or child safety restraints were used. Remember that infant car seats often are not secured properly within the vehicle and can become dangerous missiles when a collision occurs. Improperly restraining an infant or child can lead to serious injury, especially when small children are placed in adult seat belts.

An older person whose bones may be weakened may also be more easily injured in a vehicle collision or other trauma situation.

The evaluation of all trauma patients depends on the mechanism of injury. Patients involved in a significant vehicle crash often appear stable even when they have major injuries. The mechanism of injury helps guide you toward the most appropriate care. If you cannot determine the mechanism of injury, question the patient, relatives, or bystanders

---

BOX 10-1

Mechanisms of Injury Considered To Be High-Risk for Hidden Injury

- Ejection of driver or passenger from a vehicle
- Driver or passenger in the same passenger compartment where another patient died
- A fall of more than 6 m (20 ft)
- Vehicle roll-over
- High-speed vehicle collision
- Vehicle–pedestrian collision
- Motorcycle crash
- Patients who are unresponsive or who have an altered mental status
- Penetrating trauma to the head, chest, or abdomen

REVIEW QUESTIONS

MECHANISM OF INJURY

1. All patients receive a focused history and physical examination. True or False?

2. Why should EMTs reconsider the mechanism of injury?

3. Less force is required to seriously injure infants and children than for adults. True or False?

1. True
2. Things aren't always as they appear. Patients who appear to be stable may have significant injuries. The mechanism of injury may suggest that particular attention is required to care for the patient.
3. True

to learn more about how the injury occurred. Ask bystanders questions such as: "Can you tell me exactly what happened?" "How far did the patient fall?" "How fast was the car going when it hit the child on her bicycle?"

If you are unsure about the mechanism of injury, assume that it is significant and perform a rapid trauma assessment.

EVALUATING PATIENTS WITH SERIOUS INJURIES OR MECHANISMS OF INJURY

All unresponsive patients, trauma patients with a significant mechanism of injury, and patients with multiple body system trauma should receive a rapid trauma evaluation. This evaluation assesses for any life-threatening conditions.

Both before and during your trauma assessment, ask responsive trauma patients to describe their symptoms. A patient who called EMS because of a specific problem usually directs you to evaluate that injury first. Do not assess only the specific injury without carefully considering the patient as a whole. Patients with multiple injuries usually focus on their most painful injury, which is not necessarily the most serious injury.

Trauma patients with head injuries or suspected head injuries should be considered to have spinal injuries. All unresponsive patients should be treated as if they have a spinal injury. The mechanism of injury may also suggest a potential spine injury even if the patient has no complaints of head, neck, or back pain. You must stabilize or immobilize the spine before and during the entire assessment process. Specific techniques for spinal stabilization and immobilization are discussed in Chapter 28, "Injuries to the Head and Spine."

EMTs who work in **multitiered response systems** should request advanced life support (ALS) personnel for patients who are seriously injured or who have a high-risk mechanism of injury. If a patient is entrapped and possibly at the scene for some time, the ALS team may come to the scene. In systems that have an established EMS intercept protocol for ALS, such as helicopter or other ALS service, the process should be initiated as early as possible.

As the preceding chapter explains, you consider the patient's priority for rapid transportation in the initial assessment, and you should reconsider this priority if the patient who earlier appeared stable begins to become unstable. Expedite the transport of the patient to the appropriate facility in a safe, rapid manner.

During this process, continue to interact with the patient and evaluate mental status while gathering pertinent information.

PERFORMING THE RAPID TRAUMA ASSESSMENT

As you inspect and palpate the patient for injuries, use the acronym **DCAP–BTLS** to remember the eight components you are looking for:

- D—Deformities
- C—Contusions
- A—Abrasions
- P—Penetrations or punctures
- B—Burns
- T—Tenderness
- L—Lacerations
- S—Swelling

Deformities occur when bones are broken, causing an abnormal position or shape. *Contusions* are bruises. *Abrasions* occur when the top layers of the skin are scraped away, such as when a child scrapes the skin from the knee after falling from a bike. *Penetrations or punctures* involve an object penetrating the skin, such as a gunshot wound, stab wound, or stepping on a nail. *Burns* can result from exposure to heat, chemicals, electricity, or radiation. *Tenderness* is sensitivity to touch. *Lacerations* are cuts in the surface of the skin. *Swelling* is a response of the body to injury and makes the area look larger than usual.

The rapid trauma assessment should be performed in 60 to 90 seconds. If a life threat is found during this phase of assessment, direct additional crew members to care for that condition while you continue the entire assessment.

The following approach uses a head-to-toe order of assessment. The evaluation is the same for adults, infants, and children. Children may cooperate better, however, if obviously painful areas are examined last.

First evaluate the patient's head. Rapidly evaluate the whole head and face. Assess the skull for DCAP–BTLS (Fig. 10-2). Feel for any unstable areas on the face.

Immediately move to the neck, and, in addition to DCAP–BTLS (Fig. 10-3), look for **jugular vein**

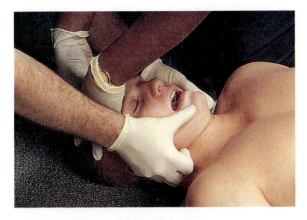

Fig. 10-2 Assess the skull for deformities while your partner manually stabilizes the patient's head.

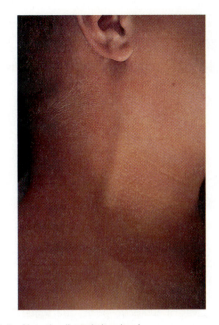

Fig. 10-4 Note the distended neck veins.

distension. The jugular veins are large veins on both sides of the neck. These veins can be distended or flat. When the patient is sitting up, you usually cannot see the jugular veins. When the patient is lying down, the veins are usually somewhat distended and can be seen. If a sitting patient's veins are visible, the veins are distended. If the veins are not visible in a patient lying down, the veins are flat. Distended jugular veins signify an increased pressure in the circulatory system (Fig. 10-4). Flat neck veins may indicate blood loss.

Assessment of the jugular veins may be difficult in children and infants because of their short necks. Vigorous crying may also produce jugular vein distension. After you evaluate the neck, have another available EMT place a cervical spine immobilization device on the patient to help maintain the head in neutral alignment (Fig. 10-5). If the cervical spine immobilization device is not applied at this time, be

sure one is applied before the patient is moved onto the long backboard.

Next, inspect and palpate the chest for DCAP–BTLS (Fig. 10-6). Contusions or abrasions over the chest wall indicate an increased risk of pulmonary injury. Also evaluate the chest for **paradoxical motion** and **crepitation**. Paradoxical motion is movement of part of the chest wall in the opposite direction from the rest of the chest wall during inhalation and exhalation. Crepitation is the sound and feel of broken bones moving against one another.

Evaluate the chest by feeling the clavicles first. Palpate the sternum and the entire rib cage for

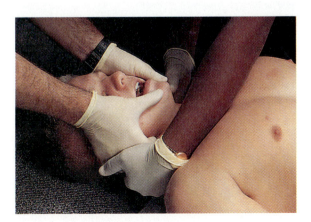

Fig. 10-3 Assess the patient's neck.

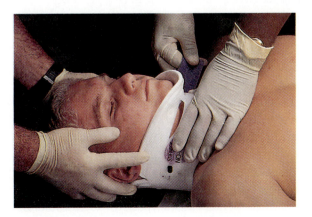

Fig. 10-5 Apply a cervical spine immobilization device after assessing the neck.

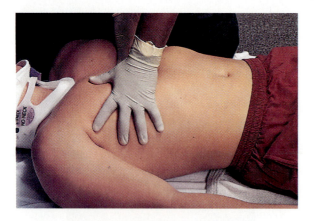

Fig. 10-6 Assess the patient's chest for DCAP–BTLS.

crepitation. Place one hand on each side of the patient's rib cage to assess for paradoxical motion. At this time, use a stethoscope in the apices, at the midclavicular line on both sides of the chest, and at the bases at the midaxillary line to determine if breath sounds are present or absent (Fig. 10-7). Determine if breath sounds are present bilaterally and if they are equal.

Next, examine the abdomen, again evaluating for DCAP–BTLS, and also determine if the abdomen is firm, soft, or distended (Fig. 10-8). The abdomen is normally soft. A firm abdomen feels rigid when you push against it. A firm abdomen can be a sign of an injury to the abdominal organs or blood collecting in the abdomen. A distended abdomen means that the abdomen appears larger than normal. Because some patients normally have a large abdomen, it may be difficult to distinguish between a normally large abdomen and an abdomen that is distended due to injury. Children may have a distended abdomen due to air swallowed during crying. To assess the abdomen, gently press with your palms against each of the four quadrants, depressing approximately 2.5 cm (1 in). You may place one hand on top of the other to assess the abdomen. The four quadrants are the right upper quadrant, the right lower quadrant, the left upper quadrant, and the left lower quadrant. The upper quadrants begin just below the ribs and end at the umbilicus. The lower quadrants begin at the umbilicus and extend to the pelvic crests (Fig. 10-9).

Assess the pelvis next, placing your hands bilaterally at the **iliac wings,** and push posteriorly first to flex the pelvis, and then push toward the midline of the patient to compress the pelvis to determine stability of the pelvis (Fig. 10-10A and B). Do not

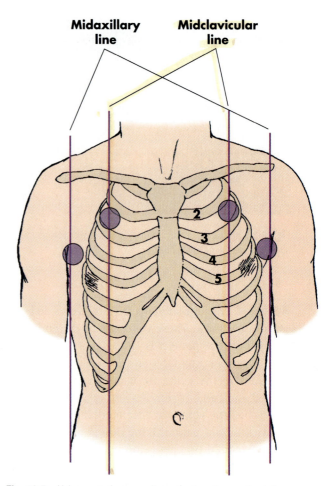

Fig. 10-7 Using a stethoscope, listen for breath sounds at four points.

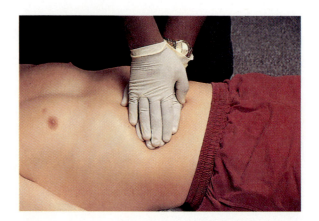

Fig. 10-8 Assess the abdomen and note whether it is firm, soft, or distended.

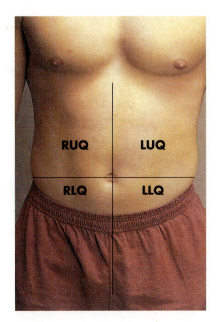

Fig. 10-9 The abdomen is divided into the upper right and left and the lower right and left quadrants.

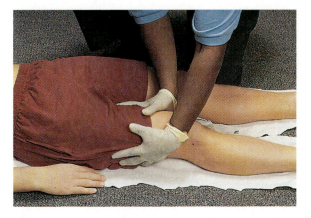

Fig. 10-11 Palpate the lower extremities with the palms of your hands.

perform flexion and compression of the pelvis if a responsive patient complains of pain in the pelvic area or if the mechanism of injury suggests that pelvic injury may have occurred. Further manipulation of an already injured pelvis may worsen the condition. For unresponsive patients and those who do not complain of pelvic pain, flex and compress the pelvis carefully. If the patient complains of pain or if the pelvis feels unstable (seems to move towards the posterior or midline during flexion and compression), do not repeat the assessment of the pelvis.

Following the pelvis assessment, evaluate the extremities beginning with the legs (Fig. 10-11). As

you evaluate both legs for injuries using DCAP–BTLS, assess also for **distal pulse, motor function,** and **sensation.** Pedal pulses can be felt either on top of the foot (Fig. 10-12) or posterior to the medial ankle. Motor function is the ability to move the feet or legs, and sensation is the ability to feel a touch against the skin (Fig. 10-13). Ask responsive patients if they can wiggle their toes and if they can feel you touching them. Do not ask patients to bend their knees or move their legs around because this movement may compromise spinal stabilization or immobilization. You may not be able to assess sensation and motor function in unresponsive patients, because these patients may or may not react to a touch on the extremities. Evaluate both arms in the same manner as the legs (Fig. 10-14).

To place a patient on the long backboard for transport, the patient must be log rolled. As one EMT assesses the patient, another EMT can be placing the long backboard beside the patient to prepare for transport. The technique for log rolling

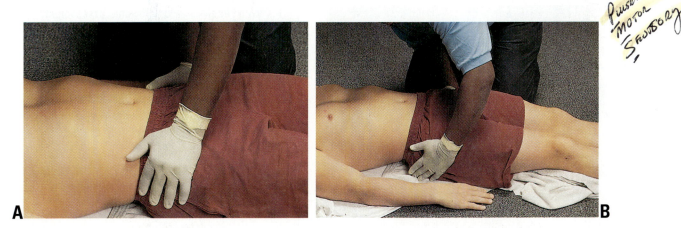

Fig. 10-10 Assess the stability of the pelvis. **A,** Flexion. **B,** Compression.

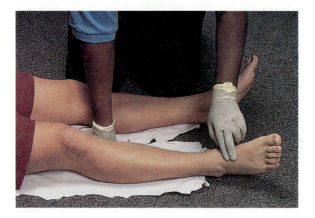

Fig. 10-12 Note the presence or absence of pedal pulses.

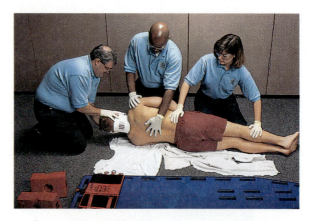

Fig. 10-15 As you log roll the patient, inspect and palpate the back for injury.

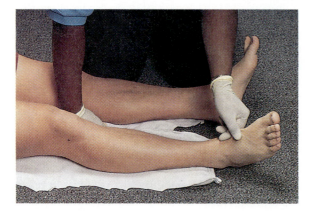

Fig. 10-13 The patient should be able to feel a light pinch if sensation is present.

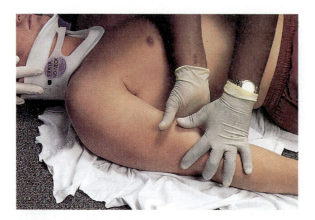

Fig. 10-14 Palpate the upper extremities with the palms of your hands.

a patient is described in Chapter 28, "Injuries to the Head and Spine." At that time you can evaluate the entire posterior of the patient from head to toe, inspecting and palpating for injuries (Fig. 10-15).

BASELINE VITAL SIGNS AND SAMPLE HISTORY

While one EMT completes the focused physical examination, another EMT can take the baseline vital signs. Chapter 5, "Baseline Vital Signs and SAMPLE History," describes the procedures for

REVIEW QUESTIONS

EVALUATING PATIENTS WITH SERIOUS INJURIES OR MECHANISMS OF INJURY

1. Who receives a rapid trauma assessment?

2. In addition to DCAP–BTLS, what else should the EMT evaluate at the patient's neck?

3. If a patient complains of pain in the pelvis, the EMT should not evaluate the pelvis by flexing and compressing. True or False?

1. All trauma patients who are unresponsive and all patients who have a significant mechanism of injury.
2. Jugular vein distension
3. True

taking vital signs. A SAMPLE history can be taken from responsive patients during the physical examination. If the patient is unresponsive, ask bystanders or family members what happened and what they know of the patient's medical history.

EVALUATING PATIENTS WITH NO SIGNIFICANT MECHANISM OF INJURY

For patients with no significant mechanism of injury—for example, a cut finger, deformed ankle, or bruised knee—begin the focused history and physical examination at the site of the injury, using the same components (DCAP–BTLS) (Fig. 10-16). Remember, however, that if the patient sustained a serious mechanism of injury, there may be underlying injuries of which the patient is not aware. Patients often are aware of only their most painful injury, which is not necessarily the most serious. If you suspect other injuries, or there is a serious mechanism of injury, perform an entire rapid trauma assessment.

Assess the patient's baseline vital signs, and take a SAMPLE history as described in Chapter 5, "Baseline Vital Signs and SAMPLE History."

A comparison of two cases will help clarify this principle. In the first case, a patient is in a motor vehicle collision resulting in severe damage to the car and tree. The patient complains only of pain in the right ankle. This patient has undergone a serious mechanism of injury and should receive an entire rapid trauma assessment. In the second case, a patient who was jogging suffered a twisted ankle when stepping off a curb. The patient did not fall and complains only of ankle pain. The physical examination for this patient can be directed toward the ankle only, because there is no mechanism of injury to require a complete trauma assessment.

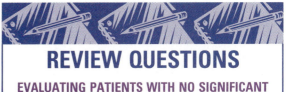

REVIEW QUESTIONS

EVALUATING PATIENTS WITH NO SIGNIFICANT MECHANISM OF INJURY

1. For a patient with an injured wrist and no significant mechanism of injury, what is the focus of the history and physical examination?

2. While evaluating a patient with a painful, swollen deformed upper right extremity, the EMT learns it was injured in a car collision. What should the EMT do?

1. Usually just the injured wrist.
2. The EMT should perform the rapid trauma assessment to evaluate the entire patient. It is always best to err on the side of overevaluation rather than underevaluation.

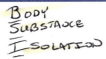
Body Substance Isolation

CHAPTER SUMMARY

MECHANISM OF INJURY

The mechanism of injury helps guide the EMT toward the appropriate care for the patient. A serious mechanism of injury should make the EMT suspect and look for hidden injuries. Infants and children can be more seriously injured than adults with the same amount of force.

EVALUATING PATIENTS WITH SERIOUS INJURIES OR MECHANISMS OF INJURY

All patients who have been seriously injured or who have a significant mechanism of injury should receive a rapid trauma assessment. EMTs should assess the patient from head to toe to evaluate for deformities, contusions, abrasions, penetrations or punctures, burns, tenderness, lacerations, and

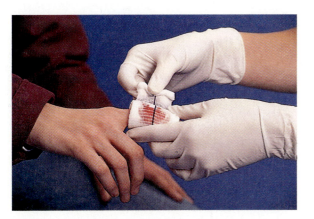
Fig. 10-16 A patient with an isolated injury like the one shown here may not need a complete rapid trauma assessment.

swelling (DCAP–BTLS). Some areas are evaluated for additional indications of injury. The neck is examined for distended jugular veins, the chest for crepitation, paradoxical motion, and equality of breath sounds, and the abdomen for rigidity or distention.

EVALUATING PATIENTS WITH NO SIGNIFICANT MECHANISM OF INJURY

Patients with no significant mechanism of injury and an isolated injury do not always require a rapid trauma assessment. EMTs may evaluate the injury only.

UNITED STATES DEPARTMENT OF TRANSPORTATION NATIONAL HIGHWAY TRAFFIC SAFETY ADMINISTRATION EMT–BASIC OBJECTIVES

Check your knowledge. The National Registry of EMTs and many state EMS agencies use the objectives below to develop EMT–Basic certification examinations. Can you meet them?

COGNITIVE

1. Discuss the reasons for reconsideration concerning the mechanism of injury.
2. State the reasons for performing a rapid trauma assessment.
3. Recite examples and explain why patients should receive a rapid trauma assessment.
4. Describe the areas included in the rapid trauma assessment, and discuss what should be evaluated.
5. Differentiate when the rapid assessment may be altered in order to provide patient care.

6. Discuss the reason for performing a focused history and physical exam.

AFFECTIVE

1. Recognize and respect the feelings that patients might experience during assessment.

PSYCHOMOTOR

1. Demonstrate the rapid trauma assessment that should be used to assess a patient based on mechanism of injury.

RAPID INITIAL ASSESSMENT   - BASE-LINE VITALS
DETAILED FOCUSSED ASSESSMENT

1) AVPU
2) DCAP BTLS
3) SAMPLE

EXAMINATION FOR MEDICAL PATIENTS

IN THE FIELD

EMTs Joe and Michelle responded to a call for a patient who was having chest pain. They completed the scene size-up and the initial assessment. The scene size-up revealed no dangers. The initial assessment revealed a 60-year-old man who stated that he was having chest pain. He was clutching his chest and appeared to be in moderate distress. The patient was alert and oriented, was breathing approximately 20 times per minute, and had a rapid, weak pulse. Joe began the focused history and physical examination. Michelle placed the patient on high-flow oxygen using a nonrebreather mask at a rate of 15 L/min and then went for the stretcher. Joe evaluated the patient by asking questions about the discomfort in his chest and his medical history.

The patient said that the pain began approximately 2 hours earlier while he was mowing his lawn. It became worse when he walked up the hill and stairs to his home. He described the pain as a tight squeezing pressure. The pain radiated down his left arm and through the middle two fingers of his left hand and to his jaw and back. The severity of the pain on a scale from one to 10 was a six at this point, but he felt that it had been an eight when he was walking up the hill. The patient that stated he had a history of cardiac disease for the past 10 years and had taken the nitroglycerin his physician had prescribed for chest pain. He told Joe that the nitroglycerin had provided some relief, and he had thought he would be fine. However, 20 minutes ago the pain returned while he was lying down resting, so he called EMS.

The patient said he had no allergies to medications, and the only medication he was taking was nitroglycerin. He said he had a mild heart attack about 2 years ago. His last oral intake was cereal and orange juice at breakfast.

After taking a set of baseline vital signs, Joe called the medical direction physician for permission to assist the patient in taking another of his prescribed nitroglycerin tablets. Joe and Michelle transferred the patient to the stretcher and then to the ambulance, and began transport. Joe assisted the patient in taking another of his nitroglycerin tablets as directed by medical direction.

Just as the focused history and physical examination for the trauma patient are designed specifically for trauma patients, the focused history and physical examination for the medical patient are designed specifically for medical patients.

In the focused history and physical examination of responsive medical patients, the patients usually can provide you with information concerning their illness. With unresponsive patients, bystanders, family members, or friends may be able to provide information about the patient's medical history or events leading to the illness.

With unresponsive patients, you may not be able to tell why they are unresponsive or decide if they have a medical problem or an injury. For these patients, you should perform a rapid assessment from head to toe using the same procedure as the focused history and physical examination for trauma patients (Fig. 11-1). Often the only difference in the assessment of unresponsive medical patients from that of trauma patients may be that the spine is not immobilized first. However, if there is any doubt about the mechanism of injury or the nature of illness in unresponsive patients, it is best to immobilize the spine.

Remember that the patient evaluation always begins with the scene size-up followed by an initial assessment (Fig. 11-2). As you approach a patient who is having difficulty breathing, focus your assessment on signs and symptoms related to respiratory distress, and provide care based on the specific assessment findings. When you approach a patient who is clenching a fist over the chest and recognize that a cardiac problem may exist, focus your

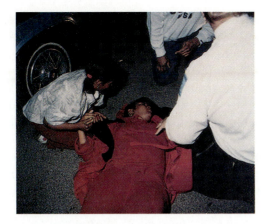

Fig. 11-1 Unresponsive patients are given a rapid assessment following the same focused history and physical examination procedure used for trauma patients.

assessment on signs and symptoms related to cardiac emergencies. You then can continue to provide appropriate care based on the findings from the focused assessment.

You do not need to complete the focused history and physical examination before you begin to treat the patient. For any patient whose illness indicates the need to use oxygen, oxygen can be administered while you are assessing the patient. Often oxygen is administered to the patient based on the findings in the initial assessment.

Patients experiencing medical emergencies are often scared, anxious, or nervous. Remember that

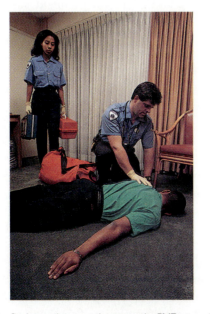

Fig. 11-2 Seeing no threats at the scene, the EMT proceeds to the initial assessment of this unresponsive patient with no history of trauma.

this situation is stressful. Treat all patients with respect. Your role is to care for patients as a whole person and not just treat their medical condition. Listen carefully to what patients tell you about their illness. Do not be judgmental about the severity of their illness—if they did not feel there was an emergency, they would not have called EMS.

RESPONSIVE MEDICAL PATIENTS

THE PATIENT'S HISTORY

Alert, responsive, adult patients usually can tell you a great deal about the nature of their illness. Infants and children may not be able to accurately describe their symptoms, although their parents may be helpful in explaining their behavior. Some older patients also may not be able to clearly describe their illness or their medical history. Listen carefully to what all patients tell you, and ask questions to clarify if you are unsure what their responses mean.

When you are gathering the history of the present illness, the **OPQRST** acronym helps you remember what questions to ask. The acronym *OPQRST* stands for *Onset, Provocation, Quality, Radiation, Severity, and Time.* These terms help define the quality of the patient's symptoms. Although the OPQRST acronym suggests a sequential order, it is not necessary for you to obtain the information in this order.

OPQRST is used primarily for a patient with a chief complaint of pain, but it also can be used to assess other conditions.

The following is an example of using OPQRST to evaluate the patient in the opening scenario, who was experiencing chest pain. All of these questions can be modified for any symptom the patient may be feeling, not just pain.

"O" signifies questions that help determine the time of onset or origin of the patient's medical problem. For example, the patient in the opening scenario has had a cardiac condition for the last 10 years. Determining the onset allows the EMT to establish a starting point for the illness. Questions to ask include: "Do you have a history of cardiac disease?" "How long have you had a cardiac condition?"

"P" signifies questions whose answers provide clues to things that provoke the medical condition. If you are assessing pain, determine what makes

(0 – 10 scale)

the pain worse (**provocation**). For the patient in the opening scenario, walking up the hill provoked more pain. Some EMTs like to think of the "P" also standing for palliative, which refers to what makes pain diminish. Therefore, "P" represents both what provokes the pain and also what is palliative. For example, the patient may tell you that lying down for a period of time helps alleviate the pain. In this case lying down is palliative because it makes the pain diminish. Other signs and symptoms can also be assessed for provocation and palliation. For example, a patient may feel more dizzy when standing up and feel less dizzy when sitting. Questions to ask include: "After the pain started, what did you do that made you feel more comfortable?" "What makes the pain more uncomfortable?" "Is there a particular position that makes the pain better or worse?"

"Q" signifies questions about the quality of the pain. When asking about the quality of the pain, be careful not to ask questions that lead the patient to a certain kind of answer. Ask patients to describe the discomfort in their own words. It is up to patients to say whether it is a sharp pain, dull pain, or stabbing pain. Questions to ask include: "Can you describe to me the pain you are feeling?"

"R" signifies questions regarding where the pain radiates. A patient with chest pain may say the pain moves up to the jaw, to the back, or down the left arm. A patient with an abdominal pain may say it radiates into the back. Not all pain radiates. However, all patients with a complaint of pain should be asked if the pain radiates or spreads anywhere else. Ask the patient questions such as: "Does the pain you are feeling in your chest spread or move anywhere else?"

"S" signifies questions about the severity of the pain. Ask the patient to describe the pain on a scale from one to 10, with one being mild discomfort and 10 being the worst pain. Patients may describe the pain at one level now but say it was at a different level when it began. Rest, position, time, and medication may reduce the severity of the pain. You can ask about the severity of any condition, not just pain. For example, patients who were vomiting could be asked how severe the vomiting was. Patients who are dizzy can be asked whether they have had dizzy spells that were worse or less severe. Ask the patient, "On a scale from one to 10—10 being the worst pain you have ever felt—how would you rank the pain at this time?" "How severe was the pain when it started?" "Has the pain gotten better or worse?" "If you've had chest pain in the past, is the pain you are feeling now more or less severe?"

"T" signifies questions about the duration of time since the patient felt it necessary to call EMS because of the symptoms. These questions are different from questions that are asked of the patient concerning the initial onset of signs and symptoms associated with the illness, which may have been weeks, months, or years ago. A patient who has had an illness for sometime may contact EMS concerning that specific illness because of changes in the type or severity of the discomfort. For example, a patient who has had heart disease for the last 3 years may contact EMS after starting to feel chest pain that is not relieved by rest as it usually is. Patients with various conditions may find that they tolerate the condition for a period of time prior to calling for EMS. For example, a patient who is weak and dizzy may have been weak and dizzy for several days, although now the patient's condition has become more severe. Questions to ask include: "How long have you been experiencing this chest pain?" "If you've been feeling sick for the last 3 days, what happened to make you call EMS now?"

After or while assessing the components of OPQRST, you also can take the **SAMPLE history** as described in Chapter 5, "Baseline Vital Signs and SAMPLE History." Remember: "S" stands for signs and symptoms, "A" for allergies (predominately to medications), "M" for history of current medications being taken, "P" for pertinent past medical history, "L" for last oral intake of fluids or solids, and "E" for the events leading to the illness. This information need not be acquired in that order. Both acronyms are just ways to remember what questions need to be asked, and the steps need not be followed in exact order.

RAPID ASSESSMENT

After gathering this information, move to the **rapid assessment** which is a head-to-toe examination of the patient. The focused history and physical examination of medical patients is guided by their chief complaint. It is often unnecessary to assess patients head to toe when they have a medical problem. For example, you may gain little beneficial information from examining a patient's arm if the patient is complaining of breathing difficulty. Assess the pertinent areas of the body relevant to the complaint.

When the patient complains of head pain, assess

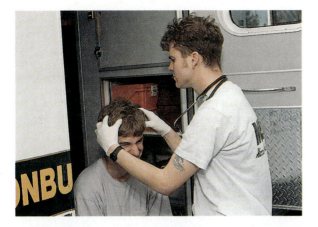

Fig. 11-3   Inspect and palpate the head of patients with head pain for signs of trauma. Remember to evaluate the need for cervical immobilization.

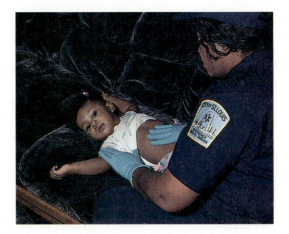

Fig. 11-5   Palpate the four quadrants of the abdomen.

the head to see if there is any trauma of which the patient is unaware (Fig. 11-3).

If the patient is complaining of a stiff neck or neck pain with no associated trauma, evaluate the need for spinal immobilization. Remember, the patient may not associate the current complaint with an earlier injury.

Patients who complain of chest pain should have their chest exposed for evaluation. This exposure makes it easier to auscultate breath sounds, to assess the possible use of accessory muscles to breathe, and to inspect the chest for any signs of trauma (Fig. 11-4).

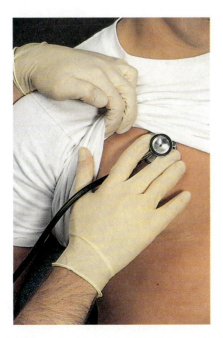

Fig. 11-4   Expose the chest to auscultate lung sounds. Look for evidence of trauma and respiratory distress as you listen.

For a patient with a chief complaint of abdominal pain, evaluate the abdomen, palpating the four quadrants (Fig. 11-5).

Patients with pelvic discomfort should be evaluated with great care. In these patients do not manipulate the pelvic region. If the patient states that there may have been trauma to the area, attempt to visualize the area, but use good judgement in doing so. Sometimes the patient has difficulty determining if the discomfort is actually pelvic or abdominal. In these situations, gently palpate the pelvis, and if there is any question about the stability of the pelvis, immobilize it.

A patient who complains of extremity pain or back pain needs that area evaluated and may, in some situations, be splinted to help reduce the discomfort. Keep in mind that the patient may have sustained an injury days or weeks earlier even though the patient now seems to be reporting a medical problem. It is always better to err on the side of providing too much care rather than to undertreat the patient.

Try to minimize the patient's discomfort by allowing the patient to assume a position of comfort unless you suspect spinal injuries. Do not repeat painful maneuvers.

VITAL SIGNS

After you have obtained a SAMPLE history and assessed OPQRST, assess the following vital signs:

- Breathing
- Circulation
- Skin
- Blood pressure
- Pupils

Chapter 5, "Baseline Vital Signs and SAMPLE History," describes the techniques for assessing vital signs.

EMERGENCY CARE

Use your good judgement as you acquire assessment information and prepare to give emergency care. With the help of other EMTs in your crew you may bring the stretcher, administer high-flow oxygen, and move the patient quickly to the ambulance while still gathering the OPQRST and SAMPLE history. Then you can begin transport and assess the baseline vital signs en route. In an EMS system in which you cannot transport the patient right away, give oxygen as early as possible to patients who need it (Fig. 11-6). Complete the OPQRST and SAMPLE history quickly, and when appropriate, perform the rapid assessment of body areas that need to be evaluated. Then provide emergency medical care based on the assessment information gained from this rapid assessment. Consult medical direction when indicated by your local protocols.

Specific interventions for medical emergencies are described in following chapters. Some patients with known medical problems may have medications to relieve their discomfort or help their condition. A patient who is having a respiratory emergency, for example, may be assisted with an inhaler. A patient who is having an allergic reaction and has an epinephrine autoinjector available may be assisted with the use of their autoinjector as part of the care you give. With other patients you may give other specific interventions for their condition. A cardiac patient may require intervention with an automated external defibrillator or nitroglycerin. A diabetic patient with altered mental status may receive oral glucose. A poisoning or overdose patient may need to be administered activated charcoal. Emergency care is always based on the patient's signs and symptoms and a thorough assessment of the patient's condition.

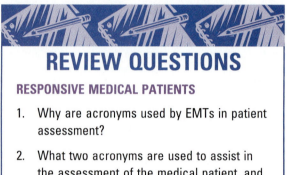

REVIEW QUESTIONS

RESPONSIVE MEDICAL PATIENTS

1. Why are acronyms used by EMTs in patient assessment?

2. What two acronyms are used to assist in the assessment of the medical patient, and what do the letters of the acronyms stand for?

3. Must EMTs follow the steps in the acronyms in exact order?

4. How should EMTs evaluate a responsive medical patient in the focused history and physical examination?

1. To assist in remembering the questions to be asked of the medical patient.
2. OPQRST (Onset, Provocation, Quality, Radiation, Severity, and Time) and SAMPLE (Signs and Symptoms, Allergies, Medications, Past pertinent medical history, Last oral intake, and Events leading up to the illness or injury)
3. No
4. Obtain the subjective information of the OPQRST and SAMPLE history before the physical examination.

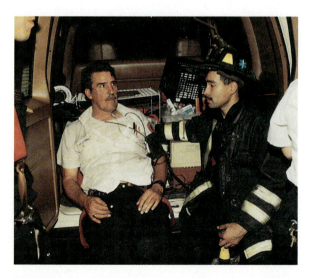

Fig. 11-6 Oxygen is an important intervention that can be given while awaiting a transport unit.

UNRESPONSIVE MEDICAL PATIENTS

For unresponsive medical patients, perform a rapid assessment using the same focused history and physical examination as for unresponsive trauma patients (Fig. 11-7). See Chapter 10, "Focused History and Physical Examination for Trauma Patients," for the specifics of the rapid trauma assessment. Assess the baseline vital signs.

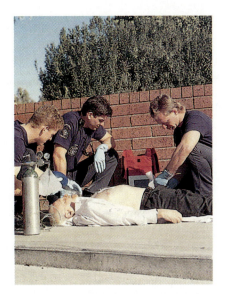

Fig. 11-7 All unresponsive patients should receive a rapid trauma assessment because the patient cannot direct you to an illness or injury.

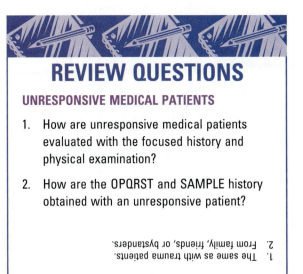

REVIEW QUESTIONS

UNRESPONSIVE MEDICAL PATIENTS

1. How are unresponsive medical patients evaluated with the focused history and physical examination?

2. How are the OPQRST and SAMPLE history obtained with an unresponsive patient?

1. The same as with trauma patients.
2. From family, friends, or bystanders.

The focused history and physical examination for trauma patients are used for all unresponsive patients because these patients cannot direct you toward their illness or injury. You may discover findings that aid you in treating the patient. Because you cannot know for certain whether the patient sustained trauma, the rapid head-to-toe assessment may provide you with valuable information.

As with any other patient, provide care based on the assessment findings. Unless the patient requires assisted ventilations, provide high-flow oxygen via a nonrebreather mask at a rate of 15 L/min.

If possible, obtain an OPQRST and SAMPLE history from family members or friends. If no one knows the patient well, try to find out what happened before the patient became unresponsive.

Because you cannot know for certain whether the patient has sustained any injury to the spine, immobilize the patient for transport to the receiving facility. Carefully monitor the patient's airway, and be prepared to suction the airway or log roll the patient if necessary.

If you can be certain there was no trauma, transport the patient in the recovery position to the receiving facility. The recovery position allows secretions to drain from the patient's mouth and helps maintain an open airway.

CHAPTER SUMMARY

RESPONSIVE MEDICAL PATIENTS

Establish a rapport with responsive patients before the physical assessment by questioning them about their illness. Take the OPQRST and SAMPLE history. The questions do not need to be asked in any specific order.

The rapid assessment may be performed based on the patient's condition, signs, and symptoms. When in doubt, perform a rapid head-to-toe assessment. Obtain baseline vital signs including breathing; circulation; skin; blood pressure; and pupils. Give care based on the patient's signs and symptoms. Provide high-flow oxygen, move the patient to the stretcher, and provide a caring attitude while transporting to the appropriate facility.

UNRESPONSIVE MEDICAL PATIENTS

Unresponsive medical patients cannot provide information to EMTs. Therefore, perform a rapid head-to-toe assessment, ask bystanders, friends, family members about the patient's condition, and provide care based on your findings. Obtain baseline vital signs in a timely manner.

All medical patients receive a focused history and physical examination. For unresponsive patients, perform an assessment similar to that of the unresponsive trauma patient. Provide care based on their signs and symptoms.

UNITED STATES DEPARTMENT OF TRANSPORTATION NATIONAL HIGHWAY TRAFFIC SAFETY ADMINISTRATION EMT–BASIC OBJECTIVES

Check your knowledge. The National Registry of EMTs and many state EMS agencies use the objectives below to develop EMT–Basic certification examinations. Can you meet them?

COGNITIVE

1. Describe the unique needs for assessing an individual with a specific chief complaint with no known prior history.
2. Differentiate between the history and physical exam that is performed for responsive patients with no known prior history and patients responsive with a known prior history.
3. Describe the unique needs for assessing an individual who is unresponsive or has an altered mental status.
4. Differentiate between the assessment that is performed for a patient who is unresponsive or has an altered mental status and other medical patients requiring assessment.

AFFECTIVE

1. Attend to the feelings that these patients might be experiencing.

PSYCHOMOTOR

1. Demonstrate the patient care skills that should be used to assist with a patient who is responsive with no known history.
2. Demonstrate the patient care skills that should be used to assist with a patient who is unresponsive or has an altered mental status.

12 DETAILED PHYSICAL EXAMINATION

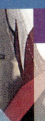

IN THE FIELD

EMTs Joe and Amanda were responding to a single-vehicle car crash involving a 20-year-old woman. They performed the scene size-up, the initial assessment, and the focused history and physical examination. The patient's chief complaint was difficulty breathing. Amanda immediately placed the patient on high-flow oxygen. The patient's respiratory rate and circulatory status were assessed; her breathing rate was 20 breaths per minute and shallow, and her heart rate was normal and strong. During the focused history and physical examination, Joe found a 1-cm (0.05-in) laceration on her forehead and a deformity of her lower left leg. The laceration was dressed and bandaged and her leg splinted. The patient was extricated from the car and transferred to the ambulance.

While en route to the hospital, Joe carefully evaluated the patient from head to toe in a more organized and methodical manner. The patient complained that her head hurt, and she was not having as much difficulty breathing. As Joe began the detailed physical examination, he found additional cuts and bruises on her right and left legs not seen earlier due to the limited light available and the patient's position. Now with the patient in the well-lighted ambulance and her clothing removed, Joe could better evaluate the patient's injuries.

The more often patients are assessed, the more information you obtain about their injury or illness. The **detailed physical examination** is designed primarily for trauma patients who may have hidden injuries that are not revealed in the initial assessment or the focused history and physical examination. The detailed assessment is also useful for unresponsive medical patients. This assessment allows you to slowly and methodically evaluate the patient from head to toe.

DETAILED PHYSICAL EXAMINATION

The detailed physical examination is a methodical head-to-toe evaluation of the patient. The detailed physical examination is similar to the focused history and physical examination of trauma patients but is more carefully and slowly performed.

PATIENTS NEEDING A DETAILED EXAMINATION

All trauma and medical patients who are unresponsive and all patients who have an altered mental status should receive a detailed physical examination. Patients with a significant mechanism of injury should also receive a detailed physical examination. During the rapid trauma assessment for unresponsive patients, you may miss details that could provide clues to the patient's condition, such as needle marks on the arm of a drug user, that would be found during a slower, more detailed physical examination.

If you are spending all your time keeping the airway clear or assisting ventilations, however, do not interrupt care for the airway, breathing, or circulation to perform a detailed physical examination.

Patients with an isolated, specific injury may not need a detailed physical examination. For a trauma patient who has a cut finger, for example, the focused history and physical examination directs you to assess and provide care for that specific injury. This patient does not need palpation of other body parts such as the abdomen, pelvis, and extremities. Most patients sustaining specific, isolated trauma do not receive a detailed physical examination.

The same holds true for many medical patients. After the focused history and physical examination, you can move directly to the ongoing assessment, described in the next chapter. A medical patient who is short of breath and in extreme distress requires assessment and care focused on the airway and oxygen. For this patient you may chose not to perform a detailed physical examination because you are likely to gain little information from palpating every body part. If you have any doubt about a situation, however, perform the detailed physical examination and explain to the patient the reason for the assessment.

EXAMINATION PROCEDURE

The detailed physical examination is similar to the focused physical examination for trauma patients because it also assesses *DCAP–BTLS:* Deformities, Contusions, Abrasions, Penetrations/Punctures, Burns, Tenderness, Lacerations, and Swelling. As you inspect and palpate the entire body surface area of the patient, evaluate these eight components again in a more detailed manner (Fig. 12-1).

The care given for the specific injuries found during the detailed physical examination is described in later chapters. This chapter describes only the skills for assessing the patient.

Beginning at the head, inspect and palpate for DCAP–BTLS. Palpate the head starting on the superior surface (top) of the head, running your hands back to the posterior occipital area (Fig. 12-2). As you bring your hands around to the patient's

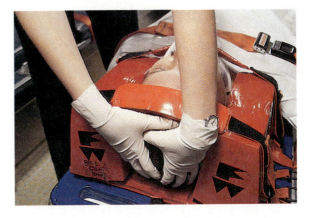
Fig. 12-2 Palpate the patient's head.

frontal area, carefully inspect and palpate; move toward the face palpating the frontal area, the zygomatic arches, the maxilla, and the mandible of the patient (Fig. 12-3). Use a penlight to check in the ears, looking for drainage (Fig. 12-4).

With the penlight, inspect the eyes of the patient, looking for any discoloration of the eye.

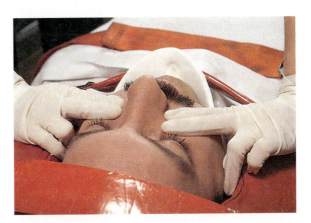
Fig. 12-3 Palpate the face.

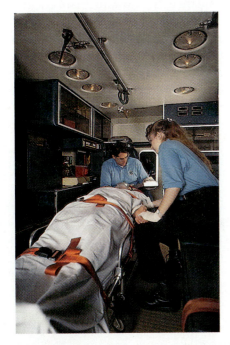
Fig. 12-1 The detailed physical examination evaluates the DCAP–BTLS components again in a more precise manner; this is usually performed during transport.

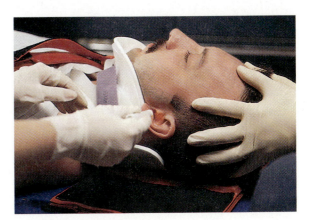
Fig. 12-4 Inspect the ears and look for blood or fluid.

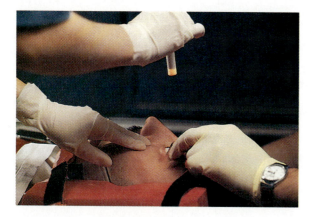

Fig. 12-5   Assess the eyes for pupillary response and any discoloration.

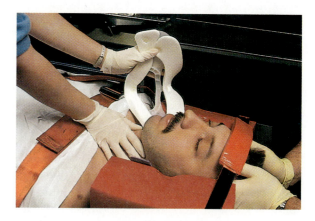

Fig. 12-7   Palpate the neck while your partner maintains manual stabilization.

Look at the pupils and assess whether they are equal in size and react to light. Also look for any foreign bodies or blood in the eyes (Fig. 12-5). Use the penlight to look in the patient's nose, inspecting for any drainage.

Open or ask the patient to open the mouth and inspect for loose teeth or any other substances that may cause obstruction, such as gum, dentures, or tobacco products. Evaluate the tongue for swelling or lacerations, and check for odors and discoloration (Fig. 12-6).

Next, evaluate the patient's neck. For a trauma patient with an immobilized spine, this is an opportunity to carefully evaluate the neck region. If the patient is already immobilized on a long backboard with a cervical spine immobilization device in place, ask your partner to manually stabilize the head while you open the cervical spine immobilization device in front, inspecting and palpating for DCAP–BTLS as well as evaluating for jugular vein distention and crepitation (Fig. 12-7). The device

should be replaced following this process.

Note: If the patient is wearing a cervical spine immobilization device that allows room for adequate palpation and inspection, you may elect to leave it in place and feel through the opening to assess the anterior neck only (Fig. 12-8).

Next, evaluate the chest, inspecting and palpating for DCAP–BTLS, crepitation, and paradoxical motion (Fig. 12-9). Determine if breath sounds are present and equal (Fig. 12-10). An easy way to perform this evaluation is to start at the clavicles and move to the sternum. While inspecting and palpating around all rib areas, move your fingers as far around their sides toward their back as possible. Ask a responsive patient to take a deep breath, or ask a crew member assisting with ventilation to squeeze the bag as you palpate on both sides. The chest should rise and fall equally on both sides. Place your stethoscope high on the anterior axillary lines, at the apices or **bilaterally** at the bases,

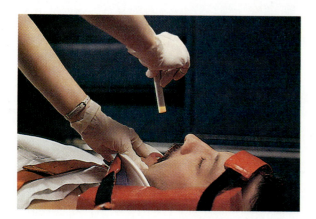

Fig. 12-6   Inspect the mouth for injury or foreign bodies.

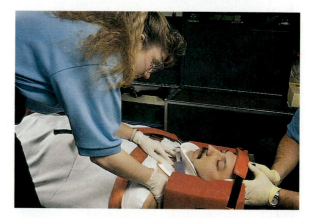

Fig. 12-8   You may be able to palpate the neck through the opening in the cervical spine immobilization device.

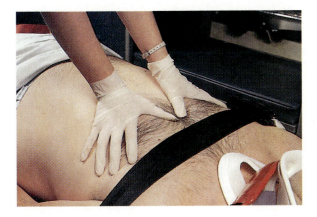

Fig. 12-9   Expose and palpate the chest, observing for paradoxical movement or deformity.

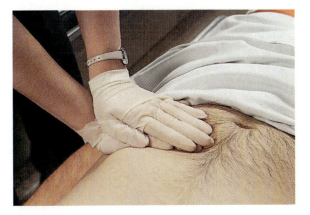

Fig. 12-11   Palpate all four quadrants of the abdomen.

evaluating the right and left sides for the presence or absence of breath sounds and for their equality.

The abdomen is evaluated next (Fig. 12-11). Because some patients are particularly sensitive about having their abdominal area touched, inform all patients what you are about to do before beginning to assess the abdomen. After placing your hand on the abdomen, allow the patient to relax the abdominal muscles so that you can better determine whether there is rigidity in the abdominal region. Position one hand on top of the other, and while looking at the patient, carefully roll the hand from the heel to the fingertips. Assess all four quadrants. During this process, evaluate for DCAP–BTLS and softness, rigidity, and distention. These areas are normally soft. While you are evaluating the abdomen, watch the patient's facial expression for grimaces. You may miss this sign if you watch only the abdominal region.

If you do not suspect that the patient has a pelvic injury based on the mechanism of injury and the patient does not complain of pain, you can also palpate the pelvis (Fig. 12-12). Place the heels of your hands bilaterally on the patient's pelvic wings. They are often more obvious in thinner individuals, but you should be able to find this point on all patients. Carefully and gently push posteriorly and then to the patient's midline to ascertain the stability of the pelvic region. If motion is present, the region is unstable. If the pelvis is unstable, do not reassess this area. Further movement of the pelvis could aggravate injuries to the spine, nerves, or blood vessels.

Finally, check the four extremities. Because you have just evaluated the pelvis, check the lower extremities first. While facing the patient, palpate each leg. Do not exert pressure with your thumbs only, but use your entire hand to assess the patient's extremities. As you move down the extremity from the pelvis, start high on the thigh of the patient's leg closest to you, and run your hands down the entire extremity (Fig. 12-13). At the end

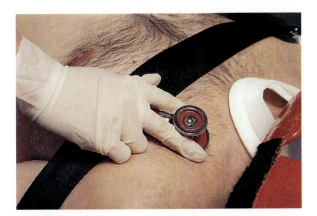

Fig. 12-10   Auscultate breath sounds.

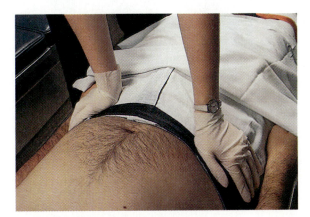

Fig. 12-12   Palpate the pelvis.

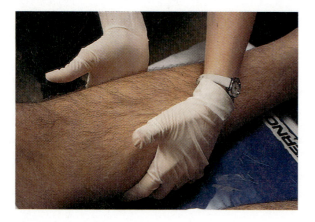

Fig. 12-13 Palpate the lower extremities and assess pulse, motor function, and sensation.

of the extremity, determine if pulse, sensation (response to touch or pain), and motor function (mobility) are present.

Note: If the patient is in extreme distress or if radial pulses were difficult to obtain, use your good judgement to determine whether to assess pedal pulses.

After checking the leg closest to you, assess the opposite leg, again including pulse, sensation, and motor function. Continue the assessment by moving to the patient's upper extremities. Evaluate one entire arm, including pulse, sensation, and motor function, and repeat with the other arm (Fig. 12-14).

If the patient is on a long backboard or stretcher en route to the hospital, do not roll the patient to evaluate the posterior region again. However, if you have not yet placed the patient on a transporting device, you may again log roll the patient to evaluate posterior injuries that may not have been revealed in the rapid trauma assessment.

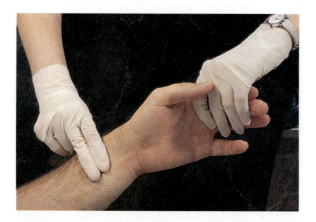

Fig. 12-14 Palpate the upper extremities and assess pulse, motor function, and sensation.

The steps of the detailed physical examination are the same for infants and children as for adults. You may wish to use a "trunk-to-head" approach, as discussed in Chapter 29, "Infant and Child Emergency Care."

The detailed physical examination ideally should be performed in the back of the ambulance while en route to the appropriate facility. If you are not transporting the patient yet or are waiting for additional help, you may perform the detailed physical examination on the scene.

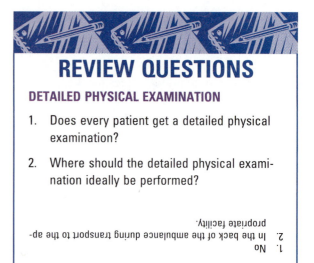

REVIEW QUESTIONS

DETAILED PHYSICAL EXAMINATION

1. Does every patient get a detailed physical examination?

2. Where should the detailed physical examination ideally be performed?

2. In the back of the ambulance during transport to the appropriate facility.

1. No

ASSESSING VITAL SIGNS

Following the detailed physical examination, evaluate the patient's vital signs again. For some patients, these may be the first set of vital signs obtained. If a patient's condition requires all of your attention to care for life-threatening injuries, do not waste time measuring the blood pressure, pulse, and respirations. If a patient is bleeding into the airway, for example, it is much more important to suction and maintain that open airway than it is to take the blood pressure.

CHAPTER SUMMARY

DETAILED PHYSICAL EXAMINATION

The detailed physical examination is an organized head-to-toe evaluation of the patient. Not all patients receive a detailed physical examination. A detailed physical examination is best performed in the back of the ambulance en route to the appropriate facility. This assessment builds on the steps of the focused history and physical examination for trauma patients in the rapid trauma assessment. This allows you to look for anything that might not have been revealed in the rapid assessment. The detailed physical examination may be omitted when, for example, there is a need to continuously maintain the airway of the patient to assist in ventilation or to assist in the circulatory support efforts of the patient. Patients who are not likely to receive a detailed physical examination include those with simple trauma, such as a cut finger, or a medical patient such as a patient with chest pain.

ASSESSING VITAL SIGNS

Evaluate the vital signs whenever the patient's condition allows. Sometimes you may not be able to evaluate vital signs because the patient's airway, breathing, or circulation require your immediate attention.

UNITED STATES DEPARTMENT OF TRANSPORTATION NATIONAL HIGHWAY TRAFFIC SAFETY ADMINISTRATION EMT–BASIC OBJECTIVES

Check your knowledge. The National Registry of EMTs and many state EMS agencies use the objectives below to develop EMT–Basic certification examinations. Can you meet them?

COGNITIVE

1. Discuss the components of the detailed physical exam.
2. State the areas of the body that are evaluated during the detailed physical exam.
3. Explain what additional care should be provided while performing the detailed physical exam.
4. Distinguish between the detailed physical exam that is performed on a trauma patient and that of the medical patient.

AFFECTIVE

1. Explain the rationale for the feelings that these patients might be experiencing.

PSYCHOMOTOR

1. Demonstrate the skills for performing the detailed physical exam.

13 ONGOING ASSESSMENT

KEY TERM

Ongoing assessment: The final step of the patient assessment process; repeats the initial assessment and focused assessment during transport.

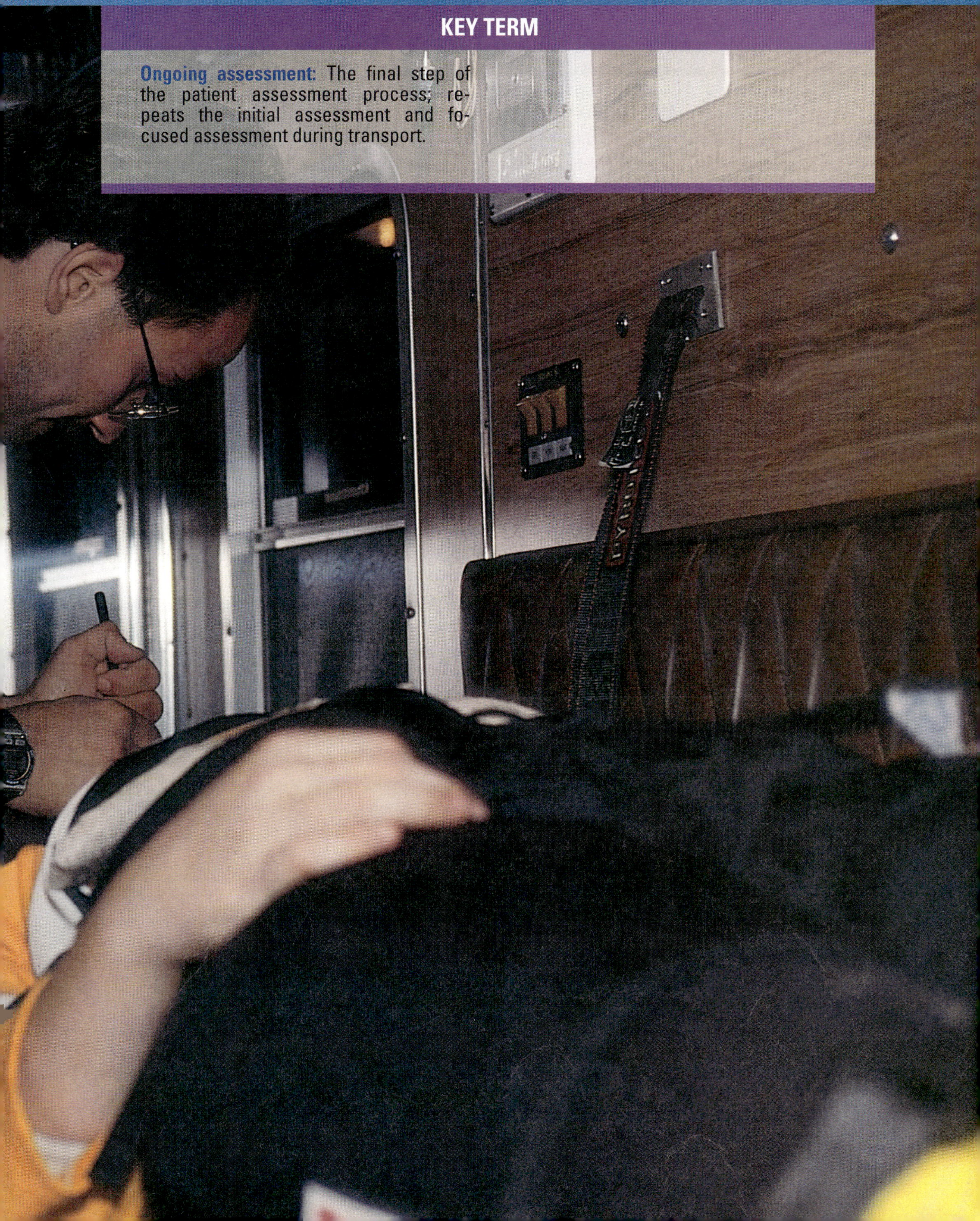

IN THE FIELD

The EMTs Jake and Amanda were dispatched to a street where a man had fallen from a ladder. On arrival at the scene, they found no hazards and determined the scene was safe. Their initial assessment revealed a 23-year-old man who was alert and oriented, had a patent airway, was breathing in an unlabored manner (at 14 breaths per minute), and had a strong regular pulse. The focused history and physical examination for this trauma patient revealed injuries to his right arm and right leg. They splinted the extremities prior to transport, and the patient was fully immobilized because of the mechanism of injury. The detailed physical examination was performed once the patient was in the ambulance and transport had begun.

As Jake and Amanda transported the patient to the hospital, Amanda performed an ongoing assessment. The transport time was approximately 45 minutes. Because the patient remained stable during this time, Amanda performed three assessments, one every 15 minutes. Throughout the transport, she continually spoke to the patient, monitoring his mental status. From the way the patient interacted, she knew the airway was clear; she monitored the patient's respiratory rate and quality. Every 15 minutes she checked the patient's pulse for rate and quality and obtained a blood pressure measurement. She noted the patient's skin color, temperature, and condition and kept Jake informed about the patient's status. Amanda contacted the receiving emergency department to notify them of the patient's status.

She also checked the flow of oxygen to the patient and all other interventions she and Jake had performed. Approximately 5 minutes before arriving at the receiving facility, Amanda reevaluated the patient for each of the components of the ongoing assessment.

Once you have responded to a call, evaluated the scene, assessed and cared for the patient, and begun transport to the appropriate facility, the patient must be continuously evaluated.

This reassessment occurs during the **ongoing assessment.** The purpose of the ongoing assessment is to reevaluate the patient's condition and to check each intervention for adequacy. Frequent evaluations allow you to notice subtle changes in the patient's condition.

Reevaluating patients also allows you to observe trends in their condition that you should document and relay to the receiving facility. Trends in a patient's mental status, blood pressure, or other vital signs can provide valuable information to the healthcare professionals who will assume care of the patient.

COMPONENTS OF THE ONGOING ASSESSMENT

Once you have responded to a call and are en route to the appropriate facility, continuous evaluation of the patient must take place. The ongoing assessment repeats the initial assessment and the focused assessment and includes an assessment of all interventions performed. Box 13-1 summarizes the elements of the ongoing assessment.

For stable patients, the ongoing assessment should be repeated and the results recorded every 15 minutes. For unstable patients, the assessment should be repeated and the results recorded every 5 minutes or less.

Stable patients are those medical or trauma patients who have simple, specific injuries. For

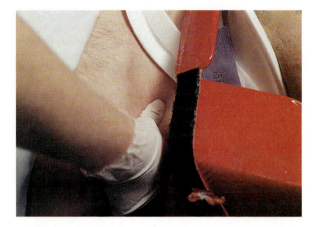

Fig. 13-1 If the patient is unresponsive, check the response to painful stimuli to establish mental status.

example, for a stable patient who injured an ankle playing softball, repeat and record the assessment every 15 minutes. A patient with a history of nausea and vomiting and no other associated injuries may also be considered to be stable.

Unstable patients are those medical patients in severe distress or trauma patients who have sustained a significant mechanism of injury, even if they appear to be stable.

Patients generally receive the ongoing assessment in the back of the ambulance en route to the receiving facility. If the EMS unit is a nontransporting unit or is awaiting additional personnel, the ongoing assessments should be performed on scene. Ongoing assessments are generally performed after the detailed physical examination. Even though not every patient receives a detailed physical examination (as discussed in the previous chapter), all patients receive ongoing assessments.

REPEAT THE INITIAL ASSESSMENT

The ongoing assessment begins by repeating the components of the initial assessment. First, reassess the mental status of the patient (Fig. 13-1). You should constantly be interacting with the patient throughout the transport. This interaction allows you to observe the mental status of the patient and note any changes for either better or worse.

Always ensure that the patient has an open and patent airway and that there is nothing in the mouth that might obstruct the airway (Fig. 13-2). Again, if you are interacting with a responsive patient en route to the hospital, you can continuously monitor the mental status and the patency of the airway at the same time by talking to the patient.

The third component is to monitor the breathing for rate and quality. With experience you can do this while a responsive patient is resting comfortably on the stretcher during transport to the facility.

Evaluate the pulse for rate and quality. If a radial pulse is palpable, use it for the ongoing assessment. However, for those patients with barely palpable radial pulses, evaluate the carotid pulse. Children's pulses are assessed the same as an adult patient's. Infants' pulses should be assessed at the brachial artery.

Next, evaluate the patient's skin color, temperature, and condition. The skin may be evaluated as

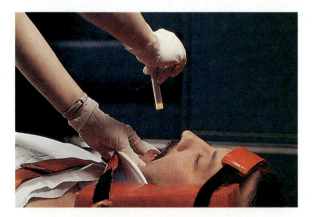

Fig. 13-2 Inspect the mouth for injury or the presence of foreign bodies.

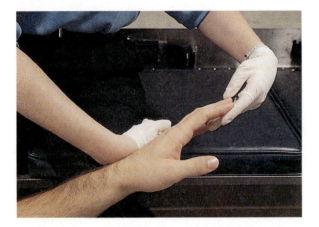

Fig. 13-3 Assess skin temperature and condition as part of your ongoing assessment of vital signs.

you obtain the patient's radial pulse. Note and document any deviations from normal or changes from your previous assessment (Fig. 13-3). Checking skin color allows you to assess perfusion as in the initial assessment. With children less than 6 years of age, assess perfusion by checking capillary refill as in the initial assessment.

Although there is no need for a separate step to assess again for major bleeding as you did in the initial assessment, because it is unlikely that the patient will suddenly start bleeding now, you should confirm that major bleeding that was assessed and controlled earlier is still being controlled. Do this assessment as part of checking the effectiveness of all interventions, as described in a later section in this chapter.

Finally, reestablish the patient's priority for transport. Ideally, all patients would remain stable or improve during transport. In reality, sometimes the patient's condition takes a turn for the worse. Therefore, reestablish the patient's priority. For example, a patient having mild chest discomfort is provided oxygen, evaluated, and transported. During transport this patient's pain may increase or the patient may go into cardiac arrest, becoming a priority patient. The transport then changes from a comfortable, unhurried ride to a quick but cautious ride with lights and siren to expedite the transport.

REPEAT VITAL SIGNS AND FOCUSED ASSESSMENT

The ongoing assessment also requires EMTs to reassess and record the patient's vital signs. The vital signs described in Chapter 5, "Baseline Vital Signs and SAMPLE History", are all evaluated as part of this process, at least every 15 minutes for stable patients and every 5 minutes or less for unstable patients. These vital signs are documented in the prehospital care report and relayed to the staff at the receiving facility.

The ongoing assessment also repeats the focused assessment of the patient's specific complaint or injury. For a patient with a specific injury and no major mechanism of injury, reevaluate that injury site specifically. For a medical patient with a respiratory problem, focus the assessment on the patient's respiratory status. The focused assessment is described in detail in Chapter 10, "Focused History and Physical Examination for Trauma Patients," and Chapter 11, "Focused History and Physical Examination for Medical Patients."

Some patients may have life-threatening conditions that require all of your attention. If you are so busy maintaining an open airway by suctioning, you may not ever have time to assess the patient's vital signs. The ongoing assessment for a patient with life-threatening injuries is almost constant.

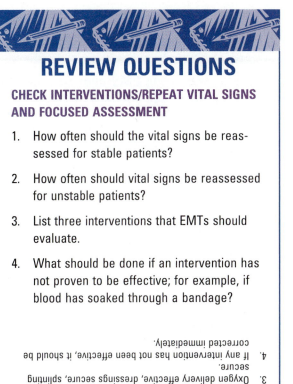

REVIEW QUESTIONS

CHECK INTERVENTIONS/REPEAT VITAL SIGNS AND FOCUSED ASSESSMENT

1. How often should the vital signs be reassessed for stable patients?

2. How often should vital signs be reassessed for unstable patients?

3. List three interventions that EMTs should evaluate.

4. What should be done if an intervention has not proven to be effective; for example, if blood has soaked through a bandage?

1. At least every 15 minutes.
2. Every 5 minutes or less.
3. Oxygen delivery effective, dressings secure, splinting secure.
4. If any intervention has not been effective, it should be corrected immediately.

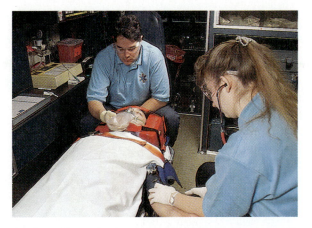

Fig. 13-4 Ensure that the nonrebreather bag remains inflated and the oxygen flow to the patient is adequate.

CHECK INTERVENTIONS

Finally, evaluate interventions that have been performed as part of the patient care process. Ensure the adequacy of oxygen delivery or artificial ventilation. For patients receiving oxygen, ensure that the oxygen flow rate is set at 15 L/min and the oxygen is adequately flowing, that the oxygen mask is a nonrebreather, that the reservoir bag is remaining inflated, and that enough oxygen remains in the cylinder for the duration of the trip (Fig. 13-4). If the patient would not tolerate a mask and has a nasal cannula in place, make sure the prongs are placed correctly in the patient's nose, that the rate is set at 6 L/min, and that the oxygen is flowing adequately as described previously. If the patient is being artificially ventilated, make sure the ventilations are adequate by watching the chest rise and monitoring the patient's vital signs.

Other interventions to assess include ensuring that bleeding is still being controlled, that splints are still effectively immobilizing injured extremities, and that straps on a long backboard are secure

but not tight enough to injure the patient. All interventions you perform should be reevaluated during the ongoing assessment.

Any intervention that is no longer meeting the needs of the patient must be corrected immediately. For example, if the splint that you applied to the patient's forearm has become too loose and is no longer immobilizing the arm, secure the splint again until the arm is properly immobilized.

Approximately 5 minutes from the receiving facility, repeat the ongoing assessment a final time to document the patient's condition at the time of arrival at the receiving facility. Relay all information to the staff about trends in the patient's condition.

CHAPTER SUMMARY

All patients receive an ongoing assessment, which repeats the components of the initial assessment and focused assessment. Stable patients need to be evaluated at least every 15 minutes during transport. Unstable patients should have the ongoing assessment performed every 5 minutes or less.

The ongoing assessment is an opportunity to check interventions that were performed before and during transport. Document and communicate this information to the receiving facility. Prior to arrival at the appropriate receiving facility, perform all the components of the ongoing assessment one last time to complete the prehospital care report, and provide this information to the receiving facility.

UNITED STATES DEPARTMENT OF TRANSPORTATION NATIONAL HIGHWAY TRAFFIC SAFETY ADMINISTRATION EMT–BASIC OBJECTIVES

Check your knowledge. The National Registry of EMTs and many state EMS agencies use the objectives below to develop EMT–Basic certification examinations. Can you meet them?

COGNITIVE

1. Discuss the reasons for repeating the initial assessment as part of the ongoing assessment.
2. Describe the components of the ongoing assessment.
3. Describe trending of asssessment components.

AFFECTIVE

1. Explain the value of performing an ongoing assessment.

2. Recognize and respect the feelings that patients might experience during assessment.
3. Explain the value of trending assessment components to other health professionals who assume care of the patient .

PSYCHOMOTOR

1. Demonstrate the skills involved in performing the ongoing assessment.

14 COMMUNICATIONS

IN THE FIELD

At the start of their shift, EMTs Jane and Roy completed their vehicle check as they did every morning and headed to the day room to examine a new piece of equipment. As Roy was reading its instructions, they were dispatched to the home of a man who was not breathing. Once in the unit, Roy contacted dispatch on the mobile radio. Dispatch advised Jane and Roy of the location of the call and gave a brief patient report. Roy reported that they were en route. The dispatcher acknowledged the time.

Upon arriving at the scene, Roy and Jane again notified dispatch and recorded the time. Once at the patient's side, Roy began the initial assessment, and Jane notified dispatch of their arrival at bedside. The original information dispatch had relayed was incorrect. Despite the best efforts of the dispatcher to gather accurate information from the man's wife, in her panic she did not think her husband was breathing. The man was breathing, but he was experiencing difficulty.

When Jane talked to the patient's wife, she noted the woman's facial expression and body language showed her fear. In a calm, reassuring voice, Jane described what was happening to the woman's husband and took the SAMPLE history. After reassuring the wife, Jane helped Roy finish the focused assessment. They provided care based on their assessment findings and prepared the patient for transport. The patient's wife was assisted into the front passenger seat and her seat belt was fastened. As they departed the scene, Jane notified dispatch of their destination and said that the unit was en route to the hospital.

In the patient compartment, Roy continued the ongoing assessment and contacted the hospital by radio to give them a brief report. At the hospital, Dr. Hector listened carefully to the radio report and recorded the information.

Upon arrival at the hospital, Jane notified dispatch and recorded the time. While transferring the patient to Room 3, Roy gave a verbal report to Nurse Jones, who would be taking care of the patient. While Jane restocked the ambulance and changed the linens, Roy completed the prehospital care report.

As they returned to the station, they notified dispatch that they were in service and available.

Communication is the transmission of information, ideas, and skills through language, body movements, gestures, and expressions. To communicate effectively with patients and other healthcare professionals, EMTs must understand communication processes and procedures. These processes and procedures include the EMS communications systems, radio components, verbal communications, and the concepts of interpersonal communication.

EMTs are constantly communicating with crew members, other EMS providers, law enforcement officers, and other public safety workers. EMTs communicate with families and patients, who are often in crisis or at their worst times. Understanding body language, tone of voice, and how best to communicate can make your role as an EMT more effective.

COMMUNICATION SYSTEMS AND COMPONENTS

This chapter is intended as an overview of communications. Because EMS systems vary, you need to become familiar with your local system, equipment, and communication protocols and procedures. Usually the components of the communication system for prehospital care include a base station, mobile two-way radios, portable radios, digital radio equipment, and telephones. You need a basic understanding of each of these components.

COMMUNICATION COMPONENTS

The **base station** is a radio at a stationary site with superior transmission and receiving capabilities, such as a hospital, mountain top, dispatch center, or other public safety agency. In most communication systems, a remote console controls the base station radio. The dispatcher at the remote console does not need to be at the base station but is connected to it by microwave or telephone links (Fig. 14-1).

The mobile two-way radio is a transceiver that can transmit and receive and is typically mounted in the vehicle. It generally has several channels. Most vehicle-mounted radios range from 25 to 50 watts and have a typical transmission range of 10 to 15 miles. A portable radio is a hand-held transceiver that typically has an output of 1 to 5 watts and a range of approximately 1 to 5 miles (Fig. 14-2). As described in Chapter 8, "Scene Size-Up," you always determine if additional help is needed during the scene size-up. If so, request this help using the vehicle radio because it has a greater range than hand-held portable radios.

EMS systems often use a repeater system. A **repeater** is a remote receiver that receives a transmission from a low-power portable or mobile radio on one frequency and then transmits the signal at a higher power, often on another frequency. Through the use of repeaters, an EMS system can communicate over a large geographical area (Fig. 14-3).

Some communication systems use digital radio equipment with a series of **encoders and decoders**

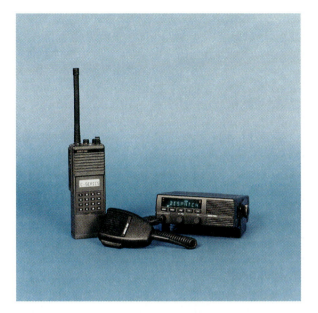

Fig. 14-2 A vehicle-mounted mobile two-way radio and a portable radio.

that block out radio transmissions not intended for that unit. In some systems this is called a *private line* or *channel guard*, which uses a combination of encoders and decoders. This method allows the system to reduce extraneous radio traffic. When using

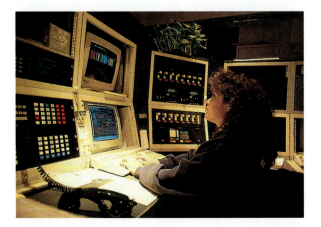

Fig. 14-1 The dispatcher at the remote console controls the base station radio by microwave or telephone links.

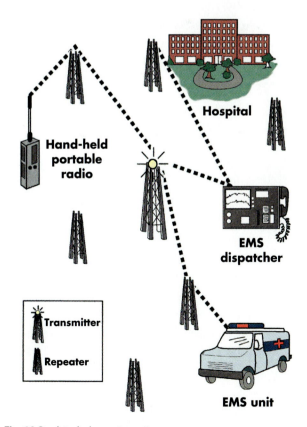

Hand-held portable radio

Hospital

EMS dispatcher

Transmitter

Repeater

EMS unit

Fig. 14-3 A typical repeater system.

a radio with channel guard, you must disable this function before transmitting to avoid transmitting over other users who might be on the same frequency at the time. The channel guard typically is disabled automatically when the microphone is lifted. Be sure to become familiar with the operation of the equipment in your own system.

Telephones are also a very important link in prehospital communications systems. The telephone may be used to consult with the medical direction physician and is an ideal mode for reporting confidential information. Cellular telephones are being used increasingly in EMS systems. They are valuable equipment for communicating with the medical direction physician while at the patient's bedside. In some systems, phone lines and/or radio transmissions may be recorded and thus become part of the documentation of the call. Unrecorded radio or phone transmissions may lead to medical or legal concerns if they are not documented.

All radio channels in the United States are regulated by the Federal Communications Commission (FCC). The FCC assigns various radio channels to different agencies. The FCC also licenses radio operators and designates which radios they may use.

The FCC regulates and routinely monitors radio transmissions to ensure that they meet the proper guidelines. You may find it helpful to review FCC regulations, which are available either in the EMS system or from the Government Printing Office.

SYSTEM MAINTENANCE

Inspect and test your communications system regularly as outlined in your local protocol. Batteries in portable radios should be charged and rotated as described by local policies. Radios must be serviced by a qualified technician. Some services use a preventive maintenance program in which a technician tests the system periodically. Any radio difficulty should be reported to your supervisor immediately. Most services have a procedure or policy to follow in the event of a communications failure.

PROCEDURES FOR RADIO COMMUNICATIONS

When speaking on the radio, follow the principles listed in Box 14-1.

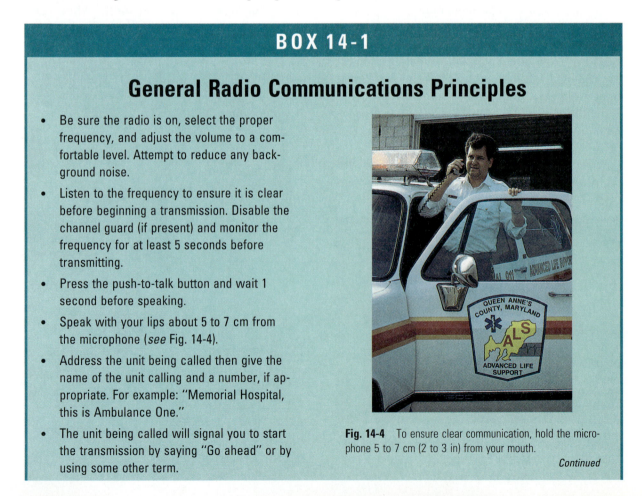

BOX 14-1

General Radio Communications Principles

- Be sure the radio is on, select the proper frequency, and adjust the volume to a comfortable level. Attempt to reduce any background noise.

- Listen to the frequency to ensure it is clear before beginning a transmission. Disable the channel guard (if present) and monitor the frequency for at least 5 seconds before transmitting.

- Press the push-to-talk button and wait 1 second before speaking.

- Speak with your lips about 5 to 7 cm from the microphone (*see* Fig. 14-4).

- Address the unit being called then give the name of the unit calling and a number, if appropriate. For example: "Memorial Hospital, this is Ambulance One."

- The unit being called will signal you to start the transmission by saying "Go ahead" or by using some other term.

Fig. 14-4 To ensure clear communication, hold the microphone 5 to 7 cm (2 to 3 in) from your mouth.

Continued

- The phrase "Stand by" means that you should wait until you receive a go-ahead from the receiving unit before continuing.

- Speak clearly and slowly. Although a monotone voice may seem dull and less human, it is more easily understood over the radio.

- Keep all transmissions brief. If the transmission takes longer than 30 seconds, stop at that point and pause for a few seconds to let emergency traffic use the frequency if necessary.

- Use clear everyday language, not codes. Remember that not all codes are consistent among services and hospitals. Much confusion can occur if codes are used. Some services, however, do use codes. When codes are used, it is important that the receiver and the sender understand the codes.

- Avoid meaningless phrases such as "Be advised."

- Courtesy is always assumed. There is no need to continually say please or thank you.

- When giving a number that may be confused, give the individual digits.

- Most EMS channels are considered by the FCC to be public channels. Scanners are very popular, and the public may be monitoring your radio transmissions with dispatch, other units, and hospitals. To help maintain patient confidentiality, do not use the patient's name on the radio.

- Be impartial and objective with all reports. EMTs may be sued for slander if a person's reputation is injured by something they say, including what is said in radio transmissions.

- Avoid words that are difficult to hear, such as "yes" and "no"; instead say "affirmative" and "negative."

- In some systems you need to indicate when the radio transmission has ended, typically by saying "over" at the end of each transmission. Always confirm that your information was received and understood.

- In your radio report, do not offer a diagnosis of the patient's condition. Instead, report objective assessment findings and the treatment provided.

- Because the radio channels may be shared with other agencies, the EMS channels should be used for EMS communication only.

- Radio communications are generally recorded for legal purposes. If a telephone is used, taping does not always occur and a record may not be available. Check on the system used in your area.

COMMUNICATION WITH DISPATCH

Radio communications are an essential component of the EMS response. You use the radio system to communicate with dispatch about the location of your EMS unit, your receipt of a call, and your status on the call. The first communication typically is the dispatcher notifying you of an emergency, usually over the radio. This communication may also be done through pagers, by telephone, or other means.

Once you receive a call, acknowledge the call and notify the dispatcher when the unit is en route to the scene. In some areas, other agencies also need to be notified that you are responding to a call. Local protocol dictates what agencies must be notified that you are responding.

As you arrive at the scene, notify the dispatcher that your unit has arrived. The dispatcher records the time and can later give you this information if you need it to complete your patient care report.

You should notify the dispatcher of the actual arrival time at the patient's side.

Notify the dispatcher at each of the stages of a call. In most systems the dispatcher records these times. Box 14-2 lists the administrative information that should be recorded.

COMMUNICATION WITH MEDICAL DIRECTION

Keep in mind that the medical direction physician may not be the service medical director. The EMT must follow local and regional protocols for communicating with the medical direction physician. After completing your patient assessment and providing immediate emergency care to the patient, contact the medical direction physician as needed. You may also consult with the medical direction physician about additional interventions and to provide a report (Fig. 14-5). The medical direction physician may be at the receiving hospital

BOX 14-2

Administrative Information

Notify the dispatcher when:

- Receiving the call
- Responding to the call
- Arriving at the scene
- Arriving at the patient's side
- Leaving the scene for the receiving facility
- Arriving at the receiving facility
- Leaving the hospital for the station
- Arriving at the station

or a different site. The medical direction physician is a valuable resource and an objective expert who can assist you in giving the best possible care to the patient.

To be effective, your report to the medical direction physician must be concise, organized, and pertinent. Because the medical direction physician may recommend additional interventions based on your report, the information you communicate must be accurate. Any time you receive orders from the medical direction physician, repeat them back exactly as you hear them. Anytime that the orders are not clear to you or you feel that they may be inappropriate, do not hesitate to ask questions that will help clarify the orders. If you do not understand the order or if you think that the order is

inappropriate for the patient, tell the medical direction physician. Discuss your concern and allow the medical direction physician an opportunity to repeat or clarify the orders.

If you are transferring the patient to the site where the medical direction physician is located, your communication with the receiving hospital now may be completed. If you are transferring the patient to a facility other than the one where the medical direction physician is located, you may need to update the receiving facility along the way, unless this update will be completed by the medical direction physician. Provide ongoing patient information while en route. If the receiving facility is in a different location from the medical direction physician, notify the receiving facility personnel about the patient's status. Communication must be concise, clear, and pertinent to best mobilize the resources of the receiving facility. In addition, proper, concise communication gives you more time to care for the patient while en route to the receiving facility.

A standard medical reporting format has been developed for EMTs to organize the report (Box 14-3).

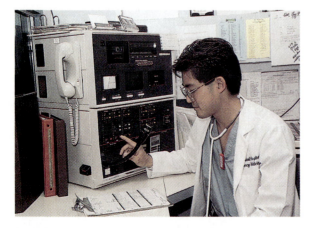

Fig. 14-5 Communicate with your medical direction physician when necessary for consultation and to provide a report on the status of your patient.

BOX 14-3

Standard Medical Reporting Format

- Patient's age and gender
- Chief complaint
- History of present illness
- Pertinent past medical history
- Mental status
- Assessment findings
- Vital signs
- Emergency care given
- Response to emergency care
- Estimated time to load the patient for transport
- Estimated travel time from the scene to the hospital
- Opportunity for questions from the receiving facility or medical direction physician

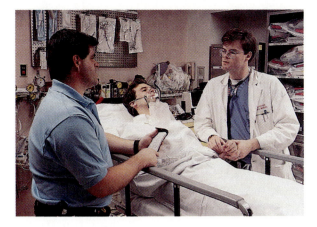

Fig. 14-6 A complete and concise report should be given to the receiving facility staff at bedside.

Early notification is important for the receiving facility. The staff there may use this information to prepare or notify specialty teams that may care for the patient or to prepare additional services for the patient.

VERBAL COMMUNICATION

Once you arrive at the hospital, give a concise but complete report to the staff who will care for the patient (Fig. 14-6). Your verbal report helps provide continuity of care for the patient. Also give this verbal report in the standard medical reporting format.

INTERPERSONAL COMMUNICATION

GENERAL PRINCIPLES

To be effective in your communications you need to understand the fundamentals of interpersonal communications. These fundamentals include the ability to communicate in a personally effective and socially appropriate manner.

EMTs must be able to understand people and situations, beginning with the general impression of the scene and the patient. As you size-up the scene, observe the patient, family, and bystanders displaying emotional expressions. You must be able to interpret these expressions to communicate effectively with them.

Once you interpret the situation, you need a communication goal and a plan to elicit information and to determine what information to provide to the patient, family, or bystanders. Based on your assessment of the scene, the patient, family, and

bystanders, you determine the best method of communicating with the patient.

To be an effective communicator, you must understand the surroundings and the situation, as well as expected behaviors in the situation. For ex-

---

REVIEW QUESTIONS

PROCEDURES FOR RADIO COMMUNICATIONS

1. A _____ is the dispatch radio transmitter and receiver located at a remote site, often controlled through a remote console.

2. A mobile two-way radio implies that the device is _____-mounted.

3. A portable radio has an output of 1 to 5 watts, and therefore the range is _____.

4. A _____ allows an EMS system to communicate over a large geographic area by rebroadcasting low-power signals on a different frequency at a higher power.

5. Encoders and _____ allow EMTs to block out transmissions not intended for their EMS unit.

6. To ensure that the report is clear and concise, EMTs should follow the _____ format.

7. When using digital radio equipment, the EMT should disable the channel guard and listen for a minimum of _____ seconds before transmitting.

8. "Stand by" means that the EMT should _____ before transmitting.

9. EMS channels should be used for _____ communications only.

1. Base station
2. Vehicle
3. 1 to 5 miles
4. Repeater system
5. Decoders
6. Standard medical reporting
7. Five
8. Wait until receiving a go-ahead.
9. EMS

ample, if you are confronted with a family whose loved one has died, you must know how to handle the situation and know the most appropriate way of communicating with the family.

In addition, you need to understand the importance of choosing the appropriate words for your communication. This involves knowing how to say the right thing at an appropriate time and knowing what behavior is appropriate with your message. For example, you usually need to use a different level of language, including simple terms, when speaking with children.

Understand also that body language plays an important role in communication. It is not only what you say but how you position yourself, using body language, that sends a message. Body language is important when you communicate with patients, family members, bystanders, or other health professionals. As you communicate with others, they receive a message from your posture, facial expressions, and tone of voice. These actions may contradict your intended verbal message.

Imagine, for example, an EMT trying to show empathy for a patient while at the same time facing the family with the arms folded across the chest, looking around, and not concentrating on the family member who is speaking. These nonverbal clues send a message that the EMT is disinterested in what this person has to say. Although this may not be the case, the family member perceives it as a lack of caring or even respect. Some people may even interpret this behavior as hostility.

When you understand the communication process, you can become a better communicator. To become a better communicator, observe and analyze your own communication skills and look for areas needing improvement. If you want to improve your communication skills, the key is practice. As with other aspects of emergency care, the EMT should seek additional education to become a better communicator.

TIPS FOR EFFECTIVE COMMUNICATION

If the patient is anxious, be supportive to help the patient regain or maintain self control. Follow these guidelines for supportive communication:

1. *Verbalize your support.* Let the patient see that you recognize he/she is an individual with needs.
2. *Be a good listener when the patient needs to talk.* Accept the patient's feelings as legitimate, regardless of any personal bias.
3. *Offer a reassuring touch.* Provide a therapeutic touch on the arm, the hand, or the shoulder, but only if you and the patient both are comfortable with touching.
4. *Be respectful.* Show respect and compassion in your communications at all times.
5. *Separate personal bias.* Keep your personal attitudes to yourself.
6. *Be silent when appropriate.* Silence is also a very useful tool in interpersonal communications. Silence gives the patient a chance to think, and with it you can display your caring without words.

SPECIAL POPULATIONS

Communicating with special populations sometimes requires different communication techniques. Special populations include the elderly, infants and children, non-English–speaking patients, and patients with certain physical disabilities.

Elderly patients may pose a challenge for you if you do not often deal with this population. Elderly patients deserve respect. Do not assume that because they are elderly, these patients cannot hear you. It is true that some patients have auditory or visual deficiencies. As you introduce yourself to patients, assess their ability to hear you. If you are in doubt, ask. Consider how fast you are speaking, in case the patient may not be able to comprehend you because of your rate of speech. Slow down and allow the patient time to process your questions. In addition, it may be important to use simple terms when speaking with elderly patients.

Dealing with an ill or injured child poses a special problem. These calls are often very emotional for the provider. For communication to be effective, you must constantly communicate with the child and the family. Use a calm, reassuring voice and age-appropriate language. Be sure to explain everything that you are doing and be honest (Fig. 14-7).

When you encounter a non-English–speaking patient, try to find a bystander, family member, or friend at the scene who can communicate with the patient. Through the use of an interpreter, you may be able to gain essential information. The interpreter's information may not be 100% accurate and may be incomplete. Be sure that your questions for the interpreter are clear. Some information may be lost in translation. Ask only one question at a time. Speak to both the patient and the interpreter. Do not rush either the interpreter or the patient.

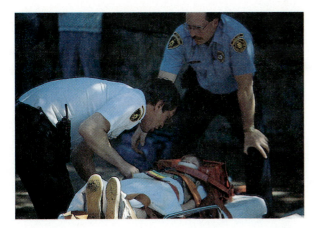

Fig. 14-7 Speak to children in a calm, reassuring voice. Explain everything you are doing, and be honest.

Communicating with a physically challenged patient can be difficult. Patients with sensory challenges, such as hearing-impaired patients, pose a special challenge. Using an interpreter or writing notes may be beneficial for communicating with these patients. This process can be slow and frustrating, especially when you are trying to gain information quickly. Be patient because showing frustration with this or any patient will not help the situation.

Communicating with these physically challenged patients can present a unique challenge. With understanding, practice, and patience, you can learn to communicate more effectively with these patients.

REVIEW QUESTIONS

INTERPERSONAL COMMUNICATION

1. When communicating with elderly patients, speak _____ and wait for a response.

2. When communicating with infants and children, speak with a _____ voice.

3. When speaking with a patient who speaks a foreign language, you may find a(n) _____ helpful.

1. Slowly
2. Calm, reassuring
3. Interpreter

CHAPTER SUMMARY

COMMUNICATION SYSTEMS AND COMPONENTS

Communication is the transmission of ideas, skills, and information. Communication includes radio communications and verbal communications.

EMTs must have knowledge of the components of their radio communication system to use them effectively. The components of a typical EMS communication system include the base station, vehicle-mounted mobile two-way radios, and hand-held portable radios. In some systems, a repeater system is used to rebroadcast low-power transmissions at a higher power on another frequency. Some EMS systems also use digital radio equipment. Through the use of encoders and decoders, transmissions not intended for a particular unit are blocked out. Land lines such as the standard telephone and cellular mobile telephones may also be useful.

PROCEDURES FOR RADIO COMMUNICATIONS

The standard medical reporting format assists the EMT in providing a clear and concise report. The elements of the standard medical report include the patient's age and sex, chief complaint, history of present illness, pertinent past medical history, mental status, assessment or physical findings, vital signs, emergency care given, response to emergency care, estimated time of loading the patient for transport, estimated travel time from the scene to the hospital, and opportunity for questions or instructions from the receiving facility or medical direction physician.

INTERPERSONAL COMMUNICATION

Interpersonal communication is extremely important to EMTs. You must be able to assess the surroundings and choose the appropriate way to best communicate with the patient. Body language plays an important role in communication. You must be aware of the message sent by body actions and facial expressions in conjunction with the verbal message.

Communicating with special populations provides unique challenges. EMTs should practice this skill. With understanding, patience, and practice you can become a more effective communicator.

UNITED STATES DEPARTMENT OF TRANSPORTATION NATIONAL HIGHWAY TRAFFIC SAFETY ADMINISTRATION EMT–BASIC OBJECTIVES

Check your knowledge. The National Registry of EMTs and many state EMS agencies use the objectives below to develop EMT–Basic certification examinations. Can you meet them?

COGNITIVE

1. List the proper methods of initiating and terminating a radio call.
2. State the proper sequence for delivery of patient information.
3. Explain the importance of effective communication of patient information in the verbal report.
4. Identify the essential components of the verbal report.
5. Describe the attributes for increasing effectiveness and efficiency of verbal communications.
6. State legal aspects to consider in verbal communications.
7. Discuss the communication skills that should be used to interact with the patient.
8. Discuss the communication skills that should be used to interact with the family, bystanders, and individuals from other agencies while providing patient care, and the difference between skills used to interact with the patient and those used to interact with others.

9. List the correct radio procedures in the following phases of a typical call:
   To the scene
   At the scene
   To the facility
   At the facility
   To the station
   At the station

AFFECTIVE

1. Explain the rationale for providing efficient and effective radio communications and patient reports.

PSYCHOMOTOR

1. Perform a simulated, organized, concise radio transmission.
2. Perform an organized, concise patient report that would be given to the staff at a receiving facility.
3. Perform a brief, organized report that would be given to an ALS provider arriving at an incident scene at which the EMT–Basic was already providing care.

KEY TERMS

Administrative information: The elements of the minimum data set related to the prehospital care call.

Minimum data set: The essential elements of patient and administrative data required for accurate and complete prehospital data collection.

Patient information: The elements of the minimum data set related to the patient's clinical condition and the emergency medical care provided.

Patient narrative: The section of a prehospital care report that allows EMTs to document patient information using a standard medical reporting format.

Prehospital care report: A form used to document the events occurring during a patient encounter, including the minimum data set of patient and administrative information.

Trending: The process of comparing serial recordings of a patient's vital signs or other assessments to note changes.

IN THE FIELD

EMTs Jane and Roy responded to the home of Mr. Bonita, a 73-year-old man who was experiencing chest pain and shortness of breath. After sizing up the scene, they began their initial assessment. During the initial assessment, Mr. Bonita informed Roy that he did not want to be transported to the hospital. Mrs. Bonita was adamant, however, saying he had to go to the hospital. Mr. Bonita allowed Jane to assess his vital signs and was cooperative during the focused history and physical examination.

As a competent adult, Mr. Bonita had the right to refuse medical care. Jane explained to him the consequences of refusing treatment and transport to the hospital. She told him that chest pain could be an indication of a fatal condition. Despite the severe warnings, Mr. Bonita still refused to be transported. While Jane was explaining the rationale for being transported, Roy contacted medical direction. He reported the situation to Dr. Bluestone. Dr. Bluestone spoke with Mr. Bonita and tried to talk him into going to the hospital; Mr. Bonita still refused.

Roy began to complete the prehospital care report. He documented the patient's age, gender, chief complaint, and the findings at the scene. He noted that the patient was sitting in a chair clutching his fist to his chest. He documented the findings of the physical examination and the vital signs. He documented the conversation regarding the refusal of treatment and transport, including the consultation with Dr. Bluestone.

After Roy had completed his documentation, he explained the form to Mr. and Mrs. Bonita. He asked Mr. Bonita to sign the section of the report regarding the refusal, and Mrs. Bonita signed the form as a witness.

Before they left the scene, Jane and Roy assured Mr. Bonita that if he changed his mind, they would be happy to return. They also urged him to seek immediate medical attention from his own doctor if he would not go the hospital. It was difficult to leave a patient with a significant medical illness, but it was his right to refuse care.

The **prehospital care report** documents the nature and extent of the emergency medical care EMTs provide. These reports are important medical and legal documents. Healthcare providers use the information in the report to monitor changes in patients' conditions. In particular, the **trending** of the patient's mental status and vital signs is extremely important to the physicians and nurses who take over the patient's care. Trending means comparing present information about a patient's status with previously recorded information to detect changes. Often trending compares pulse, respirations, and blood pressure over a specific time period.

The information in the prehospital care report can also be used for quality improvement of emergency medical care (Fig. 15-1). A good quality im-

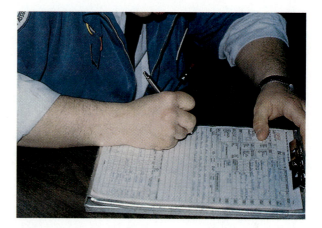

Fig. 15-1 Accurate and complete documentation in the prehospital care report contributes to quality improvement and helps to protect an agency from litigation.

provement process establishes a review process to address educational needs and helps protect the agency from litigation.

MINIMUM DATA SET

Prehospital care is constantly evolving. With recent changes in healthcare and the reform of the healthcare system, EMS systems may have to prove that they truly do affect patients' lives. This proof must be established through studies of patient outcomes, which depend heavily on patient records.

As an EMT, you must record patient and administrative information during every call to document the emergency medical care you provide. A **minimum data set** of information to be collected and reported has been established to ensure that accurate and pertinent information is recorded. The minimum data set includes the patient information

you gather from your initial contact with the patient to your arrival at the receiving facility.

The minimum data set has two categories of information: **patient information** and **administrative information.** In addition to the elements of the minimum data set, each patient record should have a unique record number. The local, regional, or state EMS system usually has a specific format for collecting this data. Box 15-1 identifies the elements of the patient information. State or local data collection may vary somewhat from this information. Be sure you understand your state, regional, or local reporting requirements.

In addition to patient information, other information is collected for administrative purposes. Box 15-2 identifies the administrative elements of the minimum data set. Again, you need to know your local or state reporting requirements.

Often this data is completed using check boxes or "bubbles" on the prehospital care report. When completing this type of form, be careful to fill in the box completely and avoid stray marks.

BOX 15-1

Patient Information Components

- Age and gender
- Chief complaint
- Cause of injury
- Preexisting conditions
- Signs and symptoms present
- Injury description
- Level of responsiveness (AVPU)
- Pulse rate
- Respiratory rate
- Systolic blood pressure in patients 3 years of age or older
- Skin perfusion (capillary refill for patients less than 6 years of age)
- Skin color, temperature, and condition
- Procedures performed on the patient
- Medications administered
- Response to treatment, including medications

BOX 15-2

Administrative Components of the Minimum Data Set

- Incident location
- Type of location
- Date incident reported
- Time incident reported
- Date the EMS unit notified
- Time the EMS unit notified
- Time unit responded
- Time of arrival at the scene
- Time of arrival at the patient
- Time the EMS unit left the scene
- Time of the EMS arrival at destination
- Time of transfer of patient care
- Time the EMS unit back in service
- Use of lights and siren to and from the scene
- Crew members responding

All recorded data must be accurate, especially the times. Work together with your EMS crew to keep accurate records. EMTs working together as a team should set their watches with the clock of the dispatcher and each other. This way, the times documented are accurate and valuable for trending. Times should be recorded in a 24-hour format on patient records, which is clearer and less likely to be mistaken than the 12-hour format with a.m. and p.m. suffixes.

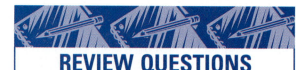

REVIEW QUESTIONS

MINIMUM DATA SET

Determine which of the following data elements are in the administrative section and which are in the patient information section of the minimum data set. Place an "A" for administrative and a "P" for patient information.

1. _____ Age and gender of the patient

2. _____ Location of the incident

3. _____ Use of lights and siren

4. _____ Cause of the patient's injury

5. _____ Time of arrival at the scene

6. _____ Patient's injury description

7. _____ Medications administered to the patient

8. _____ Time of arrival at the patient

9. _____ Procedures performed on the patient

10. _____ Time back in service

1. P
2. A
3. A
4. P
5. A
6. P
7. P
8. A
9. P
10. A

THE PREHOSPITAL CARE REPORT

FUNCTIONS OF THE PREHOSPITAL CARE REPORT

The prehospital care report is a medical and legal document (Fig. 15-2). An effective report documents the status of the patient on arrival at the scene, all emergency medical care provided, and patient changes up to arrival at the receiving facility.

> # ALERT
> The prehospital care report is a legal document. The document and the information on the form are considered confidential. Be familiar with state and local laws affecting your documentation.

All information in the prehospital care report must be objective. Objective information is information that is measurable or verifiable. At the scene of a motor vehicle collision, for example, you may see a broken windshield. This information is objective.

Subjective information is not verifiable but comes from a person's point of view. If a bystander states that the vehicle was traveling too fast, that information is subjective. Any subjective information included in a report must be clearly distinguished from objective information. One method of distinguishing between the two types of information is to enclose the information in quotation marks and write down the name of the person who made the statement.

Because you should focus on objective information, avoid statements such as "Patient was intoxicated." Such statements are difficult to defend. It is better to describe the signs and symptoms observed. For example, "The patient had slurred speech, confusion, and difficulty walking."

The prehospital care report helps ensure the continuity of patient care. Ideally, emergency department physicians and nurses read the report to verify what care was provided and also to note trends in the patient's vital signs and condition. If the patient is admitted to the hospital, the staff on the unit will also use this information.

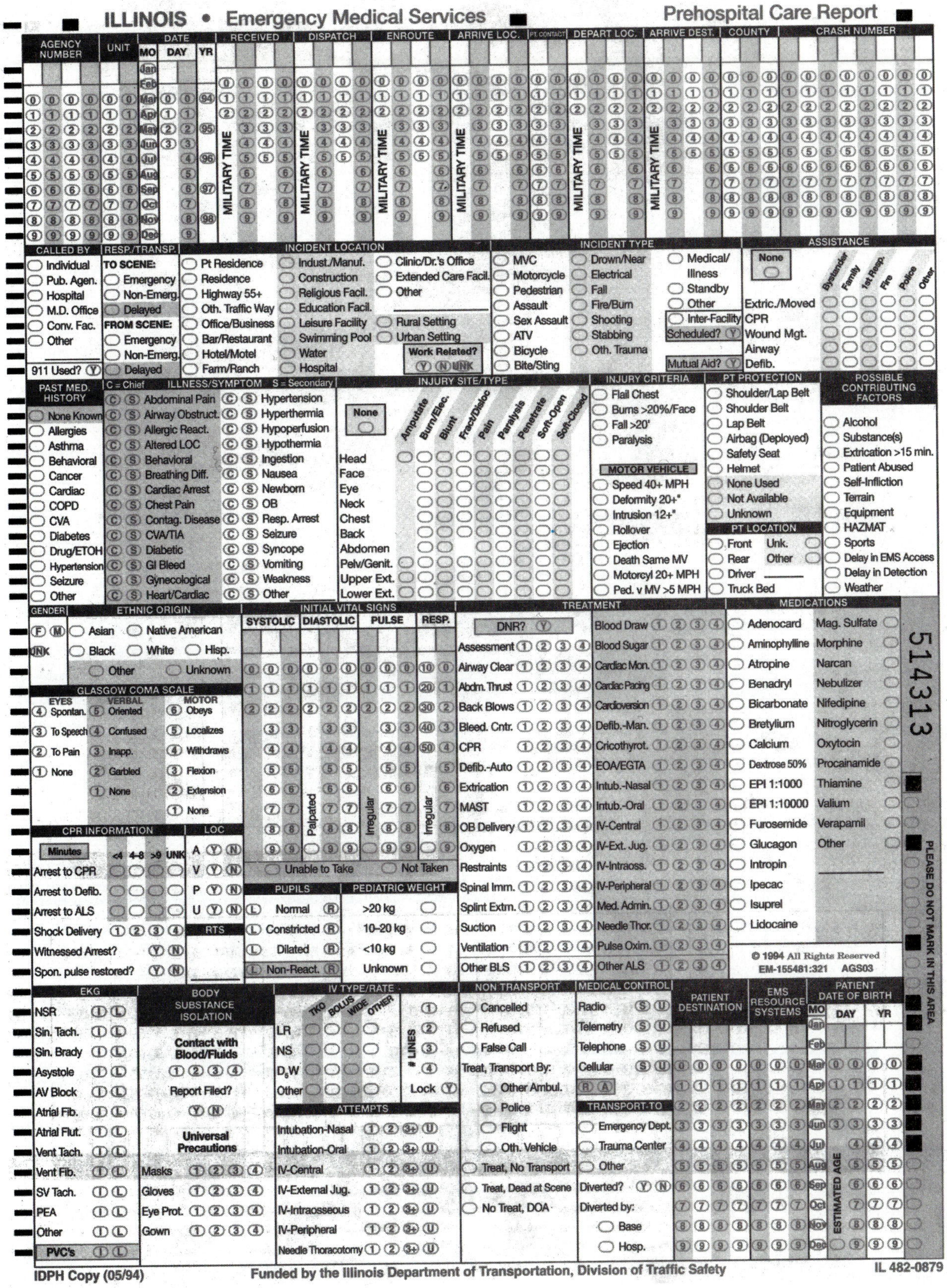
ILLINOIS • Emergency Medical Services

Prehospital Care Report

AGENCY NUMBER | UNIT | DATE MO DAY YR | RECEIVED | DISPATCH | ENROUTE | ARRIVE LOC. | PT CONTACT | DEPART LOC. | ARRIVE DEST. | COUNTY | CRASH NUMBER

Jan Feb Mar Apr May Jun Jul Aug Sep Oct Nov Dec — 94 95 96 97 98 — MILITARY TIME

CALLED BY: Individual, Pub. Agen., Hospital, M.D. Office, Conv. Fac., Other, 911 Used? (Y)

RESP./TRANSP.: TO SCENE: Emergency, Non-Emerg., Delayed; FROM SCENE: Emergency, Non-Emerg., Delayed

INCIDENT LOCATION: Pt Residence, Residence, Highway 55+, Oth. Traffic Way, Office/Business, Bar/Restaurant, Hotel/Motel, Farm/Ranch, Indust./Manuf., Construction, Religious Facil., Education Facil., Leisure Facility, Swimming Pool, Water, Hospital, Clinic/Dr.'s Office, Extended Care Facil., Other, Rural Setting, Urban Setting, Work Related? (Y) (N) (UNK)

INCIDENT TYPE: MVC, Motorcycle, Pedestrian, Assault, Sex Assault, ATV, Bicycle, Bite/Sting, Drown/Near, Electrical, Fall, Fire/Burn, Shooting, Stabbing, Oth. Trauma, Medical/Illness, Standby, Other, Inter-Facility Scheduled? (Y), Mutual Aid? (Y)

ASSISTANCE: None; Bystander, Family, 1st Resp., Fire, Police, Other — Extric./Moved, CPR, Wound Mgt., Airway, Defib.

PAST MED. HISTORY: None Known, Allergies, Asthma, Behavioral, Cancer, Cardiac, COPD, CVA, Diabetes, Drug/ETOH, Hypertension, Seizure, Other

ILLNESS/SYMPTOM (C = Chief, S = Secondary): Abdominal Pain, Airway Obstruct., Allergic React., Altered LOC, Behavioral, Breathing Diff., Cardiac Arrest, Chest Pain, Contag. Disease, CVA/TIA, Diabetic, GI Bleed, Gynecological, Heart/Cardiac, Hypertension, Hyperthermia, Hypoperfusion, Hypothermia, Ingestion, Nausea, Newborn, OB, Resp. Arrest, Seizure, Syncope, Vomiting, Weakness, Other

INJURY SITE/TYPE: None; Amputate, Burn/Elec., Blunt, Fract/Disloc, Pain, Paralysis, Penetrate, Soft-Open, Soft-Closed — Head, Face, Eye, Neck, Chest, Back, Abdomen, Pelv/Genit., Upper Ext., Lower Ext.

INJURY CRITERIA: Flail Chest, Burns >20%/Face, Fall >20', Paralysis; MOTOR VEHICLE: Speed 40+ MPH, Deformity 20+", Intrusion 12+", Rollover, Ejection, Death Same MV, Motorcyl 20+ MPH, Ped. v MV >5 MPH

PT PROTECTION: Shoulder/Lap Belt, Shoulder Belt, Lap Belt, Airbag (Deployed), Safety Seat, Helmet, None Used, Not Available, Unknown

PT LOCATION: Front, Unk., Rear, Other, Driver, Truck Bed

POSSIBLE CONTRIBUTING FACTORS: Alcohol, Substance(s), Extrication >15 min., Patient Abused, Self-Infliction, Terrain, Equipment, HAZMAT, Sports, Delay in EMS Access, Delay in Detection, Weather

GENDER: (F) (M) UNK — ETHNIC ORIGIN: Asian, Native American, Black, White, Hisp., Other, Unknown

GLASGOW COMA SCALE: EYES: (4) Spontan., (3) To Speech, (2) To Pain, (1) None; VERBAL: (5) Oriented, (4) Confused, (3) Inapp., (2) Garbled, (1) None; MOTOR: (6) Obeys, (5) Localizes, (4) Withdraws, (3) Flexion, (2) Extension, (1) None

CPR INFORMATION: Minutes <4 4-8 >9 UNK — Arrest to CPR, Arrest to Defib., Arrest to ALS, Shock Delivery (1)(2)(3)(4), Witnessed Arrest? (Y)(N), Spon. pulse restored? (Y)(N)

LOC: A (Y)(N), V (Y)(N), P (Y)(N), U (Y)(N); RTS

INITIAL VITAL SIGNS: SYSTOLIC, DIASTOLIC, PULSE, RESP. — Palpated, Irregular, Irregular, Unable to Take, Not Taken

PUPILS: (L) Normal (R), (L) Constricted (R), (L) Dilated (R), (L) Non-React. (R)

PEDIATRIC WEIGHT: >20 kg, 10–20 kg, <10 kg, Unknown

TREATMENT: DNR? (Y); Assessment, Airway Clear, Abdm. Thrust, Back Blows, Bleed. Cntr., CPR, Defib.-Auto, Extrication, MAST, OB Delivery, Oxygen, Restraints, Spinal Imm., Splint Extrm., Suction, Ventilation, Other BLS, Blood Draw, Blood Sugar, Cardiac Mon., Cardiac Pacing, Cardioversion, Defib.-Man., Cricothyrot., EOA/EGTA, Intub.-Nasal, Intub.-Oral, IV-Central, IV-Ext. Jug., IV-Intraoss., IV-Peripheral, Med. Admin., Needle Thor., Pulse Oxim., Other ALS — (1)(2)(3)(4)

MEDICATIONS: Adenocard, Aminophylline, Atropine, Benadryl, Bicarbonate, Bretylium, Calcium, Dextrose 50%, EPI 1:1000, EPI 1:10000, Furosemide, Glucagon, Intropin, Ipecac, Isuprel, Lidocaine, Mag. Sulfate, Morphine, Narcan, Nebulizer, Nifedipine, Nitroglycerin, Oxytocin, Procainamide, Thiamine, Valium, Verapamil, Other

© 1994 All Rights Reserved EM-155481:321 AGS03

514313

PLEASE DO NOT MARK IN THIS AREA

EKG: NSR, Sin. Tach., Sin. Brady, Asystole, AV Block, Atrial Fib., Atrial Flut., Vent Tach., Vent Fib., SV Tach., PEA, Other, PVC's — (I) (L)

BODY SUBSTANCE ISOLATION: Contact with Blood/Fluids (1)(2)(3)(4); Report Filed? (Y)(N); Universal Precautions: Masks, Gloves, Eye Prot., Gown (1)(2)(3)(4)

IV TYPE/RATE: TKO, BOLUS, WIDE, OTHER — LR, NS, D_5W, Other; # LINES (1)(2)(3)(4); Lock (Y)

ATTEMPTS: Intubation-Nasal, Intubation-Oral, IV-Central, IV-External Jug., IV-Intraosseous, IV-Peripheral, Needle Thoracotomy — (1)(2)(3+)(U)

NON TRANSPORT: Cancelled, Refused, False Call, Treat, Transport By: Other Ambul., Police, Flight, Oth. Vehicle; Treat, No Transport; Treat, Dead at Scene; No Treat, DOA

MEDICAL CONTROL: Radio, Telemetry, Telephone, Cellular (S)(U); (R)(A)

TRANSPORT-TO: Emergency Dept., Trauma Center, Other; Diverted? (Y)(N); Diverted by: Base, Hosp.

PATIENT DESTINATION | EMS RESOURCE SYSTEMS | PATIENT DATE OF BIRTH MO DAY YR | ESTIMATED AGE

IDPH Copy (05/94) — Funded by the Illinois Department of Transportation, Division of Traffic Safety — IL 482-0879

Fig. 15-2 **A,** Example of a prehospital care report—front side.

Continued

Illinois • Emergency Medical Services   **NARRATIVE**

SERVICE NAME		SERVICE #		TODAY'S DATE

INCIDENT LOCATION	HOSPITAL DESTINATION

PATIENT INFO

PATIENT LAST NAME	FIRST	M.I.	HOME PHONE #	AGE	DATE OF BIRTH

STREET ADDRESS

CITY	STATE	ZIP CODE	LEGAL GUARDIAN

ALLERGIES (MEDS)   ○ NONE KNOWN

CURRENT MEDICATIONS   ○ NONE KNOWN   ○ BROUGHT W/PT.

CHIEF COMPLAINT

NARRATIVE

NARRATIVE 1 OF _____

TIME	P	R	B/P	TEMP	BS	RHYTHM	TREATMENT	DOSE	ROUTE	02 SAT.	COMMENTS

LEFT	LUNG SOUNDS	RIGHT	SKIN TEMP		SKIN MOISTURE		SKIN COLOR		ABDOMEN	
			Initial — Last		Initial — Last		Initial — Last		Initial — Last	
☐ ☐	CLEAR	☐ ☐	☐ NORMAL ☐		☐ NORMAL ☐		☐ NORMAL ☐		☐ NORMAL ☐	
☐ ☐	RHONCHI	☐ ☐	☐ COOL ☐		☐ MOIST ☐		☐ PALE ☐		☐ SOFT ☐	
☐ ☐	RALES	☐ ☐	☐ COLD ☐		☐ DRY ☐		☐ CYANOTIC ☐		☐ RIGID ☐	
☐ ☐	WHEEZES	☐ ☐	☐ HOT ☐		☐ WET ☐		☐ FLUSHED ☐		☐ DISTENDED ☐	
☐ ☐	DIMINISHED	☐ ☐	☐ WARM ☐				☐ JAUNDICED ☐		☐ TENDER ☐	
☐ ☐	ABSENT	☐ ☐					☐ MOTTLED ☐			
							☐ ASHENED ☐			

SIGNATURE OF PERSON RECEIVING PATIENT

X _____

CREW SIGNATURES

DRIVER   COMPLETED REPORT

CREW MEMBER 1 _____ ☐D ☐R

CREW MEMBER 2 _____ ☐D ☐R

CREW MEMBER 3 _____ ☐D ☐R

CREW MEMBER 4 _____ ☐D ☐R

(Signatures should correspond with license numbers on back of data sheet.)

┌─────────────────┐
│   514313   │
└─────────────────┘

Service/Provider Copy

Fig. 15-2 B, Example of a prehospital care report—back side.

The prehospital care report may also be used as an educational tool. Future students can learn through presentations of real cases how different kinds of situations are handled. Properly completed prehospital care reports can be used to demonstrate the proper technique of documentation. The confidentiality of the information should be preserved in this process.

EMS administrators also use prehospital care reports for billing information. Some EMS services bill patients or insurance companies for services. Often these funds help keep the ambulance service operating. EMS administrators also compile statistics regarding the EMS service.

Researchers also use prehospital care reports to evaluate the effectiveness of prehospital care and to obtain information regarding the treatment given by EMTs. All data must be accurate and complete to be of value to these researchers.

Evaluation and continuous quality improvement are additional uses of the prehospital care report. Systems evaluate the care that EMTs give to determine both positive aspects of care provided and improvements that are needed.

TRADITIONAL FORMAT

Prehospital care reports exist in several formats. The traditional form contains boxes or bubbles you check off or fill in. These forms are very useful for data collection and quality improvement. In addi-

tion to the check boxes or bubbles, most prehospital care reports have a section for writing a **patient narrative.** This patient narrative should be written in the standard medical reporting format described in Chapter 14, "Communications." Box 15-3 lists the components of the standard medical reporting format.

If your service uses a report form that includes a patient narrative section, follow these general principles for completing this section:
1. Describe facts; don't try to reach conclusions.
2. Record important observations about the scene, such as the presence of a suicide note or weapon, and avoid radio codes.
3. Use abbreviations only if they are standard and your EMS agency has an approved abbreviation list. If you do not know the correct abbreviation, do not make up one; write out the complete word or phrase. Box 15-4 lists some standard medical abbreviations. The use of abbreviations, although necessary, should be limited.

In addition to using appropriate and accurate abbreviations, take care to spell words correctly, especially medical words. If you do not know how to spell a word, find out or use another word. For every assessment, record the time of the assessment and all findings.

The prehospital care report must be written legibly and neatly for several reasons. A sloppy, poorly written report implies the care may have been sloppy and poor, and illegible handwriting and signatures do not protect the writer from legal action. Well-written, neat reports invite reading. The staff of the receiving facility are more likely to read and pay attention to a report that is neat and well written. Ideally, use printed letters rather than cursive handwriting, which can be difficult to read even when neat (Fig. 15-3).

OTHER FORMATS

Instead of the traditional "pen-and-ink" format, some EMS systems use a computerized record method in which information is filled in on an electronic clipboard or similar device. As new technology becomes available, EMTs will see more changes in data collection and patient reporting methods. You will learn these methods in your individual service.

DISTRIBUTION

Distribution of the prehospital care report in your EMS system depends on local and state protocols and procedures. Often the prehospital care re-

---

BOX 15-3

Standard Medical Reporting Format

- Patient's age and gender
- Chief complaint
- History of present illness
- Pertinent past medical history
- Mental status
- Assessment or physical findings
- Vital signs
- Emergency care provided
- The patient's response to emergency care
- The disposition of the patient

BOX 15-4

Common Medical Abbreviations

A

Abdomen	abd
After	p̄
Alcohol	EtOH
As necessary	PRN
Aspirin	ASA
At	@

B

Bag-Valve-Mask	BVM
Before	ā
Bilateral breath sounds	BBS
Blood pressure	BP

C

Cardiac care unit	CCU
Cervical immobilization device	CID
Chief complaint	CC
Complains of	c/o
Conscious, alert, and oriented	CAO
Cubic centimeter	cc

D

Date of birth	DOB
Dead on arrival	DOA
Decreased	↓
Discontinue	D/C

E

Equal	⊖
Emergency department	ED
Endotracheal	ET
Endotracheal tube	ETT
Estimated time of arrival	ETA
Every	q

F

Female	♀

G

Gun shot wound	GSW
Gynecologic	GYN

H

Hazardous materials	Haz-mat
Heart rate	HR
History	Hx
Hypertension	HTN

I

Immediately	stat
Increased	↑
Intensive care unit	ICU

J

Jugular vein distension	JVD

K

Kilogram	kg

L

Left	Ⓛ
Less than	<
Liter	L
Long backboard	LBB
Loss of consciousness	LOC

M

Male	♂
Mercury	Hg
Milligram	mg
Milliliter	mL
Millimeter	mm
Millimeters of mercury	mm Hg
Months old	m/o
Multiple casualty incident	MCI

N

Nasal cannula	NC
Nausea and vomiting	N/V
Negative	⊖
Nitroglycerin	NTG
No known allergies	NKA
No known drug allergies	NKDA
Not applicable	N/A
Nothing by mouth	NPO

O

Obstetrics	OB
Operating room	OR
Oxygen	O_2

P

Patient	pt
Past medical history	PMHx
Penicillin	PCN
Percent	%
Positive	⊕
Prior to arrival	PTA
Pupils equal and react to light	PEARL

R

Registered nurse	RN
Respirations	resp
Right	Ⓡ
Rule out	R/O

S

Shortness of breath	SOB
Short spine board	SSB
Signs and symptoms	S/S
Sublingual	SL

T

Transport	Tx
Treatment	Rx

V

Vital signs	VS

W

Warm and dry	W/D
Water	H_2O
With	c̄
Without	s̄

Y

Year old	y/o

Use Blue/Black Ink - Press Firmly

SERVICE NAME		SERVICE #	INCIDENT #	TODAY'S DATE
COMMUNITY AMBULANCE		02165	95-1379	03 16 95

INCIDENT LOCATION
123 MAIN STREET

P A T I E N T   I N F O

PATIENT LAST NAME	FIRST	M.I.	PHONE	AGE	DATE OF BIRTH	SEX
SMITH	JANE	C.	555-1212	68	02 04 27	F

STREET ADDRESS: 123 MAIN STREET
SOCIAL SECURITY NUMBER: 123-45-6789   MEMBERSHIP ○ Yes ⊗ No

CITY	STATE	ZIP CODE
ANYTOWN	PA	15123

INSURANCE CODE #

PRIVATE PHYSICIAN: DR. MARTINEZ

○ BILL TO (COMPANY or NAME)   PHONE

MEDICAID #

ADDRESS N/A   STREET

MEDICARE #

GROUP INSURANCE #

CITY   STATE   ZIP CODE

OTHER INSURANCE #

MILEAGE
OUT 24652
SCENE 24656
DEST 24666
IN 24678

CHIEF COMPLAINT   CHEST PAIN/DISCOMFORT

CURRENT MEDICATIONS   ○ NONE KNOWN   NTG, LANOXIN 0-125 mg., TENORIUM

ALLERGIES (MEDS)   ⊗ NONE KNOWN   NKDA

PAST MEDICAL HISTORY   ○ MI   ○ CHF   ○ COPD   ⊗ ↑BP   ○ DIABETES   ○ CANCER   ○ NONE KNOWN   ⊗ OTHER   ANGINA

NARRATIVE

68 Y/O ♀ c/o CHEST PAIN/DISCOMFORT, IN MODERATE DISTRESS
(HPI) PT. STATED THAT THE ONSET OF THE PAIN WAS WHILE WALKING. NO
CHANGE IN PAIN ON PALPATION OR RESPIRATION. PT. DENIES RADIATION
OF PAIN. ALSO DENIES SHORTNESS OF BREATH, NAUSEA OR VOMITING.
PT. DESCRIBES THE PAIN AS CRUSHING IN NATURE. SEVERITY OF PAIN
RATED AS A 6 ON A 1-10 SCALE. PT. STATED THAT THE PAIN BEGAN
1 HOUR PRIOR TO EMS NOTIFICATION. (PMHX) HIGH BLOOD PRESSURE, ANGINA.
(MEDS) NTG, LANOXIN 0.125mg. & TENORIUM 10mg. NKDA (PE) PT. CAO x 3,
ASSESSMENT OF CHEST UNREMARKABLE. LUNGS CLEAR & Ⓢ. ABDOMEN SOFT,
NON-TENDER. SKIN PINK, WARM & DRY. GOOD PULSES, SENSATION & MOTOR
FUNCTION ALL EXTREMITIES. Ⓝ SACRAC OR PERIPHERAL EDEMA. VITAL SIGNS AS
NOTED BELOW. (RX) PT. WAS ALLOWED TO REMAIN IN A POSITION OF COMFORT.
INITIAL ASSESSMENT COMPLETED. OXYGEN ADMINISTERED @ 15 LPM VIA
NON-REBREATHER. FOCUSED HISTORY AND PHYSICAL EXAM COMPLETED.
DR. JOHNSON @ COMMUNITY CONSULTED. ORDERS FOR ⊤ SL NTG TABLET.
PT. PLACED ON STRETCHER INTO AMBULANCE. ASSISTED WITH THE ADMINISTRATION
OF NTG. PT. STATED PAIN WAS RELIEVED. V/S REASSESSED. TRANSPORTED
TO COMMUNITY HOSPITAL c̄ ON-GOING ASSESSMENTS EN ROUTE.

⊗ Narrative 1 of 1

TIME	P	R	B/P	RHYTHM	TREATMENT	PROVIDER ID #	RESPONSE/COMMENTS
1000					ASSESSMENT, O₂	067133	15 LPM VIA NON-REBREATHER
1005	88	18	128/76		FOCUSED Hx, P.E. VITALS	062247	
1008					STRETCHER	CREW	POSITION OF COMFORT
1010	88	16	128/76		VITALS/CONSULT	067133	ORDERS = ⊤ SL NTG
1012					ASSISTED NTG	062247	PT. FELT RELIEF
1014	86	16	120/70		VITALS	062247	
1019	86	16	122/74		VITALS	062247	PT. PAIN FREE NOW

Bonnie Brown
Signature of Person Receiving Patient   Time

DR. JOHNSON   1234
Command Physician   ID#

Crew Signatures:
A#1
A#2
A#3
A#4

☐ Service Copy

Fig. 15-3   The prehospital care report should be neat and accurate.

port uses multipart carbonless paper or forms with carbon paper between copies. Typically the original is turned over to the EMS service, and the first copy of the form is given to the receiving facility. Another copy is generally used for state or local statistics.

DOCUMENTATION OF PATIENT CARE ERRORS

When an error occurs in patient care, do not try to cover it up. As always, document what did or did not happen and what steps, if any, were taken to correct the situation.

Falsification of information in a prehospital care report can lead not only to suspension or revocation of an EMT's certificate or licensure but also to poor patient care. Other healthcare providers would have a false impression of the assessment findings or treatments given and may render additional, perhaps incorrect, care based on this false information.

For example, document vital signs only if the vital signs are actually taken. Some EMTs are tempted to falsify vital signs because they are required to obtain a set every 5 or 15 minutes, but they are sometimes too busy taking care of the pa-

tient to complete all sets. In such a case, document the care provided and explain that there was insufficient time to take additional vital signs.

On occasion an EMT may forget to give a treatment such as oxygen. Even though the patient may have needed the treatment, never falsely state that the patient was given any treatment not actually given.

Falsification of patient information is a very serious problem. The information may lead to improper care in the receiving facility and patient death or disability, as well as disciplinary action.

CORRECTION OF DOCUMENTATION ERRORS

If you make an error while completing a report, it is not necessary to start over. In the patient narrative section, correct errors by drawing a single horizontal line through the error, initialing it, and writing the correct information beside it (Fig. 15-4). Do not try to obliterate the error, which could then be interpreted as an attempt to cover up a mistake. If you are using a prehospital care report that includes check boxes or bubbles and you make an error, follow local protocol for correcting the error.

Errors discovered after the report form is sub-

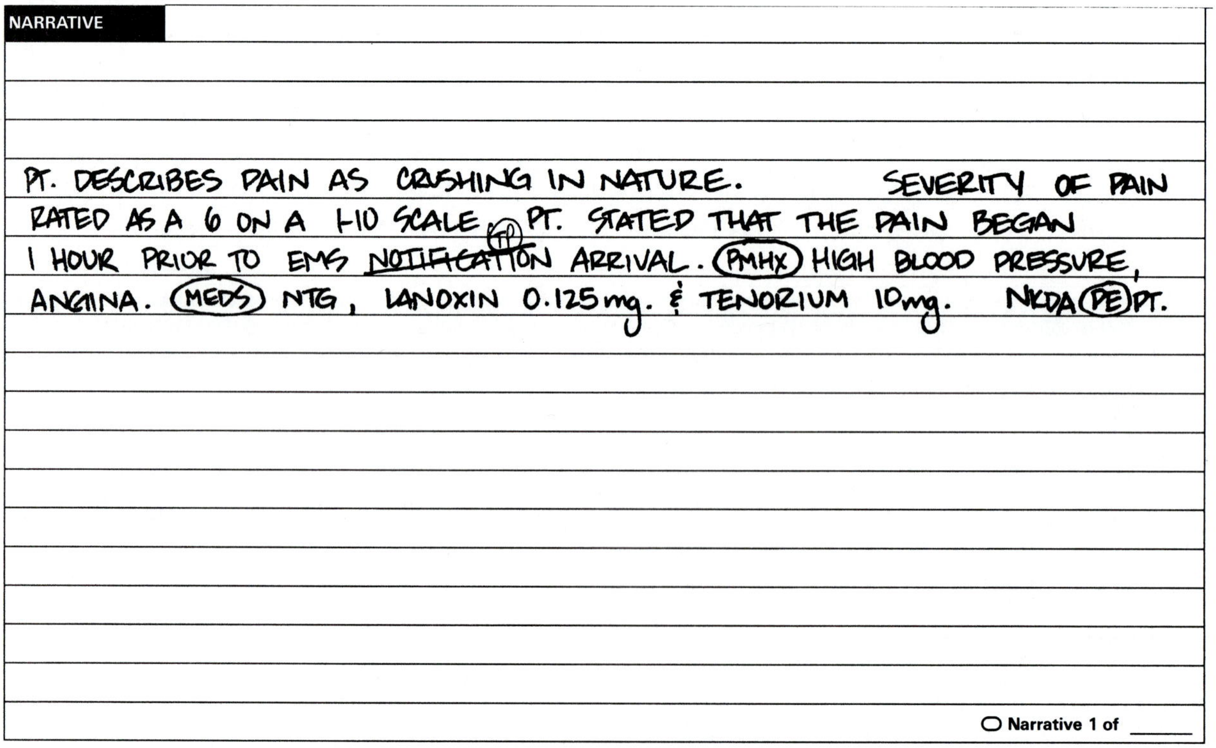

Fig. 15-4 A properly corrected error in a prehospital care report.

ing and dating it, and adding a note with the correct information. If information was omitted, add a note with the correct information, the date, and your initials. A copy of the addendum also should be provided to the receiving facility.

DOCUMENTATION OF PATIENT REFUSAL

All competent adults have the right to refuse treatment for themselves and others in their care, such as minors. This refusal of treatment can create a difficult situation. You may feel the patient should be treated and transported, but the patient has certain rights that must be respected.

Before leaving a scene where the patient is refusing treatment or transport, try several times to persuade the patient to come with you to a hospital. If the patient refuses, you must ensure the patient is making a rational, informed decision and is not being influenced by alcohol or other drugs or by the effects of illness or injury. Consult on-line medical direction to help determine the patient's competency. Chapter 3, "Medical/Legal and Ethical Issues," discusses the issue of consent more fully.

If the patient is competent, inform the patient why treatment and transport to a hospital are nec-

---

REVIEW QUESTIONS

THE PREHOSPITAL CARE REPORT

1. When completing the patient narrative, EMTs should use the _____ format.

2. In addition to being a medical document, the prehospital care report is a _____ document.

3. An EMT who does not know the appropriate abbreviation should do what?

4. To correct an error, draw a line through the error and _____.

1. Standard medical reporting
2. Legal
3. Spell out the word
4. Initial the line

---

mitted can be corrected by an addendum. This correction preferably is entered in a different color ink, drawing a single line through the error, initial-

---

PATIENT REFUSAL OF SERVICES

This is to certify that I, _____
am refusing:

○ TREATMENT
○ TRANSPORT
○ OTHER: _____

I acknowledge that I have been informed of the risk(s) involved and hereby release the ambulance attendant(s), the ambulance service, the medical command physician, and the medical command facility from all responsibility for any ill effects which may result from this action.

_____   _____
Signature of patient   Date

_____   _____   _____   _____
Witness   Date   Witness   Date

Fig. 15-5   Refusal section of a prehospital care report.

essary and what may happen without treatment. Contact medical direction, following your local protocol. The medical direction physician may talk to the patient to help with the patient's decision.

If the patient still refuses, document your assessment findings and the emergency medical care given, and then have the patient sign a refusal form. Also document that you have informed the patient of the adverse effects that may result from not accepting care and/or being transported, including possible death. Have a family member, police officer, or bystander sign the form as a witness. If the patient refuses to sign the refusal form, have a family member, police officer, or bystander sign the form saying that the patient refused to sign (Fig. 15-5).

Report the patient care the same as if the patient had been transported. Include the care you wished to provide to the patient. Before leaving the scene, tell the patient about other ways to receive care, such as by the family transporting the patient to the hospital with the ambulance following or by the ambulance transporting the patient to a physician's office. State your willingness to return if the patient's condition worsens or the patient decides to receive treatment and transport. This statement should also be documented.

SPECIAL SITUATIONS

MULTIPLE CASUALTY INCIDENTS

In multiple casualty incidents, when you must move on to care for another patient before you have completed the prehospital care report, you need to fill out the report later. Your local multiple casualty incident plan should have some means for quickly recording important medical information temporarily, such as with a triage tag. Pertinent information can be recorded on the triage tag, which is later used to complete the prehospital care report. Your EMS system should have guidelines for the completion of prehospital care reports at multiple casualty incidents.

SPECIAL SITUATION REPORTS

Special situation reports are used to document unusual occurrences. They may also be used to make reports to local authorities or to amplify and supplement the primary prehospital care report. A special report may be used in cases of abuse or neglect, hazardous materials incidents, and wounds obtained from violence or crime scenes.

BOX 15-5

Special Report Situations

- Infectious disease exposure
- Injury to EMTs or bystanders
- Equipment damage or malfunction
- Vehicle crashes involving the response unit
- Patient refusals
- Abuse or neglect
- Crime scenes
- Hazardous materials incidents

Special reports should be submitted in a timely manner. Like a prehospital care report, the special report should be accurate and objective. Keep a copy for your own records. Once completed, the report and copies are submitted according to local protocol. Box 15-5 lists additional potential situations for special reports.

REVIEW QUESTIONS

DOCUMENTATION OF PATIENT REFUSAL/SPECIAL SITUATIONS

1. All competent patients have the right to _____ medical care.

2. If the patient refuses medical care, you should consult _____.

3. A refusal should be signed by the _____ and a _____.

4. A special report is used to document _____.

5. Like a prehospital care report, the special report should be written _____.

1. Refuse
2. Medical direction
3. Patient, witness
4. Unusual occurrences
5. Accurately and objectively

CHAPTER SUMMARY

MINIMUM DATA SET

Through use of the minimum data set, EMS systems can prove their efficacy. The minimum data set contains administrative and patient information.

THE PREHOSPITAL CARE REPORT

The prehospital care report is used to document all aspects of an emergency response. It is a legal document as well as a medical document. It is used for continuity of healthcare, billing, statistics, research, education, and evaluation.

The report must be legible and accurate. Avoid misspelled words, and use only approved abbreviations. All information on the prehospital care report should be objective. Any subjective information should be clearly indicated as such.

DOCUMENTATION OF PATIENT REFUSAL

All competent adult patients have the right to refuse care. If a competent patient refuses care, you should contact medical direction and document the refusal. Offer to return if the patient later decides to accept treatment and transport, and have the patient sign a refusal form.

In cases of refusal, the prehospital care report should be completed as if the patient had been transported. Document all findings and the advice given to the patient.

SPECIAL SITUATIONS

When special situations occur, you must document them. Special reports are used to make reports to the authorities or to document damage to or malfunction of equipment.

Like any prehospital care report, the special report should be submitted in a timely manner. It should be legible and free of spelling errors.

UNITED STATES DEPARTMENT OF TRANSPORTATION NATIONAL HIGHWAY TRAFFIC SAFETY ADMINISTRATION EMT–BASIC OBJECTIVES

Check your knowledge. The National Registry of EMTs and many state EMS agencies use the objectives below to develop EMT–Basic certification examinations. Can you meet them?

COGNITIVE

1. Explain the components of the written report and list the information that should be included in the written report.
2. Identify the various sections of the written report.
3. Describe what information is required in each section of the prehospital care report and how it should be entered.
4. Define the special considerations concerning patient refusal.
5. Describe the legal implications associated with the written report.
6. Discuss state and/or local record and reporting requirements.

AFFECTIVE

1. Explain the rationale for patient care documentation.
2. Explain the rationale for the EMS system gathering data.
3. Explain the rationale for using medical terminology correctly.
4. Explain the rationale for using an accurate and synchronous clock so that information can be used in trending.

PSYCHOMOTOR

1. Complete a prehospital care report.

MEDICAL/BEHAVIORAL EMERGENCIES

An EMT is frequently challenged by being the first healthcare provider called upon to care for another human being during their time of crisis. The needs of the patient may range from a behavioral problem, a medical illness, or even a problem related to pregnancy. Any condition that challenges a human being from birth to death may result in a call for assistance from a prehospital provider. Showing compassion, maintianing a calm demeanor, and when challenged with a life-threatening situation, falling back upon the ABCs always helps to keep the EMT on track. Finally, it's important to recognize that some problems go beyond our limitations and the best we can do is just that—to do our best and provide whatever additional resources seem to be in the best interest of the patient, whether that is expeditious transport to a hospital or requiring mutual aid from another healthcare provider.

Paul M. Paris, MD, FACEP
*Professor and Chief, Division
of Emergency Medicine
University of Pittsburgh
School of Medicine*

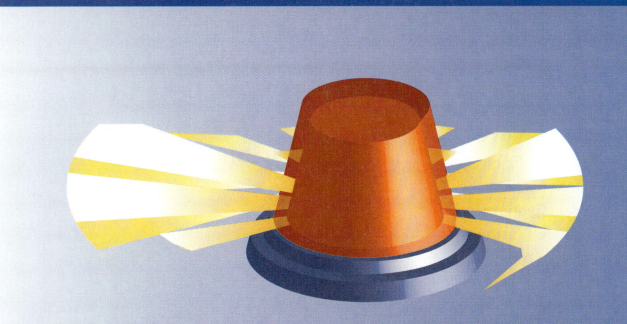

DIVISION FOUR

16 GENERAL PHARMACOLOGY

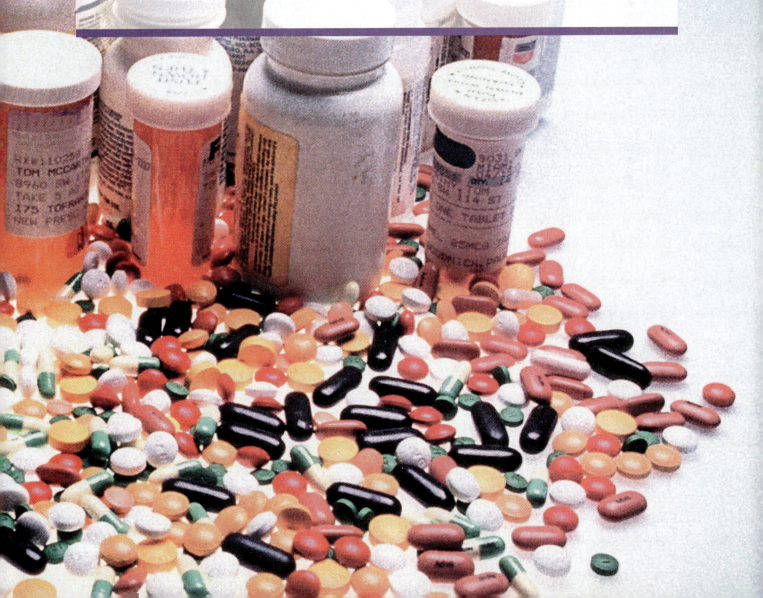

KEY TERMS

Contraindication: A situation in which a medication should not be used.

Dose: The amount of medication that should be administered.

Drug: Any substance that alters the body's functioning when taken into the body.

Generic name: The name of a medication listed in the *U.S. Pharmacopeia,* the official name assigned to the medication. The generic name is usually a simple form of the chemical name.

Indication: The condition for which a medication may be used.

Inhalation: A route of administration for medications in the form of a fine mist or a gas that are absorbed by the capillaries of the lungs.

Mechanism of action: How a medication affects the body.

Pharmacology: The science of drugs and study of their origin, ingredients, uses, and actions on the body.

Route of administration: The way the medication is administered to the patient.

Sublingual route: Putting a medication under the patient's tongue.

Trade name: The name assigned by the company that sells a medication. Trade names are copyrighted and carry the copyright symbol.

IN THE FIELD

"**M**edic 5201, respond to 1413 Charles Street for a 5-year-old boy, possible aspirin overdose." The EMT–Basics Glenn and Terri were quickly en route to the scene. On their arrival, they found the boy sitting in a chair in the living room. His mother showed them a 100-tablet bottle of aspirin that was half empty. She said that it was a new bottle she bought last week and that Johnny must have taken it from the medicine chest some time in the last hour. She wasn't sure if he had actually swallowed all of the pills missing from the bottle. He had not vomited, she said.

After assessing Johnny and finding him alert and oriented with stable vital signs, Terri called the receiving hospital for medical direction and asked if activated charcoal would be indicated for this patient. The physician ordered 25 g of activated charcoal to be administered orally. Terri repeated the order back to the physician: "That's 25 grams of activated charcoal to be administered orally."

When the order was confirmed, Terri and Glenn helped Johnny drink the activated charcoal and began transport to the emergency department. Because activated charcoal is most effective when administered within 30 minutes of ingestion, the EMT's ability to quickly administer activated charcoal proved beneficial to Johnny's medical care.

EMTs encounter many situations when a patient may benefit from a medication. Whether the medication is something that you have on the EMS unit or something that has been prescribed by the patient's physician, it is critical that you understand when, how, and why to administer medications. Just as medications can be life-saving, they can also be lethal. Administering the wrong medication, the wrong dose of the right medication, or the right medication at the wrong time are all potentially life-threatening actions. EMTs can successfully administer certain medications when they are familiar with the medications and have the approval of medical direction.

Pharmacology is the science of drugs and includes the study of their origin, ingredients, uses, and actions on the body. A **drug** is any substance that alters the body's functions when taken into the body. Medications are drugs used in medicine to prevent or treat disease or medical conditions. In medicine, the words *drug* and *medication* are often used interchangeably. This chapter describes the basics of medication information, action, and administration. Specific medications and their indica-

TABLE 16-1	Medications Described in Other Chapters
Medication	**Chapter**
Oxygen	Chapter 7 (The Airway)
Prescribed inhaler	Chapter 17 (Respiratory Emergencies)
Nitroglycerin	Chapter 18 (Cardiovascular Emergencies)
Oral glucose	Chapter 19 (Diabetes and Altered Mental Status)
Epinephrine autoinjector	Chapter 20 (Allergies)
Activated charcoal	Chapter 21 (Poisoning and Overdose)

tions, contraindications, routes, doses, and side effects are discussed in other chapters along with the conditions for which the medications are used. See Table 16-1 for chapter references for specific medications.

MEDICATION INFORMATION

TYPES OF MEDICATIONS

EMT–Basics should be familiar with two different categories of medications. First are medications carried on the EMS unit. These medications are administered to patients who fit established criteria following consultation with medical direction. EMT–Basics typically carry activated charcoal, oral glucose, and oxygen with them on the EMS unit. EMT–Intermediates and EMT–Paramedics carry an expanded number of medications with them on their EMS units.

The second category consists of physician-prescribed medications that patients already have in their possession. You may assist patients to administer these medications with approval from medical direction (obtained by direct voice contact with the physician over the radio or phone, or through a written protocol or standing order). These medications include nitroglycerin, epinephrine auto-injector, and prescribed inhalers. Patients may require assistance with their medications for a variety of reasons. For example, a patient may be experiencing chest pain and be unable to walk to the bedroom to obtain the bottle of nitroglycerin (Fig. 16-1). The EMT–Basic who is familiar with the name, route, dose, effects, and other specific information about nitroglycerin can properly assist the patient with this medication.

Patients may also have in their possession a vast assortment of other physician-prescribed medications or over-the-counter medications. EMT–Basics should not aid in the administration of any of these medications. If there is ever any question, consult medical direction for advice.

MEDICATION NAMES

Any one medication may be identified by various names. Two of these names are particularly important to the EMT. The **generic name** is the name listed in the *U.S. Pharmacopeia*, a government publication listing all medications used in the United States. This name is the official one assigned

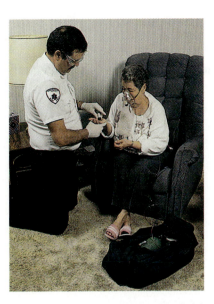

Fig. 16-1 Patients may require assistance with administration of their medications.

to the medication. The generic name is usually a simple form of the chemical name, which is a longer and more precise description of the medication's chemical composition.

Medications are also frequently referred to by their **trade name**. The trade name is the name given by the company that makes and sells the medication. Trade names are copyrighted and have the trademark symbol ® following them. Because more than one manufacturer may market the same medication, there can be multiple trade names for the same medication, even though that medication has only one generic name. Trade names are generally capitalized (Fig. 16-2).

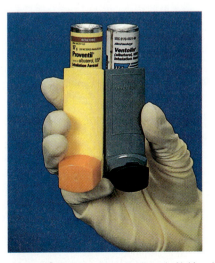

Fig. 16-2 Proventil® (Schering Corp., Kenilworth, N.J.) and Ventolin® (Allen and Hanburys, Research Triangle Park, N.C.) are the trade names for albuterol.

TABLE 16-2	Generic and Trade Names of Selected Common Medications		
Generic Name	**Trade Name**	**Form**	
Activated Charcoal	SuperChar® InstaChar® Actidose® LiquiChar®	Suspension	
Oral Glucose	Glutose® Insta-glucose®	Gel	
Oxygen	—	Gas	
Albuterol (inhaler)	Proventil® Ventolin®	Fine powder for inhalation/liquid/ vaporized fixed-dose nebulizer	
Isoetharine (inhaler)	Bronkosol®	Fine powder for inhalation/liquid/ vaporized fixed-dose nebulizer	
Metaproterenol (inhaler)	Alupent®	Fine powder for inhalation/liquid/ vaporized fixed-dose nebulizer	
Nitroglycerin	Nitrostat® Nitrolingual®	Compressed powders or tablets/ Sublingual Spray	
Epinephrine autoinjector	Adrenalin	Liquids for injection	

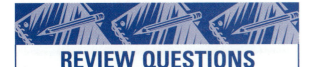

MEDICATION FORMS

Medications exist in a variety of forms. Each form has advantages and disadvantages related to the ease of administration and the onset of action. Medications you may administer as an EMT–Basic exist in the form of compressed powders or tablets, liquids for injection, gels, suspensions, fine powder for inhalation, gases, sublingual spray, or vaporized liquids. Table 16-2 lists several medications, by generic name, trade name, and medication forms that EMT–Basics must be familiar with.

MEDICATION ADMINISTRATION

You must know several essential pieces of information about a specific medication before you can administer it appropriately. These include indications and contraindications, dose, administration routes, and medication actions.

INDICATIONS AND CONTRAINDICATIONS

An **indication** is the most common use of a medication for treating a specific illness or condition. Indications are signs or symptoms for when a medication is used. For example, chest pain in a patient with a history of cardiac disease may be an indication for the administration of nitroglycerin.

A **contraindication** is a situation in which a medication should not be used. These are situations when a specific medication has been shown to be of little benefit or of potential harm for the patient. For example, certain medications should not be given to children.

The **dose** is the amount of the medication that should be administered. Some medication doses depend on the age of the patient, the weight of the patient, and some have a standard dose for all patient ages and weights.

ADMINISTRATION ROUTES

The **administration route** is the way the medication will be administered to the patient. EMT–Basics must be familiar with the four primary routes: oral, sublingual, inhalation, and intramuscular injection. The administration route depends on the type of medication, the desired site of action, and how quickly the medication must reach its location. Box 16-1 describes the four administration routes.

You can administer medications only by the order of a licensed physician. A written protocol or verbal order must be obtained prior to administration. Before administering any medication, check the label for its expiration date, check that the fluid is clear (if a liquid) and free of sediments or crystals,

BOX 16-1

Routes of Administration

Oral

The oral route is generally safe, easy, and economical. Medications administered orally are absorbed through the digestive tract in the stomach, intestines, or colon. Because the medication must travel through the digestive tract to the site where it will be absorbed, the onset of action for these medications is relatively slow. Patients must also be alert to have medications administered orally. If the patient is unresponsive or the onset of action for the medication must be rapid, oral administration is not a good option. Oral glucose and activated charcoal are examples of medications that are administered orally. The oral route is a good choice for cooperative, alert children. Medical direction will advise you how to adjust a dose of activated charcoal for a child. The use of oral medications is discussed in Chapter 21, "Poisoning and Overdose," and Chapter 19, "Diabetes and Altered Mental Status."

Sublingual

The sublingual route means placing the medication under the patient's tongue. The medication should not be swallowed but allowed to dissolve. The medication is rapidly absorbed into the capillaries under the tongue. The digestive tract is bypassed, so the onset of action is more rapid. Nitroglycerin is an example of a medication that is administered sublingually. The use of sublingual nitroglycerin is discussed in Chapter 18, "Cardiovascular Emergencies."

Inhalation

Some medications can be administered by inhalation. Inhaled medications take the form of a fine mist or a gas that is absorbed by the capillaries in the lungs, administered from a device called an *inhaler.* The onset of action is rapid. Patients may need your assistance to administer a physician-prescribed inhaler, as is commonly used for asthma and other conditions. Asthma is a common medical problem for children, and often older children have a prescribed inhaler. You assist a child with a prescribed inhaler in the same manner as an adult. Oxygen is also an inhaled medication. The use of prescribed inhalers is discussed in Chapter 17, "Respiratory Emergencies."

Intramuscular

Intramuscular injections are the introduction of a medication deep into a large muscle, where it is absorbed into the blood stream. Although intramuscular injections are not common in prehospital settings, epinephrine can be administered this way by EMT–Basics via an autoinjector. The specific technique is discussed in Chapter 20, "Allergies."

and check for the appropriate concentration. If there is any problem with the medication, do not administer the medication and consult medical direction. The liquid in an autoinjector may be obscured from view by the container, and the clarity cannot be evaluated. Always use extreme caution when dealing with medications.

> **ALERT**
> When a physician orders the administration of a medication, always repeat the name of the medication, the dose, and the route back to the physician for confirmation.

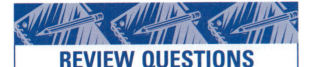

REVIEW QUESTIONS

MEDICATION ADMINISTRATION

1. _____ are the reasons that a medication is used. EMT–Basics should also be familiar with the _____ of a medication so it is not administered when it should not be.

2. Oral, sublingual, _____, and intramuscular injections are all administration _____ for medications.

3. When a medication is given by mouth, it is said to be given _____. Sublingual administration means the medication is placed under the patient's _____.

4. Match the following medications in column A with the administration route in column B:

A. Medication	B. Administration
Nitroglycerin _____	Route
Oxygen _____	A. Oral
Epinephrine auto-injector _____	B. Inhalation
	C. Sublingual
Activated charcoal _____	D. Injection

5. Medications can be administered without consulting medical direction or without a written order if the patient is in acute distress. True or False?

5. False
4. C, B, D, A
3. Orally; tongue
2. Inhalation; routes
1. Indications; contraindications

MEDICATION ACTIONS

ACTIONS

Medications affect the body in a variety of ways. The **mechanism of action** is how the medication affects the body. Different medications produce their desired effects in different ways. For example, some medications work on the muscles of the heart, whereas others work on the nervous system. Some medications stimulate actions, and others depress actions. The mechanisms of action for the medications administered by EMT–Basics are discussed in the chapters relevant to their use (*see* Table 16-1).

SIDE EFFECTS

The side effects of a medication are its undesirable actions. Any action other than the one desired is considered a side effect. Some side effects can be serious. Side effects for some medications are predictable. Nausea and vomiting, for example, are common side effects for numerous medications. Being aware of these potential side effects helps prepare you to deal with their onset. Specific side effects for medications administered by EMT–Basics are discussed along with the medications in the appropriate chapters.

REASSESSMENT STRATEGIES

Any time a medication is administered, patients must be carefully monitored for effects and side effects. EMTs should note the patient's condition before the medication is administered, and note the dose, time, and route of administration. Evaluate the patient's vital signs and physical condition before and following administration. Watch carefully for the desired actions and any undesirable side effects.

Continue these reassessments as part of the ongoing patient assessment. It is important to know if a medication has had the desired effect on the patient. For example, if a patient has chest pain and you assist the patient with a nitroglycerin tablet, reevaluate the chest pain. If the pain is only partially relieved, the medical direction physician may order another nitroglycerin tablet to be administered. The patient's response to medications—like all interventions—should be relayed to the receiving hospital and documented in the patient care report. Box 16-2 lists the information necessary to document in your report after administering medication.

BOX 16-2

Medication Administration Information to Document

- Who ordered the medication? Note the physician's name and the time of the order.
- What medication was administered? Name the medication by its generic or trade name.
- What time was the medication administered?
- What was the dose?
- What was the route (ie, injection, oral, inhalation, or sublingual)? For injections, also note the site (eg, left thigh).
- Note the vital signs before the medication was administered.
- Evaluate the patient's response to the medication. Be sure to note any changes in vital signs, mental status, and relief from pain or distress.

REVIEW QUESTIONS

MEDICATION ACTIONS

1. The mechanism of action is the way a _____ affects the body.

2. _____ are undesirable actions of medications.

3. Because some side effects are _____, the EMT–Basic must be prepared to deal with them.

4. EMT–Basics should document the patient's _____ and the_____ and/or _____ of medications in the patient care report as well as reporting them to the receiving facility.

4. Response; effects; side effects
3. Common or predictable
2. Side effects
1. Medication

CHAPTER SUMMARY

MEDICATION INFORMATION

EMT–Basics can administer two kinds of medications to patients: the patient's own physician-prescribed medication, or medications carried on the EMS unit. A medication is any substance that alters the body's functions. Medications are commonly used in medicine to treat or prevent a disease or medical condition. Medications carried by EMT–Basics include oxygen, oral glucose, and activated charcoal. Medications that can be administered (or assisted with) by the EMT–Basic include prescribed nitroglycerin, epinephrine autoinjector, and inhalers. Advanced EMTs such as EMT–Intermediates or EMT–Paramedics may carry additional medications on their EMS unit.

Medications are referred to by a variety of names. Most important to the EMT–Basic are the generic name and the trade name. Medications also come in a variety of forms. The form and the route determine the onset of action.

MEDICATION ADMINISTRATION

An indication for a medication is the situation in which it may be used. A contraindication is a situation in which it should not be used. The dose is the amount of the medication that should be administered. Some medication dosages vary based on criteria such as the patient's age or weight.

The administration route is the way in which a medication is given. Administration routes for medications used by the EMT–Basic include oral, sublingual, inhalation, and intramuscular injection. Medications can be administered by an EMT–Basic only by the order of a licensed physician. EMT–Basics should repeat medication orders back to the physician to confirm the correct dose, route, and medication.

MEDICATION ACTIONS

The mechanism of action is how the medication affects the body. Side effects of medications are any action other than the desired one. Many medications have common, predictable side effects. EMT–Basics should reassess the patient for the response to any medication given. This action should be part of the ongoing patient assessment. Any medication administered, as well as its effects and side effects, should be reported to the receiving hospital and documented in the prehospital care report.

UNITED STATES DEPARTMENT OF TRANSPORTATION NATIONAL HIGHWAY TRAFFIC SAFETY ADMINISTRATION EMT–BASIC OBJECTIVES

Check your knowledge. The National Registry of EMTs and many state EMS agencies use the objectives below to develop EMT–Basic certification examinations. Can you meet them?

COGNITIVE

1. Identify which medications are carried on the unit.
2. State the medications carried on the unit by the generic name.
3. Identify the medications that the EMT– Basic may assist the patient with administering.
4. State the medications the EMT–Basic can assist the patient with by generic name.
5. Discuss the forms in which medications may be found.

AFFECTIVE

1. Explain the rationale for the administration of medications.

PSYCHOMOTOR

1. Demonstrate general steps for assisting a patient with self-administration of medications.
2. Read the labels and inspect each type of medication.

17 RESPIRATORY EMERGENCIES

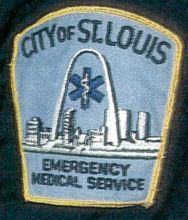

IN THE FIELD

As EMTs Jeff and Mike entered the Johnsons' home, they could immediately tell that the patient, Mr. Johnson, was in respiratory distress. They could hear loud wheezing from the patient across the room. He was sitting in a chair, leaning forward, unable to say more than a few words without taking a breath. After the initial assessment, Jeff talked to Mrs. Johnson to obtain the patient's history, because Mr. Johnson could barely speak. Mike placed Mr. Johnson on oxygen via a nonrebreather mask at a rate of 15 L/min and then began the focused history and physical examination.

After learning that Mr. Johnson had been prescribed an inhaler by his physician, Jeff called medical direction to see if Mr. Johnson could have a dose based on his condition. Mike finished taking the patient's vital signs. His heart rate was 115, his respiratory rate was 28, and his skin was cool and moist. Jeff and Mike knew that the inhaler could help Mr. Johnson breathe easier, but they also knew that they must be careful to make sure that it was delivered appropriately.

With approval from medical direction, Mr. Johnson was given one dose of medication from his inhaler in the home, and a second dose later in the back of the ambulance. After two doses, he was able to speak in whole sentences and breathe much easier. Mr. Johnson was much more comfortable through the 20-minute ambulance ride than he would have been if he had not received any medication until he arrived at the emergency department.

Over 200,000 people die every year from respiratory emergencies. As an EMT, you frequently will encounter people with difficulty breathing. One large city reported that 12% of its ambulance calls were responses for people experiencing respiratory emergencies—three times the number of ambulance calls for heart attacks. Anyone who has experienced respiratory difficulty knows that the inability to breathe adequately is terrifying. Respiratory emergencies also are common in children and are frightening for both child and parent. Respiratory distress is a true medical emergency.

After reviewing the airway and respiratory system, this chapter describes breathing assessment, the signs and symptoms of breathing difficulties, and the emergency medical care for respiratory emergencies.

RESPIRATORY SYSTEM REVIEW

This section briefly reviews the anatomy and physiology of the respiratory system. For more detail, see Chapter 4, "The Human Body."

Every cell in the body needs oxygen to live. Air containing oxygen is breathed into the lungs and is then delivered to the body tissues.

ANATOMY

Air enters the body through the nose and mouth, where it is filtered, warmed, and humidified. The air travels through the pharynx (throat), which is divided into the nasopharynx and the oropharynx. The nasopharynx lies behind the nose, and the oropharynx lies at the back of the mouth.

Air passes through the trachea, then the bronchi, and eventually into the alveoli. The trachea (windpipe) begins at the cricoid cartilage, the firm cartilage ring forming the lower portion of the larynx (voice box). The trachea is protected by a leaf-shaped structure, the epiglottis, which prevents food and liquid from entering the trachea during swallowing. The trachea divides into two bronchi, the major branches into the lungs (Fig. 17-1). The bronchi subdivide into smaller and smaller air passages that end at the alveoli, the thin-walled air sacs where respiration takes place.

There are two main sets of muscles to aid in the mechanics of breathing: the diaphragm and intercostal muscles. Inhalation begins with the contrac-

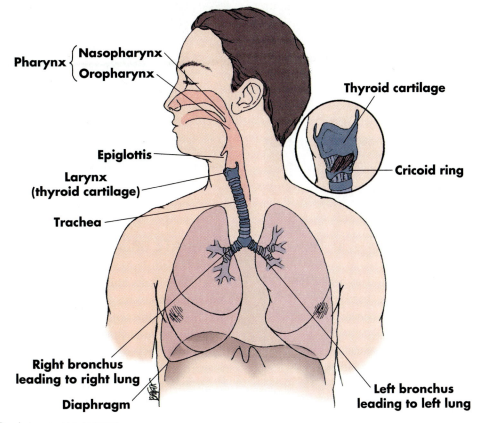

Pharynx { **Nasopharynx**
Oropharynx

Thyroid cartilage

Epiglottis

Larynx
(thyroid cartilage)

Cricoid ring

Trachea

Right bronchus
leading to right lung

Left bronchus
leading to left lung

Diaphragm

Fig. 17-1   Respiratory system anatomy.

tion of the diaphragm (moving it downward) and the intercostal muscles (pulling the ribs up and out). This causes the size of the thoracic cavity to increase, pulling air into the lungs through the nose and mouth. Inhalation is an active process.

Exhalation begins with the relaxation of the intercostal muscles and the diaphragm. As the muscles relax, the size of the thoracic cavity decreases, and air is forced out through the mouth and nose. Exhalation is usually a passive process. Sometimes air can be exhaled actively, such as with sneezing or coughing.

Because of anatomic differences, infants and children are more prone to breathing problems. Infants and children have smaller air passages that can be more easily occluded. The tongue is much larger in proportion to the size of the mouth and takes up more space. The trachea is narrower and more flexible. To avoid kinking of the airway, you must properly position these patients for ventilation. The chest wall is less developed, and infants and children depend more on the use of their diaphragms and less on their relatively weak intercostal muscles to breathe. Infants depend so heavily on

the use of their diaphragms that they are sometimes referred to as "belly-breathers." Even in normal breathing, an infant's stomach moves as the diaphragm expands and contracts. Children and infants are prone to respiratory infections and diseases and commonly experience respiratory problems.

Older patients also commonly have respiratory emergencies. Older patients are more likely to have chronic respiratory problems and may also have diminished lung capacities.

PHYSIOLOGY

In the lungs, the alveoli and capillaries exchange oxygen and carbon dioxide. As oxygen-rich air enters the alveoli, blood returning from the body with low concentrations of oxygen and high concentrations of carbon dioxide flows through the capillaries surrounding the alveoli. The oxygen is transferred from the alveoli into these capillaries. Carbon dioxide is transferred from the capillaries into the alveoli and then is exhaled. The newly oxygenated blood then returns to the heart and is pumped through the body. The oxygen is given up to the cells from the capillaries, and the cells give up carbon dioxide to the capillaries. The blood is then collected in the veins and returned to the heart to be pumped again to the lungs for oxygenation and release of carbon dioxide.

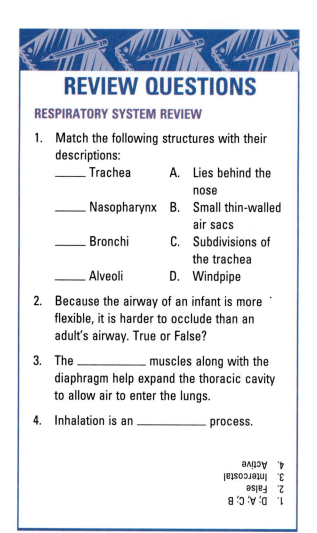

REVIEW QUESTIONS

RESPIRATORY SYSTEM REVIEW

1. Match the following structures with their descriptions:

   _____ Trachea   A. Lies behind the nose

   _____ Nasopharynx   B. Small thin-walled air sacs

   _____ Bronchi   C. Subdivisions of the trachea

   _____ Alveoli   D. Windpipe

2. Because the airway of an infant is more flexible, it is harder to occlude than an adult's airway. True or False?

3. The _____ muscles along with the diaphragm help expand the thoracic cavity to allow air to enter the lungs.

4. Inhalation is an _____ process.

1. D; A; C; B
2. False
3. Intercostal
4. Active

BREATHING ASSESSMENT

The patient's breathing is evaluated very early in patient assessment for a good reason. No one can tolerate inadequate breathing for very long, and you must act quickly to intervene in these instances. An understanding of normal, adequate breathing is basic to understanding the signs and symptoms of breathing difficulty. Breathing adequately is characterized by a normal rate, rhythm, quality, and depth.

BOX 17-1

Normal Respiratory Rates

- Adult   12–20 breaths per minute
- Child   15–30 breaths per minute
- Infant   25–50 breaths per minute

ADEQUATE BREATHING

Healthy adults breathe between 12 and 20 times a minute. Infants and children breathe at a faster rate to compensate for greater metabolic needs. Box 17-1 lists the normal ranges of respiratory rate for adults, infants, and children.

In addition to the normal rate, the rhythm of breathing should be steady and regular. There should be an even interval between each breath. For a review of how to determine breathing rate and regularity, see Chapter 5, "Baseline Vital Signs and SAMPLE History."

When air enters the lungs, both lungs should expand equally. The movement of air in and out of the lungs can be heard through the chest wall with a stethoscope. By listening to the chest wall with a stethoscope, you can assess whether breath sounds are present, and if they are present, whether they are equal. Breath sounds should be equal on both sides of the chest. Figure 17-2 shows stethoscope placement on the chest wall for listening to breath sounds.

The chest wall normally expands equally on both sides. By watching the chest wall, or placing your hands on both sides of the chest wall when the patient inhales, you can assess whether both sides of the chest are rising and falling equally.

Breathing normally takes place with little effort. As the chest wall expands, air easily enters into the thoracic cavity without use of accessory muscles. The use of accessory muscles is discussed later in this chapter.

Finally, the depth of breathing affects how much air is entering the lungs. How deeply a patient is breathing is called *tidal volume*, which is a measure of how much air enters the lungs with each respiration. The patient should not appear to be breathing deeply or shallowly.

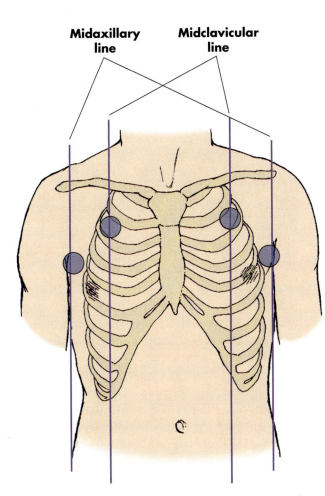

Midaxillary line   Midclavicular line

Fig. 17-2 Points of stethoscope placement for assessment of breath sounds.

BREATHING DIFFICULTY

A patient may have inadequate breathing in terms of the rate, rhythm, quality, or depth of breathing. If any of these factors is inadequate, the patient has a respiratory problem.

A breathing rate outside of the normal rate ranges may indicate inadequate breathing. Patients who are breathing too fast or too slow may not be receiving adequate oxygen to support the body's functions, or they may not be exhaling enough carbon dioxide, causing a dangerous build-up.

An irregular breathing rhythm can be a sign of a serious medical problem and needs to be evaluated by a physician.

The quality of breathing may also indicate a breathing difficulty. Unequal breath sounds, sounding different from one side of the chest to the other, can be caused by trauma, illness, or obstruction. In any case, unequal breath sounds are a sign that too little air is reaching one lung. Breath sounds can also be diminished, or not as loud as we

would expect, in one or both lungs. This condition may also be a sign that not enough air is reaching the lungs. Unequal expansion of the chest wall can also be a sign of a serious respiratory problem. Any of these conditions is a sign of a true medical emergency.

Patients may also have increased effort when breathing. Accessory muscles, the muscles of the abdomen and neck, are used when patients are having difficulty drawing enough air into their lungs by using only the diaphragm and intercostal muscles. The use of accessory muscles generally is a sign of inadequate breathing. Infants and children, however, may use their accessory muscles even when breathing normally. Any patient who has excessive use of accessory muscles, nasal flaring (flaring of the nostrils in an attempt to draw in more air), or retractions above the clavicles, between the ribs, or below the rib cage, is showing a sign of inadequate breathing.

The depth of breathing may also indicate that a patient is not breathing adequately. A patient who is breathing too deeply or too shallowly has an altered tidal volume. That affects the amount of oxygen that is available to the body.

The signs and symptoms of breathing difficulty are numerous and can be as obvious as a change in respiratory rate or as subtle as restlessness. Watch for these signs to provide the appropriate emergency medical care for correcting the problem and helping the patient breathe more effectively. Patients may be experiencing difficulty breathing due to an airway problem, a problem with the mechanics of breathing such as the function of the diaphragm, or an illness that affects the respiratory system. The signs and symptoms of breathing difficulty are listed in Box 17-2. Patients may have one or two of these signs or symptoms or any combination of them together.

You can observe the signs of respiratory distress, but shortness of breath is a symptom the patient may tell you about, for example, "I can't catch my breath." Shortness of breath is not something you can see or assess—the patient must communicate it to you. Some patients may be unable to speak because they are working too hard to breathe, or they may be able to say only a word or two before they need to breathe again.

Changes in breathing rate or pattern can signify that a patient is not receiving enough oxygen. Other signs of inadequate oxygenation are altered mental status, restlessness, and increased pulse rate

BOX 17-2

Signs and Symptoms of Difficulty Breathing

General

- Shortness of breath
- Restlessness or anxiety
- Patient position (preference for sitting up)
- Altered mental status
- Abdominal breathing (diaphragm only)
- Increased or decreased breathing rate
- Increased pulse rate (increased or decreased pulse rate in infants and children)

Visual

- Skin color (blue-gray, pale, flushed), temperature (cool), or condition (clammy) changes
- Unusual anatomy (barrel chest)
- Retractions/use of accessory muscles

Auditory

- Noisy breathing
- Inability to speak due to breathing efforts
- Coughing
- Irregular breathing rhythm
- Unequal breath sounds

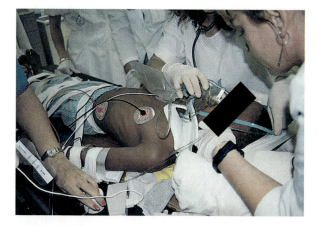

Fig. 17-3 Note the retractions between the ribs of this near-hanging victim.

(increased or decreased pulse rate in infants and children). Changes in skin color inside the eyelids or around the mucous membranes from the normal pink to blue or pale are another sign that the patient is not receiving enough oxygen.

The use of accessory muscles, chest wall retractions (Fig. 17-3), and nasal flaring (Fig. 17-4) are all signs that a patient is working very hard to breathe. Infants and children may use their accessory muscles even in normal breathing, but excessive use of accessory muscles indicates a respiratory problem. A seesaw pattern of breathing, in which the chest and the abdomen move in opposite directions, especially in infants and children, is another sign of difficulty.

Patients usually assume a position of comfort,

which allows them to breathe the easiest. Patients with difficulty breathing often insist on sitting up.

Some types of respiratory disease result from incomplete exhalation, causing air to be trapped in the lungs. Such diseases often change the chest's shape over time, making it look barrel shaped. A patient with a barrel chest most likely has been experiencing a respiratory disorder for many years (Fig. 17-5). These patients may tell you that they have a history of emphysema, bronchitis, or chronic obstructive pulmonary disease.

Normal breathing is silent. Any patient who has noisy breathing has a respiratory or airway problem. Noisy breathing can result in many different sounds. Patients can make snoring or gurgling noises, crowing noises, or have audible wheezing. **Stridor** is a harsh sound heard during breathing (usually inhalation) that indicates an upper airway obstruction. The obstruction may be caused by narrowed passageways due to swelling, mucous, disease, or the presence of a foreign body. Stridor often indicates that there is a potentially life-threatening airway problem, especially in children. Different breathing sounds have been given various names, but these names are not as important as recognizing that the patient is having difficulty breathing and needs oxygen and constant reassessment.

People near the moment of death occasionally have gasping respirations for a few breaths. These respirations are sudden, short inspirations with long pauses in between. These are called *agonal respirations* and should not be confused with normal breathing. If a patient has no pulse and has agonal respirations, begin cardiopulmonary resuscitation.

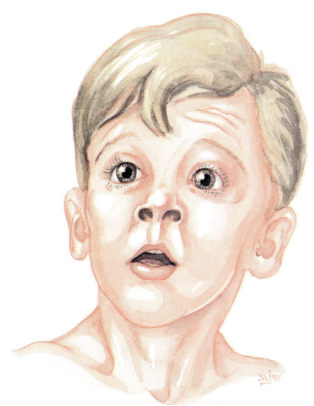

Fig. 17-4 Nasal flaring is a sign of difficult breathing.

FOCUSED HISTORY AND PHYSICAL EXAMINATION

During the focused history and physical examination for medical patients, ask patients pertinent questions about their medical history and the history of the present illness. In the SAMPLE history, find out more about the patient's present illness by using the acronym *OPQRST*. Ask patients about the *O*nset of the breathing difficulty, ask if they have a history of respiratory problems and how long they have had them. Ask patients about *P*rovocation— what makes the distress worse? Ask about the *Q*uality of the distress—what does the pain feel like? Do they feel a sharp stabbing pain with breathing or feel unable to catch their breath? *R*adiation generally refers to pain, so if there is pain when the patient breathes in or out, ask if it moves anywhere else. *S*everity is usually rated on a scale from one to 10, with one denoting only mild distress, and 10 meaning the worst distress the patient has ever felt. Severity may change with time and level of activity. Ask what *T*ime the distress started, or how long the distress has lasted. This is valuable information to relay to the receiving facility and when consulting medical direction.

Also ask the patients if they have taken any

medication to relieve the distress. If so, ask when they took the medication and whether it helped relieve the distress. Be sure to report to the receiving hospital any medications the patient has

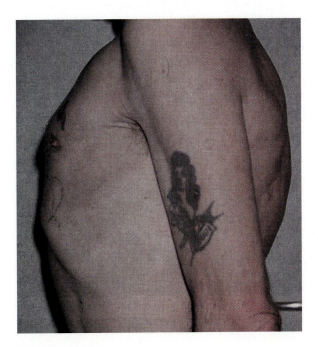

Fig. 17-5 Barrel chest.

taken and their effect. Ask the patients if they have an inhaler prescribed for respiratory distress. The use of prescribed inhalers is discussed later in this chapter.

Patients also may suffer from breathing difficulty related to a traumatic event. The elements of the assessment are the same, but a rapid trauma assessment must be completed and the patient immobilized if the mechanism of injury suggests potential injury to the spine.

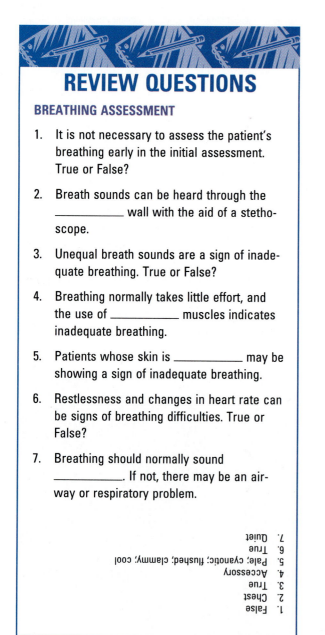

REVIEW QUESTIONS

BREATHING ASSESSMENT

1. It is not necessary to assess the patient's breathing early in the initial assessment. True or False?

2. Breath sounds can be heard through the _____ wall with the aid of a stethoscope.

3. Unequal breath sounds are a sign of inadequate breathing. True or False?

4. Breathing normally takes little effort, and the use of _____ muscles indicates inadequate breathing.

5. Patients whose skin is _____ may be showing a sign of inadequate breathing.

6. Restlessness and changes in heart rate can be signs of breathing difficulties. True or False?

7. Breathing should normally sound _____. If not, there may be an airway or respiratory problem.

7. Quiet
6. True
5. Pale; cyanotic; flushed; clammy; cool
4. Accessory
3. True
2. Chest
1. False

EMERGENCY MEDICAL CARE

OXYGEN

Oxygen is the first medication to administer to any patient in respiratory distress. Oxygen should be given to the patient as soon as possible after you recognize that the patient is having difficulty breathing.

Place a nonrebreather mask on the patient with oxygen flowing at a rate of 15 L/min (Fig. 17-6). Use a nasal cannula only for patients who cannot tolerate a mask on their face. Chapter 7, "The Airway," describes the technique for placing a patient on oxygen via a nonrebreather mask or nasal cannula. If there are any special patient considerations, such as specific respiratory diseases or a patient who is already on oxygen at home, contact medical direction for guidance.

Infants and children have less tolerance for an interruption in their oxygen supply. Whenever possible, infants and children who are breathing but have respiratory distress should be allowed to remain with their parents and to sit in a position they choose. Removing children from their parents only causes further distress, worsening the respiratory emergency. Have parents assist in keeping their children calm. Children in general do not like having an oxygen mask placed over their faces and may fight against leaving it in place. Parents can also assist by holding the oxygen supply close to the child's mouth and nose.

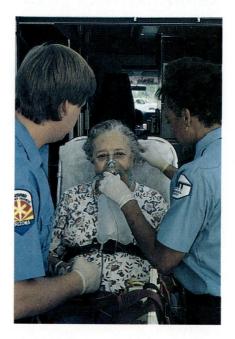

Fig. 17-6 Use a nonrebreather mask to deliver oxygen at 15 L/min.

POSITION AND TRANSPORT

Patients having respiratory emergencies can quickly deteriorate into respiratory or cardiac arrest. Patients who are experiencing respiratory difficulty need to be transported rapidly to the emergency department. Patients should be transported in the position they find the most comfortable. Most patients experiencing difficulty breathing cannot tolerate lying flat on their back and prefer to sit upright.

ARTIFICIAL VENTILATION

Be prepared to ventilate patients who may stop breathing or who cannot maintain adequate breathing on their own. If the patient is making gurgling noises and cannot clear the secretions from the airway, use suction. See Chapter 7, "The Airway," for additional information on airway obstructions and suction.

As an EMT you have a variety of methods to artificially ventilate a patient, including mouth-to-mask, bag-valve-mask, and flow-restricted oxygen-powered ventilation devices. (Patients who are intubated also require artificial ventilation; *see* Chapter 33, "Advanced Airway Techniques," for further information.) Always use body substance isolation precautions when ventilating a patient.

When artificially ventilating a patient, continually assess the adequacy of those ventilations. In adequately ventilated patients, the chest rises and falls equally with each breath delivered. Make sure the rate is appropriate for the patient's age. Ideally, the patient's heart rate and skin color, temperature, and condition should return to normal as you provide the oxygen the body was lacking. In patients in cardiac arrest or with other serious underlying medical conditions, the heart rate may not return to normal and the skin may not be perfused despite adequate ventilation.

Inadequate ventilations do not make the chest rise enough, if at all. The heart rate may be too slow or too fast or not improve with further ventilation. If the ventilations do not seem to be adequate, take steps to correct the procedure being used for ventilation. See Chapter 7, "The Airway," for a detailed description of the procedures used to ventilate patients.

INHALERS

With patients who have a prescribed inhaler, you may be able to assist with its use. During the focused history and physical examination, ask patients if they have an inhaler prescribed by a physician. Inhalers are not carried on the Basic Life Support EMS unit, but you can assist patients in using a prescribed inhaler after consulting medical direction.

Prescribed inhalers administer a variety of medications (Fig. 17-7). Most of these medications belong to a class of drugs known as *beta-agonist bronchodilators*. These medications are delivered to the tissues of the lungs as the patient inhales from the inhaler. The medication is absorbed into the tissues of the lungs, generally dilating the bronchioles to decrease resistance inside the airways. Prescribed inhalers are also sometimes called *metered-dose inhalers*. The device delivers a set amount of medication with each push of the cartridge. Generic names for the medication in inhalers include albuterol, isoetharine, and metaproteranol. Trade names for these medications are numerous, including Proventil, Ventolin, Bronkosol, Bronkometer, Alupent, and Metaprel. Other medications (mostly steroids for lung inflammation) are also available in inhalers. Always consult medical direction before assisting a patient with administration. Some inhalers may not be appropriate for use for a patient in severe respiratory distress.

Chapter 16, "General Pharmacology," explains how medications are used based on their indications. The indications for the use of prescribed inhalers must include the following criteria:

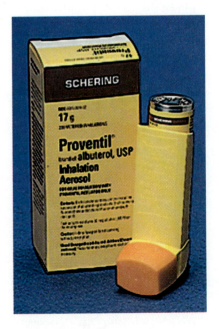

Fig. 17-7 Typical inhaler device.

1. Patients have the signs and symptoms of a respiratory emergency. Patients may exhibit any of the signs described earlier or complain of any of the symptoms of respiratory distress.
2. Patients must have their own physician-prescribed inhaler.
3. You must obtain specific authorization from medical direction to aid patients in inhaled medication administration. This authorization may be in the form of on-line medical direction (speaking directly to the physician on the phone or radio) or off-line medical direction (protocols or standing orders).

The use of a prescribed inhaler is contraindicated (ie, not recommended for use) in a patient who is not oriented enough to use the device properly. A patient who is not oriented may be unable to inhale the medication deeply enough into the lungs to be effective. Patients should also not use an inhaler that was prescribed for someone else. Although they may feel their illness is similar to that of someone else who has a prescribed inhaler, a thorough evaluation by a physician is necessary to know if an inhaler would be helpful for the patient. Assisting a patient with inhaled medication is also contraindicated in situations with a lack of approval, either on- or off-line, from medical direction. Finally, the use of an inhaler is contraindicated if the patient has already taken the maximum recommended dose before you arrived. The maximum recommended dose for an inhaler is determined by the number of inhalations ordered by the medical direction physician or the number of inhalations stated on the prescription.

Patients with a prescribed inhaler usually are familiar with its use. Patients may require assist-ance to administer their medication (Fig. 17-8). Principle Box 17-1 describes how to administer medication from a prescribed inhaler.

If the patient has a spacer device to use with the inhaler, it should be used. Spacers are attachments between the inhaler and the patient that allow for more effective use of the medication. In some situations, a patient may not be able to inhale deeply enough to breathe in all of the medication in one breath. Spacers are used to contain the medication after it is released from the metered dose inhaler until the patient can inhale it (Fig. 17-9).

Many children have respiratory diseases that may require the use of an inhaler. Few children less than 6 or 7 years of age can use inhalers correctly because of the coordination required. Children more than 12 years of age commonly use inhalers, sometimes with spacers. Middle school and high school children commonly use inhalers, generally without spacers. The indications and contraindications for use of inhalers are the same for an ill child as for an adult.

Side effects are undesired effects of a medication. The side effects of prescribed inhalers include increased pulse rate, tremors, nervousness, and sometimes nausea. Side effects should always be documented in the prehospital care report and reported to the receiving facility.

Patients must be reassessed after any intervention. Vital signs should be assessed before and after administering any medications and after the focused history and physical examination are repeated. Details of the administration of the medication should be communicated to the receiving facility staff and documented in the prehospital care report. For more information about communication and documentation, see Chapter 14, "Communications" and Chapter 15, "Documentation."

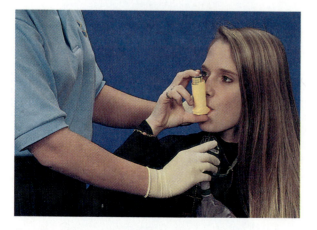

Fig. 17-8 Have the patient inhale deeply and hold his or her breath so the medication can be absorbed.

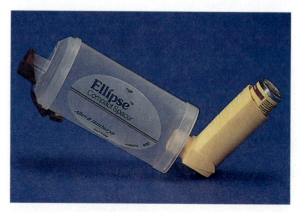

Fig. 17-9 An inhaler with a spacer.

PRINCIPLE 17-1
Assisting Patients With a Prescribed Inhaler

1. Have an on- or off-line order from medical direction.

2. Assure that the medication has been prescribed for the patient, that the medication is designed to be inhaled, and that the patient is alert enough to use the inhaler.

3. Check the expiration date of the inhaler.

4. Ask the patient if any doses have already been taken, and compare that with the prescribed dose.

5. Ensure that the inhaler is at room temperature or warmer. If the inhaler is cold, it may not deliver an accurate dose when the medication is delivered. Consult medical direction.

6. Shake the inhaler vigorously several times, and remove any protective caps.

7. Remove the oxygen mask from the patient, have the patient exhale deeply, pushing as much air from the lungs as possible. If the patient has a nasal cannula in place, it does not need to be removed for administration of the inhaler.

8. Have the patient place the lips around the mouthpiece, which is the opening of the inhaler.

9. Have the patient begin to inhale slowly and deeply, and depress the hand-held inhaler.

10. Have the patient hold his or her breath for as long as is comfortable so the medication can be absorbed.

11. Replace the oxygen mask on the patient.

12. Record the time, dose, medication, vital signs, and any change in the patient's condition after assisting with the medication.

13. Allow the patient to breathe a few times, and repeat a second dose if ordered by medical direction.

REVIEW QUESTIONS
EMERGENCY MEDICAL CARE

1. Patients who are having difficulty breathing do not require immediate intervention because they can tolerate this condition for long periods of time. True or False?

2. _____ is the first medication that should be delivered to all patients with respiratory distress.

3. Artificial ventilations need to be assessed for adequacy the same as a patient's own breathing would be assessed. True or False?

4. Prescribed inhalers should not be used in the emergency medical care of children. True or False?

5. List at least three of the side effects of inhalers.

1. False
2. Oxygen
3. True
4. False
5. Increased pulse rate; tremors; nervousness; nausea

CHAPTER SUMMARY

RESPIRATORY SYSTEM REVIEW

Air passes through the mouth, nose, pharynx, trachea, and bronchi, and into the alveoli. Once in the alveoli, oxygen enters the bloodstream through the capillaries and then is delivered to the cells of the body. The cells of the body give carbon dioxide to the capillaries. From there, carbon dioxide is returned to the alveoli. Infants and children have smaller airways and larger tongues, and, therefore, their airways can become occluded more easily. Older patients often have underlying respiratory diseases.

BREATHING ASSESSMENT

The assessment of breathing is vitally important so that you can intervene if breathing is inadequate.

Adequate breathing means that the lungs and chest wall expand equally on both sides, adequate air is entering the lungs, the depth of breathing is adequate, and it takes little effort to breathe. There are many signs of inadequate breathing, including irregular rhythm, poor quality, and the use of accessory muscles. If a patient has any signs or symptoms of difficulty breathing, immediate action should be taken to correct the problem. Assessment includes the focused history and physical examination, and the SAMPLE history using *OPQRST*.

EMERGENCY MEDICAL CARE

Oxygen should be delivered to all patients with respiratory problems. Artificial ventilations must also be assessed for adequacy. Inhalers can be used if the patient has a prescription from the physician, the patient is alert enough to use it, permission has been received from medical direction, and signs and symptoms of respiratory distress are present. Side effects include nervousness, tremors, and increased heart rate. Older children often have inhalers. The indications and procedures for use in children are the same as for adults.

UNITED STATES DEPARTMENT OF TRANSPORTATION NATIONAL HIGHWAY TRAFFIC SAFETY ADMINISTRATION EMT–BASIC OBJECTIVES

Check your knowledge. The National Registry of EMTs and many state EMS agencies use the objectives below to develop EMT–Basic certification examinations. Can you meet them?

COGNITIVE

1. List the structure and function of the respiratory system.
2. State the signs and symptoms of a patient with breathing difficulty.
3. Describe the emergency medical care of the patient with breathing difficulty.
4. Recognize the need for medical direction to assist in the emergency medical care of the patient with breathing difficulty.
5. Describe the emergency medical care of the patient with breathing distress.
6. Establish the relationship between airway management and the patient with breathing difficulty.
7. List the signs of adequate air exchange.
8. State the generic name, medication forms, dose, administration, action, indications, and contraindications for prescribed inhalers.
9. Distinguish between the emergency medical care for the infant, child, and adult patient with breathing difficulty.
10. Differentiate between upper airway obstruction and lower airway disease in the infant and child patient.

AFFECTIVE

1. Defend EMT–Basic treatment regimens for various respiratory emergencies.
2. Explain the rationale for administering an inhaler.

PSYCHOMOTOR

1. Demonstrate the emergency medical care for breathing difficulty.
2. Perform the steps for facilitating the use of an inhaler.

18 CARDIOVASCULAR EMERGENCIES

Angina: The discomfort felt when the heart does not receive enough oxygen. It is commonly experienced after exertion, and the patient usually feels better with rest and/or medication.

Diastolic blood pressure: The measurement of the pressure in an artery when the ventricles are at rest.

Electrodes: The remote pads that are attached to the defibrillator with lead wires and attached to the patient to monitor the electrical activity within the heart.

Ischemia: A decreased oxygen supply to an area of tissue.

Peripheral: A term referring to the extremities.

Pulse: The pressure wave felt in an artery when the left ventricle contracts.

Systolic blood pressure: The measurement of the pressure in an artery when the ventricles are contracting.

Ventricular fibrillation: A chaotic electrical rhythm in the ventricles. There is no ventricular contraction or pumping of blood through the heart, and therefore no pulse.

Ventricular tachycardia: Three or more heart beats in a row at 100 beats or more per minute originating in the ventricles and overriding the normal pacemaker of the heart. In this state, the atria and ventricles do not work together. A pulse may or may not be present.

IN THE FIELD

EMTs Martin and Vanita were dispatched to the home of a 65-year-old woman who was responsive, breathing, and experiencing chest pain. En route to the scene they considered what information they needed to obtain when they arrived. Had anything caused the chest pain? What kind of pain was it? Did anything help relieve the pain? When did the pain start? Did the patient have a history of heart disease?

On arrival, Vanita immediately noticed the patient was sweating profusely and her breathing was labored. The patient said she felt a crushing sensation in her chest, and the tightness was making it difficult for her to catch her breath. Vanita questioned the patient and discovered that she had a history of heart disease and that the pain had started approximately 4 hours ago and did not subside after resting. She had taken one of her own nitroglycerin tablets but experienced no relief.

As Martin took the patient's vital signs and administered high-flow oxygen with a nonrebreather mask, Vanita decided that the patient would benefit by taking an additional nitroglycerin tablet. She contacted the medical direction physician and received an order to assist with the nitroglycerin. The patient felt some relief. They continued monitoring her vital signs and began transport immediately.

Cardiac emergencies are the most prominent type of medical emergency in the United States today. Cardiovascular disease leads to over 600,000 deaths in the United States each year, with half of those deaths attributed to coronary artery disease. Up to 50% of heart attack victims suffer a cardiac arrest, and up to 50% of these arrests occur outside the hospital. Many of these victims can be saved if EMS systems can provide early CPR and early defibrillation.

REVIEW OF THE CIRCULATORY SYSTEM

ANATOMY

The heart is more than just a muscle. The heart contains specialized tissue that generates electrical impulses on its own. These electrical impulses can be seen with the use of a cardiac monitor.

The heart has four chambers. The two upper (superior) chambers are the atria, and the two lower (inferior) chambers are the ventricles. The right atrium receives oxygen-poor blood from the veins of the body and the heart and pumps oxygen-poor blood to the right ventricle. The right ventricle pumps the blood to the lungs via the pulmonary artery to become saturated with oxygen. The blood flows from the lungs into the left atrium via the pulmonary veins, and the left atrium pumps the blood into the left ventricle. The left ventricle pumps the oxygen-rich blood out through the aorta to the body. Valves in the heart between each of the chambers and major blood vessels prevent the backflow of blood (Fig. 18-1).

BLOOD VESSELS

Arteries carry blood away from the heart to the rest of the body. The aorta is the major artery that originates from the heart; it lies in front of the spine in the thoracic and abdominal cavities. The aorta divides at the level of the navel into the iliac arteries, which supply the pelvis and lower extremities with oxygen-rich blood. The pulmonary artery originates at the right ventricle and carries the oxygen-poor blood to the lungs. The coronary arteries supply the heart muscle with blood (Fig. 18-2).

The carotid arteries are the major arteries located in the neck, and they supply the head with blood. The pulsations of these arteries can be felt on either side of the neck. The artery of the upper arm is the brachial artery, and its pulsations can be palpated on the inside of the arm between the elbow and the shoulder. This artery is used for assessing blood pressure using a blood pressure cuff

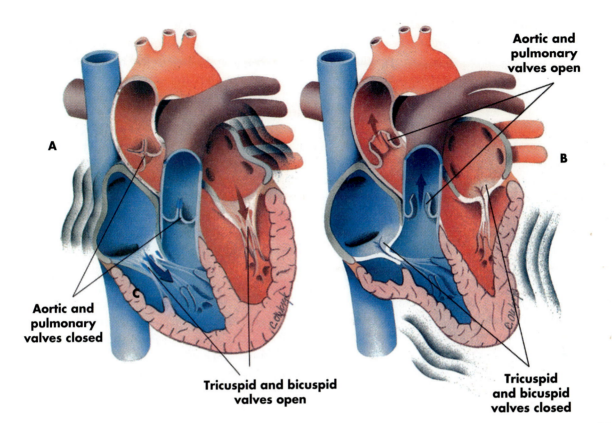

Aortic and pulmonary valves open

A

B

Aortic and pulmonary valves closed

Tricuspid and bicuspid valves open

Tricuspid and bicuspid valves closed

Fig. 18-1   Blood flow through the heart. **A,** The atria pump blood into the ventricles. **B,** The ventricles pump blood to the lungs and rest of the body.

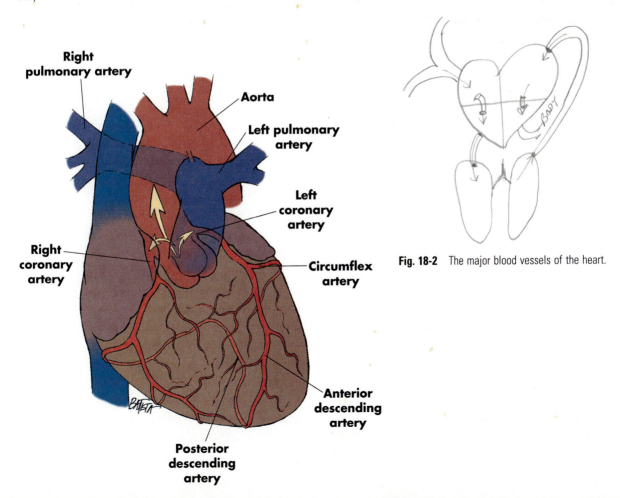

Right pulmonary artery

Aorta

Left pulmonary artery

Left coronary artery

Right coronary artery

Circumflex artery

Anterior descending artery

Posterior descending artery

Fig. 18-2   The major blood vessels of the heart.

(sphygmomanometer) and a stethoscope. The major arteries of the lower arm are the radial arteries, and their pulsations can be felt at the thumb side of the wrist. The femoral arteries are the major arteries of the thigh and supply the groin and the lower extremities with blood. Pulsations from these arteries can be palpated in the groin area. The arteries of the lower leg and foot include the posterior tibial artery, which can be palpated on the posterior surface of the medial malleolus, and the dorsalis pedis, which can be palpated on the anterior surface of the foot (Fig. 18-3).

Arterioles are the smallest branches of arteries, and lead into the capillaries. Capillaries are the tiny blood vessels that connect arterioles to venules. They are found in all parts of the body and allow for the exchange of oxygen, nutrients, and waste with body cells. The venules are the smallest branches of veins, which lead away from the capillaries and into the veins.

The major function of the veins is to carry blood back to the heart. The pulmonary vein carries oxygen-rich blood from the lungs to the left atrium to be pumped to the body. The vena cava has two branches: the inferior vena cava, which carries oxygen-poor blood from the lower half of the body and the torso; and the superior vena cava, which carries oxygen-poor blood from the head and arms. Blood flows from both branches into the right atrium.

BLOOD COMPOSITION

Blood is composed of red blood cells, white blood cells, plasma, and platelets. Red blood cells give the blood its color and carry oxygen to organs and carbon dioxide away from organs. White blood cells are part of the body's defense against infections. Plasma, the largest component of the blood, is the fluid that carries the blood cells and nutrients. Platelets are cells that are essential for the formation of blood clots as part of the body's way to stop bleeding. Table 18-1 summarizes the functions of blood components.

PHYSIOLOGY

When the left ventricle contracts, sending a wave of blood through the arteries, a pulse can be felt. The **pulse** can be palpated anywhere an artery passes near the skin surface and over a bone. The preferred sites to palpate **peripheral** pulses are at the extremities: radial artery in the wrist, the brachial artery in the upper arm, and the posterior tibial artery or the dorsalis pedis artery, both located in the foot. The most common central sites for palpating pulses are the carotid artery in the neck and the femoral artery in the groin area (Fig. 18-4).

When blood pressure is assessed, the **systolic** value (top number) is the pressure in the artery when the ventricles contract. The **diastolic** value (bottom number) is the pressure in the artery when the ventricles are at rest.

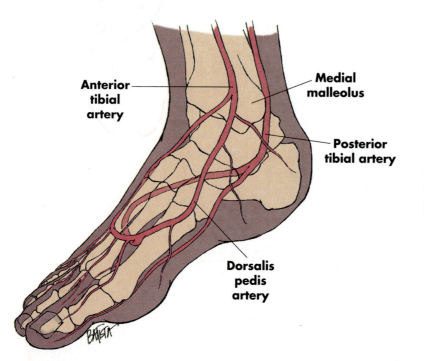

Fig. 18-3 The posterior tibial pulse can be palpated on the posterior surface of the medial malleolus. The dorsalis pedis pulse can be palpated on the anterior surface of the foot.

Anterior tibial artery

Medial malleolus

Posterior tibial artery

Dorsalis pedis artery

TABLE 18-1	Blood Component Functions
BLOOD COMPONENT	**FUNCTION**
Red blood cells	Give blood its color Carry oxygen to organs Carry carbon dioxide away from organs
White blood cells	Part of body's immune system Help fight infection
Plasma	Fluid that carries the blood cells and nutrients
Platelets	Essential for the formation of clots

When a person has inadequate circulation, sometimes due to a reduction in total blood volume, the organs and tissues do not receive enough oxygen. The vital processes of the body are progressively depressed. This state is also known as *shock* (hypoperfusion). Shock may be characterized

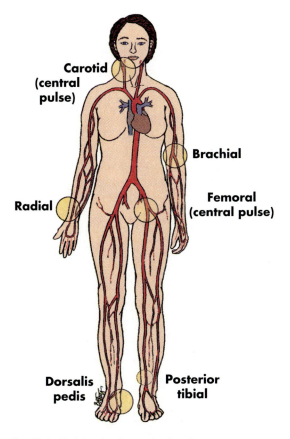

Fig. 18-4   Peripheral and central pulse sites.

Carotid (central pulse)

Brachial

Radial

Femoral (central pulse)

Dorsalis pedis

Posterior tibial

BOX 18-1

Signs and Symptoms of Shock (Hypoperfusion)

- Rapid and weak pulse
- Pale or cyanotic skin
- Cool, clammy skin
- Rapid and shallow breathing
- Restlessness and anxiety
- Mental dullness, confusion
- Nausea, vomiting, and thirst
- Low or decreasing blood pressure (usually a late sign)
- Subnormal temperature

ALERT

Blood pressure remains normal early in shock as the body tries to compensate. Low blood pressure is a late sign of shock (hypoperfusion), and rapid transport is required. Never rely solely on blood pressure, normal or low, to determine whether a patient has the signs and symptoms of shock.

by a wide range of signs and symptoms, which are listed in Box 18-1.

Chapter 25, "Bleeding and Shock," provides more detailed information and treatment guidelines for patients with the signs and symptoms of shock.

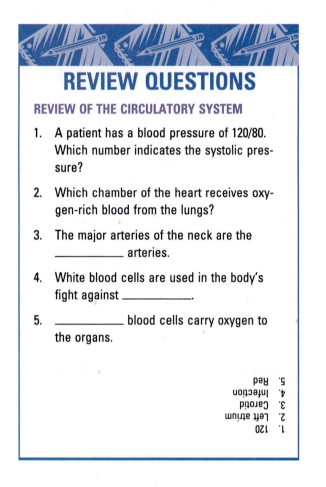

REVIEW QUESTIONS

REVIEW OF THE CIRCULATORY SYSTEM

1. A patient has a blood pressure of 120/80. Which number indicates the systolic pressure?

2. Which chamber of the heart receives oxygen-rich blood from the lungs?

3. The major arteries of the neck are the _____ arteries.

4. White blood cells are used in the body's fight against _____.

5. _____ blood cells carry oxygen to the organs.

1. 120
2. Left atrium
3. Carotid
4. Infection
5. Red

CARDIAC COMPROMISE

Patients with chest discomfort, shortness of breath, anxiety, indigestion, and nausea may be experiencing **angina** or a heart attack. The chest discomfort results from **ischemia,** an area of heart muscle that is not receiving enough oxygen. Angina is a condition that produces chest discomfort upon exertion or activity that usually goes away with rest and/or nitroglycerin. No actual damage is done to the heart muscle. A heart attack, on the other hand, is a condition in which there is blockage in one of the blood vessels of the heart. The muscle tissue beyond the blockage is oxygen-deprived and tissue damage occurs. In most cases, you

can not know how severe the actual problem is but should give treatment based on the patient's signs and symptoms. With either angina or a heart attack, the patient is experiencing some type of cardiac compromise, ranging from minor reversible discomfort to extreme discomfort that is a result of major damage to the heart muscle.

Specific signs and symptoms of cardiac compromise are listed in Box 18-2. Respiratory pain is usually a sharp, stabbing pain that increases with respiration or movement and is generally localized to a specific area. Cardiac pain usually does not change with movement or palpation and is described as a crushing or pressure pain. Cardiac pain may occur also in the shoulder, neck, and/or jaw area or may move from one area to another (radiating pain). Patients often deny that the pain they are experiencing might be due to a heart problem.

ASSESSMENT

The initial assessment of a patient with cardiac compromise includes forming a general impression and assessing the patient's airway, breathing, and circulation, and the patient priority. High-flow oxygen should be administered. If the patient is

BOX 18-2

Signs and Symptoms of Cardiac Compromise

- Squeezing, dull pressure or pain in the chest that commonly radiates to the arms, neck, jaw, or upper back
- Sudden onset of sweating
- Difficulty breathing
- Anxiety or irritability
- Feeling of impending doom
- Abnormal and sometimes irregular pulse rate (high or low)
- Abnormal blood pressure (different from the patient's normal blood pressure)
- Epigastric pain or discomfort in the abdomen (severe indigestion)
- Nausea or vomiting

responsive and has a known history of cardiac problems, perform the initial assessment and the focused history and physical examination. Place the patient in the position of comfort and assess the baseline vital signs. If the patient is complaining of chest pain or discomfort, ask the *OPQRST* questions:

- *Onset.* When did the pain begin? Once it started, how long did it take to reach its highest level?
- *Provocation.* What were you doing when it started? What makes it worse or better? Does it hurt on inspiration or expiration?
- *Quality.* Describe the pain. What does the pain feel like?
- *Radiation.* Does the pain move anywhere such as the arms, neck, jaw, or back?
- *Severity.* How bad is the pain? On a scale of one to 10, 10 meaning the worst pain you've ever felt, what do you rate it? (Ask the same question after care is provided. This results in a trending of patient information.)
- *Time.* How long have you had the pain; has it been steady or did it come and go?

The answers to these questions provide important information to the receiving facility about the patient and may help the medical direction physician determine the seriousness of the situation and whether the pain is cardiac in nature.

Ask if the patient has a prescription for nitroglycerin and if the nitroglycerin is nearby now. If the patient has nitroglycerin available and the patient's systolic blood pressure is greater than 100 mm Hg, you may assist the patient with taking one dose after consulting medical direction, as described in the next section.

EMERGENCY MEDICAL CARE

Emergency medical care for the patient experiencing chest pain may include CPR and automated external defibrillation, oxygen and positioning, and nitroglycerin. These procedures are described in the following sections.

OXYGEN AND POSITIONING

As soon as you have determined that the responsive patient may be experiencing cardiac compromise, place the patient in a position of comfort and give high-flow oxygen via a nonrebreather mask at a rate of 15 L/min. Patients often feel more comfortable sitting up than lying down when they are experiencing chest pain or difficulty breathing.

NITROGLYCERIN

If you learn in the focused history that the patient has a prescription for nitroglycerin, you may assist the patient in taking one dose after receiving an order from medical direction.

Nitroglycerin (generic name) is commonly called *nitro*. EMT–Basics can assist with the administration of nitroglycerin in the tablet and sublingual spray forms (0.3–0.4 mg) (Fig. 18-5). Nitroglycerin acts to dilate blood vessels and to decrease the workload of the heart, therefore producing some relief to patients experiencing chest pain or discomfort. These actions may result in a decrease in blood pressure.

Table 18-2 lists vital information about nitroglycerin. It is extremely important to know the indications, contraindications, side effects, dosage, actions, and administration techniques of any medication with which you assist the patient.

Before assisting a patient with nitroglycerin, find out what that patient's prescribed dosage is and how many doses (if any) the patient has taken before your arrival, by what route it was taken, and what effect it has had. If the patient has more nitroglycerin, perform a focused assessment, assess all vital signs, and ensure that the systolic blood pressure is greater than 100 mm Hg. Contact medical direction.

Assure that the nitroglycerin is for the right pa-

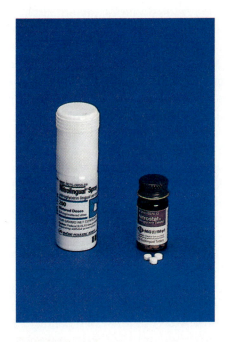

Fig. 18-5 Nitroglycerin in tablet and sublingual spray forms.

TABLE 18-2		Nitroglycerin	
INDICATIONS	**CONTRAINDICATIONS**	**MECHANISM OF ACTION**	**SIDE EFFECTS**
Signs and symptoms of cardiac chest pain **AND**	Patient has systolic blood pressure < 100 mm Hg **OR**	Relaxes vascular smooth muscle to increase coronary blood flow	Lowers blood pressure
Patient has physician-prescribed sublingual tablets or spray **AND**	Patient does not have own nitroglycerin that is prescribed by a medical doctor **OR**	Causes decrease of blood return to the heart to decrease the heart's workload	Headache
EMT–Basic has approval from medical direction physician	Patient has a head injury or is not mentally alert **OR**		Pulse rate changes (may drop dramatically)
	Patient is an infant or child **OR**		Burning sensation on or under the tongue
	Patient has already taken the maximum prescribed dosage prior to EMT–Basic arrival		

tient, the right route of administration (sublingual), the right dose (0.3–0.4 mg), and the right medication (nitroglycerin spray or tablet). Always check the expiration date of the medication, and inform the medical direction physician if it is expired. Nitroglycerin tablets tend to lose their potency quickly once the bottle has been opened and exposed to light. If nitroglycerin is not a part of standing orders, obtain an order from the medical direction physician to assist with the administration of nitroglycerin. The patient must be responsive and alert. You may assist with up to three doses (one dose every 3–5 min) if the patient has no relief, if the systolic blood pressure remains above 100 mm Hg, and if each dose is authorized by the medical direction physician.

Put the patient in a seated position then assist with the nitroglycerin. If the blood pressure drops after administering the nitroglycerin, place the patient in Trendelenburg's (with feet up) position. Reassess the vital signs and chest pain, and if there is no change, you can assist with a second dose 3 to 5 minutes later after consulting medical direction. Once again, reassess vital signs and chest pain. If still symptomatic, consult medical direction for authorization for a third dose. Continue to reassess the patient en route to the receiving facility, and notify the medical direction physician of any changes in the patient's condition. Treat the patient for the signs and symptoms of shock if the blood pressure drops below 100 systolic. It is critical to record all findings, assessments, and treatments on the prehospital care report, including the medication's time of administration, route, and dose as well as all vital signs (*see* Technique 18-1. Administration of Nitroglycerin). Do not wait to begin transport until after all three doses of nitroglycerin have been administered.

If the patient does not have nitroglycerin, or if the patient has nitroglycerin but the systolic blood pressure is less than 100, do not use the nitroglycerin but continue with the focused assessment. Nitroglycerin acts to dilate blood vessels, thereby increasing the area in which the blood circulates in the body. The blood pressure may drop because less blood is returning to the heart. If a patient takes too much nitroglycerin, the blood pressure may become very low. The patient may experience light-headedness and feel faint. This effect happens more often in elderly and dehydrated patients. Therefore, always monitor the blood pressure and treat for the signs and symptoms of shock if the pressure drops below 100 systolic. Prompt transport is necessary with all cardiac patients, because their condition may worsen suddenly.

See Chapter 15, "Documentation," for more de-

tailed information to document when administering a medication.

BASIC LIFE SUPPORT

All chest pain patients you encounter do not become cardiac arrest patients, but you should always be prepared for that possibility. When a cardiac arrest patient needs to be cared for, you must know basic life-support measures. Always request advanced cardiac life support (ACLS) back-up, if it is available, to continue the chain of survival. As defined by the American Heart Association, the

TECHNIQUE 18-1
Administration of Nitroglycerin

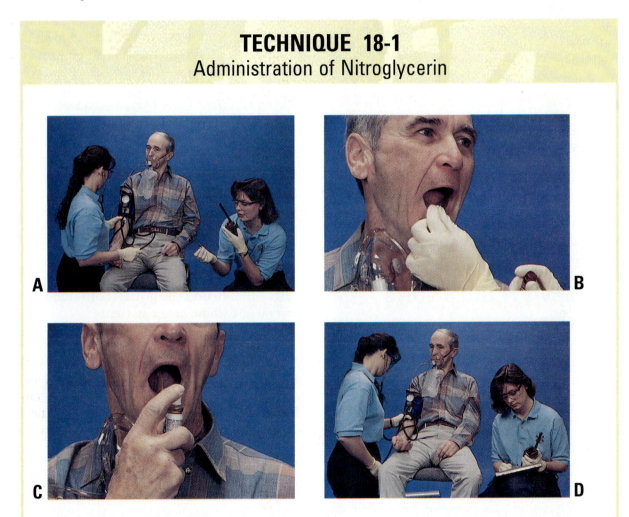

Fig. 18-6   A, Follow appropriate body substance isolation precautions and assess the patient's vital signs. Consult medical direction. Nitroglycerin can be absorbed through the EMT's skin if gloves are not worn, producing a headache. **B, Ask the patient to lift the tongue, and place one tablet under the tongue. C,** If the patient uses nitroglycerin spray, spray one dose (one spray) under the tongue. Have the patient quickly close the mouth. **The patient may be able to place the tablet or spray under the tongue.** Instruct the patient to keep the mouth closed with the tablet under the tongue until it is dissolved and absorbed. The tablet should not be chewed or swallowed. Take the patient's blood pressure within 2 minutes. Record the name of the patient, the name of the medication, the time of administration, the dosage of the drug, and the name of the medical direction physician. **D, Reassess all vital signs and the effect of the medication on the patient's chest pain; record this information.** Contact the medical direction physician with any changes in the patient's condition or to assist with another dose.

chain of survival is a series of critical interventions that includes early access to EMS, early CPR, early defibrillation, and early ACLS.

EMTs rarely perform one-person CPR in the field, except in situations when a partner is getting equipment or is driving to the receiving facility. With a two-person crew, if an arrest occurs en route to the facility, the driver should stop the unit, request back-up, and then assist you with basic life support and defibrillation as needed.

Two-person CPR is an important part of your education. You must also be familiar with the use of automated external defibrillator (described later in this chapter), the use of bag-valve-mask devices with oxygen attached, the use of flow-restricted, oxygen-powered ventilation devices, techniques of lifting and moving patients, suctioning the airway, the use of airway adjuncts, body substance isolation precautions, and techniques for interviewing bystanders and family members to obtain facts related to cardiac arrest events (*see* Chapters 5 through 7).

REVIEW QUESTIONS

CARDIAC COMPROMISE

1. The *O* and the *S* in the patient interviewing technique, *OPQRST*, stand for _____ and _____.

2. A patient with cardiac chest pain may be sweating profusely. True or False?

3. If a patient complains of indigestion, cardiac chest pain is not the problem and can be ruled out. True or False?

4. If the systolic blood pressure is greater than 100 mm Hg and the patient has a prescription, the EMT–Basic may assist the patient with taking _____ after contacting medical direction.

1. Onset; severity 2. True 3. False 4. Nitroglycerin

You must stay current with these principles and techniques and practice them so that you are ready for any situation that may present itself.

THE AUTOMATED EXTERNAL DEFIBRILLATOR

The successful resuscitation of a patient in cardiac arrest outside the hospital depends on the chain of survival including early access, early CPR, early defibrillation, and early ACLS. Early access includes the recognition of an emergency and the response to it. Early CPR includes an effort to open the airway and provide mechanical ventilations and compressions as soon as possible, often by a trained bystander. Early defibrillation includes the recognition and treatment of **ventricular fibrillation**, the most common lethal electrical disturbance in the heart (arrhythmia), and other shockable rhythms. Early ACLS includes providing advanced airway control and intravenous medications rapidly. The resuscitative effort is a continuum of care beginning at a basic level and progressing toward an advanced level as soon as possible. The AED allows for early defibrillation and higher-level care to patients much sooner from basic life-support providers. **Defibrillation is the primary intervention that makes the greatest difference in survival of cardiac arrest patients.**

Many EMS systems across the country have demonstrated that EMS providers can save the lives of cardiac arrest patients who are in ventricular fibrillation with the use of the AED. These EMS systems have added defibrillation to the role of the EMT and, in some cases, to the role of the first responder.

OVERVIEW OF THE AUTOMATED EXTERNAL DEFIBRILLATOR

The AED was developed in the early 1980s and has gained widespread application in the United States. Healthcare providers have been using defibrillation, an electric shock to the heart, for decades as the primary treatment of life-threatening electrical disturbances in the heart. By combining computer technology with the defibrillator, much of the human decision-making and possibility for error has been reduced. The use of an AED can be learned in a short period of time. In the future, these machines may be available in every shopping mall, airport, or hotel, and their use taught in advanced CPR courses.

There are two types of AEDs: fully automatic and semiautomatic. A fully automatic external defibrillator requires the EMT simply to hook up two defibrillatory patches to the patient's chest, connect the leads, and turn on the AED. A semiautomatic external defibrillator requires the EMT to attach the patches and leads to the patient's chest, turn on the AED, and press a button to analyze the rhythm; its computer-synthesized voice then advises you what steps to take based on its analysis of the patient's cardiac rhythm. You then deliver the shocks manually by pressing a button, if advised (Fig. 18-7).

To administer a shock, the AED's computer must detect a life-threatening electrical disturbance in the heart, which is generally a condition known as *ventricular fibrillation.* This patient has no pulse or respirations, and the heart is simply "quivering" inside the chest (Fig. 18-8). The rhythm has electrical activity but does not cause a mechanical pumping action of the heart to produce a pulse.

There are other rhythms that the AED will shock, but these are seldom present on arrival of EMS. One of them, **ventricular tachycardia**, is three or more beats in a row at a rate of 100 beats or more per minute that originate in the ventricles (Fig. 18-9). This rhythm may or may not produce a detectable pulse. This rhythm occurs frequently at the onset of arrest but generally deteriorates quickly to ventricular fibrillation. Both rhythms can be shocked by an AED, but the key is that the patient must be pulseless and apneic before the machine can even be attached to the patient.

Depending on whether the specific AED machine has a screen that shows the patient's rhythm, you may never know or see the patient's rhythm. Therefore, your primary concerns are the absence

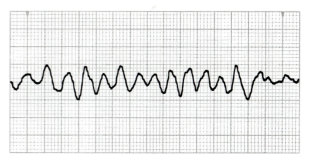

Fig. 18-8   Ventricular fibrillation.

ALERT
The AED should be attached only to patients who are unresponsive and do not have a carotid pulse to avoid delivering inappropriate shocks to patients who actually have a pulse. Shocking a patient with a pulse may put that patient into ventricular fibrillation or into asystole (an unshockable lack of rhythm with no electrical impulses).

or presence of a carotid pulse and following the directions of the AED. Remember that the machine can not detect pulses, only electrical activity within the heart. The electrical activity may or may not be producing a pulse.

These machines are very accurate in detecting both shockable rhythms and rhythms not needing shocks. A correct and accurate analysis by the AED depends on properly charged defibrillator batteries and proper maintenance of the defibrillator. The few documented cases of inappropriate shocks occurring are attributed to human error, such as using the device on a patient with a pulse or activating it in a moving vehicle, and mechanical error, such as low batteries.

CPR should be stopped when the patient's heart rhythm is being analyzed by the AED or shocks are being delivered. Anyone touching the patient, stretcher, or anything attached to the patient may also receive a shock. It is dangerous to be close to the patient when the AED is used. For example, even contact with oxygen tubing that is touching the patient can transmit the high-voltage shock. Do

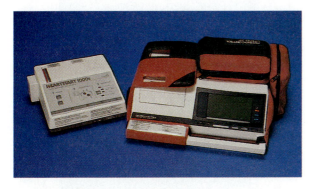

Fig. 18-7   Fully automatic (*left*) and semiautomatic (*right*) external defibrillators.

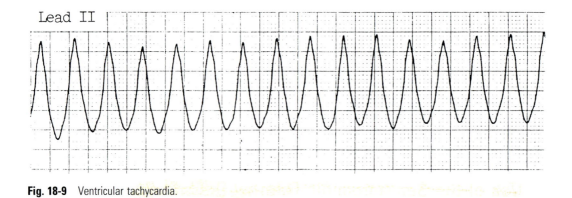

Lead II

Fig. 18-9 Ventricular tachycardia.

not touch the patient when the rhythm is being analyzed because movement may cause discrepancies in the analysis of the rhythm. You should stop CPR and artificial ventilations and stop the ambulance. Defibrillation is a higher priority than CPR, so it is beneficial to the patient to stop CPR to use the AED. CPR may be stopped for up to 90 seconds when three consecutive shocks are delivered. Resume CPR only after the first three shocks are delivered, or when the AED indicates a "no shock" situation.

ADVANTAGES OF THE AUTOMATED EXTERNAL DEFIBRILLATOR

There are many advantages for the use of the AED. The speed of operation is very fast—usually the first shock can be delivered to the patient within 1 minute of arrival at the patient's side. The remote defibrillation uses adhesive pads, making it a "hands-off" process that is safer than conventional ACLS defibrillators. The **electrodes** are larger and easier to place. Some models have an optional rhythm monitoring capability.

OPERATION OF THE AUTOMATED EXTERNAL DEFIBRILLATOR

Always take appropriate body substance isolation precautions. On your arrival at the scene, perform the initial assessment, and if appropriate use the AED.

If an unresponsive medical patient has no pulse, perform CPR and use the automated external defibrillator (AED) for patients who are at least 12 years of age *or* weigh at least 41 kg (90 lbs). If the patient is younger than 12 years of age or weighs less than 41 kg (90 lbs), consult medical direction or follow local protocol regarding use of the AED.

Technique 18-2 describes the steps for AED using a common type of machine. Many AEDs have built-in tape recorders; follow local protocol for taping while using the AED. Figure 18-10 shows the AED with the cables and adhesive pads attached.

Figure 18-12 illustrates a standardized algorithm for AED use.

To use the fully automatic external defibrillator, follow the same procedure. The machine will initiate the shocks automatically. The machine will state "clear the patient" before delivering shocks, or will state "no shock indicated" when appropriate. Follow standard operating procedures in all cases (Box 18-3).

The AED generally is not used for patients less than 12 years of age or patients weighing less than 41 kg (90 lbs). The airway and artificial ventilation are of prime importance in these patients. In young children, cardiac arrest usually results from respiratory compromise, not from cardiac problems. Patients weighing less than 41 kg (90 lbs) may

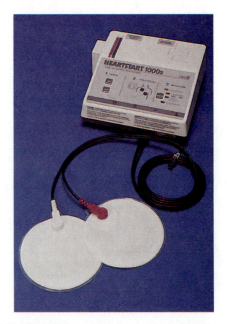

Fig. 18-10 The AED is connected to two pads that are applied to the patient's chest.

TECHNIQUE 18-2
Use of the Semiautomatic External Defibrillator

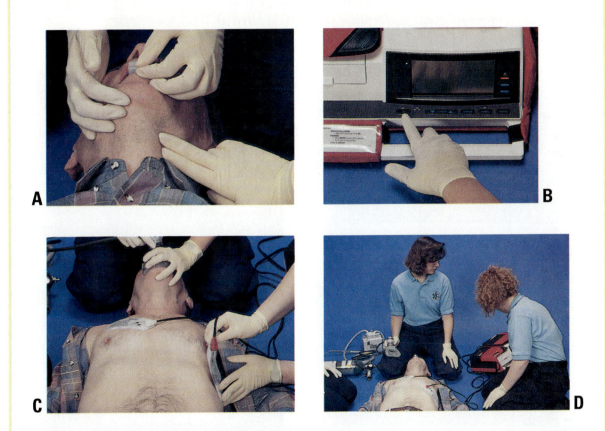

Fig. 18-11   Follow appropriate body substance isolation precautions. **A, Perform the initial assessment and confirm the patient is in cardiac arrest. Stop CPR if it is in progress and verify apnea and pulselessness.** Resume CPR. If you are the only EMT present, proceed with the use of the AED. **B, Turn on the AED's power.** If the machine has a tape recorder, turn it on. **C, Attach the device to the patient. One electrode is placed to the right of the upper portion of the sternum below the clavicle. The other electrode is placed over the ribs to the left of the nipple with the center in the midaxillary line.** Most electrodes include diagrams showing correct placement. **D, Stop CPR, clear everyone away from the patient, and initiate analysis of the rhythm.**

Continued

TECHNIQUE 18-2
Use of the Semiautomatic External Defibrillator

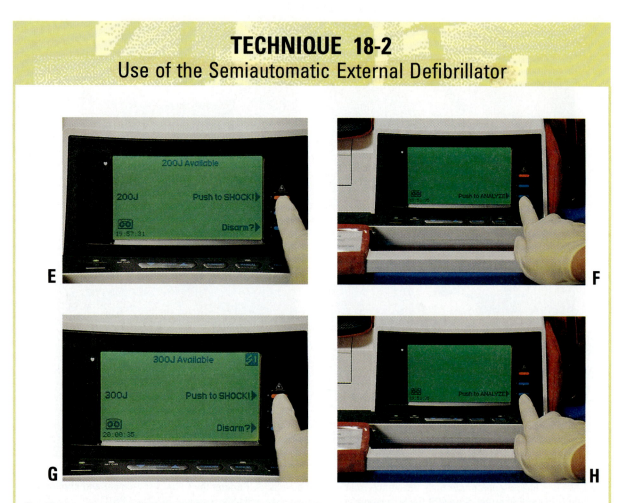

Fig. 18-11 *Continued* **E,** If the machine advises a shock, deliver the first shock (generally 200 J); if not, go to step L. **F,** Reanalyze the rhythm. **G,** If the machine advises another shock, deliver a second shock (at 200–300 J); if not, go to step L. **H,** Reanalyze the rhythm.

TECHNIQUE 18-2
Use of the Semiautomatic External Defibrillator

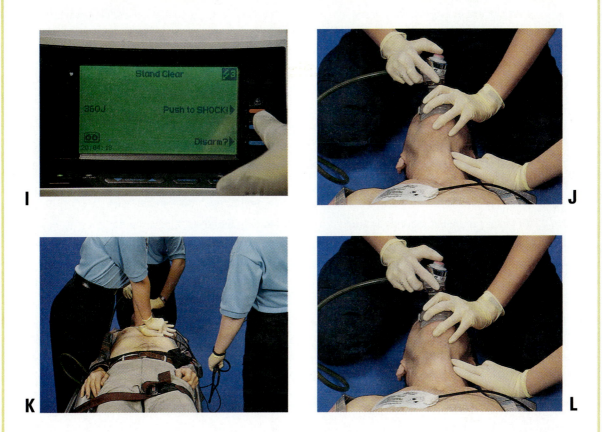

Fig. 18-11 *Continued* **I, If the machine advises another shock, deliver a third shock (at 360 J); if not, go to step L. J, Check the patient's pulse.** If the patient has a pulse, check breathing. If the patient is breathing adequately, provide high-flow oxygen via a nonrebreather mask and transport the patient. If the patient has a pulse and is not breathing adequately, provide artificial ventilations with high-flow oxygen and transport. If the patient does not have a pulse, resume CPR for 1 minute. At the direction of the AED, deliver one more cycle of up to three stacked shocks (at 360 J), and reassess the pulse. If there is no pulse, consult medical direction as to whether to deliver a third set of shocks on scene or en route. **K, Transport the patient with appropriate interventions including CPR, artificial ventilations, or high-flow oxygen as necessary.** If there is a pulse, transport the patient with appropriate emergency medical care. **L, If the machine advises "no shock," check the patient's pulse.** If there is a pulse, check breathing and treat appropriately for adequate or inadequate breathing by ventilating with a bag-valve-mask or providing high-flow oxygen, and transport the patient. If there is no pulse, perform CPR for 1 minute, and then recheck the pulse. Reanalyze the rhythm if there is still no pulse. If "no shock" is again advised and there is still no pulse, resume CPR for 1 minute. Analyze the rhythm a third time. If shock is advised, deliver up to two sets of three stacked shocks separated by 1 minute of CPR, consult the medical direction physician, and transport the patient with appropriate interventions. If "no shock" is advised and the patient still has no pulse, resume CPR. If no ACLS personnel are on scene, transport the patient.

BOX 18-3

Standard Operating Procedures for the Automated External Defibrillator

- If no ACLS personnel are on scene, the patient should be transported when:
  A. Pulse is regained.
  B. Six shocks are delivered (consult the medical direction physician to administer additional sets of shocks on scene or en route).
  C. The machine gives three consecutive messages (separated by 1 minute of CPR) that no shock should be delivered.

- One EMT operates the defibrillator, and the other one performs CPR.

- After opening the airway and confirming an arrest, defibrillation comes first. Don't hook up oxygen or do anything that delays analysis of the rhythm or defibrillation. The first shock should be delivered within 60 seconds of arrival at the patient's side.

- All contact with the patient must be avoided during analysis of rhythm and delivery of shocks. Never analyze the rhythm in a moving vehicle. Stop the vehicle before analyzing it.

- State "clear the patient" before delivering shocks, and verify that everyone is clear.

- No defibrillator can function correctly without properly working batteries. Check the batteries at the beginning of each shift, and carry extra batteries.

- Be familiar with the specific AED devices used in your EMS system.

- If alone when you approach a cardiac arrest victim, use the AED after assessing the ABCs, rather than initiating CPR.

- En route to the receiving facility, as long as the AED advises a shock, continue shocking the patient with sets of three stacked shocks separated by 1 minute of CPR, until the patient regains a pulse or the machine advises "no shock." Stop the vehicle to analyze and to shock.

- Additional shocks may be delivered at the approval of the medical direction physician.

---

receive too high an electrical charge for their size, resulting in damage to the heart.

If the patient does not regain a pulse and there is no available ACLS back-up, deliver a total of six shocks <u>on scene</u> and then prepare to transport. The medical direction physician may advise you to stay on scene if ACLS providers are en route. If additional shocks are ordered en route by the medical direction physician, the vehicle must be stopped completely before the defibrillator can analyze the rhythm. Use of the AED is never safe or appropriate in a moving ambulance.

Ventricular fibrillation may recur following successful shocks. If you are en route with a patient who has been resuscitated but is unresponsive, check pulses every 30 seconds. If at any time the patient becomes pulseless, stop the vehicle and analyze the rhythm. Deliver up to three stacked shocks if indicated, and continue the resuscitation according to your local protocol.

If you are en route with a responsive patient having chest pain who becomes unresponsive, apneic, and pulseless, then stop the vehicle, attach the AED, analyze the rhythm, deliver up to three shocks if indicated, and continue the resuscitation according to your local protocol.

If a situation arises in which you are the only EMT with an AED, take body substance isolation precautions, perform an initial assessment to verify apnea and pulselessness, turn on the AED power, attach the device to the patient, initiate analysis of the rhythm, and deliver a shock if necessary. Follow the local protocol for the remainder of the treatment. Defibrillation should always be the first step before CPR. Do not leave the patient to contact medical direction or to call for assistance until the

Automated External Defibrillation (AED) Algorithm

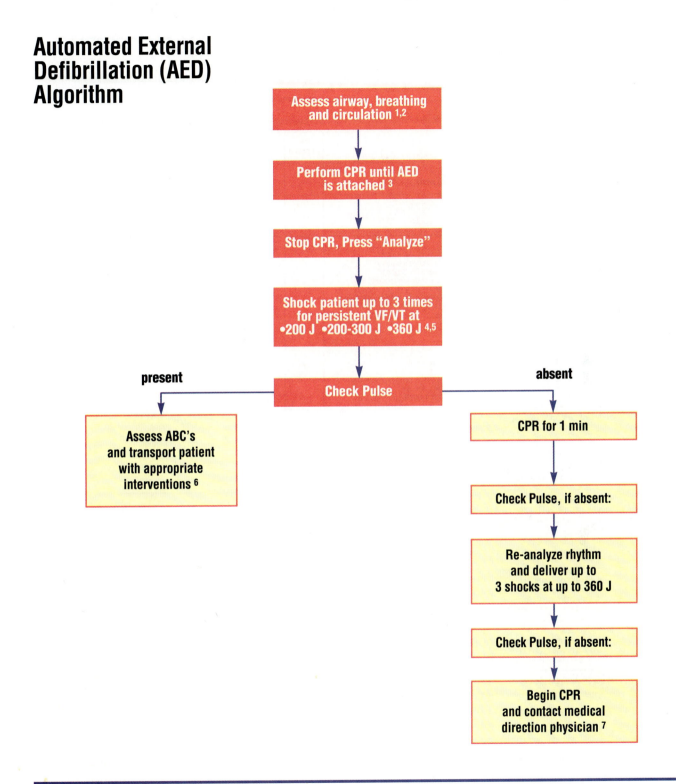

Assess airway, breathing and circulation [1,2]

Perform CPR until AED is attached [3]

Stop CPR, Press "Analyze"

Shock patient up to 3 times for persistent VF/VT at
•200 J •200-300 J •360 J [4,5]

present

Check Pulse

absent

Assess ABC's and transport patient with appropriate interventions [6]

CPR for 1 min

Check Pulse, if absent:

Re-analyze rhythm and deliver up to 3 shocks at up to 360 J

Check Pulse, if absent:

Begin CPR and contact medical direction physician [7]

1. Use appropriate body substance isolation precautions

2. If CPR was started before your arrival, stop CPR to confirm apnea and pulselessness

3. If you are the only rescuer, proceed to the use of the AED

4. Pulse checks are not required after shocks 1, 2, 4 and 5 unless "no shock indicated" advised.

5. If "no shock indicated" is advised at any time by AED, check pulse. If pulse is absent, perform CPR for 1 minute, recheck pulse and re-analyze the rhythm. After three consecutive "no shock indicated" messages, continue CPR and transport the patient. Re-analyze the rhythm per your local protocol.

6. If pulse is present and respirations are adequate, transport with high flow oxygen via non-rebreather. If pulse is present and respirations

are not adequate, provide high flow oxygen via bag-valve-mask.

7. The medical direction physician may ask you to transport the patient or to stay and provide up to 3 additional shocks at up to 360 J. *

* When en route to the receiving facility, the vehicle must be stopped to analyze the rhythm or to deliver shocks.

Fig. 18-12 Algorithm for AED use.

Automated Defibrillators: Operator's Shift Checklist

Date _____ Shift _____ Location _____

Mfr/Model No. _____ Serial No. or Facility ID No. _____

At the beginning of each shift, inspect the unit. Indicate whether all requirements have been met. Note any corrective actions taken. Sign the form.

	OK as Found	Corrective Action/ Remarks
1. Defibrillator Unit Clean, no spills, clear of objects on top, casing intact		
2. Cables/Connectors a. Inspect for cracks, broken wire, or damage b. Connectors engage securely and are not damaged*		
3. Supplies a. Two sets of pads in sealed packages, within expiration date* f. Monitoring electrodes* b. Hand towel g. Spare charged battery* c. Scissors h. Adequate ECG paper* d. Razor i. Manual override module, key, or card* e. Alcohol wipes* j. Cassette tape, memory module, and/or event card plus spares*		

4. Power Supply
a. Battery-powered units
  (1) Verify fully charged battery in place
  (2) Spare charged battery available
  (3) Follow appropriate battery rotation schedule per manufacturer's recommendations
b. AC/battery backup units
  (1) Plugged into live outlet to maintain battery charge
  (2) Test on battery power and reconnect to line power		

5. Indicators*/ECG Display a. Remove cassette tape, memory module, and/or event card* b. Power-on display c. Self-test OK d. Monitor display functional* e. "Service" message display off* f. Battery charging; low battery light off* g. Correct time displayed; set with dispatch center		
6. ECG Recorder* a. Adequate ECG paper b. Recorder prints		
7. Charge/Display Cycle a. Disconnect AC plug – battery backup units* b. Attach to simulator c. Detects, charges, and delivers shock for VF d. Responds correctly to nonshockable rhythms e. Manual override functional* f. Detach from simulator g. Replace cassette tape, module, and/or memory card *		
8. Pacemaker* a. Pacer output cable intact b. Pacer pads present (set of two) c. Inspect per manufacturer's operational guidelines		
Major Problem(s) Identified (Out of Service)		

*Applicable only if the unit has this supply or capability

Signature _____

Fig. 18-13 Example of an AED operator checklist.

"no shock indicated" command is given, the pulse returns, three shocks are delivered, or help arrives. Pulse checks are not performed after shocks one, two, four, and five. A pulse check should be performed after shock three and after shock six.

Always follow the local protocol for the use of AED. Each EMS system has guidelines for continu-ing education and the use of AED. Use of the defib-rillator does not require ACLS personnel to be at the scene, although they should be notified as soon as possible. Whether you should remain on scene to wait for ACLS or transport the patient depends on the local protocol and the transport time.

For safety reasons, do not use the defibrillator

near water or in the rain. The defibrillator is an electrical device. If the patient is lying in water and you are standing in the water beside the patient, the electrical shock will travel from the patient to you through the water. Move the patient to the ambulance if there is no closer dry place available and remove any wet clothes from the patient. The patient also should not be touching any metal. The electrical discharge from the defibrillator would travel through the patient and through the metal to anyone touching it.

POSTRESUSCITATION CARE

If the patient does not regain a pulse at the completion of the AED protocol, follow local protocol regarding transport with CPR, ACLS back-up, or continued use of the defibrillator. If a pulse does return, ensure a patent airway and transport the patient with basic life support maintained (*see* Chapter 7, "The Airway," and Chapter 6, "Lifting and Moving Patients"). Keep the defibrillator attached to the patient en route to the receiving facility. Perform the focused assessment and reassessment en route.

Document all findings in your report. Be sure to document each step performed, any changes in patient condition, and any responses to interventions. Document all vital signs before and after use of AED. Document all interactions with bystanders and any information obtained regarding the patient. The prehospital care report is a vital part of the emergency medical care.

AUTOMATED EXTERNAL DEFIBRILLATOR MAINTENANCE

Defibrillators require regular maintenance. The EMS system should have a maintenance schedule for each unit. A checklist, "Operator's Shift Checklist for Automated Defibrillators," must be completed on a daily basis by EMT–Basics (Fig. 18-13). The most common cause of defibrillator failure is improper device maintenance, usually battery failure. Battery replacement schedules should be maintained for each unit.

The American Heart Association publishes a variety of guidelines and additional information on AEDs. Follow these guidelines.

AUTOMATED EXTERNAL DEFIBRILLATOR SKILLS

You must maintain your AED skills. EMS systems usually require a skill review every 90 days to reassess competency. Medical direction is a required component of systems that use AEDs. Successful learning of automated external defibrillation in an EMT–Basic course does not permit usage of the device without approval by state regulations and local medical direction. Every event in which AED is used must be reviewed by the medical director or designated representative. Reviews of events using the AED may be accomplished by a written report and a review of the voice-electrocardiogram tape recording made by the AED machine or the solid-state memory modules and magnetic tape recordings stored in the device. Quality improvement involves both the individuals using AED and the EMS system in which the AEDs are used.

EMS delivery systems should have all the necessary links in the chain of survival, medical direction, an audit or quality improvement program in place, and mandatory continuing education with skill competency reviews for EMS providers.

REVIEW QUESTIONS
THE AUTOMATED EXTERNAL DEFIBRILLATOR

1. The preferred immediate treatment for most patients in cardiac arrest is _____.

2. The AED should be used only with patients who are _____, _____, and _____.

3. It is okay to touch the patient during a defibrillation because the electrical charge is not high enough to shock you. True or False?

4. The pulse should be checked between all shocks. True or False?

5. A common mechanical failure of the defibrillator is _____ failure.

1. Defibrillation
2. Unresponsive; pulseless; apneic (nonbreathing)
3. False
4. False
5. Battery

CHAPTER SUMMARY

EMTs must be prepared to assess and manage patients experiencing cardiac emergencies. Rapid defibrillation is the major determinant of survival of patients in cardiac arrest caused by ventricular fibrillation and ventricular tachycardia.

REVIEW OF THE CIRCULATORY SYSTEM

The heart contains four chambers: two atria and two ventricles. The right atrium receives blood from the veins of the body and pumps it to the right ventricle. The right ventricle pumps this oxygen-poor blood to the lungs. The left atrium receives blood from the lungs and pumps it to the left ventricle. The left ventricle pumps this oxygen-rich blood to the body. The heart muscle is composed of specialized tissue that generates electrical impulses.

Arteries carry blood from the heart to the rest of the body. Arterioles are the smallest branches of arteries and lead to the capillaries, where gas and nutrient exchange takes place in the body. Veins carry blood from the body back to the heart. Blood is composed of red blood cells, white blood cells, platelets, and plasma.

A patient's pulse can be palpated when the left ventricle contracts, forcing blood through the arteries. The blood pressure is a measurement of the pressure of blood in the arteries. The systolic pressure measures the pressure in the artery when the left ventricle contracts. The diastolic pressure measures the pressure in the artery when the left ventricle is at rest.

Inadequate circulation produces a state in the body known as *shock* (hypoperfusion). The signs and symptoms of shock include pale, cyanotic, and cool, clammy skin, rapid and shallow breathing, restlessness, thirst, anxiety or mental dullness, nausea and vomiting, and low or decreasing blood pressure.

CARDIAC COMPROMISE

The signs and symptoms of cardiac compromise may include a squeezing, dull pressure that commonly radiates to the arms, neck, jaw, and/or upper back, the sudden onset of sweating, difficulty breathing, anxiety or irritability, a feeling of impending doom, abnormal pulse rate, abnormal blood pressure, epigastric pain or discomfort, and nausea and vomiting.

Emergency medical care for the cardiac patient includes the initial assessment of the airway, breathing, and circulation. Automated external defibrillation and CPR are indicated for medical patients at least 12 years of age or at least 41 kg (90 lbs). CPR and rapid transport is indicated for medical patients less than 12 years of age or less than 90 pounds (41 kg).

Responsive patients with a known cardiac history should receive a focused history and physical examination and be placed in the position of comfort. Important questions to ask regarding the chest pain include <u>O</u>nset, <u>P</u>rovocation, <u>Q</u>uality, <u>R</u>adiation, <u>S</u>everity, and <u>T</u>ime. The patient may be assisted with the administration of nitroglycerin after consulting medical direction.

Nitroglycerin acts to relax blood vessels and decrease the workload of the heart. Before you can administer it, the patient must exhibit signs and symptoms of chest discomfort and have prescribed nitroglycerin; you also need authorization from the medical direction physician. Do not give nitroglycerin to an infant or child, patients with decreased blood pressure (systolic blood pressure less than 100 mm Hg) or a head injury, or a patient who has already taken the recommended dosage. With authorization, you may administer the tablet or spray under the patient's tongue after putting on gloves. Reassess all vital signs, report any changes to the medical direction physician, and document the actions and effects of the drug.

THE AUTOMATED EXTERNAL DEFIBRILLATOR

The successful prehospital resuscitation of a patient in cardiac arrest depends on a series of critical interventions known as the *chain of survival*, including defibrillation. The fully automatic external defibrillator operates without action by the EMT–Basic, except to attach the patches and leads and turn on the power. The semiautomatic defibrillator requires the EMT–Basic to push a button to initiate the shocks. These devices have a computer microprocessor that evaluates the patient's rhythm and confirms the presence of a rhythm for which shock is indicated. The defibrillator administers shocks for certain rhythms that are producing electrical activity within the heart but producing no mechanical pumping (pulse) of the heart muscle.

Advantages of the AED include:
- The speed of operation is very fast, with the first shock usually delivered to the patient within 1 minute of arrival at the patient's side.

- The defibrillation occurs through the use of adhesive pads, and the electrodes have a larger pad surface area and are more easily placed than paddles.
- Some models have an optional rhythm monitoring capability.

Standard operating procedures include the following:

- If ACLS personnel are not on the scene, the patient should be transported after regaining a pulse, six shocks are delivered, or the machine gives three consecutive messages (separated by 1 min of CPR) that no shock should be delivered.
- One EMT–Basic operates the defibrillator, and the other one performs CPR.
- Defibrillation comes first (do not hook up oxygen or do anything that delays analysis of the rhythm or defibrillation).
- All physical contact with the patient must be avoided during analysis of rhythm and delivery of shocks. Stop the vehicle and state "Clear the patient" before delivering shocks.
- Check the batteries at the beginning of each shift, and carry extra batteries.
- EMT–Basics must be familiar with the specific AEDs used in the EMS system.
- Follow local protocols.

Medical direction is a required component of systems that use defibrillators. Successful completion of automated external defibrillation in an EMT–Basic course does not permit usage of the device without approval by state regulations and local medical direction. Every event in which AED is used must be reviewed by the medical director or a designated representative. AED skills must be maintained. EMS systems usually require a skill review every 90 days to reassess competency. Figure 18-12 summarizes the technique for use of an AED.

UNITED STATES DEPARTMENT OF TRANSPORTATION NATIONAL HIGHWAY TRAFFIC SAFETY ADMINISTRATION EMT–BASIC OBJECTIVES

Check your knowledge. The National Registry of EMTs and many state EMS agencies use the objectives below to develop EMT–Basic certification examinations. Can you meet them?

COGNITIVE

1. Describe the structure and function of the cardiovascular system.
2. Describe the emergency medical care of the patient experiencing chest pain/discomfort.
3. List the indications for automated external defibrillation.
4. List the contraindications for automated external defibrillation.
5. Define the role of the EMT–Basic in the emergency cardiac care system.
6. Explain the impact of age and weight on defibrillation.
7. Discuss the position of comfort for patients with various cardiac emergencies.
8. Establish the relationship between airway management and the patient with cardiovascular compromise.
9. Predict the relationship between the patient experiencing cardiovascular compromise and basic life support.
10. Discuss the fundamentals of early defibrillation.
11. Explain the rationale for early defibrillation.
12. Explain that not all chest pain patients result in cardiac arrest and do not need to be attached to an automated external defibrillator.
13. Explain the importance of prehospital ACLS intervention if it is available.
14. Explain the importance of urgent transport to a facility with Advanced Cardiac Life Support if it is not available in the prehospital setting.
15. Discuss the various types of automated external defibrillators.
16. Differentiate between the fully automated and the semiautomated defibrillator.
17. Discuss the procedures that must be taken into consideration for standard operation of the various types of automated external defibrillators.
18. State the reasons for assuring that the patient is pulseless and apneic when using the automated external defibrillator.
19. Discuss the circumstances which may result in inappropriate shocks.
20. Explain the considerations for interruption of CPR, when using the automated external defibrillator.
21. Discuss the advantages and disadvantages of automated external defibrillators.

22. Summarize the speed of operation of automated external defibrillation.
23. Discuss the use of remote defibrillation through adhesive pads.
24. Discuss the special considerations for rhythm monitoring.
25. List the steps in the operation of the automated external defibrillator.
26. Discuss the standard of care that should be used to provide care to a patient with persistent ventricular fibrillation and no available advanced cardiac life support.
27. Discuss the standard of care that should be used to provide care to a patient with recurrent ventricular fibrillation and no available ACLS.
28. Differentiate between the single rescuer and multi-rescuer care with an automated external defibrillator.
29. Explain the reason for pulses not being checked between shocks with an automated external defibrillator.
30. Discuss the importance of coordinating ACLS trained providers with personnel using automated external defibrillators.
31. Discuss the importance of postresuscitation care.
32. List the components of postresuscitation care.
33. Explain the importance of frequent practice with the automated external defibrillator.
34. Discuss the need to complete the Automated Defibrillator: Operator's Shift Checklist.
35. Discuss the role of the American Heart Association (AHA) in the use of automated external defibrillation.
36. Explain the role medical direction plays in the use of automated external defibrillation.
37. State the reasons why a case review should be completed following the use of the automated external defibrillator.
38. Discuss the components that should be included in a case review.
39. Discuss the goal of quality improvement in the use of automated external defibrillation.
40. Recognize the need for medical direction of protocols to assist in the emergency medical care of the patient with chest pain.
41. List the indications for the use of nitroglycerin.
42. State the contraindications and side effects for the use of nitroglycerin.

Check your knowledge. The National Registry of EMTs and many state EMS agencies use the objectives below to develop EMT–Basic certification examinations. Can you meet them?

43. Define the function of all controls on an automated external defibrillator, and describe event documentation and battery defibrillator maintenance.

AFFECTIVE

1. Defend the reasons for obtaining initial training in automated external defibrillation and the importance of continuing education.
2. Defend the reason for maintenance of automated external defibrillators.
3. Explain the rationale for administering nitroglycerin to a patient with chest pain or discomfort.

PSYCHOMOTOR

1. Demonstrate the assessment and emergency medical care of a patient experiencing chest pain/discomfort.
2. Demonstrate the application and operation of the automated external defibrillator.
3. Demonstrate the maintenance of an automated external defibrillator.
4. Demonstrate the assessment and documentation of patient response to the automated external defibrillator.
5. Demonstrate the skills necessary to complete the Automated Defibrillator: Operator's Shift Checklist.
6. Perform the steps in facilitating the use of nitroglycerin for chest pain or discomfort.
7. Demonstrate the assessment and documentation of patient response to nitroglycerin.
8. Practice completing a prehospital care report for patients with cardiac emergencies.

KEY TERMS

Altered mental status: A state of mind that is not normal for the patient; a condition in which the patient is not oriented to person, place, or time (not necessarily all three together).

Diabetes mellitus: A disease that prevents insulin from being produced. Without insulin, the body cannot break down sugar into usable forms of energy.

Glucose: A form of sugar that is converted into usable energy.

Hypoglycemia: Low level of sugar in the blood.

Insulin-dependent: A diabetic patient who requires injections of insulin for the body to use sugar. Not all diabetics require insulin injections.

Seizure: Rapid discharge of nerve cells in the brain, typically causing muscular contractions that create erratic movements of the body or an otherwise unexplained change in mental status.

IN THE FIELD

EMTs Carl and Mike were dispatched to a scene where a patient was reported by bystanders to be intoxicated, combative, and hostile. While they were en route to the call, the dispatcher reported that police were on the scene and the patient appeared to be intoxicated and was being restrained by the police.

After ensuring scene safety, Carl began his initial assessment of the patient. As he approached the patient, his general impression was that the patient was approximately 30 years old and had an altered mental status. He was informed by a bystander that the patient had a rapid onset of symptoms. The patient's airway was clear, and his breathing was rapid, irregular, and deep. His pulse was rapid, and his skin was clammy. Carl identified him as a high-priority patient and began the focused history and physical examination for a medical patient. He discovered that the patient was wearing a medical condition bracelet stating that he was an insulin-dependent diabetic. The patient was alert but disoriented. He knew his name but did not know where he was or any details of his medical history. He kept insisting he was fine and wanted to go home.

Mike and Carl knew the patient needed immediate attention in an emergency department. Because they knew oral glucose could be helpful in this case, they contacted medical direction. Mike obtained an order and administered one tube of oral glucose. Within minutes of administering the oral glucose, the patient became more oriented and knew where he was and why he was there, but was unable to recall the events immediately before the arrival of the ambulance. Mike and Carl transported the patient to the receiving facility for further evaluation.

Altered mental status is revealed when a patient's verbal or nonverbal response shows that he or she is not alert and aware of the situation. Altered mental status can occur in a wide variety of illnesses. Although it is sometimes possible to identify the most likely cause of a patient's altered mental status, knowing the cause is not as important as providing appropriate care for the patient's signs and symptoms.

CAUSES OF ALTERED MENTAL STATUS

The many possible causes of altered mental status include both medical and traumatic situations. Diabetes and seizures are common medical causes of altered mental status, and head injuries are a common cause in trauma patients.

DIABETIC EMERGENCY

Diabetes mellitus is a common disease in the United States, with 2% to 5% of the total popula-

tion estimated to have diagnosed or undiagnosed diabetes. EMTs often see emergencies related to diabetes.

Diabetes prevents the body from turning glucose into usable forms of energy. **Glucose** is a basic sugar that is present in some form in most foods. The body uses insulin to convert glucose into usable energy. In diabetes, the body either does not produce enough insulin, or the insulin does not work well enough to allow the body to process the glucose into energy.

Diabetes affects each individual differently. Some individuals need regular injections of insulin; others may take oral medications; some may control their diabetes with diet; and still others are not even aware they have diabetes.

If a patient with a history of diabetes develops an altered mental status over several minutes, chances are the patient is very ill. This rapid onset typically occurs if the patient misses a meal after taking insulin. Diabetics usually have a routine medication and eating schedule. **Insulin-dependent** diabetics inject the insulin into their bodies. If the person does not eat, the insulin will draw on other stores of sugar in the body tissues. This causes a severe and sudden drop in blood sugar levels, called **hypoglyce-mia,** resulting in an altered mental status. This can also occur if the person vomits following eating after taking insulin. There may not have been enough time for the body to absorb the meal. Strenuous physical activity uses the available sugar from a meal, leaving less for the insulin to use. In some cases, there is no identifiable precipitating factor for the diabetic emergency.

Patients in a diabetic emergency may appear intoxicated. They may be staggering, have slurred speech, or be completely unresponsive. Due to the altered mental status, it may seem as though the patient is intoxicated or taking drugs, as in the opening scenario in which the police thought the patient was intoxicated. Unfortunately, this is how some patients in diabetic emergencies are perceived and treated. Through careful patient assessment, however, you may be able to tell if the patient is experiencing a diabetic emergency or is under the influence of alcohol or another drug. If the patient is unresponsive, you may not be able to determine the cause.

In a diabetic emergency the heart rate is usually increased. The skin is cold and clammy.

Sometimes a patient in a diabetic emergency may not have any of the above signs or symptoms. Low blood sugar levels usually cause uncharacteristic behavior. The patient may appear normal physiologically, but he or she may seem hostile or agitated. Anxiety may also be part of the behavior change. In extreme cases, the patient can become combative, again a result of low blood sugar.

The patient may also be hungry. This is the natural response of the body to low blood sugar levels. Seizures may occur in diabetic patients due to the effect of low blood sugar levels on the central nervous system.

Look for any medications around the patient. Insulin is usually found in the refrigerator, and other diabetic medications may be kept elsewhere in the patient's home or vehicle. Box 19-1 lists some common medications that a diabetic patient may be using.

A patient with an altered mental status and a history of diabetes usually requires some form of medication and may require other emergency interventions. Emergency medical care is described later in this chapter.

SEIZURES

Seizures are another common cause of an altered mental state. A **seizure** is a convulsive movement of the body or an altered mental state caused by a random discharge of the brain's electrical impulses. Seizures can range from an episode in which the patient just seems to stare ahead blankly to convulsions in which the entire body is in motion. Not all seizures are life-threatening emergencies. For example, seizures in children who have a chronic seizure disorder are rarely life-threatening. Febrile seizures, which are commonly seen in children, are caused by fever. Medical direction can help guide the appropriate care for these patients.

BOX 19-1

Common Diabetic Medications

Insulin (injection)
- Humulin

Oral Medications
- Diabinese
- Orinase
- Micronase

BOX 19-2

Common Causes of Seizures

- Fever
- Infection
- Poisoning
- Intoxication
- Hypoglycemia
- Head trauma
- Decreased levels of oxygen
- Epilepsy uncontrolled by medication
- May be idiopathic (no known cause)

The length of a seizure may range from seconds or many minutes. In general, the longer a seizure lasts, the greater the chances of complications such as vomiting or inadequate respiration.

Seizures can be caused by many conditions. Box 19-2 lists some of the common causes.

After a seizure, a patient may be in a postictal state in which he or she seems asleep and almost unresponsive. The brain has suffered a massive discharge of energy, and the body is recovering for a short time after the seizure. The postictal state may also include agitation or combativeness. Although a seizure and the postictal state are often frightening events for bystanders, chronic seizure patients may be familiar with what occurs and may refuse treatment after they have become responsive. A seizure is especially frightening for the patient, family, and bystanders when it occurs for the first time or unexpectedly. Encourage all seizure patients to be evaluated in the emergency department by a physician.

OTHER POSSIBLE CAUSES

In addition to diabetic emergencies and seizures, there are many other causes of altered mental status. Box 19-3 lists some common causes.

Certain poisons or drugs interfere with the normal functions of the central nervous system or may cause hallucinations or psychotic behavior. A poison to which the patient was exposed may also be a threat to you. Take appropriate body substance isolation precautions and call for a hazardous materials team if necessary.

Infections may also affect mental status. Severe infections can affect the brain directly or spread toxic substances through the bloodstream. Ask the patient or family members about the patient's recent medical condition. A recent history of fever may indicate an infection.

Head trauma may cause altered mental status due to temporary or permanent damage to the central nervous system. Being deprived of oxygen can have a similar effect. It is often difficult to determine the cause of a patient's altered mental status, but the basic emergency care for altered mental status is the same regardless of the cause.

BOX 19-3

Common Causes of Altered Mental Status

- Low blood sugar
- Seizure
- Poisoning
- Intoxication
- Infection
- Head trauma
- Decreased oxygen levels
- Hypothermia or hyperthermia

REVIEW QUESTIONS

CAUSES OF ALTERED MENTAL STATUS

1. List at least three possible causes of altered mental status.

2. Diabinese is an oral medication used to control diabetes mellitus. True or False?

3. Insulin is usually stored in the refrigerator, and is an injectable medication used to control diabetes mellitus. True or False?

4. A patient acting intoxicated does not need medical evaluation. True or False?

5. There is no need to consider the possibility of a diabetic emergency when evaluating a combative patient. True or False?

6. A patient with diabetes who is taking insulin can miss eating all day and be fine. True or False?

1. Low blood sugar; poisoning; seizure; infection; head trauma; decreased oxygen levels; intoxication; hypothermia; hyperthermia
2. True
3. True
4. False
5. False
6. False

EMERGENCY CARE OF PATIENTS WITH ALTERED MENTAL STATUS

The primary goal of emergency care for a patient with altered mental status is maintaining a patent airway. This can be accomplished by any of the techniques described in Chapter 7, "The Airway." Always have suction equipment readily available. Artificial ventilation may be required for patients showing cyanosis or who are not breathing adequately on their own. Altered mental status may not be caused by an underlying medical condition. Trauma is also a possibility. Do not assume that every patient with altered mental status has an underlying medical problem. All patients experiencing altered mental status should be encouraged to see a physician in the emergency department to determine the cause of this condition.

ASSESSMENT

As always, perform an initial assessment of a patient with altered mental status. This includes looking around the scene for clues and medications, while also checking the patient's airway, breathing, and circulation. Proceed to the focused history and physical examination. Box 19-4 lists the major points to note about the patient in addition to the usual information obtained in the SAMPLE history.

The focused history and physical examination help determine what treatment may be required for the patient. Ask patients if they remember what happened (some will not recall). If you can, find out when the symptoms began and their duration. Are there any associated symptoms such as cold, clammy skin, or a rapid heartbeat? Look for signs of trauma. An isolated head injury may be revealed only by subtle signs that could easily be overlooked in a hectic situation. Ask if the episode has stopped or has remained unchanged. Note if any seizures have occurred along with the altered mental status and whether a fever is present. Assess the scene for any additional clues. All these parts of the focused history and physical examination can help you and medical direction determine what treatment is necessary.

Assess baseline vital signs and obtain a SAMPLE history. Patients with altered mental status should be considered unstable, and their vital signs monitored every 5 minutes. Check the patient and setting for medical identification tags or signs of medications that may indicate the patient has diabetes. The specific management for patients with altered mental status and a known history of diabetes is discussed later in this chapter.

AIRWAY MANAGEMENT

Never overlook the airway when caring for a patient with altered mental status. Depending on the severity of the altered mental status, the airway may be patent or the patient may need an airway adjunct and artificial ventilation.

Assess the airway for patency first. Maintain the airway as discussed in Chapter 7, "The Airway." Look and listen for signs and symptoms of impending respiratory distress. Listen for gurgling or snoring respirations. In some altered mental status patients the tongue may obstruct the airway. In some patients who are unresponsive and have no gag reflex, oral secretions may be occluding the airway. Suctioning and placing the patient in the recovery position (if no spinal injury is suspected) are important for maintaining a patent airway.

BOX 19-4

Focused History for Patients with Altered Mental Status

- Onset
- Duration
- Associated symptoms
- Evidence of trauma
- Seizures
- Fever

ALERT

Remember to reassess the airway of a patient with altered mental status. It is easy to become caught up in other aspects of patient care and forget the basic principles of airway management and patient assessment.

Next, check breathing, including the rate and quality. You may have to assist the patient with ventilation or completely take over ventilations. If the rate and quality are within the limits described in Chapter 5, "Baseline Vital Signs and SAMPLE History," then oxygen should be delivered via a nonrebreather mask. If the rate of breathing is slow or the depth shallow, you must assist the patient with artificial ventilations.

TREATMENT FOR DIABETIC EMERGENCY

The assessment of a patient with altered mental status and a known history of diabetes is the same as for any patient with altered mental status. In addition, try to determine the time of the diabetic patient's last meal and whether he or she has taken

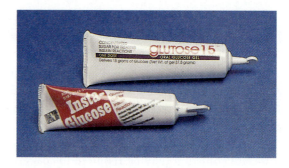

Fig. 19-1 Types of oral glucose.

any medication recently. Diabetic patients often have other associated illnesses such as heart disease or elevated blood pressure (hypertension).

Determine whether the patient can swallow. If

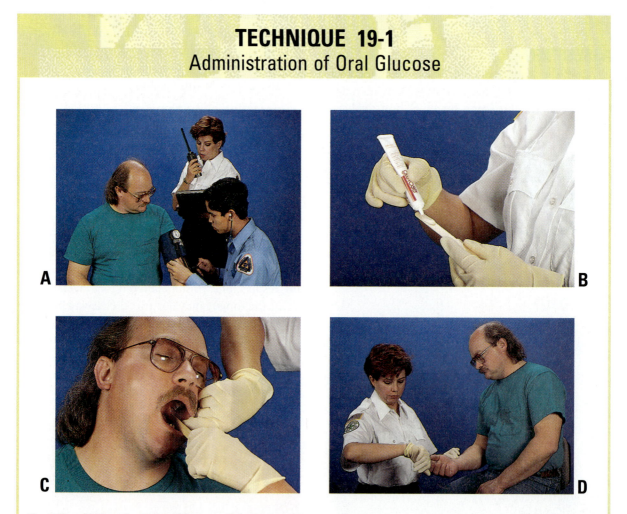

TECHNIQUE 19-1
Administration of Oral Glucose

Fig. 19-2   Perform the focused history and physical examination. Administer oral glucose only when the patient has the signs and symptoms of altered mental status and a known history of diabetes controlled with medication. **A, Consult on-line or off-line medical direction for authorization to administer oral glucose.** Ensure that the patient is responsive and able to swallow. **B, Administer the full tube of glucose (C), between the patient's cheek and gum, allowing the mucous membranes to absorb the glucose. D, Perform an ongoing assessment.**

he or she can swallow, oral glucose administration may be authorized by medical direction.

In prehospital settings, EMT-Basics can administer oral glucose to patients with altered mental status and a known history of diabetes. Oral glucose is not indicated for every patient with altered mental status—only those with a known diabetic history. Glucose administration can reverse the diabetic emergency and possibly save the patient's life. An order from medical direction is needed to proceed with oral glucose administration.

Oral glucose has several different trade names, including Glutose 15 and Insta-glucose. Figure 19-1 shows some types of oral glucose. You should be familiar with the type of oral glucose used by your EMS service.

Oral glucose is contraindicated for patients who cannot protect their own airway. Any patient who is unresponsive should not receive oral glucose, because an unresponsive patient often has a diminished or absent gag reflex. Similarly, the patient may be unable to swallow for other reasons, thus complicating maintenance of the airway and preventing the administration of oral glucose.

The medication comes in a tube in gel form. The proper dose is one complete tube. Technique 19-1 describes how to administer oral glucose.

It is imperative that a thorough examination of the patient be performed. Oral glucose is used only when a known history of diabetes is present along with altered mental status. For example, a patient may have altered mental status after falling and sustaining head trauma, with the injury causing the altered mental status. In this case, oral glucose is not indicated. In another situation, a patient in a diabetic emergency may have suffered head trauma from a fall caused by having low blood sugar.

Oral glucose works to reverse the patient's altered mental status by increasing the blood sugar. There are no significant side effects of the medication. The greatest danger in using oral glucose is the risk of aspiration. By assessing the patient carefully first, you can prevent this from occurring.

Reassess the patient continually. When necessary, assist the patient in maintaining a patent airway. Perform ongoing assessments every 5 minutes because these patients are considered unstable.

REVIEW QUESTIONS

EMERGENCY CARE OF PATIENTS WITH ALTERED MENTAL STATUS

1. Airway control is a low priority in treating patients with altered mental status. True or False?

2. It is appropriate to skip the initial assessment of the patient with an altered mental status and a history of diabetes and proceed directly to the focused history and physical examination. True or False?

3. If the patient has a good gag reflex, chances are the airway can be controlled by the patient. True or False?

4. Use of the _____ airway is required along with a _____ to adequately provide ventilation for the altered mental status patient.

5. Oral glucose comes in a box that has to be mixed with water, then given to the patient to swallow. True or False?

6. Medical direction is not required to give oral glucose. True or False?

7. The patient must be unresponsive for the oral glucose to be effective. True or False?

8. Oral glucose works by alleviating the patient's hunger. True or False?

1. False
2. False
3. True
4. Oral or nasal; bag-valve-mask, pocket mask, or oxygen-powered ventilation device
5. False
6. False
7. False
8. False

CHAPTER SUMMARY

CAUSES OF ALTERED MENTAL STATUS

There are many causes of altered mental status. A common cause is a diabetic emergency occurring because of low amounts of sugar in the blood. The diabetic patient with low blood sugar may seem intoxicated and is sometimes treated by others as such. Seizures are another cause of altered mental status. When EMTs arrive, the patient typically is past the active seizure and is in a postictal state. Altered mental status caused by a seizure should resolve over time as the patient recovers. Altered mental status can also be caused by poisoning, intoxication, infection, head trauma, or decreased oxygen levels.

EMERGENCY CARE OF PATIENTS WITH ALTERED MENTAL STATUS

The emergency care for all patients with altered mental status is to protect the airway first. Assess the ABCs. Support ventilation as needed and ad-minister oxygen. Remember to complete a focused history and physical examination, and do not assume that a medical condition is the cause of the altered mental status. Most seizure patients require only supportive care, with special attention to maintaining a patent airway. Encourage all patients with a history of altered mental status to seek immediate evaluation by a physician. All patients with ongoing altered mental status should be transported to an appropriate facility.

If the patient has altered mental status and a history of diabetes, consult medical direction for authorization to administer oral glucose.

UNITED STATES DEPARTMENT OF TRANSPORTATION NATIONAL HIGHWAY TRAFFIC SAFETY ADMINISTRATION EMT–BASIC OBJECTIVES

Check your knowledge. The National Registry of EMTs and many state EMS agencies use the objectives below to develop EMT–Basic certification examinations. Can you meet them?

COGNITIVE

1. Identify the patient taking diabetic medications with altered mental status and the implications of a diabetic history.
2. State the steps in the emergency medical care of a patient taking diabetic medicine with an altered mental status and a history of diabetes.
3. Establish the relationship between airway management and the patient with altered mental status.
4. State the generic and trade names, medication forms, dose, administration, action, and contraindications for oral glucose.
5. Evaluate the need for medical direction in the emergency medical care of diabetic patients.

AFFECTIVE

1. Explain the rationale for administering oral glucose.

PSYCHOMOTOR

1. Demonstrate the steps in the emergency medical care for the patient taking diabetic medicine with an altered mental status and a history of diabetes.
2. Demonstrate the steps in the administration of oral glucose.
3. Demonstrate the assessment and documentation of patient response to oral glucose.
4. Demonstrate how to complete a prehospital care report for patients with diabetic emergencies.

20 ALLERGIC REACTIONS

IN THE FIELD

EMTs Tony and Lisa responded to a 911 call for an unresponsive man lying outside a house. The man was lying beside a hedge, with lawn tools nearby. Tony quickly assessed the patient and found that he was awake and oriented but had hives and was having extreme difficulty breathing. Lisa placed the patient on high-flow oxygen via a nonrebreather mask. The patient had a rapid pulse, and his skin was cool and clammy. The patient stated he was allergic to bee stings, and he thought he may have been stung on his shoulder. Bees were flying around the scene. His wife said he had an epinephrine autoinjector in the house.

During the focused examination, Tony found a red, swollen area on the patient's left shoulder. Because they suspected that the patient was having a reaction to a bee sting, Lisa contacted medical direction. The patient's wife brought the autoinjector, and Lisa received orders to help the patient administer it. Shortly thereafter, the patient began to breathe easier, and Tony and Lisa prepared to transport him to the hospital.

In the opening scenario, the EMTs administered potentially life-saving medication to a patient having an allergic reaction. Allergic reactions can range from a simple rash to life-threatening airway or circulatory compromise. Patients experiencing an allergic reaction are treated based on the signs and symptoms found during assessment.

ASSESSMENT OF ALLERGIC REACTIONS

An **allergic reaction** is an individual's exaggerated immune response to a substance with which the body comes in contact. Many possible substances can produce an allergic reaction. Insect bites or stings, foods, plants, and medications are all common **allergens**, substances that commonly cause allergic reactions. Patients can be allergic to a wide variety of other substances (Fig. 20-1).

CAUSES OF ALLERGIC REACTIONS

Insect bites or stings cause pain and localized swelling in most people. A small percentage of the population, however, has a much more severe reaction to bee or wasp venom. This allergic reaction can be life threatening.

Foods such as crustaceans (shrimp and shellfish) and peanuts may also cause an allergic reaction in some people. People who know they have a food allergy usually try to avoid eating that type of food.

However, sometimes they may be unaware that they have eaten a meal prepared with that food, until they have a reaction.

Plants also cause allergic reactions in humans. Most people are familiar with the common allergy to poison ivy, for example. This allergic reaction results in local blistering of the skin as a result of contact with the oil on the plant's leaves. If a person ingests any plant to which the person is allergic, a more serious allergic reaction may result.

Medication allergies are another large class of allergic reactions. People who know that they have an allergy to certain medications often wear medical condition alert bracelets or necklaces to let others know of their allergy in the event of an emergency. For example, allergic reactions to antibiotics such as penicillin or sulfa compounds commonly occur. Almost anything in the environment can cause an allergic reaction. Chemicals, dust, and pollen also are common allergens.

SIGNS AND SYMPTOMS OF ALLERGIC REACTIONS

In general, most allergic reactions are characterized by basic signs and symptoms that you can learn to recognize and treat accordingly.

Because hypoperfusion often occurs in severe allergic reactions, assess the patient's skin. The skin is a good indicator of perfusion. As the allergic reaction begins to affect the entire body, the patient may experience a warm tingling feeling or numb-

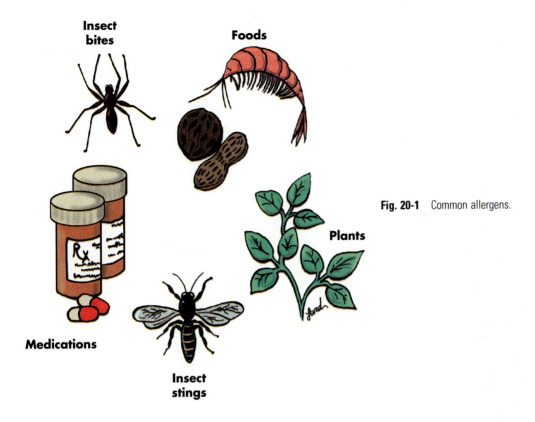

Insect bites

Foods

Plants

Medications

Insect stings

Fig. 20-1 Common allergens.

ness in the face, mouth, chest, feet, and hands. Sometimes, the patient notices the reaction radiating from the site of exposure. For other patients, the allergic reaction occurs systemically. This systematic reaction means that from the single source of exposure, the reaction spreads throughout the entire body. The skin is itchy, red, or flushed, and hives may develop (Fig. 20-2). The body reacts with swelling of the face, neck, hands, feet, and tongue. The swelling occurs due to the body's attempt to attack the allergen with its natural defense mechanisms.

Attention to the respiratory system is critical in an allergic reaction. The patient may feel a tightness in the throat or chest due to the swelling of the face and neck. Associated signs and symptoms are coughing, rapid and labored breathing, noisy breathing, hoarseness, stridor, and wheezing. At times, the reaction is so great that the wheezing may be heard without a stethoscope. Respiratory distress is usually the most serious complication in an allergic reaction. If swelling of tissues in the respiratory system is severe, the patient may have very quiet breath sounds. This reaction is caused by little air moving in and out of the lungs.

The heart responds to the allergen as well. Hypoperfusion usually occurs in cases of severe aller-

gic reaction. The heart responds to the hypoperfusion by increasing the heart rate in an effort to maintain the blood pressure. The reaction causes the peripheral vascular network to relax and expand, which results in low blood pressure.

Not all allergic reactions are this severe. A mild reaction may include itchy, watery eyes, a runny nose, and a headache. In severe reactions, the patient may have a feeling of impending doom as the reaction spreads over the entire body and may act nervously or apprehensively. The patient may feel very uncomfortable and behave oddly. Figure 20-3 illustrates common signs and symptoms of an allergic reaction.

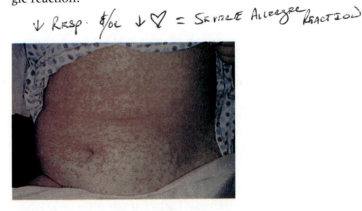

Fig. 20-2 Rash caused by an allergic reaction.

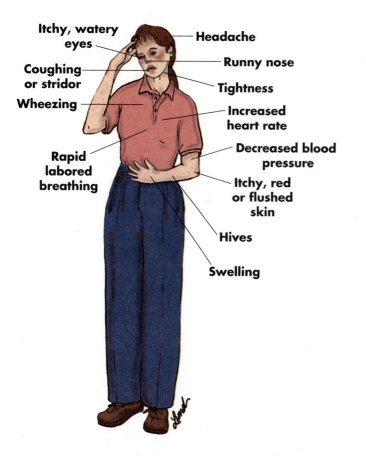

Itchy, watery eyes

Coughing or stridor

Wheezing

Rapid labored breathing

Headache

Runny nose

Tightness

Increased heart rate

Decreased blood pressure

Itchy, red or flushed skin

Hives

Swelling

Fig. 20-3   Common signs and symptoms of allergic reactions.

Remember that the first and best sign of hypoperfusion is a change in the mental status of the patient. The altered mental status is not caused by a diabetic emergency or other causes described in Chapter 19, "Diabetes and Altered Mental Status," but instead is caused by decreased blood pressure, which causes poor blood flow and decreased gas exchange and oxygen to the tissues.

Any assessment findings that reveal hypoperfusion or respiratory distress may indicate a severe allergic reaction. The emergency medical care for mild and severe allergic reactions is discussed in the next section of this chapter.

EMERGENCY CARE FOR PATIENTS WITH ALLERGIC REACTIONS

Responsive patients with severe allergies often recognize the allergic reaction and can tell you what is wrong. They may have come in contact with the allergen in the past and are therefore aware of the symptoms. They may complain of difficulty breathing and may exhibit signs and symptoms of hypoperfusion.

Form a general impression of the patient in the initial assessment. If the patient shows signs and symptoms of respiratory compromise or hypoperfusion, a true medical emergency exists, and the patient should be transported to the hospital immediately.

Perform the focused history and physical examination to gain vital information. Find out about the patient's history of allergies. Try to find out to what _INGESTED_ and how the patient was exposed. Was the patient bitten or stung, or did the patient ingest something? Ask the patient to describe the symptoms and any previous reaction. Determine the progression of the reaction to inform the medical direction physician. Place the patient on high-flow oxygen via a nonrebreather mask.

Assess the baseline vital signs, and take a SAMPLE history. Determine if the patient has a prescribed epinephrine autoinjector available. Prepare the epinephrine autoinjector, and contact medical direction. Epinephrine autoinjectors are used for patients with signs and symptoms of an allergic reaction and respiratory compromise or hypoperfusion, with permission from medical direction. If the patient has more than one autoinjector, bring additional ones with you when you transport the

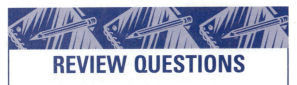

REVIEW QUESTIONS

ASSESSMENT OF ALLERGIC REACTIONS

1. A patient was stung by a bee and shortly thereafter developed swelling of the eyes and tongue. The patient is also having trouble breathing. This patient requires emergency treatment. True or False?

2. Hives can be a sign of an allergic reaction. True or False?

3. Every patient stung by an insect will have a severe allergic reaction. True or False?

4. The patient experiencing an allergic reaction has an altered mental status due to hypoperfusion. True or False?

5. The patient experiencing an allergic reaction may feel anxious or scared. True or False?

1. True
2. True
3. False
4. True
5. True

---

patient. The administration of the autoinjector is discussed later in this chapter.

Reassess and record the patient's vital signs every 5 minutes. If the patient does not have an autoinjector, transport immediately to a medical facility. This situation is a true medical emergency.

For the patient who has an allergic reaction without the signs or symptoms of hypoperfusion or respiratory distress, continue the examination with a focused assessment. Do not treat with epinephrine unless the patient is wheezing or has signs of respiratory compromise or hypoperfusion.

AIRWAY MANAGEMENT

In severe allergic reactions the patient may have signs and symptoms of airway or respiratory distress. This distress may range from simple breathing difficulty to complete respiratory arrest. The reaction may proceed rapidly or take some time. With increased swelling of airway tissues, the condition of the airway deteriorates. The patient's condition can continue to change. Continue to assess the patient for airway obstruction and manage as necessary. The basic principle is to continually monitor the patient for change. The patient must be treated aggressively with oxygen. The airway should be managed according to the principles presented in Chapter 7, "The Airway."

ADMINISTRATION OF MEDICATION

Epinephrine is a medication used to dilate the bronchioles to help the patient breathe easier by preventing the obstruction of the airway due to constriction and swelling of tissues. Epinephrine also causes the blood vessels to constrict thereby increasing blood pressure, which improves the patient's mental status and the delivery of oxygen and nutrients to all parts of the body.

Patients who have had problems with severe allergic reactions in the past may have a prescribed epinephrine autoinjector in case of allergic reactions. An autoinjector is a device that administers a preset dose of the medication in a safe manner and is designed for the patient's own use. Use of the epinephrine autoinjector is relatively simple. The label on the autoinjector lists the generic name of epinephrine and the trade name of Adrenalin. Box 20-1 lists the criteria for the use of the epinephrine autoinjector.

There are no contraindications when the epinephrine autoinjector is used in a life-threatening situation. The medication is in liquid form administered via an automatically injectable needle and syringe system (Fig. 20-4). The dosage for the adult

---

BOX 20-1

Criteria for Use of the Epinephrine Autoinjector

All criteria must be met

- Emergency medical care for a patient with the assessment findings of a severe allergic reaction (respiratory distress or hypoperfusion).

- Medication has been prescribed for this patient by a physician.

- Medical direction authorizes use for this patient.

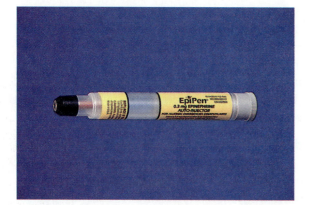

Fig. 20-4 Epinephrine autoinjector.

is one autoinjector, which contains 0.3 mg of epinephrine. An infant or child autoinjector generally contains about one half the adult dose. *(0.15mg)*

Epinephrine has some side effects. The heart rate increases and the skin may become pale. Dizziness, chest pain, and headache are typical complaints, as well as nausea and vomiting. Excitability and anxiousness are also common. All of these are common and expected side effects of epinephrine administration. Be prepared to suction as necessary in the case of vomiting. Technique 20-1 describes how to administer the epinephrine autoinjector.

TECHNIQUE 20-1
Use of the Epinephrine Autoinjector

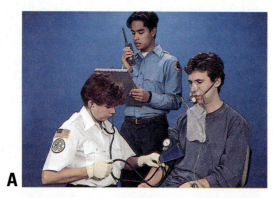

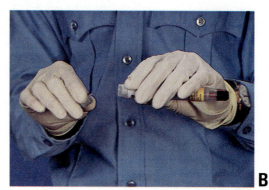

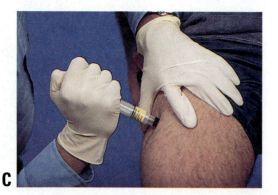

Fig. 20-5 A, Have on-line or off-line authorization from medical direction to use the autoinjector. Obtain the patient's prescribed autoinjector. Make sure that the prescription is for the patient experiencing the allergic reaction. Check that the medication is not discolored or crystallized. Check the expiration date. **B, Remove the safety cap on the autoinjector.** If possible, remove clothing from the injection site. If removing the clothing would take too much time, the autoinjector can be administered through clothing. **C, Place the tip of the autoinjector at a 90° angle against the lateral portion of the patient's thigh midway between the waist and knee.** Push the injector firmly against the thigh until the injector activates. Hold the injector in place for at least 10 seconds or until the medication is injected. Record the intervention and the time of injection. Dispose of the injector in a biohazard container or other container designated for needles. Reassess the patient and document any changes in the patient's condition. *TAKE INJECTOR TO ER*

decreasing blood pressure. Consult medical direction when any change occurs. The physician may order an additional dose of epinephrine if the patient has a second autoinjector. Treat the signs and symptoms of hypoperfusion, and prepare to initiate basic life support if the patient suffers cardiac arrest, including cardiopulmonary resuscitation and use of the automated external defibrillator, if indicated. Provide supportive care for the patient including oxygen.

CHAPTER SUMMARY

ASSESSMENT OF ALLERGIC REACTIONS

The causes of allergic reactions are numerous. Allergic reactions can be as mild as a runny nose or itchy eyes, and as severe as airway obstruction resulting from airway swelling and constriction. The allergic reaction can proceed rapidly and can be life threatening.

EMERGENCY CARE FOR PATIENTS WITH ALLERGIC REACTIONS

Airway management is necessary for the patient suffering from an allergic reaction. When indicated, the epinephrine autoinjector is the drug of choice to treat allergic reactions. The drug works by dilating the bronchioles and constricting the blood vessels. There are no contraindications for use of the autoinjector when the patient's life is in danger. Proper airway management and use of the autoinjector will assist the patient suffering from a severe allergic reaction.

REVIEW QUESTIONS

EMERGENCY CARE FOR PATIENTS WITH ALLERGIC REACTIONS

1. Adrenalin is the medication in an epinephrine autoinjector. True or False?

2. In a patient having a severe allergic reaction, the airway is controlled only after use of the autoinjector. True or False?

3. Medical direction does not need to be contacted for use of the autoinjector. True or False?

1. True
2. False
3. False

Regardless of whether the patient did or did not receive the epinephrine, you must continuously reassess the patient. Perform an ongoing assessment of the patient's mental status, airway, breathing, and circulation along with the vital signs every 25 minutes. Begin transport as soon as possible, without delay for any reason. These patients can rapidly deteriorate. Constant monitoring and reassessment are the most important prehospital interventions.

Continue to observe the patient for decreasing mental status, increasing breathing difficulty, or

UNITED STATES DEPARTMENT OF TRANSPORTATION NATIONAL HIGHWAY TRAFFIC SAFETY ADMINISTRATION EMT–BASIC OBJECTIVES

Check your knowledge. The National Registry of EMTs and many state EMS agencies use the objectives below to develop EMT–Basic certification examinations. Can you meet them?

COGNITIVE

1. Recognize the patient experiencing an allergic reaction.
2. Describe the emergency medical care of the patient with an allergic reaction.
3. Establish the relationship between the patient with an allergic reaction and airway management.
4. Describe the mechanisms of allergic response and the implications for airway management.
5. State the generic and trade names, medication forms, dose, administration, action, and contraindications for the epinephrine autoinjector.
6. Evaluate the need for medical direction in the emergency medical care of the patient with an allergic reaction.
7. Differentiate between the general category of those patients having an allergic reaction and those patients having an allergic reaction and requiring immediate medical care, including immediate use of epinephrine autoinjector.

AFFECTIVE

1. Explain the rationale for administering epinephrine using an autoinjector.

PSYCHOMOTOR

1. Demonstrate the emergency medical care of the patient experiencing an allergic reaction.
2. Demonstrate the use of epinephrine autoinjector.
3. Demonstrate the assessment and documentation of patient response to an epinephrine injection.
4. Demonstrate proper disposal of equipment.
5. Demonstrate completing a prehospital care report for patients with allergic emergencies.

IN THE FIELD

EMTs Dave and Sara responded to a 911 call for a 6-year-old male patient who reportedly ingested some of his mother's seizure medication. The dispatcher had no further information. When Sara and David arrived on the scene, they found the boy being held by his father, sitting on a chair in the kitchen. The boy was awake and responding to questions. The father said they found him eating pills from a bottle in his mother's purse. The parents were unsure how many pills the child had eaten.

While Sara began the examination and assessed vital signs, Dave called medical direction with the information they had gathered and the name of the medication the child had taken, Dilantin. The medical direction physician ordered 25 g of activated charcoal to be administered to the child. Dave explained the treatment to the boy and his father and encouraged him to drink the activated charcoal. En route to the hospital, Dave closely monitored the patient for changes in mental status. Because vomiting is a common side effect of poisoning, he was prepared to suction if necessary. Because the nearest hospital was 20 minutes away, the early administration of activated charcoal made a difference in the outcome and further treatment of the child.

Poisoning emergencies are common in both adults and children. Thousands of children are poisoned every year in and outside the home. Curious children may place objects in their mouth and may drink fluids such as household cleaners. Adults can be poisoned by unintentional means or by deliberately taking a poison or overdosing on a drug or medication.

A **toxin** is any substance, including medications, that, through its chemical action, can harm a person. "Poison" is a general term used by lay people for substances with toxic effects that were not intended to enter the body, such as cleaning products. For example, most people do not think of aspirin as a poison, but in larger-than-recommended doses it has toxic effects and can cause a poisoning. An overdose is the intentional or accidental use of too much medication.

Early prehospital management of poisoning and overdose patients greatly increases the likelihood of their successful recovery.

HISTORY OF POISONING

When you encounter a possible poisoning or overdose patient, begin with the basic steps of patient assessment. Protect yourself from contact with body fluids by using body substance isolation precautions. Conduct the initial assessment the same as for all other situations, paying particular attention to the airway, breathing, and circulation. Conduct the focused history and physical examination, and obtain a SAMPLE history. Assess the patient's baseline vital signs. Perform a detailed physical examination when appropriate, as described in the patient assessment chapters. Ongoing assessments are performed every 5 minutes for patients who are unstable and every 15 minutes for stable patients.

The patient assessment process is adapted in several ways for poisoning and overdose patients.

In some cases of poisoning or overdose, the toxin is known. Responsive and oriented patients may tell you to what they were exposed. In other cases, you must act like a detective and gather as much information as possible. In the history, ask questions such as the following:

- *What substance was involved?*
  Ask responsive patients to what substance were they exposed or what substance did they ingest. With unresponsive patients, check the scene for clues about the substance involved in the poisoning, looking for things such as open containers, cans, bottles, or other types of containers. Ask family members, friends, or bystanders for any information about the substance. The location of the patient can also be a valuable clue. For

example, you might suspect that a farmer who was found lying unresponsive in a field next to a crop duster has been poisoned by the insecticide used in crop dusting.

- *When did you ingest or become exposed to the substance?*
  The time since ingestion or exposure to the toxin is critical for the management of the patient. Over time, the toxic agent enters the patient's body systems, making it more difficult for a poison treatment to work. Find out if the patient ingested multiple doses or had multiple exposures, because treatment is often determined by the amount of a substance ingested or length of exposure to a substance. The amount of toxin ingested or length of exposure to some toxins can have serious implications for the patient's outcome.

- *If you ingested the poison, how much did you ingest?*
  The amount of the poison ingested can affect the course of associated illness and the treatment plan.

- *Over what time period did the poisoning occur?*
  Patients can become poisoned by medications that they have been taking every day, other medications they are taking, and a variety of other causes. A chronic poisoning over a long period of time is treated differently from a poisoning by rapid ingestion.

- *What has happened since the poisoning?*
  Has the patient tried any over-the-counter medications? Has the patient vomited? Some remedies tried at home may actually be more harmful than helpful.

- *How much do you weigh?*
  Some poisons have greater effects on small people than on larger people. The effects of many poisons vary depending on body weight.

If the patient can talk, ask specific questions and try to find out exactly what happened. The more details you can obtain, the better the chance of helping the patient. If the patient is unresponsive, gather as much information as possible from family members or friends, or even bystanders. Examine the area for clues.

Do not be judgmental toward patients who deliberately took too much of a medication or other drug. Treat these patients medically as you would any other patient suffering from poisoning. Remember, however, that patients who intended to harm themselves may attempt to harm themselves again in your presence. If the patient be-

comes violent, request additional help from law enforcement officials.

TYPES OF TOXINS

Many substances have toxic effects. Figure 21-1 shows common types of poisons. Toxins can enter the body through four routes: ingestion, inhalation, absorption, or injection. These routes of poisoning have specific assessment or treatment considerations.

INGESTED TOXINS

An **ingested toxin** is a poison that is consumed orally. Try to determine what the patient ingested. Ask questions to determine if the ingestion of poison was intentional. A person mistakenly could eat a poisonous mushroom, which is an unintentional poisoning, or deliberately could drink a chemical cleaner with the intent of committing suicide.

Some ingested poisons result in nausea, vomiting, diarrhea, and abdominal pain or cramping, but not all these signs or symptoms are present every time. A toxic substance reaches the blood stream relatively rapidly following absorption through the intestinal tract. Patients may have an altered mental status following a poison ingestion. See Chapter 19, ''Diabetes and Altered Mental Status,'' for information on assessing mental status. Look for chemical burns or unusual colors around the patient's mouth. Check for unusual breath odors, which can offer valuable clues. For example, cyanide smells like bitter almonds, and some insecticides smell like garlic or petroleum products.

The emergency medical care of patients who in-

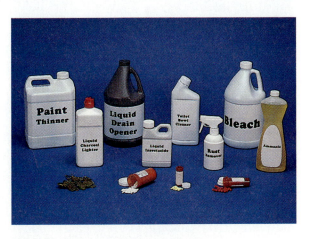

Fig. 21-1 Common types of household poisons.

gested a toxin begins with the basics. Determine if the patient has an open airway. If the patient is unresponsive, insert an oral or nasal airway to maintain an open airway. If the patient is not breathing, initiate artificial ventilations. If the patient is breathing, administer oxygen. If airway reflexes are intact and breathing is adequate, monitor the patient carefully. Poisoned patients may get worse quickly and require frequent reassessment.

With gloved hands, remove any pills, tablets, or fragments from the patient's mouth. Insert a bite block before placing your hands in an unresponsive patient's mouth. Ask a responsive patient to spit out the pills. Do not place your fingers in the mouth of an uncooperative patient who may injure you by biting. Consult medical direction once you have gathered all possible information on the patient's condition. The physician may order you to administer activated charcoal, which is a medication that binds to poisons to prevent absorption. When possible, bring containers, bottles, labels, vomitus, or pill fragments to the receiving facility with the patient. With children, also look for plants and leaves that may have been ingested. This evidence will help the staff form a treatment plan for the patient.

INHALED TOXINS

Inhaled toxins generally result in signs or symptoms of compromise related to the airway, lungs, or brain. Patients often complain of difficulty breathing. Inhaled substances can burn the lining of the airway and can lead to coughing, hoarseness, gagging, or tightness in the throat caused by airway swelling. Additional signs and symptoms of inhalation injury include chest pain, dizziness, headache,

confusion, altered mental status, weakness, syncope (fainting), and seizures. Inhaled substances can be rapidly absorbed directly into the blood stream through the lung tissue and cause generalized poisoning.

Your first concern with inhalation poisonings is the danger to you and others in the area. The inhaled poison may still be in the air you are breathing. The substance may be invisible, odorless, and tasteless, such as carbon monoxide (Fig. 21-2). Patients may complain only of general symptoms of being weak and sleepy and not know that carbon monoxide is the reason for their symptoms. If you believe there is any danger to you or others from inhaled poisons, avoid exposure until specially educated rescuers move the patient to a safe environment.

After controlling the airway, oxygen is the first treatment for inhalation poisonings. Continually monitor the patient for respiratory depression or arrest. The speed at which the poison enters the blood stream often does not give you much time to protect the patient from the toxic effects. Usually, inhaled toxins have been absorbed by the time you arrive, and your main function is to prevent further decline. Figure 21-3 illustrates some common signs and symptoms associated with inhaled toxins. Bring any containers, bottles, labels, and so on to the receiving facility with the patient to help the staff there formulate the treatment plan.

INJECTED TOXINS

Injected toxins enter the body through a puncture in the skin. Injection poisonings include insect and spider bites or stings, snake bites, and the stings

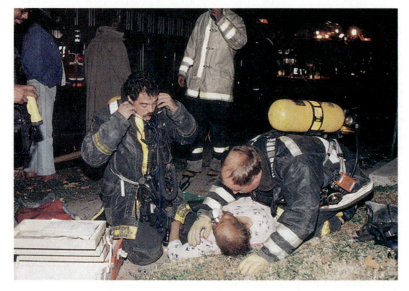

Fig. 21-2 Carbon monoxide poisoning is a serious possibility with fire victims.

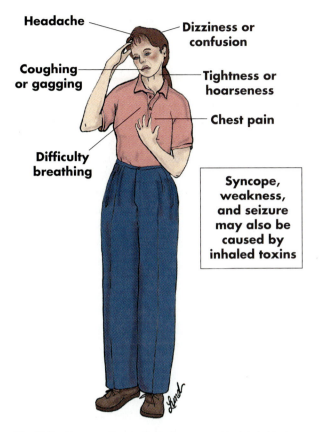

Headache

Coughing or gagging

Difficulty breathing

Dizziness or confusion

Tightness or hoarseness

Chest pain

Syncope, weakness, and seizure may also be caused by inhaled toxins

Fig. 21-3   Common signs and symptoms caused by inhaled toxins.

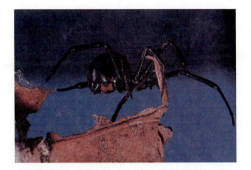

Fig. 21-4   Black widow spider.

or bites of marine animals. The large variety of possible sources often makes it difficult for you to determine what is responsible for the injection poisoning. Injection poisonings also can include the injection of a drug into a vein with a needle and syringe. Signs such as the presence of a syringe or needle puncture wounds are valuable help for determining the possible problem. Look also for bite or sting marks from animals. Carefully examine the patient's injury and the surrounding location for clues.

Your own safety is the first priority. When dealing with bites and stings, remember that whatever stung or bit the patient may still be present and able to injure you. Do not try to capture the creature for identification purposes. Figures 21-4 through 21-8 illustrate several sources of injected toxins.

The generalized signs and symptoms of injection poisoning include weakness, dizziness, chills, nausea, fever, and vomiting. Localized signs and symptoms may include swelling, redness, tingling, and burning around the injection site. The rate of absorption of the toxin depends on many factors, including location of the injection site, the type of insect or creature that caused the injury, and the blood flow to the bitten area.

The emergency medical care for injection poisonings starts with the basics and oxygen administration. Closely monitor the airway and be prepared to suction if the patient vomits. If possible, bring the agent that caused the injury to the receiving facility for identification. Do not try to catch a venomous snake or a spider for identification or tests; leave this job for the appropriate professionals. Give the receiving facility a description of the injection source, the location of the injury, the patient's signs and symptoms, and what treatments have been attempted so far. Do not use your mouth to try to suck out venom from the bite site, because this action could cause severe infection or poisoning for you. Immobilization of the bitten extremity is the readily accepted prehospital treatment. This immobilization prevents agitation and excitation of the limb, thus slowing the circulation of the poison.

ABSORBED TOXINS

An **absorbed toxin** enters the body through the skin. The absorbed poison may be obvious on the skin of the patient or may not be present. The

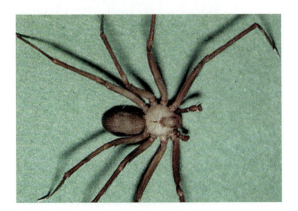

Fig. 21-5   Brown recluse spider.

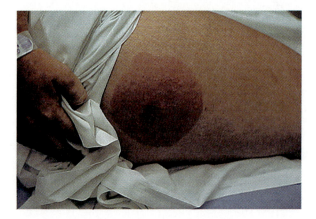

Fig. 21-6 Brown recluse spider bite after approximately 6 hours.

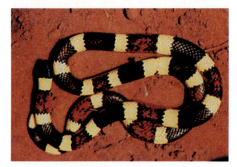

Fig. 21-7 Coral snake.

patient may be able to tell you of the event and may complain of burning, itching, or irritation around the location of the injury. The area may appear red or swollen. In some cases, no obvious signs may be present. The generalized signs and symptoms of absorbed poisoning may include weakness, dizziness, chills, nausea, and vomiting. Figure 21-9 illustrates some poisons that can be absorbed.

The emergency medical care for absorbed poisons begins with removing the substance from the patient. Always protect yourself from contamination. With powdered toxins, remove any contaminated clothing from the patient, brush off the powdered toxin, and continue care as for other absorbed poisons. With liquid toxins, remove any contaminated clothing, irrigate the site with clean water for at least 20 minutes, and proceed to transport. If an eye is involved, protect the unaffected eye and irrigate the affected eye with clean water, away from the unaffected eye, for 20 minutes. When possible, irrigate the affected area en route to the receiving facility. Contact medical direction as early as possible with the name of the poison that was absorbed.

Always contact medical direction as early as possible with the name of the poison that was ingested,

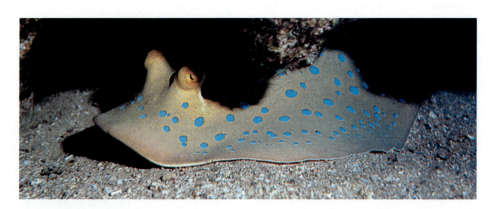

Fig. 21-8 Stingray.

BOX 21-1

Signs and Symptoms of Common Types of Poisonings

Ingested toxins

- Nausea
- Vomiting
- Diarrhea
- Altered mental status
- Abdominal pain
- Chemical burns around the mouth
- Particular breath odors

Inhaled toxins

- Difficulty breathing
- Chest pain
- Cough
- Hoarseness
- Dizziness
- Headache
- Confusion
- Seizures
- Altered mental status

Injected toxins

- Weakness
- Dizziness
- Chills
- Fever
- Nausea
- Vomiting

Absorbed toxins

- Liquid or powder on patient's skin
- Burns
- Itching
- Irritation
- Redness

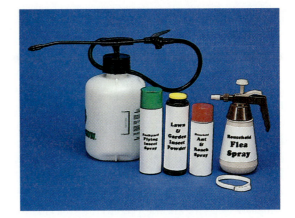

Fig. 21-9 Common toxins that can be absorbed.

absorbed, inhaled, or injected. The treatment for the poisoned patient may be a specific agent, called an *antidote*, that counteracts the effects of the poison. The receiving facility can have appropriate medications ready if they know in advance what the poison is. Box 21-1 lists the signs and symptoms for common types of poisonings.

REVIEW QUESTIONS

HISTORY OF POISONING/TYPES OF TOXINS

1. The patient's weight can determine the effect of certain poisons. True or False?

2. Injected poisonings always occur intentionally. True or False?

3. A person inhaling a poison can always smell it. True or False?

4. Always flush a skin absorption site for at least 5 minutes. True or False?

5. Always attempt to locate the snake that bit a patient so that the receiving facility can test the animal. True or False?

1. True
2. False
3. False
4. False
5. False

AIRWAY MANAGEMENT

Poisonings commonly affect the airway. Use the airway techniques described in Chapter 7, "The Airway," to manage any airway problems. The patient's airway can be compromised by tissues swelling due to an inhaled poison, or by vomiting caused by any type of poisonings.

The patient's condition can deteriorate rapidly, so continue to assess the patient for airway difficulties and manage the patient as necessary. Provide high-flow oxygen, and be prepared to use suction or assist the patient's ventilations as necessary.

USE OF ACTIVATED CHARCOAL

Medical direction may authorize **activated charcoal** for management of a poisoning victim. Acti-

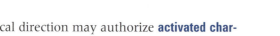

Fig. 21-10 Two types of activated charcoal.

TECHNIQUE 21-1
Administration of Activated Charcoal

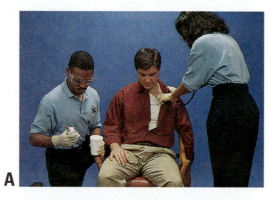

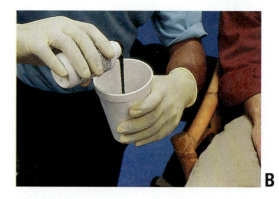

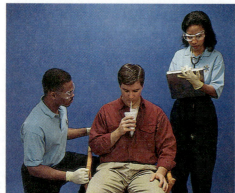

Fig. 21-11 Obtain an order from medical direction (either on- or off-line) to administer activated charcoal. **A, Shake the container thoroughly to suspend the medication in the fluid. B, Pour the liquid into a container.** Because the medication looks like mud, covering the container with a lid and using a straw may make it easier for the patient to drink it. Inform the patient of the drug's action and the potential side effects. **C, Persuade the patient to drink the full dose.** If the patient takes a long time to drink the medication, the charcoal will settle; shake or stir the liquid again. **Record the intervention and the time.**

vated charcoal is used only for ingested toxins. Activated charcoal works by binding to certain poisons, preventing them from being absorbed into the body. Not all brands of activated charcoal are the same, so consult medical direction about which brand to use.

Activated charcoal is the generic name for the medication. Trade names include InstaChar, Actidose, and LiquiChar (Fig. 21-10).

The indication for activated charcoal is a patient with the clinical signs and symptoms of ingested poisoning. Activated charcoal binds to poison in the stomach and therefore is not effective for poisoning by injection, inhalation, or absorption. Contraindications for activated charcoal are the patient having an altered mental status, being suspected of ingesting an acid or alkali substance, being unable to swallow, or having seizures. Activated charcoal is an oral medication; if the patient cannot swallow, it cannot be administered.

The early administration of activated charcoal can improve the patient's outcome considerably. To use activated charcoal, contact medical direction and provide information about the patient's route of poisoning and the poison ingested.

Activated charcoal is premixed in water and supplied in plastic bottles containing 25 g of activated charcoal. Powder forms are available but are seldom used in the field because they are messy and difficult to mix in a critical situation. The dose for adults and children is typically 1 g of activated charcoal per kg of body weight. On average, adults receive 25 to 50 g, and infants and children receive 12.5 to 25 g. Technique 21-1 describes the key steps for administering activated charcoal.

The side effects of activated charcoal include black stools and vomiting. Be prepared to suction if the patient vomits.

If the patient vomits after the administration of activated charcoal, repeat the dose once, following orders from medical direction. As after all interventions, reevaluate the patient frequently. Be prepared for possible deterioration.

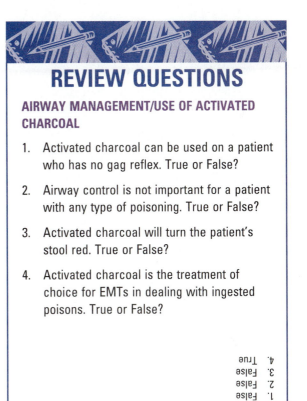

REVIEW QUESTIONS

AIRWAY MANAGEMENT/USE OF ACTIVATED CHARCOAL

1. Activated charcoal can be used on a patient who has no gag reflex. True or False?

2. Airway control is not important for a patient with any type of poisoning. True or False?

3. Activated charcoal will turn the patient's stool red. True or False?

4. Activated charcoal is the treatment of choice for EMTs in dealing with ingested poisons. True or False?

1. False
2. False
3. False
4. True

CHAPTER SUMMARY

The four basic types of toxic exposures are: ingestion, inhalation, injection, and absorption. The symptoms vary depending on the type of poisoning. Airway control is always important, and the patient often may deteriorate. Vomiting is a common side effect of many poisons. Be prepared to assist ventilations or suction as necessary.

Activated charcoal is often used in the management of ingested poisonings. Its use requires medical direction. The activated charcoal works by binding to certain poisons, preventing them from being absorbed into the body. Activated charcoal is administered orally. The usual adult dose is 25 g to 50 g; the usual infant or child dose is 12.5 g to 25 g.

UNITED STATES DEPARTMENT OF TRANSPORTATION NATIONAL HIGHWAY TRAFFIC SAFETY ADMINISTRATION EMT–BASIC OBJECTIVES

Check your knowledge. The National Registry of EMTs and many state EMS agencies use the objectives below to develop EMT–Basic certification examinations. Can you meet them?

COGNITIVE

1. List various ways that poisons enter the body.
2. List signs/symptoms associated with poisoning.
3. Discuss the emergency medical care for the patient with possible overdose.
4. Describe the steps of emergency medical care for the patient with suspected poisoning.
5. Establish the relationship between the patient suffering from poisoning or overdose and airway management.
6. State the generic and trade names, indications, contraindications, medication form, dose, administration, actions, side effects, and reassessment strategies for activated charcoal.
7. Recognize the need for medical direction in caring for the patient with poisoning or overdose.

AFFECTIVE

1. Explain the rationale for administering activated charcoal.

2. Explain the rationale for contacting medical direction early in the prehospital management of the poisoning or overdose patient.

PSYCHOMOTOR

1. Demonstrate the steps in the emergency medical care for the patient with possible overdose.
2. Demonstrate the steps in the emergency medical care for the patient with suspected poisoning.
3. Perform the necessary steps required to provide a patient with activated charcoal.
4. Demonstrate the assessment and documentation of patient response.
5. Demonstrate proper disposal of administration of activated charcoal equipment.
6. Demonstrate completing a prehospital care report for patients with a poisoning/overdose emegency.

22 ENVIRONMENTAL EMERGENCIES

IN THE FIELD

Pittsburgh River rescue services responded to a 911 call for a child who had fallen into the Allegheny river. The water in April was still very cold. Four-year-old Taylor had been playing in a riverside park when he slipped and fell into the dark, fast-moving water. His father had run to grab him but saw his son's body slip below the surface. Bystanders held him back from jumping into the water to save his son. They knew he wouldn't be able to rescue his son alone and would likely become a victim himself.

The rescue team arrived within minutes of the call. En route, Tom and Larry donned dry suits and SCUBA tanks—they knew they would have to go in for the boy. The rest of the team, including EMT-Basic Everitt, met them at the river's edge. Tom entered the water 12 minutes after the boy was last seen. He had difficulty but finally found the tiny body in the murky water.

Although the boy had no pulse and had been immersed for almost 20 minutes, Everitt knew that Taylor had a chance. He remembered from his EMT-Basic class that patients submerged in cold water can survive for a long time. He managed the airway and ventilated the cold, blue, rigid little body as his partner started cardiopulmonary resuscitation.

When they arrived at the hospital, the patient still had no pulse, but his color was a little better. The physician worked feverishly to resuscitate the little boy. Two days later Taylor woke up in the intensive care unit. He had recovered fully.

Work and recreational activities often take us outdoors. Unfortunately, the outdoor environment often presents hazards. Environmental emergencies include injuries that are caused by heat and cold, water, and bites and stings from animals, insects, marine life, and reptiles. EMT-Basics in all localities respond to such situations. Recognizing the signs and symptoms of environmental emergencies is necessary for giving effective prehospital care.

THERMOREGULATORY EMERGENCIES

To work effectively, the human body must maintain a relatively constant internal temperature. Alterations in the temperature of the body cause profound changes in vital chemical functions and can be life threatening. Increasing or decreasing the temperature of the body or a body part leads to injuries that are **thermoregulatory emergencies**.

TEMPERATURE REGULATION IN THE BODY

To understand cold and heat injuries, you need to understand how the body regulates temperature. There is a delicate balance between the heat generated in the body and the heat lost from it. The body is like a furnace. It takes in fuel in the form of food and "burns" it to produce energy. This process generates heat. Heat is lost to the environment in five ways: conduction, convection, evaporation, radiation, and respiration (Fig. 22-1).

Conduction is the transfer of heat directly from one object to another. If you sit on metal bleachers outside at a football game on a cold day, you lose heat through conduction to the metal. An injured patient who is lying on the ground in the winter loses heat by conduction into the earth. You can reduce conductive heat loss by placing insulating material such as a blanket between the patient and the ground.

Convection is the loss of heat through moving air or liquid. Blowing on hot soup cools it by convec-

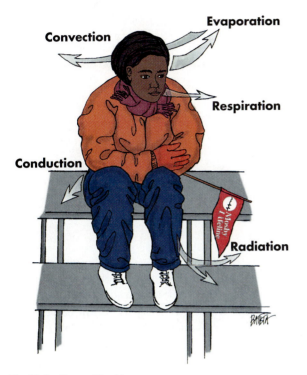

Fig. 22-1 Types of heat loss.

tion. We lose body heat faster when the wind is blowing—on a cold day this is called wind chill. You can decrease convective heat loss in cool weather by covering patients with a blanket.

Heat loss due to **evaporation** occurs when a liquid changes into a gas. The body uses this process to lose excess heat through sweat evaporating from the skin. Rubbing alcohol feels cool when applied to the skin because it evaporates quickly.

Your body constantly **radiates** heat outward into the air and to nearby colder objects. Most of this heat is in the form of infrared energy, which is what enables objects to be "seen" with night-vision goggles. Clothing and blankets reduce some radiant heat loss, but there is little you can do to significantly reduce heat loss due to radiation.

Air breathed into the body must be humidified and warmed to body temperature to be used by the lungs. This warm, humidified air is then exhaled, carrying heat out of the body. This constant cycle of inhalation, warming and humidifying, and exhaling expends much energy and leads to tremendous heat loss. In some regions EMTs may warm and humidify oxygen using special equipment to prevent this form of heat loss. If your EMS system warms and humidifies oxygen, follow your local protocol.

When faced with falling body temperatures, the body tries to maintain its temperature. This maintenance is accomplished by minimizing heat loss. The body constricts the peripheral blood vessels so less heat is lost from the skin by convection and conduction. The body also produces heat by shivering.

When faced with rising temperatures, the body tries to maintain its temperature by losing heat. The blood vessels dilate so that more warm blood reaches the skin where heat can be lost through conduction and convection. The body produces sweat to lose heat as the sweat evaporates. The body continues to lose heat by radiation and respiration as usual.

EXPOSURE TO THE COLD

GENERALIZED HYPOTHERMIA

Technically, anytime the body temperature falls below normal (37°C; 98.6°F), the patient is **hypothermic**. In any locality you may encounter a patient with a body temperature that is too low. Clinically, hypothermia is a progression of events from mild hypothermia as the body begins to cool to more severe late hypothermia that occurs as a patient's body temperature lowers significantly.

Predisposing Factors. The most common cause of generalized hypothermia is exposure to a cold environment. The temperature does not need to be extraordinarily cold for hypothermia to occur. In fact, the most dangerous temperature range is 40 to 50°F (5°–10°C), because in this range people often underestimate the danger of hypothermia and do not dress warmly enough. Other common factors contributing to hypothermia include water, ice, and snow. Less common causes include metabolic, neurological, traumatic, toxic, and infectious processes.

Alcohol use is a complicating factor in many hypothermic patients. Alcohol affects judgment and decision making, often resulting in a patient not seeking shelter from the cold. Alcohol also causes the blood vessels in the extremities to dilate, actually increasing heat loss even though the patient may not be aware of the loss.

Water conducts heat from the body much faster than air, and submersion in water can rapidly decrease body temperature. Immersion hypothermia should be suspected anytime the patient has been in the water.

BOX 22-1

Predisposing Factors for Generalized Hypothermia

- Cold environments
- Immersion in water
- Age (elderly and the very young)
- Alcohol
- Shock
- Head or spinal cord injury
- Burns
- Generalized infection
- Diabetes
- Hypoglycemia
- Some medications and poisons

ALERT

Look for signs of hypothermia in the following situations:
Patient who has ingested ethanol (alcohol)
Patient with general poor health
Drug overdoses and poisoning
Major trauma
Outdoor resuscitation
Chilly homes of elderly patients

The most important sign of hypothermia is a decrease in the mental status and motor function of the patient (Box 22-2). In hypothermic patients the level of responsiveness indicates the degree of hypothermia. This assessment is important because the treatment of hypothermia is based on the patient's mental status.

Cool skin in the extremities is an unreliable sign of hypothermia because blood flow to the extremities is normally decreased to prevent heat loss. To assess the patient's general temperature, place the back of your hand under the patient's clothing and against the abdomen. Cool abdominal skin is a sign of a generalized cold emergency.

The old and the young are particularly susceptible to hypothermia. Older patients lose insulating fat, and the body may not respond as efficiently to an increased need for heat production. Medications that some elderly patients take may interfere with the normal ability to respond to temperature changes. Young patients have a relatively large surface area for their small size and very little fat for insulation. The younger the child, the less likely the child is to seek protection by getting out of the cold or putting on more clothes. Infants have immature temperature regulation mechanisms.

Underlying medical conditions also predispose the patient to hypothermia. When the body is using energy to compensate for other injuries, it cannot generate enough heat to prevent hypothermia. Box 22-1 lists major predisposing factors for generalized hypothermia.

Signs and Symptoms of Generalized Hypothermia. You should consider the possibility of hypothermia whenever the patient has obviously been exposed to the cold. Remember, even in relatively warm conditions, hypothermia is possible. Hypothermia occurs in a progression, beginning with a slight drop in body temperature. The signs and symptoms of early hypothermia are very subtle, such as shivering and loss of sensation, and become more dramatic, such as dizziness and memory loss, as the hypothermia becomes more profound.

BOX 22-2

Mental Status and Motor Function Changes Caused by Hypothermia

- Poor coordination
- Memory disturbances
- Reduced or absent sensation of touch
- Mood changes
- Joint or muscle pain
- Poor judgement (for example, the patient may actually remove clothing)
- Less communicative
- Dizziness
- Speech difficulties

TABLE 22-1	Vital Signs in Hypothermia	
SIGN	**EARLY HYPOTHERMIA**	**LATE HYPOTHERMIA**
Pulse	Rapid	Slow and barely palpable Irregular
Blood pressure	Normal	Low or absent
Breathing	Rapid	Shallow, slow, absent
Skin	Red	Pale, cyanotic Stiff and hard
Pupils	Reactive	Sluggish

When the body temperature drops, a normal response is to increase heat production by shivering. Shivering is an effective method of the body for generating heat, but it is not always present in hypothermic patients. Usually the body stops shivering as the body temperature drops below 90°F (32°C). These patients may have a stiff or rigid posture. Children and infants and many elderly patients have small muscle mass that cannot generate very much heat by shivering.

The hypothermic patient's vital signs change as body temperature drops. Initially, the body attempts to increase heat production, and the heart rate and breathing increase. If the hypothermia progresses, the vital signs deteriorate as the patient's body attempts to prevent heat loss. Table 22-1 lists these changes.

Hypothermia affects the patient's level of responsiveness and ability to make rational decisions. Some hypothermic patients appear to be intoxicated, may be confused, and may exhibit poor judgment. Some hypothermic patients become so confused that they remove all of their clothing in extremely cold weather.

While assessing a patient who has been exposed to the cold, you should ask the patient or bystanders the questions listed in Box 22-3.

Emergency Care for Patients With Generalized Hypothermia. Generalized hypothermia occurs in three progressive stages:
1. Alert and responsive
2. Responding inappropriately or unresponsive
3. No signs of life

The treatment at each stage is different, as described in the following sections, but some general principles apply in all stages (Principle 22-1).

There are two ways that hypothermic patients are rewarmed: actively or passively. Passive rewarming uses the patient's own heat production to return the body temperature to normal. For passive rewarming to occur, you must first prevent further heat loss by removing the patient from the cold environment. Then allow the patient's normal body functions to raise the body temperature. Although this process is slow, it is very safe for patients with mild hypothermia. Active rewarming, on the other hand, adds heat to the patient. In the field, active rewarming techniques include the use of warmed oxygen and heat packs. In the hospital,

BOX 22-3

Questions for Patients Exposed to the Cold

- What was the source of the cold (water, snow, etc.)?
- Where were you (cool apartment, homeless, outdoors, etc.)?
- Did you experience any loss of consciousness?
- Are the effects general (affecting the entire body) or local (affecting a specific body part)?

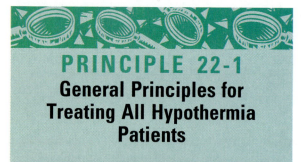

PRINCIPLE 22-1
General Principles for Treating All Hypothermia Patients

1. Remove the patient from the cold environment, and protect the patient from further heat loss.
2. Remove any wet clothing, and cover the patient with a blanket.
3. Handle the patient with extreme care. Avoid rough handling.
4. Administer high-flow oxygen. If possible, the oxygen should be warmed and humidified, using special equipment. If your EMS system warms and humidifies oxygen, follow your local protocol.
5. Do not allow the patient to eat or drink stimulants (chocolate, coffee, tea, etc.) or alcohol.
6. Do not massage the extremities.
7. Check for a pulse for 30 to 45 seconds before starting cardiopulmonary resuscitation (CPR).

additional active rewarming techniques may include using warm intravenous fluids and flushing the stomach or abdomen with warm solution.

Emergency care for the alert patient who is responding appropriately: As described earlier, the patient's level of responsiveness is correlated with the body temperature. If the patient does not have a decreased level of responsiveness, you can actively rewarm the patient safely:

1. Cover the patient in warm blankets.
2. Place heat packs (at approximately 102°–104°F or 38°–39°C) at the groin, armpits (axilla), neck, and head. Wrap heat packs in towels to ensure that they do not burn the patient.
3. Do not allow the patient to walk or become active.
4. Transport the patient to the hospital for complete evaluation. Turn up the heat in the patient compartment of the ambulance.
5. Administer warmed and humidified oxygen, if available.

Emergency care for the hypothermic patient with decreased level of responsiveness: Any decrease in the level of responsiveness of a hypothermic patient indicates severe hypothermia. Anytime that a cold patient is not responding appropriately or is disoriented or confused, the patient may be severely hypothermic. Actively rewarming a severely hypothermic patient could cause lethal heart irregularities. Although covering the patient and turning up the heat in the ambulance does not significantly rewarm a hypothermic patient, these actions prevent further heat loss and are therefore very important. Make sure that the patient is covered with lots of dry blankets and the patient compartment of the ambulance is warm so that the patient does not continue to lose heat.

1. Cover the patient in warm blankets.
2. Give high-flow oxygen.
3. Do not allow the patient to walk or become active.
4. Turn up the heat in the patient compartment of the ambulance.

Because active rewarming of a severely hypothermic patient could cause life-threatening changes in heart rhythms, the prehospital approach to hypothermic patients with a decreased level of responsiveness is to prevent further heat loss and allow for passive rewarming. Active rewarming will be accomplished in the hospital under more controlled circumstances.

ALERT
Do not attempt to actively warm hypothermic patients with a decreased level of responsiveness; simply prevent further heat loss.

Emergency care for the hypothermic patient with no signs of life: Unresponsive hypothermic patients may have a very slow heart rate or blood pressure so low that they may appear to be dead. Hypothermic patients in cardiac arrest are a significant challenge. Consult medical direction for advice, and follow your local protocol. In general, the following recommendations apply:

1. Ensure a patent airway.
2. Ventilate the patient with 100% oxygen.

3. Assess the pulse for 30 to 45 seconds before you start CPR. If you feel no pulse, begin external chest compressions.
4. Cover the patient in warm blankets.
5. Turn the heat up in the patient compartment of the ambulance.

Depending on local medical direction, the automated external defibrillator (AED) may be used with patients who are hypothermic and show no signs of life. If the AED detects a shockable rhythm, up to three shocks may be delivered. Shocking a patient whose heart is very cold may not be effective, but out of the hospital there is no way of knowing exactly how cold a patient's heart has become. Contact medical direction, and follow local protocol regarding the use of the AED for hypothermic patients.

LOCAL COLD INJURIES

The generalized cooling of the body is a danger to life, but local cooling can present a danger to the extremities and other body tissues. Local cold injuries result from decreased blood flow in a cold part of the body or the actual freezing of a body part. Local cold injuries occur in a gradual progression: the deeper the freezing occurs, the more damage will result.

Local cold injuries are most common in the fingers, toes, ears, nose, and face. These injuries are often called *frostbite* or *frostnip*, but these terms can be confusing and should be avoided.

Predisposing Factors. A history of local cold injury may have damaged the blood vessels in an extremity, making it more susceptible to cold injuries. Smoking constricts blood vessels to extremities and also increases the likelihood of local cold injuries.

Signs and Symptoms of Local Cold Injuries. The signs and symptoms of local cold injuries causing early or superficial injury may include:
1. Pale skin with delayed capillary refill
2. Loss of feeling and sensation in the injured area
3. Skin still soft
4. Tingling sensation when rewarmed

The signs and symptoms of local cold injuries causing late or deep damage may include:
1. White or waxy skin
2. Firm or frozen feeling on palpation
3. Swelling and blisters
4. Loss of sensation in the injured area

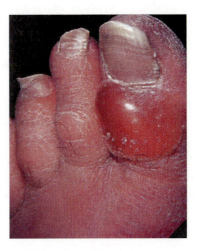

Fig. 22-2 Local cold injury after thawing.

5. If the injury has thawed or partially thawed, the skin may appear flushed with areas that are purple, pale, mottled, or cyanotic (Figs. 22-2 and 22-3).

Emergency Care for Patients With Local Cold Injuries. Rewarming of local cold injuries is extremely painful and best performed in the hospital where the patient can be given medication for the pain.
1. Remove the patient from the cold environment.
2. Protect the cold extremity from further injury. Because the tissues in the cold extremity are susceptible to additional injury, prevent unnecessary contact with that extremity.
3. Administer oxygen if you have not already done so.
4. Remove wet or restrictive clothing and all jewelry. It may be necessary for you to cut jewelry off if the extremity is swollen or if removal would cause damage to frozen tissues.

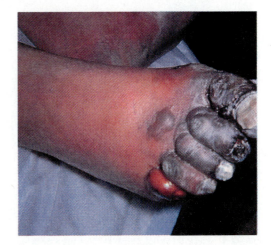

Fig. 22-3 Local cold injury after thawing.

5. Splint the extremity, and cover the injury with dry, sterile dressings.
6. There are several actions to avoid:
   - DO NOT reexpose the area to the cold.
   - DO NOT break blisters.
   - DO NOT rub or massage the area.
   - DO NOT apply heat or rewarm the area.
   - DO NOT allow the patient to walk on an affected extremity.

If you have an extremely long transport time or if transportation to a hospital is delayed, consider rewarming the injury rapidly in the field after contacting medical direction. To rapidly rewarm the area:

1. Immerse the affected part in warm (102°–104°F or 38°–39°C) water.
2. The water will become cool from the cold part that is immersed. Be sure to keep adding warm water. Continuously stir the water.
3. Continue the immersion until the skin is soft and the color and sensation have returned. Do not rub the area dry; pat gently.
4. Dress the injury with dry sterile dressings. If the injury is on the hand or foot, place dressings between the fingers and toes (Fig. 22-4).
5. Protect the injured area from refreezing. Refreezing causes more damage than allowing the injury to remain frozen. If you cannot ensure that the injury will not be refrozen, do not thaw a frozen area.

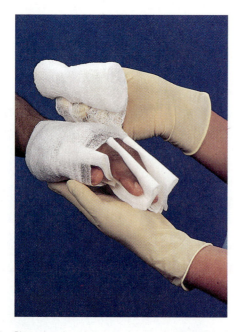

Fig. 22-4 Place dressings between the fingers affected by local cold injury.

EXPOSURE TO HEAT

Hyperthermia is present anytime a patient's internal temperature rises above normal (37°C; 98.6°F). The terms *heat stroke* and *heat exhaustion* have been used to describe the condition of generalized hyperthermia. Because there is considerable disagreement about the precise meaning of these terms, the term *hyperthermia* should be used instead.

The body can warm itself more effectively in the cold than cool itself in the heat. Delicate central nervous system tissue is extremely sensitive to high body temperatures; therefore, hyperthermia can be a severe life threat.

PREDISPOSING FACTORS

The body eliminates excess heat by increasing blood flow to the extremities, where heat can be lost from the skin, and by sweating. Heat emergencies occur most often when the environment is hot and humid. In these circumstances, the body cannot lose heat as effectively by radiation or evaporation of sweat. During exercise and vigorous activity in hot weather, the body can lose more than 1 L of sweat per hour. Sweat contains fluid and electrolytes (sodium and chloride) that are needed by the body.

BOX 22-4

Predisposing Factors for Heat Emergencies

- Hot, humid weather
- Vigorous activity
- Elderly
- Infants and newborns
- Heart disease
- Dehydration
- Obesity
- Previous history of hyperthermia
- Fever
- Fatigue
- Diabetes
- Drugs and medications

The elderly are predisposed to heat emergencies because they have less effective thermoregulatory mechanisms, may be on medications that affect their ability to eliminate heat, and may not be able to get away from a hot environment. Infants and newborns also have less effective thermoregulation. Infants are not able to get drinking water or remove clothing on their own. Preexisting medical conditions can also predispose an individual to heat injuries. Box 22-4 lists predisposing factors for heat injuries.

SIGNS AND SYMPTOMS OF GENERALIZED HYPERTHERMIA

Hyperthermia is a progression of events that occurs as the patient's internal temperature rises. A small rise in temperature is easily tolerated in most healthy patients. If the patient's temperature continues to rise, the signs and symptoms of generalized hyperthermia develop.

As in cold emergencies, altered mental status is an important assessment finding in the hyperthermic patient. As body temperature rises, the patient becomes disoriented and confused. If the temperature continues to rise, the patient will become unresponsive.

The signs and symptoms of generalized hyperthermia are:
1. Muscle cramps
2. Weakness or exhaustion
3. Dizziness or fainting
4. Rapid, pounding heart beat
5. Altered mental status
6. Moist, pale, cool, or normal skin
7. Nausea and vomiting
8. Abdominal cramps

Hot skin, whether it is moist or dry, is a sign of a dire emergency. Hot skin indicates that the body has lost its ability to eliminate heat, and the rising temperature is likely to cause extensive organ damage.

EMERGENCY CARE FOR PATIENTS WITH GENERALIZED HYPERTHERMIA

Emergency care for generalized hyperthermia in patients with moist, pale, cool, or normal skin:
1. Move the patient from the heat to a cool environment (eg, the back of an air-conditioned ambulance).
2. Administer oxygen if you have not already done so during the initial assessment.

3. Loosen or remove clothing.
4. Cool the patient by fanning.
5. Place a responsive patient in the supine position with legs elevated. Unless the patient is nauseated, give cool water to drink.
6. Place a patient who is unresponsive or is vomiting on the left side.

Emergency care for generalized hyperthermia in patients with hot skin: A heat-injured patient with hot

REVIEW QUESTIONS
THERMOREGULATORY EMERGENCIES

1. List the five ways that patients lose heat.

2. Water conducts heat from the body faster than air. True or False?

3. The most important assessment finding in evaluation of the hypothermic patient is:
   A. Level of responsiveness
   B. Skin color
   C. Shivering
   D. Exposure to extremely cold temperatures

4. Label whether the following signs and symptoms of general hypothermia are early or late signs.
   A. Slow irregular pulse _____
   B. Stiff and hard skin _____
   C. Red skin _____
   D. Rapid breathing _____
   E. Rapid pulse _____
   F. Cyanosis _____
   G. Normal blood pressure _____

5. On what assessment findings do you decide to rapidly cool a hyperthermic patient?

5. Hot skin or altered mental status
G. Early
F. Late
E. Early
D. Early
C. Early
B. Late
4. A. Late
3. A
2. True
1. Conduction; convection; evaporation; radiation; and respiration

skin or altered mental status is a serious emergency. The patient's temperature must be brought down immediately, before permanent organ damage occurs. The most effective way to drop body temperature combines convective, conductive, and evaporative heat loss. In addition to the emergency care steps listed above, you should:

1. Apply cool packs to the patient's neck, groin, and armpits.
2. Keep the patient's skin wet by applying water with a sponge or wet towels.
3. Fan the patient aggressively.
4. Transport the patient immediately to the hospital.

DROWNING AND NEAR DROWNING

Drowning is defined as death following immersion in water (or any other liquid). Near drowning occurs when a patient survives an immersion incident. Drowning is a major cause of accidental death in the United States. In most drowning deaths the victims are less than 30 years of age; many of these victims are less than 4 years of age. Risky behavior and alcohol contribute to water-related emergencies in teenagers and young adults. Lack of supervision often contributes to drowning in the very young.

Your personal safety is paramount when you respond to a water-related emergency. Water rescue is a specialized form of rescue that should be attempted only if you have had the appropriate education. In some cases you may respond to a scene in which lifeguards or bystanders have already brought a victim out of the water, allowing you to begin medical care immediately.

The incidence of spinal injuries in water-related emergencies is very high. Anytime a patient is found unresponsive in the water, you should suspect a spine injury caused by the patient having struck a diving board, an object in the water, or the bottom. Because these patients require immediate management of their life-threatening condition, you should quickly place them on a long board, secure two straps, and remove them from the water while manually stabilizing the head.

If the patient is responsive and the mechanism of injury suggests that a spinal injury may have occurred, fully immobilize the patient while still in the water. Apply a cervical spinal immobilization device, strap the patient to a long spine board with

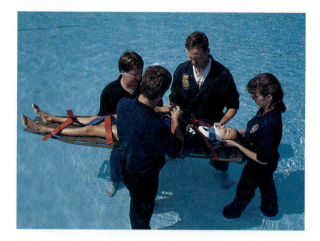

Fig. 22-5 Fully immobilize a conscious patient with a suspected spinal injury while still in the water.

3 to 4 straps, and secure the head to the board (Fig. 22-5).

EMERGENCY MEDICAL CARE OF THE NEAR-DROWNING PATIENT

1. Immobilize the spine if trauma is suspected. Whenever possible, do this in the water.
2. Ensure an adequate airway.
3. Provide oxygen and ventilate if necessary.
4. Provide external chest compressions if the patient is pulseless.
5. Suction as needed.
6. If no trauma is suspected, place the patient on the left side to allow fluids to drain from the airway.
7. If gastric distention interferes with artificial ventilation, place the patient on the left side. With suction immediately available, place your hand over the epigastric area and apply firm pressure to relieve the distention.

ALERT
DO NOT attempt to relieve gastric distention unless it interferes with artificial ventilation. There is a significant risk of aspiration.

In some cases, patients have survived after extremely long periods of submersion in cold water. Any patient who is found pulseless and apneic following submersion in cold water should be resuscitated.

BITES AND STINGS

Just about everyone has been stung by an insect at some time. For most people, these stings are merely uncomfortable. In some cases, however, a bite or sting can be life threatening because of either an injected venom or an allergic reaction. This chapter discusses the treatment of bites and stings when the patient does not have an allergic reaction. The care for a patient experiencing an allergic reaction is discussed in Chapter 20, "Allergies."

As an EMT, you should be able to treat stings from insects, scorpions, and marine life and bites from spiders and snakes (Fig. 22-6A–C). You should learn more about the kinds of bites and stings that are common in your area.

SIGNS AND SYMPTOMS

In most cases the patient (or bystanders) can tell you whether they were stung or bitten. Unfortunately, in some cases they may not know what it was that stung or bit them. Although identifying the animal or insect causing the injury may provide useful information to the receiving facility, do not put yourself at risk to obtain this information. Box 22-5 lists the possible signs and symptoms of bites and stings. Patients may have a wide variety of signs and symptoms depending on the type of bite or sting. You may see any combination of these signs and symptoms.

EMERGENCY MEDICAL CARE FOR BITES AND STINGS

1. Ensure an adequate airway, breathing, and circulation.
2. Inspect the site. If a stinger is present, scrape it out with the edge of a piece of rigid cardboard, butter knife, or plastic card such as a credit card. Do not use tweezers or forceps because these can squeeze venom out of a venom sac still attached to the stinger in the skin (Fig. 22-7).
3. If possible, wash the area gently.
4. Remove jewelry from the injured area before swelling occurs.
5. If the injury is on an extremity, position the bite or sting site slightly below the level of the patient's heart.
6. In cases of snakebites, consult medical direction regarding the use of a constricting band.
7. Observe the patient for the development of signs and symptoms of an allergic reaction and treat as needed. Chapter 20, "Allergies," provides information about allergic reactions.

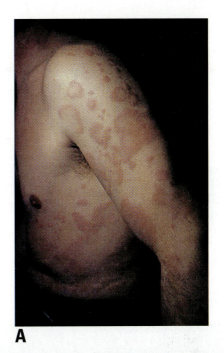

A

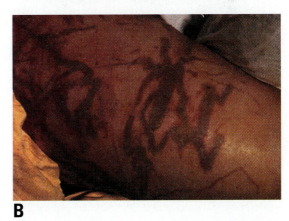

B

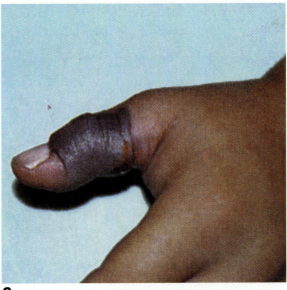

C

Fig. 22-6 Bites and stings. **A**, A wasp sting with systemic reaction. **B**, Jellyfish sting. **C**, Swelling caused by a snake bite.

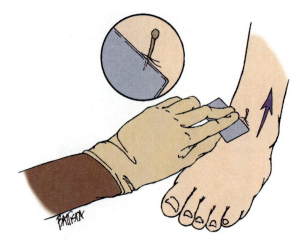

Fig. 22-7 The proper way to remove a stinger.

BOX 22-5

Signs and Symptoms of Bites and Stings

- Bite marks
- Rash
- Stinger in skin
- Local pain, redness, and swelling
- Weakness
- Dizziness
- Chills
- Fever
- Nausea and vomiting

REVIEW QUESTIONS

DROWNING AND NEAR DROWNING/BITES AND STINGS

1. How should you immobilize an unresponsive near-drowning patient with a suspected spinal injury?

2. What piece of equipment is <u>not</u> needed to treat a near-drowning patient.
   A. Suction
   B. Oxygen
   C. Ventilation equipment
   D. Reeves stretcher

3. Why should tweezers <u>not</u> be used when removing a stinger?
   A. Pinching the stinger may release venom into the wound.
   B. The stinger may break off.
   C. It hurts the patient too much.
   D. You cannot get a good hold of the stinger with tweezers.

3. A
2. D
1. Quickly place the patient on a long board with two straps, and remove the patient from the water while manually stabilizing the head.

---

to the heat causes the internal temperature of the body to increase and can also be a life-threatening situation. Anytime the patient's skin is hot to the touch, the patient must be cooled immediately.

DROWNING AND NEAR DROWNING

Drowning is a common form of accidental death and can occur anywhere there is water. Spinal injuries often accompany water-related injuries. Prompt management of the airway, breathing, and circulation with attention to suctioning are needed for a near-drowning patient.

BITES AND STINGS

Stings from insects, scorpions, and marine animals and bites from spider and snakes can occur anywhere. The patient's reaction to these injuries can range from mild discomfort to death.

CHAPTER SUMMARY

THERMOREGULATORY EMERGENCIES

Thermoregulatory emergencies occur when the patient's internal temperature is higher or lower than normal. This emergency can be serious because the body's functions depend on a constant temperature. The body must maintain a delicate balance between the amount of heat it generates and loses. Generalized hypothermia can cause a decrease in mental status and motor functions and eventually death. Local cold injuries are common to the fingers, toes, nose, ears, and face. Exposure

UNITED STATES DEPARTMENT OF TRANSPORTATION NATIONAL HIGHWAY TRAFFIC SAFETY ADMINISTRATION EMT–BASIC OBJECTIVES

Check your knowledge. The National Registry of EMTs and many state EMS agencies use the objectives below to develop EMT–Basic certification examinations. Can you meet them?

COGNITIVE

1. Describe the various ways that the body loses heat.
2. List the signs and symptoms of exposure to cold.
3. Explain the steps in providing emergency medical care to a patient exposed to cold.
4. List the signs and symptoms of exposure to heat.
5. Explain the steps in providing emergency care to a patient exposed to heat.
6. Recognize the signs and symptoms of water-related emergencies.
7. Describe the complications of near drowning.

8. Discuss the emergency medical care of bites and stings.

PSYCHOMOTOR

1. Demonstrate the assessment and emergency medical care of a patient with exposure to cold.
2. Demonstrate the assessment and emergency medical care of a patient with exposure to heat.
3. Demonstrate the assessment and emergency medical care of a near-drowning patient.
4. Demonstrate completing a prehospital care report for patients with environmental emergencies.

Abnormal behavior: A behavior exhibited by a person that is outside of the norm for the situation and is socially unacceptable; this behavior may result in harm to the person or to others.

Behavioral emergency: A situation in which a person exhibits abnormal behavior that is unacceptable or intolerable to the person, family members, or the community.

Domestic dispute: A form of violence that results from a family argument and may result in abuse of spouse or children.

Psychotic: Refers to behavior by a person who has lost touch with reality.

Reasonable force: The force necessary to keep a person from injuring him- or herself or others.

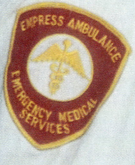

IN THE FIELD

Carlos, an EMT, responded with his crew to an emergency call of a motorcycle crash. Law enforcement personnel were requested because of the danger of oncoming traffic and the crowd of bystanders. As Carlos and his crew approached the scene, they saw no apparent dangers. No electrical lines were down, and no fluid was leaking from the motorcycle.

Expecting to find a typical trauma patient, Carlos rushed into the scene with a trauma bag. He was mentally reviewing the steps of the initial assessment as he approached the injured man lying on the ground.

The patient was positioned on his side with his back toward Carlos. As Carlos approached the man and began to assess his responsiveness, the patient suddenly turned and pulled a gun from behind him. In an instant, Carlos became a potential victim at risk from the gun pointed directly toward him.

Carlos did the only thing he could do: he calmly talked to the patient. He explained who he was and asked pertinent medical questions so that the patient knew that he was not a threat. Carlos was thankful he had contacted law enforcement prior to approaching the scene. As he spoke to the patient, law enforcement personnel arrived on the scene, approached the patient from behind, and took control of the weapon.

Carlos was then able to assess the patient and treat his injuries. It was later discovered at the hospital that the patient suffered from head trauma that produced his irrational behavior.

EMTs respond to many situations involving behavioral emergencies, from stress reactions to severe altered mental status resulting from illness or injury. Some behavioral emergencies result from psychologic problems caused by mental illness or the use of mind-altering substances, such as alcohol, illegal drugs, or prescription medications. Other emergencies result from a traumatic injury or acute illness.

You must be aware of behavioral emergencies and their causes. You must know how to handle these delicate situations and what options are available to you as a caregiver. Sometimes EMTs approach an apparently safe scene, such as a medical call, but then discover a danger present. For this reason, it is acceptable for EMS providers to contact law enforcement prior to entering any situation.

BEHAVIOR

A behavior is the manner in which a person acts or performs. All physical and mental activities of a person are behaviors. Humans behave differently for various reasons. For example, one person may be frightened of something that another person finds humorous.

A **behavioral emergency** results when a person exhibits **abnormal behavior** in a situation that results in potential harm to himself or others (Fig. 23-1). An abnormal behavior is one that is unacceptable or intolerable to the person, family members, or the community. This behavior might be the result of extreme emotion and could lead to violence. An abnormal behavior can also be caused by traumatic injuries or acute illness, such as lack of oxygen or low blood sugar.

BEHAVIORAL CHANGES

Many situational stresses, medical illnesses, and legal or illegal drugs including alcohol, may alter a person's behavior. Diabetic patients who have low blood sugar may have a change in behavior, such as aggressiveness, restlessness, or anxiety, if they do not stay on a proper diet. These patients do not have enough energy reaching their cells, and the brain suffers from the lack of nutrients, resulting in an altered mental status. Lack of oxygen and inadequate blood flow to the brain are other causes of an altered mental status, resulting in similar

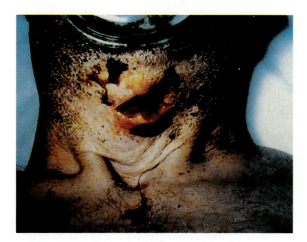

Fig. 23-1   A self-inflicted knife wound in the throat.

behavior. These conditions may also result from head or other trauma with loss of blood.

Excessive cold or heat exposure may produce a reaction in the body that changes a person's behavior. For example, a person experiencing a heat-related emergency can have a decreased level of responsiveness, can be confused and disoriented, and can experience panic. There are also many types of drugs and alcohol that produce obvious changes in behavior. People exposed to a very stressful situation also may temporarily panic.

Many behavioral changes occur in otherwise normal, healthy people when they are exposed to any extreme condition. For example, you may respond to a trauma call to find a patient who is stable. The patient might be acting unusual only because he or she has never been in a trauma situation and is scared. Family members of the patient also may be experiencing the stress of the situation and begin acting abnormally if they are scared or upset. You may end up caring for multiple patients.

Geriatric patients may be more at risk for behavioral emergencies because their bodies cannot tolerate changes as efficiently as a younger patient's. They are more susceptible to hypothermia, hyperthermia, and metabolic changes because their bodies cannot compensate easily. Many elderly patients suffer from hypothermia in cold weather, even indoors. They may forget to turn up the thermostat or may intentionally keep it set very low to save money.

Be aware of the environment in which you find the patient, and document any findings such as temperature, lack of food, lack of proper ventilation, cleanliness, and so on. These findings may be important for you and the receiving facility to properly treat the patient.

PSYCHOLOGIC CRISES

Other changes in behavior may result from mental illness and produce **psychotic** thinking or depression. A person experiencing a psychologic crises may panic easily as a result of very little stress, or may become agitated with no apparent or obvious provocation. These patients may be a danger to themselves or to others. They can be provoked to suicide or violence very easily, and their behavior can change quickly and unpredictably. Patients experiencing certain psychoses think and behave differently. A patient with paranoia may be convinced that people are plotting against them. A manic patient may be very agitated, moving and speaking rapidly without producing clear or complete sentences. A depressed patient may not want to move or answer any questions. Treat these patients gently and without sudden moves or actions to prevent scaring and agitating them.

SUICIDAL GESTURES

When you examine a patient who may be experiencing an abnormal behavior, determine

---

BOX 23-1

Risk Factors of Suicide

- Patients more than 40 years of age, widowed or divorced, alcoholic, or depressed
- Patients who have spoken of taking their own lives
- Patients with a previous history of self-destructive behavior
- Patients with recently diagnosed serious illness
- Patients in an environment where there is an unusual gathering of destructive articles (eg, guns or large amounts of pills)
- Patients who have recently lost a loved one
- Patients who were recently arrested or imprisoned
- Patients who have lost their job

whether the patient may be at risk to harm himself or herself, or others. A person who is notably depressed may be expressing thoughts of death or suicide and may seem very sad in expressions and behavior. It is important to recognize signs of depression and suicidal gestures before the patient behaves self-destructively. Box 23-1 describes some risk factors that may help you determine if a person is at risk for suicidal behavior.

The fact that patients do not have any risk factors for suicide, however, does not mean that they are not at risk, and patients who have some risk factors may not be considering suicide. Find out from fam-ily members and friends if the patient has been depressed recently. Patients may seem cheerful when you are present, but previous indications of risk factors are extremely important. Depressed patients may be too exhausted to commit suicide but may be at risk thereafter.

ASSESSMENT AND EMERGENCY CARE

SCENE SIZE-UP

The first action EMTs should take in the emergency medical care of a patient with a suspected behavioral emergency is the scene size-up. Be careful when examining the environment of the patient. The environment may be unsafe, or the patient may have an unsafe object that presents a risk. The patient may be seated in a defensive position or have fists clenched. Notice if the patient is calm or standing and yelling, and observe how the patient is moving. If you believe the scene is unsafe, do not enter. Contact law enforcement personnel as needed.

Gather information from family or bystanders about the patient's behavior prior to your arrival. Do not let the patient get between you and the nearest exit route (Fig. 23-2). Stay near doors or exits if possible. If the scene becomes unsafe and cannot be secured after you have entered and begun care, exit as quickly as possible. See Chapter 8, "Scene Size-Up," for more detailed information regarding safety.

REVIEW QUESTIONS

BEHAVIOR

1. The manner in which a person acts or per-forms is called _____.

2. Of the following, which situation would not be considered a risk factor for suicide:
   A. Divorce
   B. Loss of job
   C. Diagnosis of serious illness
   D. Previous destructive behavior
   E. 30 years of age and not married

3. Which of the following should not cause an altered mental status by itself?
   A. Low blood sugar
   B. Head trauma
   C. Excessive exposure to cold or heat
   D. Mental illness
   E. Bumping the arm and getting a bruise

4. A behavioral emergency exists when the person acts in an _____ manner that may be a threat to himself or herself or others.

5. A person acting sad or depressed may be experiencing _____ tendencies.

1. Behavior
2. E
3. E
4. Abnormal
5. Suicidal

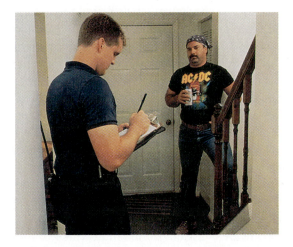

Fig. 23-2 Do not allow any participant in a dispute to position himself between you and the door or exit route.

BOX 23-2

Signs of Potential Patient Violence

- Sitting on edge of seat, as if ready to move
- Clenched fists
- Yelling and using profanity
- Standing or moving toward EMT
- Throwing things
- Holding onto a potentially dangerous object
- Any behavior that makes the EMT uneasy

You may need to remove the patient from the surroundings and from bystanders to be able to perform the assessment. For example, an adolescent with peers present may not answer questions correctly for fear of embarrassment or may not want to admit a problem in front of friends.

If the patient was or is displaying destructive behavior toward himself or herself or others, or if you feel threatened or sense that the situation may get out of control and you require additional assistance, contact law enforcement. Box 23-2 lists the signs of potential violence.

As you enter a situation, approach patients from the head (if supine) rather than the side or the foot in case they may have a weapon.

ALERT
Use caution! Any object near the patient may become a dangerous object if the patient intends to do harm.

Often violence erupts in a **domestic dispute**. If you suspect abuse to a spouse or child, ensure that law enforcement assistance is requested.

ALERT
Stay near doors and exits. Do not let the patient block your route of escape if the situation becomes out of control.

COMMUNICATION AND EMERGENCY MEDICAL CARE

After determining that the scene is safe, introduce yourself and explain to the patient why emergency medical services are there (if they are not the ones who called EMS). Then, assess the patient for injury or illness. If there is a medical problem, perform the appropriate interventions while explaining everything to the patient. Assess how the patient actually feels and if the patient expresses suicidal tendencies.

You may ask questions to try to determine whether the unusual behavior has a medical or psychologic cause, although too much prying may provoke some individuals into aggressive behavior. Ask basic questions to assess the patient, such as the following: "What is your name, the date, your address?" "How do you feel?" "Would you like some help with your problem?" "Do you have a history of diabetes, heart disease, etc?" Usually the answers to simple questions such as these can help you determine the psychologic status of the patient.

Observe the patient's appearance, activity, speech, and orientation for time, person, and place. If you suspect a drug overdose, take any drugs or medications found at the scene to the medical facility with the patient. Always treat the patient with respect and dignity. If the patient displays disturbed thinking, however, do not make statements that agree with them.

In cases of domestic disputes in which you may suspect abuse of a spouse or child, request assistance from police. Document any abuse observed or your reasons for suspecting abuse, and report that information to the receiving medical facility. You must know the laws in your state regarding the documentation and reporting of suspected abuse.

CALMING THE PATIENT

Try to calm the patient if they are upset, and do not leave the patient alone unless there is a danger to yourself and your crew. Ask all questions in a calm and reassuring manner, and do not be judgmental toward the patient. Repeat the patient's answers to show the patient you are listening. Always acknowledge how the patient feels and do not challenge or argue with the patient. During questioning, remain a comfortable distance away from the patient, use good eye contact, and do not make sudden movements. It is imperative to remain calm. Involve family members and friends to gain a detailed history of the patient, including medical and psychiatric illnesses. Perform an initial assessment of the patient, including an evaluation of mental status and the potential for violence or suicide.

RESTRAINTS

In some situations, you will be unable to calm patients enough to approach and provide care safely. Family members often insist that patients be taken to a medical treatment facility, or insist they be treated for their safety or well-being. Patients who do not calm down and are showing destructive behavior toward themselves or others may need to be restrained before treatment and transportation (*see* Principle 23-1).

Follow your local protocols and laws regarding restraints. In many areas, restraints cannot be used without the cooperation of law enforcement or without consultation with medical direction.

Restraints can be dangerous to use. If used improperly, they can do harm to the patient. Suffocation, poor circulation distal to the restraints, poor access to the airway or injury, and poor access to the patient are some medical problems complicated by restraints.

You must document the patient's condition before and after applying restraints and conduct several assessments after application. Patients experiencing a behavioral emergency may later claim injury because of the restraints. Once again, documentation is extremely important. Use soft leather or padded cloth restraints, not metal handcuffs, so soft-tissue damage to the patient is avoided (Fig. 23-3). If applying a mask to a patient, use one that will not obstruct the airway or decrease oxygen flow, such as a surgical mask or an oxygen mask. Once restraints are applied, do not remove them. Removal should be done by the receiving facility or law enforcement. If the restraints are too tight when you reevaluate them, they should be loosened, not removed. Technique 23-1 describes one way to restrain a patient.

See Chapter 3, "Medical/Legal and Ethical Issues," for more information on legal issues regarding the use of restraints and law enforcement.

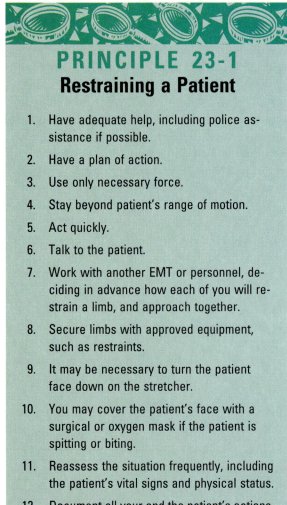

PRINCIPLE 23-1
Restraining a Patient

1. Have adequate help, including police assistance if possible.

2. Have a plan of action.

3. Use only necessary force.

4. Stay beyond patient's range of motion.

5. Act quickly.

6. Talk to the patient.

7. Work with another EMT or personnel, deciding in advance how each of you will restrain a limb, and approach together.

8. Secure limbs with approved equipment, such as restraints.

9. It may be necessary to turn the patient face down on the stretcher.

10. You may cover the patient's face with a surgical or oxygen mask if the patient is spitting or biting.

11. Reassess the situation frequently, including the patient's vital signs and physical status.

12. Document all your and the patient's actions.

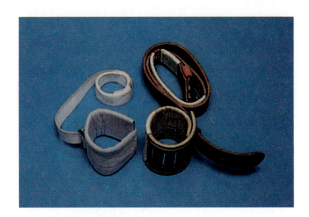

Fig. 23-3 Examples of soft restraints.

TECHNIQUE 23-1
Restraining a Patient

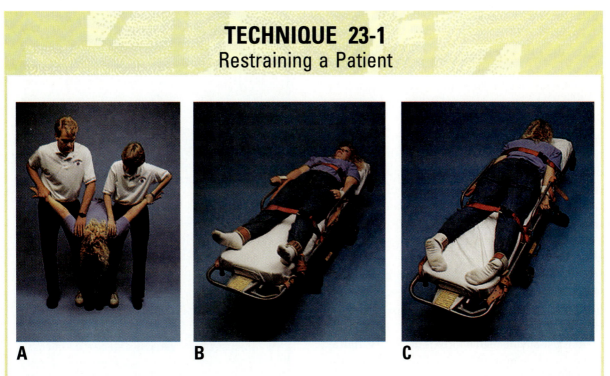

A   **B**   **C**

Fig. 23-4 A, Two EMTs approach from behind, pull the patient's arms back, and bend the patient forward at the waist to assume the control position. B, Place the patient supine or, C, prone on the stretcher with wrist and ankle restraints. Do not remove the restraints before arriving at the receiving facility. Continuously reassess the patient's vital signs and physical well-being.

REVIEW QUESTIONS

ASSESSMENT AND EMERGENCY CARE

1. The first assessment that the EMT should do is the _____ .

2. For a patient who is anxious or upset, the EMT should try to _____ the patient and not leave the patient alone.

3. Treat the patient with _____, but do not agree with _____ thinking.

4. Contact _____ if a situation becomes out of control or you need help.

5. Involve family and friends when gathering the _____ of the patient.

5. History
4. Law enforcement
3. Respect; disturbed or abnormal
2. Calm
1. Scene size-up

MEDICAL AND LEGAL CONSIDERATIONS

CONSENT

When confronted with a behavioral emergency, EMTs must determine the appropriate action to take. If an emotionally disturbed patient consents to treatment and transport, the decisions are more easily made and the legal problems are avoided or greatly reduced.

RESISTANCE TO TREATMENT

Unfortunately, emotionally disturbed patients often resist treatment or transport. The patient may threaten to harm you or others if approached. Once again, follow local protocols regarding the care of patients who refuse treatment. In general, you must decide if the patient is mentally able to make an informed decision. Consider the patient's psychologic status, level of consciousness, age, and injury. A competent adult may choose to refuse treatment even after being informed of the consequences. For example, some religions do not permit medical intervention. See Chapter 3, "Medical/Legal and Ethical Issues,'' for more information on consent.

On the other hand, adults with abnormal behavior or an altered mental status may refuse treatment after being informed of the consequences because they do not understand the seriousness of the illness or injury. Such patients may be transported without consent after you contact medical direction. To treat or transport a patient without consent often requires the assistance of law enforcement to restrain a patient. If you are unsure of the mental capabilities of the patient, you should choose to treat and transport.

USE OF FORCE

The use of force in behavioral emergencies should be limited to the force necessary to keep patients from injuring themselves or others, including yourself or other personnel. Law enforcement is usually needed if force is necessary, though sometimes you may be involved in the process also.

Many factors must be considered to determine if **reasonable force** is to be used to restrain a patient. Use only enough force to keep the patient from injuring themselves or others, and avoid physical force that may cause injury to the patient. Be aware that after a period of combativeness and aggression, some calm patients may be unknowingly provoked to cause unexpected and sudden injury to themselves and others.

A L E R T

Reasonable force depends upon:
1. **Patient's size and strength;**
2. **Type of abnormal behavior exhibited by the patient;**
3. **Gender of the patient;**
4. **Mental status of the patient;**
5. **Method of restraint used.**

DOCUMENTATION

EMTs cannot be too cautious when dealing with an emotionally unstable patient. Documentation of all abnormal behavior exhibited by the patient is extremely important (*see* Box 23-3). Because patients may accuse EMTs of sexual misconduct, always ask someone else on the scene to be a witness. If same-sex attendants are available, let them

---

BOX 23-3

Important Documentation for Behavioral Emergencies

- The position in which the patient was found
- Any aggressive or abnormal action produced by the patient
- Anything unusual the patient says, documented in direct quotations if possible
- Document every aspect of assessment and the findings in detail
- Document any restraining procedures used and assessment findings before and after their use
- Document any persons assisting or witnessing the treatment and transport of the patient

---

REVIEW QUESTIONS

MEDICAL AND LEGAL CONSIDERATIONS

1. Patients exhibiting a behavioral emergency often _____ treatment or transport.

2. If the patient is violent and cannot be calmed, the EMT may use _____, if determined by local protocol.

3. _____ of all actions is a very important aspect of the medical and legal aspects of patient care.

4. Always have a _____ present when caring for the patient with a behavioral emergency.

5. The EMT should be very cautious when dealing with an emotionally unstable patient. True or False?

1. Refuse
2. Restraints
3. Documentation
4. Witness
5. True

provide or assist you with care. You or your partner should never be alone with psychologically unstable patients.

CHAPTER SUMMARY

BEHAVIOR

EMTs must be aware that any call can become a behavioral emergency. Even if the scene size-up does not indicate an immediate danger, the situation may later become dangerous. There are many causes of behavioral emergencies.

A behavior is the manner in which a person acts or performs, including all physical and mental activity. A behavioral emergency is a situation in which a person exhibits abnormal or unacceptable behavior that is intolerable to the person, family, or community. A change in behavior may result from mental illness, situational stress, alcohol, drugs, medical illness, or a traumatic injury.

ASSESSMENT AND EMERGENCY CARE

Be aware of the danger that can arise when dealing with a behavioral emergency. Always be concerned for your own safety and then the safety of others. Under no circumstances should you risk injury to yourself or others.

Determine if patients are a danger to themselves or others and consider the need for law enforcement and restraints. Patients may have certain risk factors predisposing them to suicidal thoughts and tendencies.

First perform the scene size-up. Observe the patient's environment, attitude, and behavior. Do not let the patient get between you and the nearest door or exit route. Involve family, friends, and bystanders in obtaining the history of the patient. If the patient cannot be managed and is a threat to self or others, consider the use of restraints. Follow local protocol to get approval from medical direction or seek law enforcement assistance before using restraints. Use only reasonable force when restraining a patient. Perform several assessments after applying restraints to ensure the safety of the patient.

Be very cautious when dealing with a behavioral emergency. Emotionally disturbed patients often refuse treatment or transport. You may treat a patient without consent if you believe that the patient will harm self or others. Document all patient behaviors and witnesses for later verification if needed. Patients may accuse the EMT of sexual harassment or assault. Always try to have a witness to validate the documentation, and try not to be alone with the patient.

MEDICAL AND LEGAL CONSIDERATIONS

It is essential that you know the local protocols and laws regarding treating and transporting patients who refuse care. In general, patients who are mentally competent can elect to refuse care. Determine if the patient is mentally competent to make an informed refusal. If you are unsure, decide to treat and transport. Seek medical direction and assistance from law enforcement in difficult situations. Document all events in the situation so that you can legally defend any actions you performed or did not perform in the treatment of the patient.

UNITED STATES DEPARTMENT OF TRANSPORTATION NATIONAL HIGHWAY TRAFFIC SAFETY ADMINISTRATION EMT–BASIC OBJECTIVES

Check your knowledge. The National Registry of EMTs and many state EMS agencies use the objectives below to develop EMT–Basic certification examinations. Can you meet them?

COGNITIVE

1. Define behavioral emergencies.
2. Discuss the general factors that may cause an alteration in a patient's behavior.
3. State the various reasons for psychological crises.
4. Discuss the characteristics of an individual's behavior which suggest that the patient is at risk for suicide.
5. Discuss special medical/legal considerations for managing behavioral emergencies.
6. Discuss the special considerations for assessing a patient with behavioral problems.
7. Discuss the general principles of an individual's behavior which suggest he is at risk for violence.
8. Discuss methods to calm behavorial emergency patients.

AFFECTIVE

1. Explain the rationale for learning how to modify your behavior toward the patient with a behavioral emergency.

PSYCHOMOTOR

1. Demonstrate the assessment and emergency medical care of the patient experiencing a behavioral emergency.
2. Demonstrate various techniques to safely restrain a patient with a behavioral problem.

24 OBSTETRICS AND GYNECOLOGY

KEY TERMS

Abortion: The medical term for any delivery or removal of a human fetus before it can live on its own.

Amniotic sac: The membrane forming a closed, fluid-filled sac around a developing fetus.

Birth canal: The lower part of the uterus and the vagina.

Bloody show: The expulsion of the mucous plug as the cervix dilates, which is sometimes mixed with blood; it often occurs at the beginning of labor.

Breech presentation: The presentation of the baby's feet or buttocks first in delivery.

Caesarean section: A surgical delivery in which the muscles of the abdomen are cut and the baby is delivered through the abdomen.

Cephalic: The presentation of the baby's head first in delivery.

Cervix: The neck of the uterus.

Crowning: The stage in which the head of the baby is seen at the vaginal opening.

Fetus: An unborn, developing baby.

Meconium: The fetal stool that may be present in the amniotic fluid.

Miscarriage: Spontaneous delivery of a human fetus before it is able to live on its own.

Perineum: The area of skin between the vagina and anus.

Placenta: The fetal and maternal organ through which the fetus absorbs oxygen and nutrients and excretes wastes; it is attached to the fetus via the umbilical cord.

Presenting part: The part of the fetus that appears at the vaginal opening first.

Prolapsed cord: The situation in which the umbilical cord delivers through the vagina before any other presenting part.

Umbilical cord: The cord that connects the placenta to the fetus.

Uterus: The female reproductive organ in which a baby grows and develops.

Vagina: The canal that leads from the uterus to the external opening in females.

IN THE FIELD

EMTs Carlos and Sally were teaching an infant cardiopulmonary resuscitation (CPR) class to expectant mothers and fathers at the local YMCA. Halfway through the practice session, one of the women, further along in her pregnancy than most in the class, said she had been experiencing some contractions during the day and that her water had just broken. She said her contractions were strong and regular now. Because she was expecting her third baby, Carlos and Sally knew the delivery might occur soon. Carlos went to call dispatch for an ambulance while Sally assessed the patient.

Although Sally had never assisted with a delivery, she was well educated and knew what questions to ask. When she confirmed that the patient's water had broken and that her contractions were about 2 minutes apart, Sally and Carlos decided to prepare for delivery on the scene. The closest hospital was 45 minutes away, and the baby probably would not wait that long. Sally and Carlos, along with the patient and her husband, were a little nervous, but they knew childbirth is a natural process and is rarely an emergency for the patient or the newborn.

The delivery went well. After the baby was born, the mother, father, and healthy baby girl were all transported to the hospital for evaluation. Carlos and Sally had just participated in one of the most professionally rewarding calls an EMT can experience.

Although most babies in the United States are born in the hospital, this is not true worldwide. Most babies in the world are not born in any type of medical facility. Birth is a natural process, which usually does not require any medical intervention.

When an ambulance is called for a woman in labor there is usually adequate time for the mother to be transported to the hospital. In some cases, however, EMTs may arrive on the scene to find a woman who is so far along into labor that there is no time to get to the hospital before delivery. In situations when prehospital delivery is likely to occur, EMTs must be ready to assist the mother with the delivery.

This chapter discusses what EMTs need to understand to assist with a prehospital delivery, beginning with a description of the anatomy of the woman and the developing baby. Emergency medical care for predelivery emergencies is discussed, as well as the procedure for assisting with a normal delivery and the management of complications. Resuscitation of the newborn and care of the mother are included. The chapter ends with a dis-

cussion of gynecological emergencies and the emergency medical care required.

REPRODUCTIVE ANATOMY AND PHYSIOLOGY

The anatomy of the human female (Fig. 24-1) and the growing baby allow pregnancy and delivery to occur with few problems. The mother's **uterus** (womb) is the structure in which the baby grows and develops. The uterus is a muscular organ that eventually contracts and expels the fetus during childbirth. During pregnancy, the **cervix,** the neck of the uterus, contains a mucous plug. As the cervix dilates (widens) during labor to allow the fetus to pass through, the mucous plug becomes dislodged.

When the muscles of the uterus contract, the fetus is pushed into the **birth canal,** which consists of the lower part of the uterus and the **vagina.** The fetus is pushed through the birth canal into the outside world during childbirth.

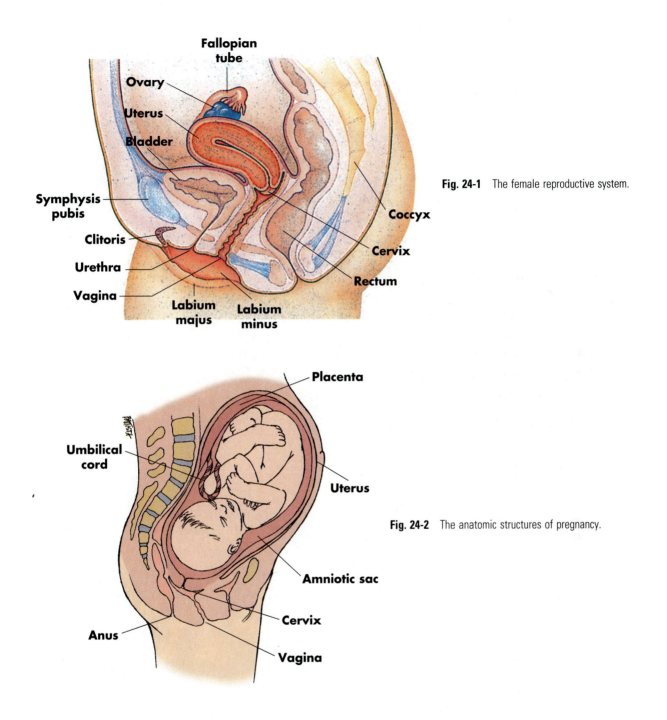

Fig. 24-1   The female reproductive system.

Fig. 24-2   The anatomic structures of pregnancy.

The **perineum** is the area of skin between the vagina and anus. This skin often tears as a result of the pressure exerted by the fetus during childbirth (Fig 24-2).

An unborn developing baby is called a **fetus.** The fetus is nourished through the **placenta.** The placenta attaches to the wall of the uterus and is composed of fetal and maternal tissue. It is attached to the baby via the umbilical cord. The placenta is an organ that develops during pregnancy. It is not present when a woman is not pregnant and is ex-

pelled from the body following childbirth. The placenta allows oxygen and nutrients to pass from the mother's bloodstream to the fetus. The placenta also allows carbon dioxide and waste products to pass from the fetus to the mother for elimination. This transfer of material from the placenta to the fetus and back to the placenta is accomplished through the **umbilical cord.**

The umbilical cord is an extension of the placenta and contains two arteries and one vein. Blood flows from the fetus to the placenta and back to the

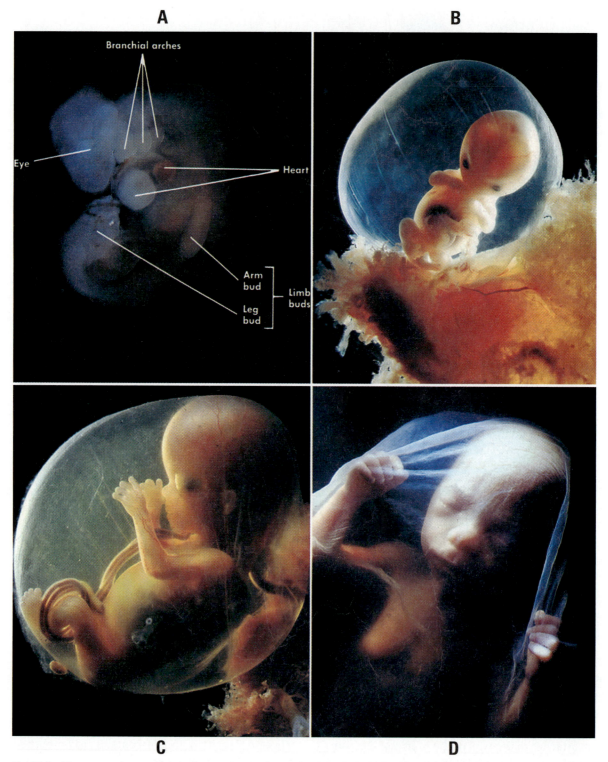

Fig. 24-3 The uterus enlarges and expands to encompass the growing fetus. **A,** At 35 days. **B,** At 49 days. **C,** After the first trimester. **D,** At 4 months.

fetus. Maternal and fetal circulatory systems are independent of each other, and blood does not flow directly from mother to the fetus.

The fetus is surrounded by a bag of fluid, which is called the **amniotic sac.** The amniotic sac contains 1 to 2 L of liquid called amniotic fluid. The amniotic fluid cushions the baby and helps protect it from injury. The amniotic sac generally ruptures before childbirth (often described by the patient as "my water broke"), and the amniotic fluid lubricates the birth canal during delivery.

The fetus grows and develops for approximately 9 months or 40 weeks. During pregnancy the mother's body changes to accommodate the growing fetus within her uterus. During pregnancy, the mother's uterus expands for the growing fetus (Fig. 24-3A through D). Her blood volume increases along with the amount of blood traveling through her heart each minute and her heart rate. Her blood pressure decreases slightly and her digestion slows.

LABOR

Labor is the process by which babies are born. Labor is generally divided into three stages, beginning with the first uterine contractions and ending when the placenta is delivered after childbirth (Fig. 24-4). Labor consists of contractions of the walls of the uterus that push the fetus through the cervix and into the birth canal.

The first stage of labor begins with regular contractions of the uterus and continues until the fetus enters the birth canal. During this stage of labor, the cervix (the opening from the uterus to the vagina) must dilate to allow the baby to pass through into the birth canal. As the cervix dilates, mucous and blood may pass through the vagina. This mucous and blood, which is the **bloody show,** is normal. Each contraction thins and shortens the cervix to prepare to allow the head of the fetus to pass. Once the cervix dilates to approximately 10 cm (4 in), the head can pass through and the second stage of labor begins.

The second stage of labor begins when the fetus enters the birth canal and ends when the baby is born. Rhythmic contractions of the uterus push the fetus through the birth canal into the vaginal opening. Most babies are born with their head as the **presenting part**—the part that appears at the vaginal opening first. **Crowning** occurs when the head bulges against the vaginal opening. When you see crowning, delivery is imminent and you should be prepared for immediate delivery (Fig. 24-5).

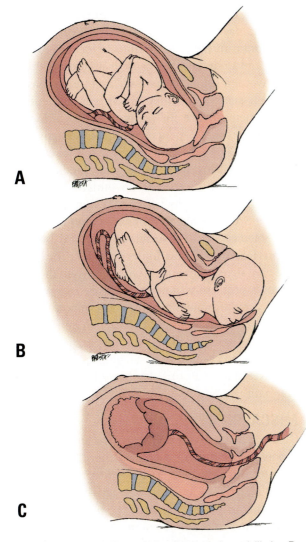

A

B

C

Fig. 24-4   The three stages of labor. **A,** contraction and dilation. **B,** baby moves through birth canal and is born. **C,** delivery of placenta.

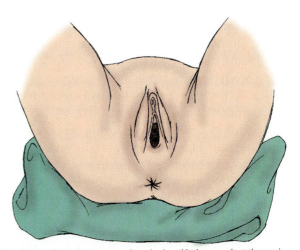

Fig. 24-5   Crowning occurs when the head bulges against the vaginal opening.

In the third stage of labor, which starts after the baby is born, the placenta, umbilical cord, and other tissues are delivered. The placenta detaches from the uterine wall and passes through the birth canal. This tissue is still connected to the fetus by the umbilical cord unless the cord has already been cut.

Labor pains occurring with each contraction are normal. Women generally experience pain when the uterus contracts and experience relief from pain as the contraction ends. A support person should be available to help the mother. The father, a friend, or another EMT should encourage her, help her to breath regularly through the contractions, and make her as comfortable as possible. The length of normal labor varies greatly among women, depending on the woman's age, previous deliveries, and other individual factors and the circumstances. The length of time a woman spends in labor generally decreases with each delivery.

CONTENTS OF THE CHILDBIRTH KIT

To assist with delivery, you need some basic supplies. You should have the equipment needed for delivery assembled in one place in preparation for assisting deliveries. Commercial obstetric (OB) kits are available and generally contain the following (Fig. 24-6):

1. Surgical scissors or a scalpel—used to cut the umbilical cord.
2. Hemostats or cord clamps—used to clamp the umbilical cord.
3. Umbilical tape or sterilized cord—used to tie the umbilical cord.
4. Bulb syringe—used to suction the infant's mouth and nose.
5. Towels—to dry the infant
6. 2 × 10 gauze sponges—to wipe the infant's mouth and nose.
7. Sterile gloves—to wear during delivery.
8. One baby blanket—to warm the infant.
9. Sanitary napkins—for the mother after delivery.
10. Plastic bag—to transport the placenta to the hospital.

You also need to be equipped with the proper personal protective equipment: gloves, gown, mask, and eye protection.

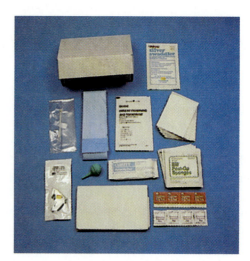

Fig. 24-6 Contents of an obstetrical kit.

PREDELIVERY EMERGENCIES

During the approximately 9 months or 40 weeks of pregnancy, complications may arise. These complications can result from trauma or medical conditions, and sometimes the cause is unknown. Pregnant women should be assessed and treated based on their signs and symptoms. In general, emergency medical care for pregnant patients is the same as for other patients with the same signs and symptoms. The following are some special considerations requiring specific emergency medical care. Always perform a scene size-up, initial assessment, and focused history and physical examination including SAMPLE history (Signs/Symptoms; Allergies; Medications; Provocation; Last oral intake; Events leading to illness/injury), and take the baseline vital signs. Remember that even when the origin of a problem is not known, care is provided based on the patient's signs and symptoms and your assessment findings. Also keep in mind that a woman's vital signs change during pregnancy. Her heart rate may be faster and her blood pressure may be lower than is normal for her when she is not pregnant.

MISCARRIAGE

A miscarriage is the delivery of the fetus before it can live independently of the mother. The medical term for this early delivery is **abortion,** but it is generally referred to as a **miscarriage** when it occurs spontaneously. A miscarriage usually occurs within the first 3 months of pregnancy. A woman experiencing a miscarriage generally has abdominal cramping that may be severe. She may be bleeding, and there may be noticeable vaginal discharge of clots and tissue.

EMERGENCY CARE FOR MISCARRIAGE

1. Treat the woman as is appropriate for her signs and symptoms.
2. Administer oxygen via a nonrebreather mask at a rate of 15 L/min.
3. Apply external vaginal pads or sanitary napkins, and bring any fetal tissue to the hospital. The amount of blood that has been lost can be estimated by keeping track of the number of sanitary napkins used.
4. Be prepared to care for the signs and symptoms of shock, and transport the mother to the hospital.
5. Emotional support is very important for the mother. Grief is normal and should be expected from both parents.

SEIZURE DURING PREGNANCY

Some women develop medical conditions during pregnancy that cause them to experience seizures. These women are generally healthy and do not have a history of a seizure disorder.

EMERGENCY CARE FOR SEIZURE DURING PREGNANCY

1. Treat the patient based on her signs and symptoms.
2. Administer oxygen via a nonrebreather mask at a rate of 15 L/min.
3. Keep the patient calm and quiet.
4. Transport the patient on her left side to reduce the pressure on her circulatory system from the fetus (Fig. 24-7).

VAGINAL BLEEDING LATE IN PREGNANCY

A number of problems can cause vaginal bleeding to occur late in pregnancy. The bleeding may or may not be accompanied by pain. Late pregnancy vaginal bleeding usually involves a problem with the placenta.

EMERGENCY CARE FOR BLEEDING LATE IN PREGNANCY

1. Treat the woman based on her signs and symptoms.
2. Administer oxygen via a nonrebreather mask at a rate of 15 L/min.
3. Place a sanitary napkin over the vaginal opening.

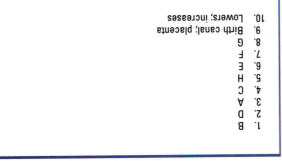

REVIEW QUESTIONS

REPRODUCTIVE ANATOMY AND PHYSIOLOGY

Match the following terms in the left column with their definitions in the right column:

1. Uterus _____	A. The passageway from the uterus through which the baby is born
2. Cervix _____	B. The organ where the baby develops
3. Birth canal _____	C. The skin between the vagina and the anus
4. Perineum _____	D. The neck of the uterus
5. Fetus _____	E. The organ that allows nutrients to pass from mother to fetus and waste from fetus to mother
6. Placenta _____	F. The fluid-filled sac that cushions the fetus
7. Amniotic sac _____	G. The connection from the placenta to the fetus
8. Umbilical cord _____	H. The unborn developing baby

9. The first stage of labor begins with uterine contractions and ends when the fetus enters the _____. The second stage of labor ends with the delivery of the baby. The third stage of labor ends with the delivery of the _____.

10. The mother's blood pressure generally _____ during pregnancy. Her heart rate usually _____.

10. Lowers; increases
9. Birth canal; placenta
8. G
7. F
6. E
5. H
4. C
3. A
2. D
1. B

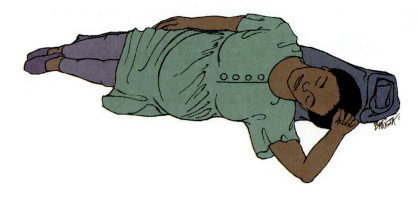

Fig. 24-7 Transporting the mother on her left side will reduce the pressure the fetus places on her circulatory system.

4. Transport the woman on her left side to the hospital.
5. Be prepared to treat the woman if there are signs and symptoms of shock.

TRAUMA

Traumatic injuries to a pregnant woman are treated the same as traumatic injuries for other patients, including the focused history and physical examination for trauma patients. Whatever treatment is best for the mother will also be the best treatment for the fetus. A few special considerations should be taken with pregnant trauma patients.

EMERGENCY CARE FOR TRAUMA IN PREGNANCY

1. Transport the mother on her left side unless you suspect a spine injury. If a spine injury is suspected and the patient is immobilized on a long backboard, the entire board can be tilted to the left by placing a blanket or padding under the right side of the backboard. This tilting reduces the pressure on the vena cava from the uterus allowing blood to return normally to the heart from the lower body (Fig. 24-8).
2. Administer oxygen via a nonrebreather mask at a rate of 15 L/min.

3. Because digestion slows during pregnancy, the pregnant patient often has food in her stomach. Expect vomiting and be prepared to suction.
4. Be prepared to care for the signs and symptoms of shock.
5. If the mother should die as a result of traumatic injuries, transport her to the hospital immediately while performing CPR. A physician may be able to perform an emergency **caesarean section,** which is a surgical delivery that may allow the baby to survive on its own. Caring for the traumatic death of pregnant patients is a controversial issue in many areas. Consult medical direction and be familiar with your local policies and protocols when dealing with this special situation.

NORMAL DELIVERY

Childbirth is not an "emergency" unless complicating factors are involved. In a normal delivery, your role as an EMT is to provide support and assistance to the mother as she delivers her child and to provide care and, if necessary, resuscitation to the newborn.

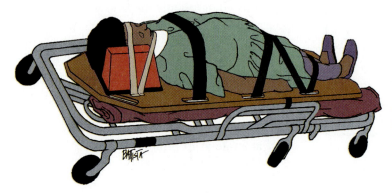

Fig. 24-8 Transport a pregnant woman on her left side. If she is immobilized on a long back board, the entire board can be tilted to the left by placing a blanket or padding under the right side.

PREDELIVERY CONSIDERATIONS

In general, it is best to transport the expectant mother to the hospital unless delivery is anticipated within 5 minutes. When deciding whether to transport or to assist in delivery on the scene, consider the following criteria:

1. *When is the baby due?* Ask the mother the baby's due date or how long she has been pregnant. Is this her first child? Does she know if she is having twins? Does she know if the baby is in a breech presentation? When assessing the SAMPLE history, ask the mother if she has had any problems with her pregnancy.

2. *Are there any contractions or pain?* Contractions occur closer together and last longer as labor progresses. Assess the duration of contractions by timing how long a contraction lasts; begin timing at the beginning of the contraction and stop timing at the end of the contraction. Assess the frequency of contractions by timing from the beginning of one contraction to the beginning of the next contraction. If the amniotic sac has ruptured, determine the color of the fluid.

3. *Is there any bleeding or discharge?* The presence of a bloody show or the rupture of the amniotic sac usually signals that labor has begun. If either of these events has occurred, ask how long ago it happened.

4. *Is the mother feeling an increasing pressure in the vaginal area?* As the baby moves into and through the birth canal, pressure is exerted against the rectum, causing the feeling of a bowel movement. If she answers yes, birth may be near. Do not allow the mother to go to the bathroom.

5. *Does the mother feel the urge to push?* As birth nears, women often feel a strong urge to push, to aid the baby through the birth canal.

6. *Is there crowning during contractions?* Explain to the patient that it is necessary to see if there is crowning with contractions. Remove enough of the patient's clothing to see the vaginal opening. Move bystanders from the scene to maintain the mother's privacy. A calm professional manner helps reduce the mother's embarrassment. If there is crowning with contractions, birth is imminent and delivery should occur at the scene.

7. *Place a gloved hand on the abdomen above the navel to assess contractions.* The abdomen feels hard during strong contractions that occur in late stages of labor.

The decision to transport the patient to the hospital is based on how near delivery appears to be. If the baby is crowning, if contractions are coming frequently (less than 2 to 3 minutes apart) with long duration (longer than 45 to 60 seconds), and if the mother feels the need to push, the baby may be born before transport is possible, and delivery should occur on scene. If the mother is not experiencing these signs and symptoms, transport should begin. The decision to transport is also based on how far away the nearest hospital is and the conditions of the highways (traffic, inclement weather, etc.).

During transport, be prepared to assist delivery. The length of time spent in labor varies among women and usually becomes shorter with each baby the woman delivers. For most women, 12 to 18 hours is an average length of labor for the first baby. Do not attempt to hold the mother's legs together or otherwise delay delivery.

PRECAUTIONS

If the decision is made to deliver on the scene, take the following precautions. Practicing body substance isolation precautions is a must when you assist in childbirth. Blood and amniotic fluid should be expected and may splash. The mother may feel the need to go to the bathroom, but should not be allowed to use the toilet. The feeling of a bowel movement is common and is caused by the baby's head pressing against the walls of the rectum. The baby may deliver while she is trying to have a bowel movement.

If delivery is expected soon and crowning has occurred, consult medical direction concerning the decision for delivery on site. If delivery does not occur within 10 minutes, consult medical direction for permission to transport.

DELIVERY PROCEDURE

Once the decision has been made to assist in delivery on the scene, take the following steps:

1. Follow body substance isolation precautions.
2. Position the mother. Have her lie with her knees flexed, drawn up, and widely separated. The buttocks may be elevated with a blanket or pillow. Make sure there is enough room (approximately 2 m [6.5 ft] of space) in front of the mother's buttocks to care for the infant initially (Fig. 24-9).
3. Create a sterile field around the vaginal opening with sterile towels or paper barriers. Towels

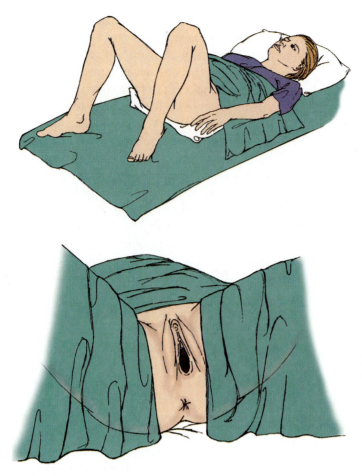

Fig. 24-9 Positioning the mother for delivery.

Fig. 24-10 A sterile field is made around the vaginal opening with sterile towels or paper barriers.

should be placed under the mother's buttocks and one under the vaginal opening. Additional towels should be placed across her thighs and abdomen (Fig. 24-10). Have towels available to replace the one under the mother, which is used to collect fluids.

4. When the infant's head appears during crowning, place gentle pressure on the perineum, over the bony part of the skull to prevent an extremely rapid delivery or explosive birth. This pressure can also help to prevent tearing of the perineum. Babies have soft spots called *fontanelles* on their heads. Do not push on these areas (Fig. 24-11).

5. If the amniotic sac has not broken, use a clamp to puncture the sac and push it away from the infant's head and mouth as it appears.

6. As the infant's head is being delivered, determine if the umbilical cord is around the infant's neck. If the cord is around the neck, attempt to loosen the cord and slip it over the baby's head. The baby cannot be delivered with the cord around its neck. If the cord cannot be removed, quickly but carefully clamp the cord in two

places, cut the cord in between the two clamps, and remove the cord from the baby's neck (Fig. 24-12).

7. Once delivered, support the head as it rotates and wipe the baby's mouth and nose. Suction the baby's mouth and nose with a bulb syringe. The bulb syringe should be compressed before placing it in the baby's mouth. Once the bulb

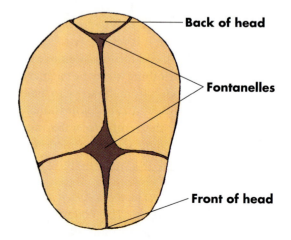

Fig. 24-11 Location of fontanelles on an infant's head.

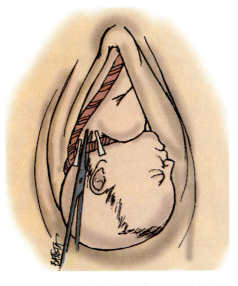

Fig. 24-12 If the umbilical cord is wrapped around the baby's neck and cannot be removed, clamp the cord in two places and cut the cord between the clamps.

syringe is in the mouth, release the bulb and allow the fluids to fill the syringe. Withdraw the syringe and release the contents of the syringe onto a towel. Suction the mouth two or three times and then suction each nostril once or twice. Do not place the bulb syringe in so far that it touches the back of the mouth and gags the baby (Fig. 24-13).

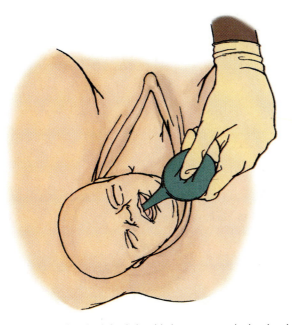

Fig. 24-13 After the infant's head is born, support the head and wipe the mouth and nose. Suction the baby's mouth and nose with a bulb syringe.

8. Guide the head downward to deliver the first shoulder, then upward to deliver the second shoulder. As the torso and body appear, support the infant with both hands.

9. As the feet are delivered, grasp the feet firmly with one hand. Newborn babies are slippery.

10. Wipe any additional blood and mucous away from the face with sterile gauze, and suction the mouth and nose again.

11. Wrap the infant in a warm blanket and place it on its side with the head slightly lower than the trunk to aid the draining of fluid from the mouth and nose. Keep the infant at the same level as the mother's vagina to prevent blood from returning through the umbilical cord to the placenta (Fig. 24-14).

12. One EMT should monitor the infant and complete care. The third stage of labor is just beginning, and a second EMT needs to continue treating the mother.

13. After pulsations in the umbilical cord cease, the cord should be clamped, tied, and then cut. Place the first clamp approximately four finger widths away from the baby, and the second clamp several inches further away from the first clamp. The cord should be cut between these two clamps (Fig. 24-15). Evaluate the cord to make sure it is not bleeding. Care for a bleeding umbilical cord is discussed later in this chapter.

14. Begin to prepare the mother and infant for transport. Prepare for delivery of the placenta.

15. As the placenta delivers, wrap it in a towel and place it in a plastic bag. Take the placenta to the hospital where it can be examined by the hospital staff for completeness. If pieces of the placenta remain attached to the uterine wall, infection or hemorrhage could result. The placenta will deliver on its own, usually within a few minutes after the birth of the baby but sometimes as much as 30 minutes later. Some EMS systems wait on the scene for the placenta to deliver, and others transport after cutting the cord. The woman will feel contractions again as the placenta delivers, and she should be encouraged to push. Never pull on the umbilical cord to try to force the placenta to deliver (Fig. 24-16).

16. After the placenta delivers, place a sterile pad over the mother's vaginal opening. Her legs can now be lowered.

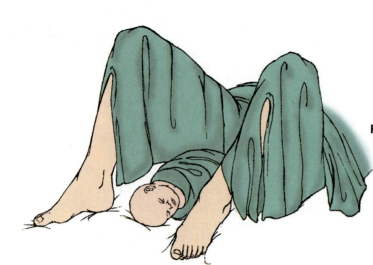

Fig. 24-14 Positioning for newborn infants.

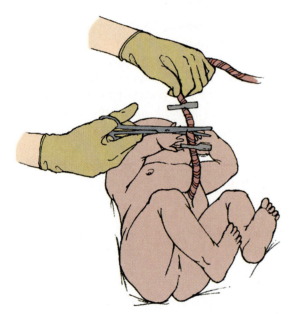

Fig. 24-15 Cut the cord between the two clamps approximately four finger widths from the baby.

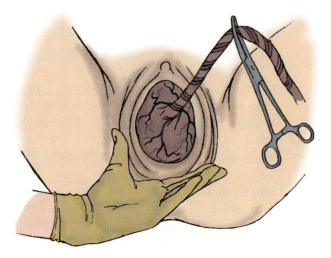

Fig. 24-16 Delivery of the placenta.

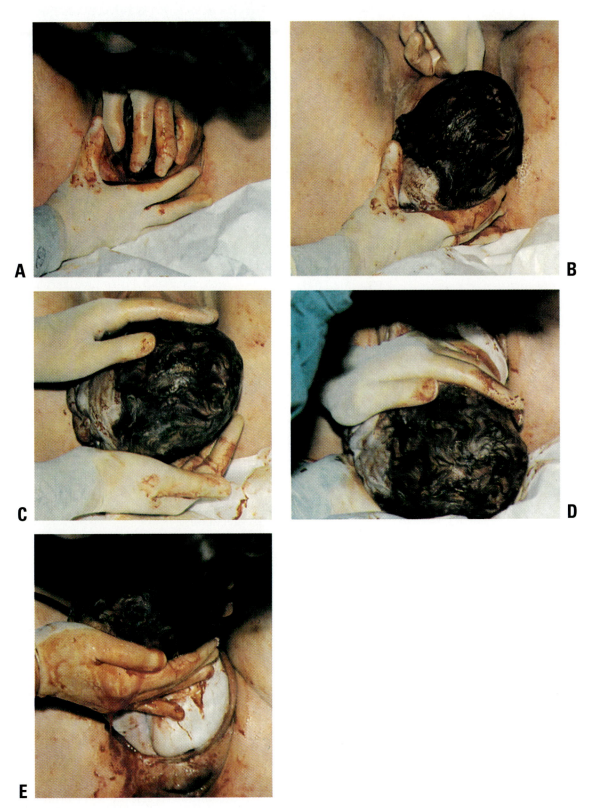

Fig. 24-17   The delivery process. **A,** Crowning. **B,** Check the neck for presence of the umbilical cord. **C,** Support the head as it rotates. **D,** Guide the head downward to deliver the shoulder. **E,** The other shoulder is delivered.

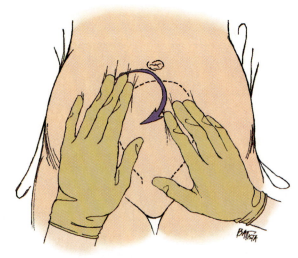

Fig. 24-18   Uterine massage to help control bleeding after delivery.

17. Record the time of delivery. Mother, infant, and placenta should be transported to the hospital.

Figure 24-17 shows the full delivery process.

Vaginal bleeding following the delivery should be expected. Up to 500 mL of blood is considered normal. More than 500 mL of blood is excessive and should be managed by massaging the uterus. Place both hands with fingers fully extended on the lower abdomen above the pubis. Gently massage or knead the area (Fig. 24-18). Bleeding should lessen with massage. Because the massage may feel uncomfortable or even painful, explain to the mother that uterine massage will help stop the bleeding. If the mother has the signs and symptoms of shock, regardless of the amount of blood lost, treat her for shock, provide high-flow oxygen, and transport immediately. Continue to massage the uterus en route to the hospital.

INITIAL CARE OF THE NEWBORN

Immediately after birth, dry the infant with a clean towel. Wrap the baby in a warm blanket and cover the head to preserve body heat. Position the infant on its side with the head slightly lower than the feet to aid fluid drainage from the mouth and nose. Repeat suctioning as necessary. Box 24-1 summarizes the care of the newborn infant.

The infant should be assessed continually. Record the assessment findings 1 minute after birth and again 5 minutes after birth. Evaluate the infant for the following:

1. *Appearance.* Note the infant's color. Is the infant's skin blue, dusky, or gray in color, or is it pink? It is normal for the infant to have some cyanosis peripherally (of the arms, hands, legs, and feet), but the trunk should not be cyanotic.

2. *Pulse.* Determine the infant's pulse rate. The pulse rate should be greater than 100 beats per minute. A slower rate may indicate inadequate oxygenation.

3. *Grimace.* Evaluate the infant's response to an irritable stimulus, such as suctioning the nose. Does the infant grimace, react vigorously, or cry, or is there little or no response? The infant should cry or grimace with this stimulus.

4. *Activity.* How much is the baby moving? The baby should have good motion in all the extremities.

5. *Respiratory effort.* Is the baby breathing on its own or crying or is the respiratory effort labored? The baby should be breathing on its own or crying.

You can remember these five assessments with the acronym *APGAR.* The APGAR scoring system is traditionally used to evaluate the infant at 1 and 5 minutes after birth (Table 24-1). Record your findings and continue to assess and treat the mother and infant as necessary. However, do not delay any treatment or transport to perform these assessments. Perform needed interventions immediately

TABLE 24-1	APGAR Scoring System		
SIGN	**0**	**1**	**2**
Appearance (Skin color)	Blue, pale	Body pink, blue extremities	Completely pink
Pulse Rate (Heart rate)	Absent	< 100/minute	> 100/minute
Grimace (Irritability)	No response	Grimace	Cough, sneeze, cry
Activity (Muscle tone)	Limp	Some flexion	Active motion
Respirations (Respiratory effort)	Absent	Slow, irregular	Good, crying

after birth; do not wait for 1 minute for the first assessment or 5 minutes for the next.

An infant who is breathing well on its own, is active and has a pink trunk, a pulse greater than 100 beats per minute, and a grimace reaction can be wrapped in dry towels and held by the mother during transport.

Infants should start breathing on their own within 20 to 30 seconds after birth. An infant who is not breathing may need to be stimulated. One method for stimulating an infant to breathe is to gently but firmly massage the infant's back in a circular motion. You may also try flicking the soles of the infant's feet. More vigorous stimulation, such as slapping the infant's buttocks, is not necessary.

The frequency of need for resuscitative measures for newborns is represented in Figure 24-19. After drying, warming, positioning, and suctioning the newborn and providing tactile stimulation, evaluate the newborn. Note that most newborns respond to these simple measures. If necessary, perform the following resuscitative measures:

1. *Evaluate the respiratory effort.* If the respirations are inadequate (slow, shallow, or absent), provide positive pressure ventilations at the rate of 60 per minute with a bag-valve-mask. If the newborn is crying, continue the assessment.
2. *Evaluate the heart rate next.* If the rate is less than 100 beats per minute, provide artificial ventilations at a rate of 60 per minute. Reassess after 30

seconds. If the rate is less than 80 beats per minute and the newborn is not responding to ventilation, start chest compressions following newborn CPR standards. If on reassessment the heart rate is above 100 and the baby's spontaneous respirations appear adequate, stop ventilations and compressions and administer free-flow oxygen. Free-flow oxygen is oxygen administered by holding an oxygen mask or tubing as close as possible to the newborn's mouth and nose.

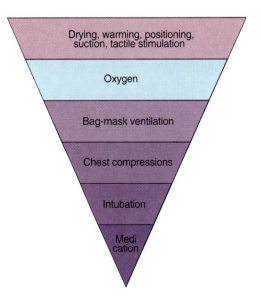

Fig. 24-19 The frequency of need for resuscitative measures is illustrated by the inverted pyramid of neonatal resuscitation.

3. *Assess the newborn's color.* If cyanosis is present on the baby's trunk with spontaneous breathing and an adequate heart rate, administer free-flow oxygen.

4. If these measures are not successful, the newborn requires advanced life-support measures and should be immediately transported to a hospital equipped for neonatal resuscitation.

Although most newborns respond to the simple measures of drying, warming, positioning, suctioning, and tactile stimulation, you must be prepared to deal with newborn resuscitation and should

practice these procedures to become comfortable with them. Contact medical direction with any questions about the resuscitation.

ABNORMAL DELIVERIES AND COMPLICATIONS

Although most women have normal deliveries, you must be prepared to manage certain possible complications. A delivery that occurs outside the hospital is not in itself an emergency. The following conditions, however, are emergencies and require immediate assistance to prevent harm or death to the mother and baby.

Most babies are born in a head-first (**cephalic**) position (Fig. 24-20). When a body part other than the head presents first, the baby may not be able to deliver without surgical intervention.

PROLAPSED CORD

Sometimes during delivery, the first presenting body part you see is the umbilical cord. This condition is called **prolapsed cord.** In this condition, the umbilical cord may be compressed between the baby's head and the wall of the birth canal. This condition can prevent an adequate oxygen supply from reaching the baby. A prolapsed cord is a true emergency, and you must act quickly (Fig. 24-21).

EMERGENCY CARE FOR PROLAPSED CORD

1. Place the mother in a position that removes pressure from the cord. The mother should be placed with her head down or her pelvis elevated to lessen pressure on the umbilical cord.

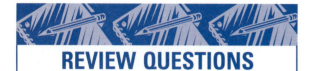

REVIEW QUESTIONS

PREDELIVERY EMERGENCIES/NORMAL DELIVERY

1. A _____ is the spontaneous delivery of the fetus before it is able to live outside of the womb.

2. Pregnant seizure patients should be transported on their _____ side to prevent pressure from the fetus on the vena cava.

3. Traumatic injuries to a pregnant patient require that the backboard be _____ to the left.

4. After the head delivers, you should check to see if the _____ is wrapped around the baby's neck.

5. The _____ usually delivers within 30 minutes of the baby and should be taken to the hospital to be checked for completeness.

6. Vaginal bleeding is expected following delivery, and up to _____ mL is considered to be normal.

7. Infants who have poor respiratory effort or slow heart beats may require _____, _____, or _____.

1. Miscarriage
2. Left
3. Tilted
4. Umbilical cord
5. Placenta
6. 500
7. Oxygen, ventilations, or chest compressions

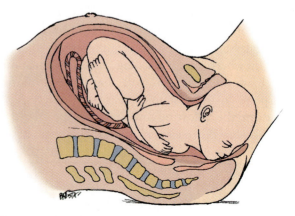

Fig. 24-20 Cephalic delivery position.

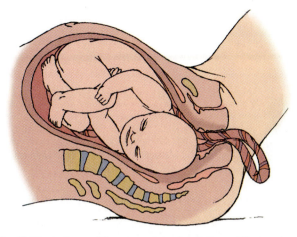

Fig. 24-21 In the condition of a prolapsed cord, the umbilical cord can be compressed between the baby's head and the wall of the vaginal canal.

2. Place the mother on high-flow oxygen via a nonrebreather mask. Encourage her to pant and to not push during contractions. Pushing would increase the pressure on the umbilical cord, restricting the blood flow from mother to infant.

3. With a gloved hand, insert several fingers into the vagina to gently push the baby off the cord. Do not attempt to replace the cord in the vagina (Fig. 24-22).

4. Maintain this position en route to the hospital.

5. If any portion of the cord is visible outside of the vagina, apply moist sterile dressings to the cord. This moisture helps prevent the cord from becoming dry and minimizes temperature changes that could cause spasm of the arteries in the umbilical cord.

6. Transport the patient to the hospital immediately.

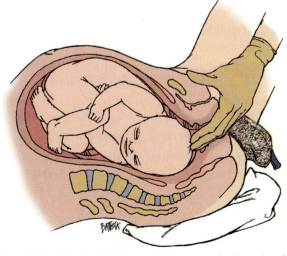

Fig. 24-22 Patient positioning and management of prolapsed cord.

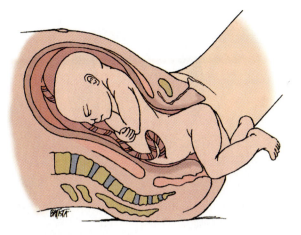

Fig. 24-23 Breech position.

BREECH PRESENTATION

A **breech presentation** is a delivery in which the head delivers last. The baby may present buttocks or both legs first. A breech delivery can be facilitated in a hospital where a surgical delivery can be performed if problems arise during the vaginal delivery. Breech presentations are the most common abnormal presentation (Fig. 24-23).

EMERGENCY CARE FOR BREECH PRESENTATION

1. Prepare the mother for delivery in the same manner as if a head-first delivery were expected.

2. Place the mother on high-flow oxygen via a nonrebreather mask.

3. Allow the delivery to occur spontaneously until the feet, buttocks, and trunk are delivered. Support the baby on the palm of one hand.

4. Guide the shoulders out of the birth canal. The head often delivers without difficulty once the shoulders have emerged.

If the head does not deliver immediately, action must be taken to prevent suffocation. The cord possibly is being compressed by the baby's head, preventing oxygenated blood from moving through the cord. The baby's attempts to breathe spontaneously could be prevented by the walls of the birth canal pressing against the face. In this case you should:

1. Place a gloved hand into the vagina with your palm facing the baby's face.

2. Make a V with your index and middle fingers on either side of the baby's nose. Push the vaginal wall away from the baby's face until the head is delivered. Do not hyperextend the baby's head while pushing the vaginal wall away from the face.

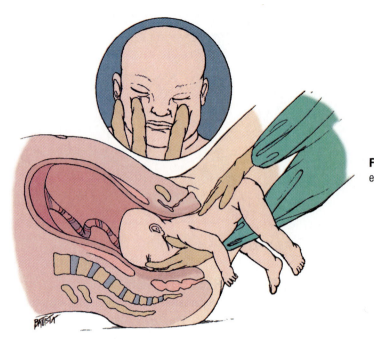

Fig. 24-24 Management of breech birth with undelivered head.

3. If the head does not deliver, transport immediately while maintaining the V position with your hand (Fig 24-24).

Do not attempt to force delivery by pulling on the trunk or legs of the infant.

LIMB PRESENTATION

In rare instances, a limb may be the presenting part. If you see an arm or leg when checking for crowning, a true emergency exists (Fig. 24-25). The baby cannot be delivered in this position. Often in these cases the cord is also prolapsed.

EMERGENCY CARE FOR LIMB PRESENTATION

1. Position the mother in the same manner as described for a prolapsed cord.

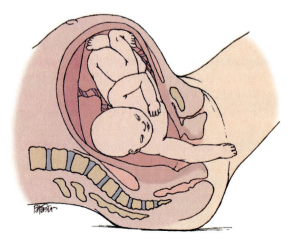

Fig. 24-25 Limb presentation.

2. Exert gentle pressure on the baby's body to prevent pressure on the umbilical cord. Maintain pressure until you arrive at the hospital.
3. Place the mother on high-flow oxygen via a nonrebreather mask.
4. Transport the patient to the hospital immediately.

MULTIPLE BIRTHS

Twins occur in one of every 80 to 90 births, and triplets occur in one of 8000 births. Although unusual, it is possible the mother may be unaware that she has been carrying more than one baby, especially if she has not had prenatal care. If the mother begins to feel strong contractions after the birth of the first baby, prepare to deliver another child. There may be one or more placentas. In general, both infants are born before the delivery of the placenta(s). Delivery is assisted in the same manner as a normal cephalic birth with the following considerations:

EMERGENCY CARE FOR MULTIPLE BIRTHS

1. Expect complications. Multiple births have a higher rate of associated complications than single births.
2. Call for assistance, and be prepared for more than one resuscitation. A second EMS crew may be needed to resuscitate the second infant.
3. After delivery of the first infant, clamp or tie and cut the umbilical cord.

4. When contractions begin again, usually within 5 to 10 minutes of the first delivery, assist the delivery of the second baby as usual. The second infant may be born before or after delivery of the placenta.
5. Clamp or tie and cut the umbilical cord of the second infant.
6. Provide maternal care as for a single birth.
7. Keep in mind that two or more babies born at one time are usually smaller and are often premature. Give premature birth care as described later in this chapter.

MECONIUM

Meconium, or *fetal stool,* may be present in the amniotic fluid. The presence of meconium is associated with fetal distress and a greater risk for infant death. The reasons meconium is sometimes present are unclear, but it may be related to stress on the infant. Amniotic fluid containing meconium is brownish-yellow or greenish in color rather than clear. The immediate danger to the baby is the possibility of breathing the meconium into the lungs, where it can cause severe respiratory problems.

EMERGENCY CARE WHEN MECONIUM IS PRESENT

1. Assist with the delivery as normal.
2. Do not stimulate the infant before suctioning the oropharynx. Stimulating the infant will cause it to breathe and possibly inhale the meconium into the lungs.
3. Suction as soon as possible.
4. Maintain an open airway.
5. Transport the infant to the hospital immediately.
6. During transport, notify the receiving facility of presence of meconium.

PREMATURE BIRTH

Infants are considered premature if they are born less than 28 weeks or 7 months after conception or weigh less than 2.5 kg (5.5 lb). Premature infants are smaller and less developed than full-term infants. Their cardiovascular and respiratory systems are often immature, and they are also more susceptible to hypothermia. Premature infants have less fat for insulation and less control of the regulation of body temperature than full-term infants. Oxygen can be administered by a face mask sized for infants or by free-flow oxygen held close to the baby's face. Special care must be taken with premature infants. Premature newborns often require resuscitation. Always attempt resuscitation, even if the infant appears too small or underdeveloped to live. You may have difficulty resuscitating such small infants because of a lack of appropriate equipment, or the baby may not respond to any resuscitative efforts due to lack of development of the lungs or other organs.

EMERGENCY CARE FOR PREMATURE BIRTHS

1. Keep the infant warm. Make sure the infant is dry and wrapped in a blanket.
2. Suction as necessary.
3. Monitor the umbilical cord to assure that there is no bleeding. If there is bleeding, place an additional clamp on the cord closer to the infant. Do not remove the first clamp.
4. Administer free-flow oxygen to the infant. Ventilate as necessary.
5. Transport the infant to a hospital equipped for neonatal resuscitation and care.

Any time you are transporting a woman who is having an abnormal delivery, you should contact the receiving hospital as soon as possible so that an obstetrician and pediatrician can be available immediately.

GYNECOLOGIC EMERGENCIES

Gynecologic emergencies can occur in women who are not pregnant. Gynecologic emergencies result from a variety of causes. Some are of unknown origin, whereas others can be explained by the anatomy and function of the female reproductive system. Three of the most common gynecologic emergencies are discussed in this chapter: vaginal bleeding, trauma, and sexual assault.

VAGINAL BLEEDING

Vaginal bleeding can result from a variety of causes, but the treatment is essentially the same for all. The bleeding may be painless, extremely painful, or anywhere in between. Unless the bleeding is caused by trauma, examination of the genitalia is unnecessary.

While obtaining a SAMPLE history, ask the patient if she may be pregnant. Ask if the blood is dark red (like menstrual blood) or bright red. Also ask her approximately how many sanitary pads have been soaked with blood, to estimate the amount of blood that has already been lost. Note any clots or tissue that were discharged with the blood.

Have the patient place a sanitary napkin over the vaginal opening, and transport her to the hospital. If she may be pregnant, treat her as described in the previous section. Bleeding may be excessive, and the signs and symptoms of shock should be anticipated. Treat the patient based on her signs and symptoms.

TRAUMA TO EXTERNAL GENITALIA

Trauma to external genitalia should be treated exactly like any other soft tissue injury. These injuries are not common but can result from straddle injuries, blunt trauma, childbirth, or sexual assault. Calm, professional care helps reassure the patient and minimize embarrassment. Explain your actions to the patient in advance. Control bleeding with local pressure using trauma dressings or sanitary napkins. Ice may be used to minimize swelling and reduce pain. Wrap a cold pack in a towel and apply to the area of trauma. Never place a dressing inside the vagina. Monitor the patient's vital signs, and give care based on her signs and symptoms.

SEXUAL ASSAULT

Sexual assault is a devastating crime with lasting physical and emotional repercussions. The crime of rape has risen 54% in just one decade, and an estimated one in 30 American women will be raped at some time in her lifetime. Although men and boys are also victims of sexual assault, girls and women are most frequently the victims of these crimes. The rapist is often someone that the victim knows.

The initial care for a sexual assault victim is the same as for other injuries. Perform a scene size-up and initial assessment. Once you have determined that no life-threatening injuries are present, proceed with special considerations for the patient. You may be the first person to encounter a victim of sexual assault, and the care you give can have lasting impact. The following measures are important when dealing with a victim of sexual assault:

1. Provide care for injuries as usual. Examine the genitalia only if profuse bleeding is occurring. Note and document any injuries in detail.
2. When possible, an EMT of the same sex as the patient should perform the examination. As always, body substance isolation precautions should be taken when there is a possibility that you will be in contact with blood or other body fluids.
3. Remain nonjudgmental during the SAMPLE focused assessment. Calm the patient as much as

possible, ask and answer questions directly, and provide reassurance that the victim is now safe.
4. Discourage the patient from bathing, urinating, douching, or cleaning wounds so that evidence is not destroyed.
5. Protect the crime scene. Preserve evidence at the scene, including clothing and weapons. Disturb the scene as little as possible so police can collect evidence. Call the police to the scene, and encourage the patient to cooperate, report the assault, and answer questions. Do not delay treatment or transport of a patient with life-threatening injuries to wait for police.
6. Transport the patient to the hospital and continue to reassure her of her safety.
7. Document what the patient says and what you directly observe.

Do not include personal opinions about the crime. All sexual assaults are potential legal cases, and your prehospital care report is a legal document. Follow local protocols for reporting sexual assaults.

Emergency medical care for victims of sexual assault should be provided in a gentle manner and only after explaining what is being done and why it is necessary.

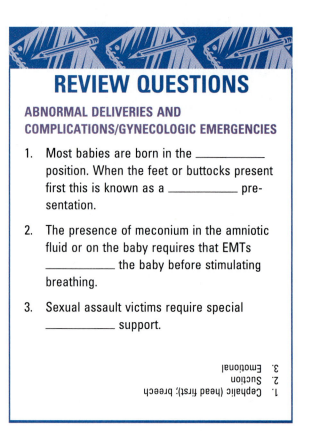

REVIEW QUESTIONS

ABNORMAL DELIVERIES AND COMPLICATIONS/GYNECOLOGIC EMERGENCIES

1. Most babies are born in the _____ position. When the feet or buttocks present first this is known as a _____ presentation.

2. The presence of meconium in the amniotic fluid or on the baby requires that EMTs _____ the baby before stimulating breathing.

3. Sexual assault victims require special _____ support.

3. Emotional
2. Suction
1. Cephalic (head first); breech

CHAPTER SUMMARY

REPRODUCTIVE ANATOMY AND PHYSIOLOGY

The uterus is the structure in which the baby grows and develops. The cervix is the neck of the uterus. The vagina is the birth canal through which the baby will be born. The perineum is the area of skin between the vagina and anus that is commonly torn during delivery.

The unborn baby is called a *fetus*. The placenta is the organ that attaches to the wall of the uterus and connects to the baby through the umbilical cord. The placenta allows nutrients and oxygen to be delivered to the baby and waste products to be delivered to the mother for elimination. The amniotic sac surrounds the fetus with protective fluid.

The mother's body changes along with the growing fetus. Her blood pressure drops, her heart rate and cardiac output rise, and her digestion slows.

Labor is the process of the baby being born. The first stage of labor begins with uterine contractions and ends when the fetus enters the birth canal. The second stage of labor begins when the fetus enters the birth canal and ends when the fetus is delivered. The third stage begins with the delivery of the baby and ends with the delivery of the placenta.

CONTENTS OF THE CHILDBIRTH KIT

The childbirth kit contains all of the necessary items to assist a mother in the delivery of her baby.

PREDELIVERY EMERGENCIES

Complications during pregnancy are not common. Emergency medical care is generally based on the woman's signs and symptoms and administering oxygen, with a few special considerations. A miscarriage is the spontaneous delivery of the fetus before it is able to live outside of the womb. Be prepared to treat the signs and symptoms of shock and to offer emotional support. Seizures can occur in previously healthy women. Keep the patient calm, and transport her on her left side. Vaginal bleeding may or may not be associated with abdominal pain. Be prepared to treat the woman for the signs and symptoms of shock. Traumatic injuries are treated the same as in other patients. Expect vomiting, and transport the patient with the backboard tilted to the left.

NORMAL DELIVERY

In general, it is best to transport the mother to the hospital while she is in labor unless the birth is imminent. During childbirth the EMT assists the mother in delivering her baby. Take body substance isolation precautions because contact with blood and amniotic fluid is common. Up to 500 mL of blood is a normal amount of vaginal bleeding following delivery. If hemorrhaging begins, uterine massage may help stop the bleeding.

Newborns should be dried, suctioned, positioned, stimulated, and warmed. Few babies require further resuscitation. Assess the baby after 1 and 5 minutes after delivery for appearance, pulse, grimace, activity, and respiratory effort (APGAR). Evaluate the baby for respiratory effort, pulse rate, and color. Resuscitative measures include chest compressions, ventilations, and free-flow oxygen.

ABNORMAL DELIVERIES AND COMPLICATIONS

Abnormal conditions include:
- Prolapsed cord—the umbilical cord is the presenting part.
- Breech presentation—the feet or buttocks are the presenting part
- Limb presentation—arm, leg, or arm and leg are the presenting parts.

Multiple births usually result in smaller babies who may require resuscitation. Meconium is fetal stool that may be present in the amniotic fluid when the fetus is under stress and can cause increased risk for respiratory complications. Premature babies require special measures to keep them warm and to prevent complications.

GYNECOLOGIC EMERGENCIES

Gynecologic emergencies include vaginal bleeding, trauma to the external genitalia, and sexual assault. Be sure to preserve evidence and provide emotional support when dealing with a sexual assault patient.

UNITED STATES DEPARTMENT OF TRANSPORTATION NATIONAL HIGHWAY TRAFFIC SAFETY ADMINISTRATION EMT–BASIC OBJECTIVES

Check your knowledge. The National Registry of EMTs and many state EMS agencies use the objectives below to develop EMT–Basic certification examinations. Can you meet them?

COGNITIVE

1. Identify the following structures: uterus, vagina, fetus, placenta, umbilical cord, amniotic sac, and perineum.
2. Identify and explain the use of the contents of an obstetrics kit.
3. Identify predelivery emergencies.
4. State indications of an imminent delivery.
5. Differentiate the emergency medical care provided to a patient with predelivery emergencies from a normal delivery.
6. State the steps in the predelivery preparation of the mother.
7. Establish the relationship between body substance isolation and childbirth.
8. State the steps to assist in the delivery.
9. Describe care of the baby as the head appears.
10. Describe how and when to cut the umbilical cord.
11. Discuss the steps in the delivery of the placenta.
12. List the steps in the emergency medical care of the mother postdelivery.
13. Summarize neonatal resuscitation procedures.
14. Describe the procedures for the following abnormal deliveries: breech birth, prolapsed cord, limb presentation.
15. Differentiate the special considerations for multiple births.
16. Describe special considerations of meconium.
17. Describe special considerations of a premature baby.
18. Discuss the emergency medical care of a patient with a gynecological emergency.

AFFECTIVE

1. Explain the rationale for understanding the implications of treating two patients (mother and baby).

PSYCHOMOTOR

1. Demonstrate the steps to assist in the normal cephalic delivery.
2. Demonstrate the necessary care procedures of the fetus as the head appears.
3. Demonstrate infant neonatal procedures.
4. Demonstrate postdelivery care of infant.
5. Demonstrate how and when to cut the umbilical cord.
6. Attend to the steps in the delivery of the placenta.
7. Demonstrate the postdelivery care of the mother.
8. Demonstrate the procedures for the following abnormal deliveries: vaginal bleeding, breech birth, prolapsed cord, limb presentation.
9. Demonstrate the steps in the emergency medical care of the mother with excessive bleeding.
10. Demonstrate completing a prehospital care report for patients with obstetrical/gynecological emergencies.

TRAUMA

A trauma call can be one of the most difficult situations an EMT may have to face. However, all the skills necessary to respond to a call—even the most trying trauma call—are available to the EMS professional who wants to push his or her level of skill and knowledge to the limit. To provide patient care in the field independently and know you can make a difference between life and death is the greatest accomplishment an EMS provider can achieve.

Martin R. Butler, EMT-I
Leading Petty Officer
Emergency Medical
Department
Naval Hospital,
Roosevelt Roads
Puerto Rico

DIVISION FIVE

25 BLEEDING AND SHOCK

KEY TERMS

Capillary refill: A measure of the perfusion of the skin; decreased capillary refill is a good indicator of shock in patients less than 6 years of age.

Circumferential pressure: Pressure put around the circumference of an extremity to control bleeding.

Epistaxis: Bleeding from the nose.

Hemorrhagic shock: Hypoperfusion that results from bleeding.

Hypoperfusion: The state that results when cells are not perfused adequately; oxygen and nutrients are not delivered and there is an inadequate removal of metabolic waste products.

Hypovolemic shock: Hypoperfusion that results from an inadequate volume of blood.

Perfusion: The process of delivering oxygen and nutrients to, and removing metabolic waste products from, the body's cells.

Pressure point: A place in an extremity where a major artery lies close to a bone; used with direct pressure and elevation to stop bleeding in an arm or leg.

Shock: Hypoperfusion.

IN THE FIELD

EMTs Sondra and Abdul were sitting down to lunch when they heard the dispatch call over the radio. "Medic 11, please respond code three, 37 Laurel Court, man fell from a ladder, bleeding severely; time out 1417." They got into the ambulance and turned on the lights and siren. Because the dispatch information said the patient was bleeding profusely, they donned gloves, gowns, eye wear, and masks as they arrived. After performing the scene size-up and determining the area was safe, they approached the patient. The patient was lying on the sidewalk, placing pressure on a gaping laceration on his right forearm. When he let go, blood spurted from the wound.

Sondra stabilized the patient's head. He was responsive but anxious when he told Abdul, "Something is wrong with me, I don't feel right." Sondra estimated that there was approximately 300 mL of blood on the sidewalk. When Abdul flexed the patient's pelvis during the rapid trauma assessment, he screamed in pain. They knew that they had to work quickly.

Sondra controlled the bleeding from the forearm with concentrated direct pressure and bandages, and placed the patient on 100% oxygen using a nonrebreather mask at a flow rate of 15 L/min. She also splinted the arm, while Abdul called medical direction and received instructions to inflate the pneumatic antishock garment (PASG). The patient was immobilized with a spine board and cervical collar and immediately transported to the local trauma center. Sondra and Abdul were pleased with the 6-minute scene time.

The patient spent 6 hours in surgery to repair his fractured pelvis and received 7 units of blood. The trauma surgeon later said the EMTs probably saved his life by controlling the external bleeding, recognizing the signs and symptoms of shock, and moving so quickly.

Consider what might have happened if the EMTs had spent too long at the scene.

Trauma calls are some of the most dramatic, emotionally charged, and challenging situations that you will face as an EMT. There is bleeding in almost all traumatic injuries. Sometimes bleeding is external and obvious; in these cases, blood can cover the patients, be splashed on the walls, or collect in puddles on the road. This is what most new EMTs may visualize when they are told about massive trauma scenes. However, blood loss is not always so obvious. When internal bleeding occurs, the patient loses blood into the body. In the opening scenario, for example, the patient lost much more blood through internal bleeding than he did through the external bleeding from his arm. An understanding of bleeding and shock situations is critically important for all EMTs.

REVIEW OF THE CARDIOVASCULAR SYSTEM

Before considering the mechanics of bleeding and blood loss, you need a basic understanding of the anatomy of the cardiovascular system. The cardiovascular system is the plumbing of the body. This system must deliver a fluid (blood) to all of the organs of the body through a network of pipes (ie, arteries, veins, and capillaries) and driven by a pump (the heart) (Fig. 25-1).

An average adult has approximately 6 L of blood in the body. Blood carries oxygen and other nutrients to every cell in the body. Blood also removes waste products, preventing the buildup of toxic chemicals in the tissues. The process of delivering

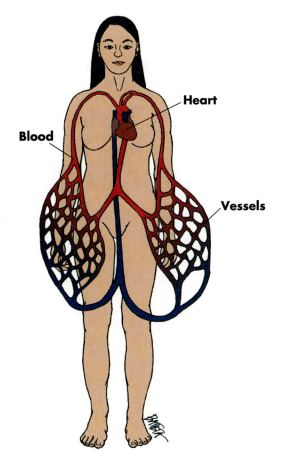

Fig. 25-1 Components of the cardiovascular system. The heart pumps blood to all organs of the body through the blood vessels.

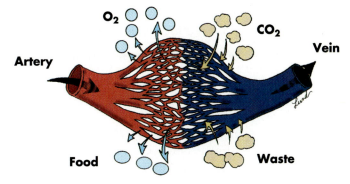

Fig. 25-2 Perfusion is the process in which the blood delivers oxygen and nutrients to and removes waste and carbon dixoide from organs.

oxygen to and removing waste from an organ is called **perfusion** (Fig. 25-2). All organs do not need to be perfused equally. The body has the amazing ability to increase or decrease the amount of blood that it delivers to specific organ systems. For example, when a person is running, the leg muscles must be richly perfused with blood; the arteries supplying these muscles dilate to increase blood flow. Simultaneously, digestion slows during exercise, so perfusion of the gastrointestinal tract is decreased.

The normal adult heart rate of 60 to 100 beats per minute pumps blood throughout the body. Even at rest, this efficient pump circulates the body's entire volume of blood in less than 1 minute. In times of emergency or stress, the heart rate can increase significantly. When beating at maximum efficiency, the heart can fill a gallon paint can in less time that it took you to read this paragraph! The resting heart rate of infants and children is faster than that of adults; the heart rate slows as a child gets older.

The relationship between blood pressure and perfusion is important. Blood is pumped to the body's organs by the pressure created by the heart. The diastolic blood pressure is the pressure in the vessels while the heart is in its relaxation phase. During contraction, the pressure rises momentarily as blood is ejected into the arteries. This intermittent pressure rise is the systolic blood pressure. Adequate blood pressure is necessary for good perfusion.

SHOCK

Every cell in the body needs a rich, continuous supply of blood to function properly. Each beat of the heart ejects blood into the arterial circulation and moves the blood quickly through the body. As each organ is perfused, the continuous delivery of fresh blood provides oxygen and nutrients and removes waste.

Any alteration in the body's ability to deliver blood to every organ is detrimental to the body. Cell death and organ failure can result from a disruption of blood flow. When patients bleed profusely, they lose blood from within the cardiovascular system. The loss of blood volume decreases perfusion to many body tissues. This situation of widespread **hypoperfusion** is called **shock**.

Shock results when the cardiovascular system cannot adequately perfuse the body's vital organs. Shock causes delicate tissues to be damaged from a lack of oxygen and a buildup of waste products. Shock is a life-threatening condition. The brain, heart, lungs, and kidneys are easily damaged by hypoperfusion. Failure of these organs causes death. You must learn how to estimate if the patient is in the early or late stage of shock and how to treat it quickly. The key to effective shock management is recognizing early signs and symptoms of shock and transporting the patient to the hospital before late shock develops.

When shock is caused by an inadequate volume of blood, it is called **hypovolemic shock.** An inadequate blood volume can be caused by dehydration, excessive vomiting or diarrhea, or internal or external blood loss. **Hemorrhagic shock** is hypoperfusion caused by bleeding only. Hypovolemic shock is the most common type of shock in trauma patients. Shock can occur for other reasons such as allergic reactions and cardiac failure.

ASSESSING SHOCK

The earliest and most subtle signs and symptoms of shock result from minute changes in the perfusion of the brain. Even small changes in the blood flow to the brain can cause slight changes in the patient's mental state. These generally are seen as restlessness, anxiety, and combativeness. It is very easy to dismiss these signs as normal stress for injured patients, but the perceptive EMT recognizes mental status changes as early signs and symptoms of shock. Mental status changes are especially im-

portant for patients with internal bleeding, because the signs and symptoms of shock may be the only indications that you have that the patient is experiencing a life-threatening blood loss. You need not determine whether the patient actually is in shock, as you should give treatment based on whether the signs and symptoms of shock are present.

> **ALERT**
> Subtle mental status changes,
> such as restlessness and anxiety,
> are the earliest signs of shock.

Many signs and symptoms of shock are related to the body's attempt to maintain perfusion following blood loss. When a patient bleeds significantly, hormones are released into the blood that cause blood vessels to constrict. The constriction of the blood vessels, called *vasoconstriction*, decreases the space that the remaining blood occupies (Fig. 25-3).

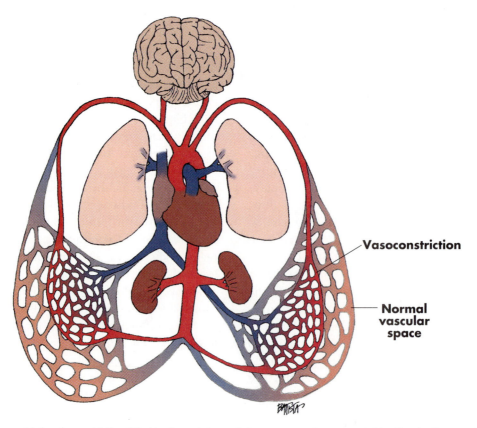

Vasoconstriction

Normal vascular space

Fig. 25-3 Vasoconstriction, the constriction of the blood vessels to nonvital organs, occurs in response to blood loss to allow more blood to reach the vital organs. This causes the skin to become pale, cool, and clammy.

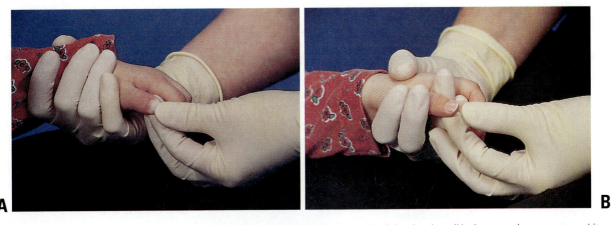

Fig. 25-4 Assessment of capillary refill. **A**, Pressing your thumb on the back of the patient's hand or the nail beds causes the area to turn white as you force blood out of the underlying capillaries. **B**, As you release pressure, the area should return to pink in less than 2 seconds.

Perfusion of the skin is decreased, and blood is diverted to vital organs such as the heart, lungs, brain, and kidneys. Decreased blood flow causes pale, cool, and clammy skin.

As the vessels in the body constrict, perfusion to the arms and legs decreases, causing weak peripheral pulses. Decreased peripheral perfusion can be evaluated by comparing the carotid or femoral pulses to the radial pulses and assessing **capillary refill.** These signs are reliable indicators of early shock in infants and children less than 6 years of age. Adults sometimes have other diseases that affect peripheral circulation, making these signs less dependable in older patients.

Capillary refill is assessed by gently pressing your thumb on the back of the patient's hand or the nail beds. This will cause the area to turn white as you force blood out of the underlying capillaries. As you release pressure, the color should return to pink in less than 2 seconds (Figs. 25-4A and B).

You should assess capillary refill only under normal room temperature conditions (approximately 70° F.) If the patient is cold, peripheral circulation will be decreased, making the capillary refill test unreliable. Even at room temperature, a pediatric patient who has been undressed may feel cold.

One of the most sensitive signs of early shock is heart rate. When a patient loses blood, the heart rate increases so that the remaining blood pumps faster. Any time a patient's pulse is faster than normal, you should consider the possibility of early shock. Some patients, especially older adults, may be receiving medications that prevent their heart rates from increasing in shock, so do not ignore other signs of shock with a normal heart rate.

The increased heart rate and vasoconstriction enable the body to maintain blood pressure even when the patient has lost a significant amount of blood. Eventually, continued blood loss will cause the blood pressure to fall. Once the patient's blood pressure drops, profound shock occurs. The early recognition and treatment of shock is the key to proper patient management.

> # ALERT
> **Decreased blood pressure is a late sign of shock. You must not wait for the blood pressure to drop before you consider and treat for shock.**

Decreased blood pressure is a late sign of shock in any patient. Infants and children have strong, healthy hearts and can maintain a normal blood pressure until they have lost over half of their blood volume. By the time that blood pressure is affected, the patient is close to death. Infants and children in shock have less reserve once they have decreased blood pressure. Do not wait to see decreased blood pressure before you treat for shock. Patients with preexisting cardiac disease, common in geriatric patients, have a limited ability to respond to blood loss and may deteriorate very quickly.

You may notice an increase in the respiratory rate as the patient attempts to oxygenate the remaining blood. As shock progresses, the breathing may become shallow, labored, and irregular.

There are some other signs and symptoms of

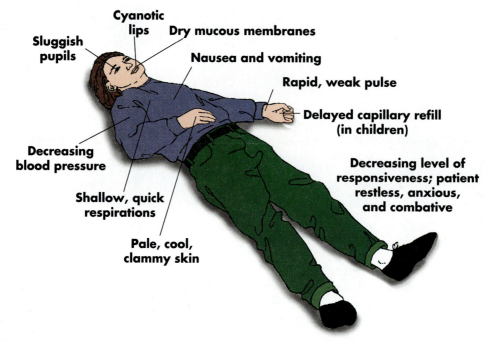

Sluggish pupils

Cyanotic lips

Dry mucous membranes

Nausea and vomiting

Rapid, weak pulse

Delayed capillary refill (in children)

Decreasing blood pressure

Decreasing level of responsiveness; patient restless, anxious, and combative

Shallow, quick respirations

Pale, cool, clammy skin

Fig. 25-5 Signs and symptoms of shock.

shock that may help you recognize a patient in danger. Although these are not always present, if you see them you should be alerted to the possibility of hypoperfusion (Fig. 25-5). When blood is diverted to vital organs, blood flow to the gastrointestinal tract is decreased and can cause nausea and vomiting. Because blood loss triggers the body's thirst mechanism, patients in shock may ask for something to drink. Because many of these patients will require surgery, do not allow them to eat or drink anything.

Capillaries in mucous membranes lie close to the surface of the skin. Paleness or cyanosis of the lips may be seen in patients in shock. As shock becomes profound, the pupils become sluggishly reactive to light. Box 25-1 summarizes the signs and symptoms of shock.

EMERGENCY CARE FOR SHOCK

After following body substance isolation precautions, the first step in treating the signs and symptoms of shock in the emergency setting is to ensure an adequate airway and ventilation. If the patient is unresponsive, manually position the airway immediately. Trauma patients may have blood, vomit, or broken teeth in their airway. Any such material must be removed or suctioned immediately. The treatment of shock and external bleeding is important, but proper airway management is always the first priority.

BOX 25-1

Signs and Symptoms of Shock

- Restlessness, anxiety, combativeness
- Increased heart rate
- Decreased capillary refill (evaluated in infants and children only)
- Pale, cool, clammy skin
- Thirst
- Decreasing level of responsiveness
- Breathing changes
- Nausea and vomiting
- Decreased blood pressure
- Cyanosis of nailbeds, lips, and mucous membranes
- Sluggishly reactive pupils

The major problem in shock is the body's inability to deliver oxygen and nutrients to the tissues. Therefore, it is very important to provide as high a concentration of oxygen as possible to the patient.

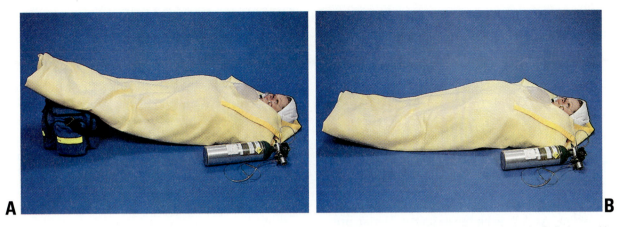

Fig. 25-6   Positioning of a patient in shock. **A**, Raising the legs will maximize the delivery of oxygenated blood to the brain. **B**, Patients with injuries to pelvis, head, chest, abdomen, neck, spine, or lower extremities should not have the legs raised.

High concentration oxygen will decrease cell death from the hypoxia caused by hypoperfusion.

The next step is to stop or slow the bleeding. Methods for controlling external and internal blood loss are described later in this chapter.

If the patient does not have suspected serious injuries to the pelvis, lower extremities, head, chest, abdomen, neck or spine, elevating the legs 20 to 30 cm (8 to 12 in) will decrease blood flow to the lower extremities and maximize the delivery of oxygenated blood to the brain (Fig. 25-6A). Lifting the legs should be avoided if the patient has such injuries because of the possibility of worsening these injuries. These patients should be immobilized in the neutral position. If the patient has injuries to the chest or abdomen, elevating the legs may actually increase bleeding or cause difficulty breathing. Patients with these injuries should be kept in the supine position (Fig. 25-6B).

It is very important to prevent body heat loss in patients in shock. When a patient feels cold, the body attempts to raise its temperature by shivering. Shivering wastes oxygen and energy that could be used for the more important task of perfusing the vital organs. The best way to prevent this problem is to cover the patient with a blanket. You should cover patients even in warm weather, because injuries decrease the body's ability to generate heat. In cold weather, also place a blanket under a patient who is lying on the ground or a cold surface.

If the patient has obvious bone or joint injuries, you should quickly splint them. Although splinting slows blood loss, do not spend too much time treating skeletal injuries. Usually, the patient will continue to bleed and the longer you spend in the field, the more blood the patient will lose.

Shock must be treated in the hospital. Many pa-

BOX 25-2

Emergency Treatment of Patients with Signs and Symptoms of Shock

- Use appropriate body substance isolation precautions including gloves, eye wear, a mask and a gown.
- Maintain an open airway.
- Provide the patient with 100% oxygen.
- Control the bleeding as much as possible.
- Elevate the patient's legs 20 to 30 cm (8 to 12 in) if the patient has no injuries to the legs, pelvis, head, chest, abdomen, neck, or spine.
- Cover the patient with a blanket to prevent heat loss.
- Splint suspected extremity fractures if time permits. Do not delay transportation of a patient in shock to splint extremity injuries.
- Transport immediately.

ALERT
The best treatment for the patient in shock is rapid transportation! You must immediately transport any patient with signs and symptoms of shock.

tients in shock require intravenous fluids, blood transfusions, and immediate surgery to repair damaged vessels. Box 25-2 summarizes the emergency care of patients with the signs and symptoms of shock.

EXTERNAL BLEEDING

BODY SUBSTANCE ISOLATION PRECAUTIONS

When treating any patient with obvious external blood loss, follow body substance isolation precautions before you approach the patient. Several infectious diseases can be transmitted by blood, so protect yourself. Because blood can spurt or splash, you should wear gloves, eye protection, mask, and a gown. Hand washing after each transport also helps decrease the possibility of infecting yourself or the next patient. Refer to Chapter 2, "The Well-Being of the EMT–Basic," for a detailed discussion of body substance isolation precautions.

REVIEW QUESTIONS

SHOCK

1. The shock that results from blood loss is called _____, and the shock that results from an inadequate blood volume is _____.

2. The earliest sign of shock is _____.

3. Capillary refill is a valuable assessment step under which circumstances?

4. _____ is a late and serious sign of shock.

5. Patients with serious injuries to the pelvis, legs, head, chest, abdomen, neck, or spine should be transported in the _____ position.

1. Hemorrhagic; hypovolemic
2. Restlessness or anxiety
3. Capillary refill is assessed in infant and children under 6 years of age, in normal room temperature.
4. Decreased blood pressure
5. Supine or neutral

ASSESSING BLOOD LOSS

The amount of blood that a patient can lose before developing shock depends on the person's size. The smaller the patient, the less blood is present in the body and the less bleeding that can occur before shock occurs. An adult suddenly losing 1 L of blood (approximately 1 qt) is considered serious. Geriatric patients cannot tolerate comparable blood loss, because their heart may be unable to respond to an increased demand. In a child, blood loss of 0.5 L is life threatening. Just 100 to 200 mL of blood loss in an infant is very dangerous.

> ## ALERT
> Remember that children bleed at the same rate as adults. Therefore, equal wounds will become life threatening much faster in smaller patients.

The severity of blood loss should be estimated based on the patient's signs and symptoms. Well-trained athletes are generally able to tolerate bleeding more easily than others, because their hearts are strong and can respond to blood loss by greatly increasing the force of contraction. Patients with underlying medical problems or elderly patients are at greater risk for complications from small amounts of bleeding, because their cardiovascular systems may not be able to compensate for a decreased amount of blood.

By quickly estimating the amount of blood that has been lost externally, you may anticipate the patient experiencing the signs and symptoms of shock and can consider immediate transport.

TYPES OF BLEEDING

In response to blood loss, the body naturally attempts to stop the bleeding by vasoconstriction and blood clotting. Severe injuries may bleed with so much force that clotting is impossible. As an EMT, you will find situations where you must control severe bleeding. The difficulty of controlling bleeding depends on the type of bleeding (Fig. 25-7).

ARTERIAL BLEEDING

When an artery is damaged, blood under high pressure spurts from a wound. If a major artery is

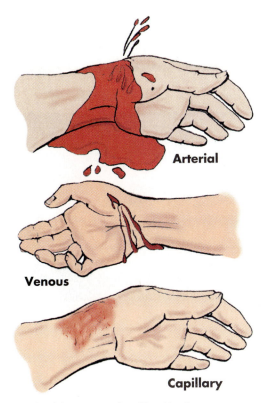

Fig. 25-7   Arterial, venous, and capillary bleeding.

damaged, the patient can quickly go into shock from blood loss and die. Fortunately, most large arteries are deep within the body and are protected from damage by surrounding tissues. External arterial bleeding is characterized by large amounts of bright red, oxygen-rich blood that may be squirting from the injury. Arterial bleeding is the most difficult to stop because of the high arterial pressure. You must act quickly to minimize significant blood loss.

VENOUS BLEEDING

In contrast to arterial bleeding, venous bleeding is dark red and flows in a steady stream from the injury. Venous bleeding may be profuse and dangerous, but it is usually easier to control because it is under much lower pressure than arterial bleeding.

CAPILLARY BLEEDING

Capillary bleeding is usually dark red and oozes from the injured site. Capillary bleeding is the least dangerous type of bleeding and normally clots by itself. The most common form of capillary bleeding occurs when the top layers of skin are scraped away. These abrasions can look grotesque but are rarely life threatening.

EMERGENCY CARE FOR EXTERNAL BLEEDING

Whatever the type of bleeding, the basic treatment is the same. First, before you make contact with the patient, take body substance isolation precautions. As always, ensure that the patient has an open airway and adequate ventilation.

CONCENTRATED DIRECT PRESSURE

Most major bleeding originates from damage to one main artery or a large vein. The most effective method of controlling this type of bleeding is concentrated direct pressure. To apply concentrated direct pressure, use your fingertip to press directly on the bleeding point. Ideally, do this with sterile gauze. If you do not have immediate access to gauze, simply apply pressure with your gloved finger. If fingertip pressure fails to stop the bleeding, remove the gauze and be sure you are applying pressure to the correct bleeding point. Technique 25-1 lists the steps for concentrated direct pressure.

DIFFUSE DIRECT PRESSURE

If the injury is large or the bleeding is not coming from one spot, more diffuse pressure is required. Diffuse direct pressure works by decreasing the

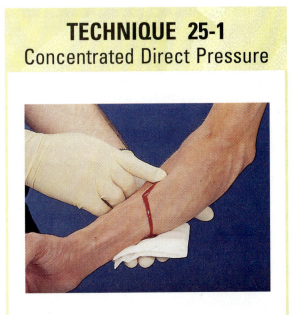

TECHNIQUE 25-1
Concentrated Direct Pressure

Fig. 25-8   Locate exactly where the bleeding is coming from. (This is often one major vessel.) **Apply direct concentrated pressure with a gloved finger and continue until you are able to apply a dressing that will keep pressure on the injury.**

TECHNIQUE 25-2
Diffuse Direct Pressure

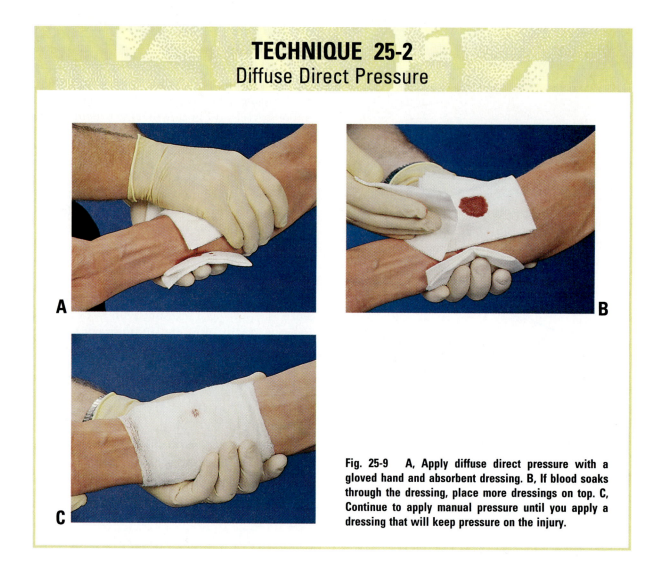

Fig. 25-9 **A, Apply diffuse direct pressure with a gloved hand and absorbent dressing. B, If blood soaks through the dressing, place more dressings on top. C, Continue to apply manual pressure until you apply a dressing that will keep pressure on the injury.**

blood flow through the arteries and veins leading to the injury. To apply diffuse direct pressure, place sterile gauze pads on the injury and apply pressure with your entire hand. If diffuse bleeding soaks through the dressings, do not remove them, but simply place more dressings on top. For gaping wounds with severe bleeding, pack the injury with sterile gauze. Technique 25-2 lists the steps for diffuse direct pressure.

When an extremity is injured, there are two techniques that are used as needed when concentrated or diffuse direct pressure alone does not stop the bleeding: *extremity elevation* and *pressure points*.

EXTREMITY ELEVATION

If there is no pain, swelling, or deformity, you should elevate the extremity. Elevation above the level of the heart will decrease blood flow and help to slow all three types of bleeding. Never move an extremity that is painful, swollen, or deformed, because there may be skeletal injuries present and this would aggravate the injury. Technique 25-3 lists the steps for elevating the extremity.

PRESSURE POINTS

Another technique to decrease bleeding is to use **pressure points** (Fig. 25-11). If the injury is to the arm, the pressure point is the brachial artery. If the injury is to the leg, the pressure point is the femoral artery. Pressing on the pressure point decreases blood flow to the extremity (Fig. 25-12). Because no extremity is supplied by a single artery, and venous bleeding is usually also present, a pressure point will slow bleeding but rarely stop it.

TECHNIQUE 25-3
Extremity Elevation

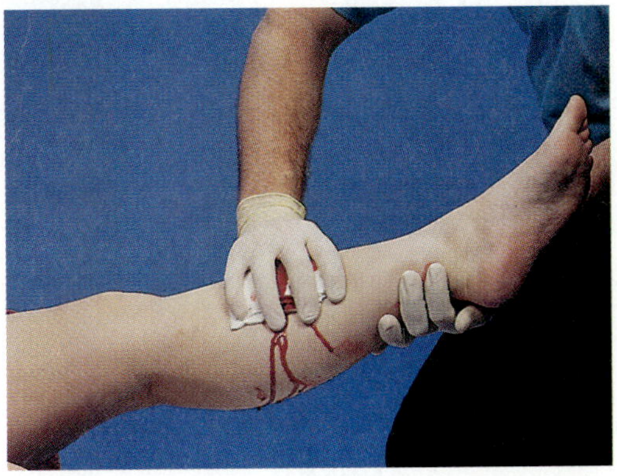

Fig. 25-10   Attempt to control bleeding by direct pressure. Check the entire extremity for other injuries; if there are signs or symptoms of skeletal injuries, do not elevate the extremity until it is splinted. **Elevate the extremity to slow external bleeding.**

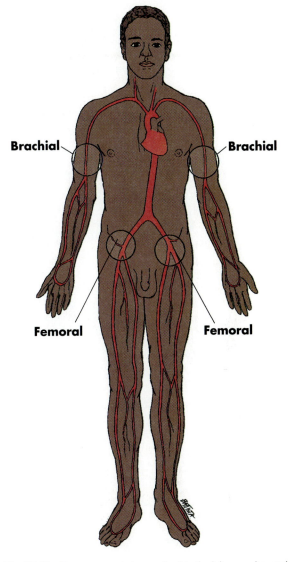

Fig. 25-11   Pressure on arteries proximal to the injury can be used to control bleeding in the extremities.

Technique 25-4 lists the steps for controlling bleeding with a pressure point.

A combination of direct pressure, elevation, and pressure points will normally stop almost all bleeding. Two other techniques that can be used to minimize bleeding associated with skeletal injuries are: *splinting* and *use of a tourniquet.*

SPLINTS

By immobilizing bone injuries with a splint, you reduce the movement of broken bone ends. These bone ends are very sharp and can cause tremendous damage to blood vessels and nerve tissue (Fig. 25-14).

Pneumatic antishock garments (PASGs), also known as *Military Anti-Shock Trousers (MAST)®*, are helpful in immobilizing the pelvis and controlling bleeding in the lower extremities. These devices are placed on the patient and inflated with air, providing **circumferential pressure** to the pelvis and lower extremities. This diffuse pressure plays an important role in restricting the movement of the pelvis and lower extremities as well as controlling bleeding at the specific injury site.

Pneumatic antishock garments are used in prehospital care for three reasons:

1. As a component of pelvic injury management when associated with the signs and symptoms of shock, to immobilize the pelvis and assist in the reduction of internal blood loss. When used for this purpose, all compartments should be inflated.
2. As a pressure dressing, to control severe bleeding caused by massive soft-tissue damage in the lower legs. When used for this purpose, only the leg compartment(s) that encompass the damaged tissue should be inflated.
3. As a splint, to immobilize bone and joint injuries of the lower legs. Only the leg compartment(s) that encompass the injury should be inflated in this instance.

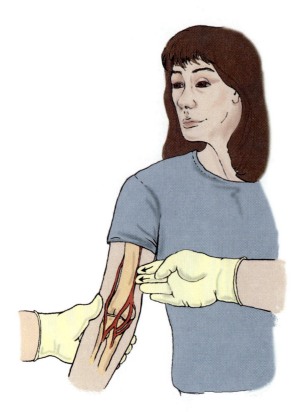

Fig. 25-12 Pressing on a pressure point decreases blood flow to the extremity.

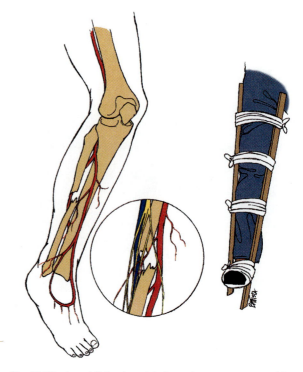

Fig. 25-14 Immobilizing bone injuries reduces movement and further injury caused by sharp bone ends.

There is controversy about the uses and effectiveness of the PASG. Regardless of the reason for use, you should consult with medical direction before applying and inflating the PASG. The PASG should not be used if there is evidence of chest injuries. Local protocol may include additional contraindications to the use of the PASG.

The PASGs come in adult and pediatric sizes. To ensure patient safety and maximum effectiveness of the device, use the size appropriate for the patient. Check that the top of the garment will not be placed above the level of the patient's lowest rib.

There are a number of techniques for applying the PASG. Because the majority of these patients have traumatic injuries, spinal immobilization is critical to the application process. Therefore, the easiest way to apply the PASG is to place the garment on the long spine board first. Technique 25-5 lists the steps for applying the PASG in pelvic injury.

The PASG is almost never deflated before the patient arrives at the hospital. If the patient experiences difficulty breathing, consult medical direction. Keep the pump and hoses connected to the trousers, and leave them with the patient at the hospital.

In addition to the PASG, other types of pneumatic pressure splints can also be used to control

TECHNIQUE 25-4
Pressure Points

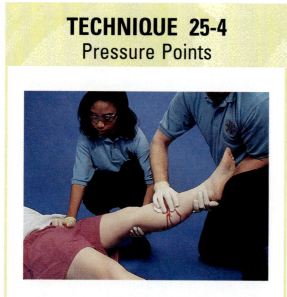

Fig. 25-13 **Attempt to stop the bleeding with direct pressure and elevation if possible. Apply manual pressure to the brachial artery or the femoral artery to decrease bleeding in the extremity.** Continue to apply pressure while transporting the patient, because release may cause bleeding to resume.

TECHNIQUE 25-5
Application of Pneumatic Antishock Garment

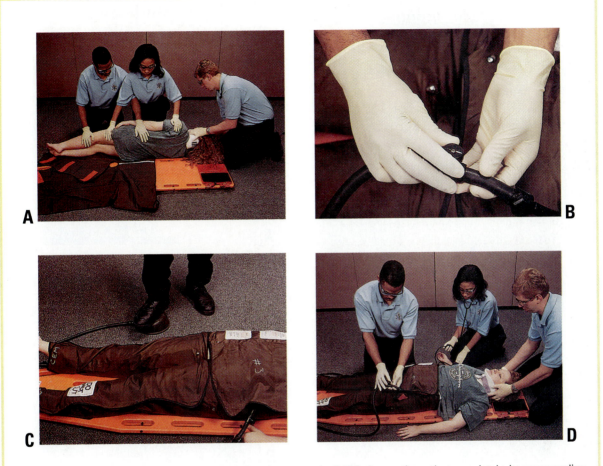

Fig. 25-15 Receive authorization from medical direction to use the PASG. Assess the patient completely, because application of the PASG will prevent further inspection of the abdomen, pelvis, and lower extremities. Remove all clothing on the patient from the waist down. Place the unfolded PASG on the long backboard, patient side up. Position the trousers slightly off center (toward the patient) and at the level of the patient's lowest rib. **A, Log roll the patient onto the backboard.** Secure the velcro straps and attach the hoses to the valves of the device. **B, Check all the valves to ensure that the proper chambers are open and closed depending on the reason for applying the device. For most devices, orienting the line on the valve parallel to the hose means the line is open. C, Inflate the chambers until the PASG provides adequate immobilization. D, Close all the valves to prevent leakage.** Repeatedly assess the trousers to make certain they remain inflated; add air if the device loses pressure.

bleeding. These are discussed in Chapter 27, "Musculoskeletal Care."

TOURNIQUETS

The last-resort method for the control of bleeding is a tourniquet. A tourniquet is rarely required, as most bleeding can be controlled with other techniques. Use of a tourniquet often causes permanent damage to muscles, nerves, and blood vessels, and therefore is a decision to be made carefully. Even in cases of complete amputation, use of a tourniquet is

rarely necessary. Principle 25-1 lists the principles of using a tourniquet to control severe bleeding.

Technique 25-6 describes one technique for applying a tourniquet.

Technique 25-7 details another tourniquet technique, using a blood pressure cuff continuously inflated. A blood pressure cuff is a convenient quick alternative to a tourniquet, because it is often easily accessible.

Always record the time of application. Some experts advocate writing the time that you applied the

PRINCIPLE 25-1
Using Tourniquets

1. Use a tourniquet only after all other methods of bleeding control are exhausted.

2. Use a wide device that will not cut or damage tissue. Never use wire, rope, a belt, or any material that will cut the underlying tissue.

3. The tourniquet must provide continuous circumferential pressure great enough to stop the bleeding.

4. Do not apply a tourniquet over a joint. Because amputation immediately proximal to the tourniquet site is likely, place it as close to the injury as possible, but avoid placing it over a joint.

5. Do not remove or release the tourniquet once it has been applied. This can cause blood clots to be released from the site and cause life-threatening complications if they lodge in the lungs. Removal of a tourniquet increases the possibility of rebleeding.

6. Record the time of application and alert other healthcare professionals that you have used a tourniquet.

7. Leave the tourniquet in plain view so that anyone who treats the patient will easily see it.

TECHNIQUE 25-6
Using a Triangular Bandage as a Tourniquet

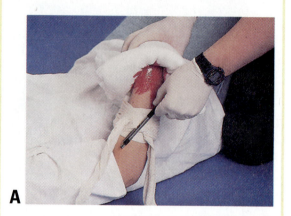

A

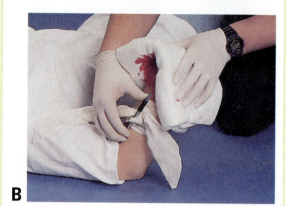

B

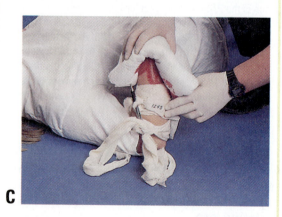

C

Fig. 25-16 Select a bandage at least 4 in wide. Wrap the bandage around the extremity twice, proximal to the bleeding but as close to the injury as possible. **A, Tie one knot in the bandage, place a stick or pen on top of the knot, and tie the ends of the bandage over the knot. B, Twist the stick (or pen) until the bleeding stops. C, Secure the stick (or pen) in position. Record the time of application.**

tourniquet on the patient's forehead. Be sure to notify emergency department personnel that a tourniquet has been applied. Also, document in your prehospital care report that you used a tourniquet.

Remember that a tourniquet is used as a last resort. The use of such a constricting band can cause tremendous tissue damage, and the extremity often must be amputated at the site of the tourniquet. Always try other methods first to control the bleeding, to decrease the possibility of permanent damage. Box 25-3 summarizes the management of external bleeding.

TECHNIQUE 25-7
Using a Blood Pressure Cuff as a Tourniquet

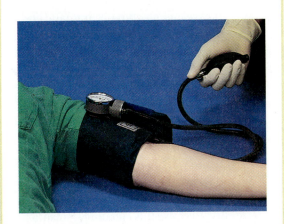

Fig. 25-17   Apply the blood pressure cuff proximal to the bleeding, but as close to the injury as possible. **Inflate the cuff until the bleeding stops.** Close the valve tightly to avoid accidental deflation and record the time of application.

BLEEDING FROM THE EARS, NOSE, AND MOUTH

Most external blood loss can be controlled by the methods described above. However, a few specific injuries deserve particular attention.

BOX 25-3

The Management of External Bleeding

- Follow body substance isolation precautions.
- Maintain an open airway and adequate ventilation.
- Use concentrated direct pressure or diffuse direct pressure.
- Elevate a bleeding extremity with no signs of skeletal injuries.
- Use the appropriate pressure point (for extremity bleeding) or pneumatic antishock garment (for lower extremity bleeding).
- Use a tourniquet only as a last resort.

Bleeding from the ears or nose can be a sign of a skull fracture. Occasionally, this blood is mixed with cerebrospinal fluid. Cerebrospinal fluid is a clear liquid that surrounds the brain and spinal cord. Cerebrospinal fluid may be coming from the ears or nose and is occasionally streaked with blood. If there is trauma to the head, bleeding from the nose and ears should be covered lightly with sterile gauze. This will decrease the risk of infection.

Facial trauma can result in profuse bleeding because of the rich supply of blood to the head and face. Many of these vessels lie close to the surface and can be easily lacerated in traumatic injuries. These injuries often look gruesome, but fortunately you can usually stop the bleeding with direct pressure. Never use the carotid arteries as pressure points or tie a tourniquet around the neck.

Bleeding from the nose, called **epistaxis,** without other significant trauma is considered a special case. Nosebleeds are often caused by blunt forces to the nose or by digital trauma (eg, nose picking). There are also some medical causes of epistaxis such as sinusitis and other respiratory tract infections, hypertension, and coagulation disorders. Nosebleeds may be life threatening in patients who are receiving blood-thinning medications, commonly taken by elderly patients or patients with heart disease.

Because you cannot easily place direct pressure on a nosebleed, there are three steps that you can take to slow the bleeding.

1. If no spinal injury is suspected, place the patient in a sitting position leaning forward. It is important to keep blood from going down the patient's throat, causing the patient to vomit. If

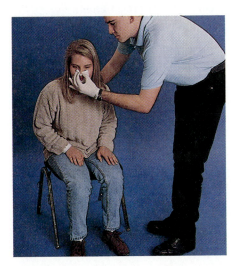

Fig. 25-18   Lean the patient forward and pinch the fleshy portion of the nostrils together to control epistaxis.

trauma is suspected, immobilize the patient as usual and be prepared for nausea and vomiting.
2. Pinch the fleshy portion of the nostrils together (Fig. 25-18).
3. Keep the patient calm and quiet.

The soft tissues in the mouth and throat can be lacerated by trauma or by eating a sharp object, such as a shell or a piece of bone. In this case, the patient generally spits out bright red blood. Transport the patient rapidly if the blood loss is severe.

With either mouth or nose bleeding, if no trauma is suspected, place the patient in the recovery position so that the blood drains out of the mouth or nose instead of into the airway where it may cause an obstruction or throat where it may be swallowed. If the patient has sustained trauma and is immobilized on a long backboard, you should tilt the entire board to the side to prevent bleeding

directly into the airway and suction the patient as needed.

INTERNAL BLEEDING

Although external bleeding is dramatic and obvious, internal bleeding can be deceptive. Not only is internal bleeding more difficult to recognize, but it is much more difficult to stop. Severe internal blood loss can quickly result in profound shock and death.

ASSESSING BLOOD LOSS

Damaged internal organs can bleed into the thoracic and abdominal cavities. Skeletal trauma can damage blood vessels and result in bleeding within the extremity. Because this bleeding is so difficult to recognize, you should suspect internal bleeding based on the mechanism of injury and the patient's signs and symptoms. The signs and symptoms of shock may be the first indicators of internal bleeding. Box 25-4 contains a list of mechanisms of injury that often result in internal bleeding.

You must be careful in your assessment to recognize the signs and symptoms of internal blood loss. Some internal bleeding is present with any musculoskeletal injury. Figure 25-19 shows the amount of blood loss associated with various injuries. You should suspect blood loss in any painful, tender, swollen extremity.

REVIEW QUESTIONS

EXTERNAL BLEEDING

1. The sudden loss of _____ liter(s) of blood is considered serious in an average adult.

2. Match the following:
   A. Arterial bleeding   1. Steady-flowing blood
   B. Venous bleeding   2. Oozing blood
   C. Capillary bleeding   3. Spurting blood

3. Place the following steps for controlling bleeding in the proper order.
   A. Pressure points
   B. Tourniquet
   C. Elevation
   D. Diffuse direct pressure
   E. Concentrated direct pressure

4. List the three steps in stopping a nose bleed.

1. 1
2. A - 3
   B - 1
   C - 2
3. E, D, A or C (either first), B
4. Place the patient in a sitting position leaning forward; pinch the fleshy portion of the nostrils together; keep the patient calm and quiet.

BOX 25-4

Mechanisms of Injury With a Possibility of Internal Bleeding

- Falls
- Motorcycle crashes
- Automobile-pedestrian collisions
- Automobile collisions
- Explosions
- Penetrating injuries

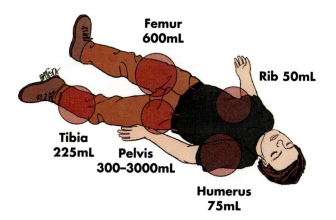

Fig. 25-19 The amount of blood loss associated with various musculoskeletal injuries.

SIGNS AND SYMPTOMS OF INTERNAL BLEEDING

There are many situations where a patient can bleed huge quantities of blood into the body. Often, there is no external indication of the bleeding. Any patient who has the signs and symptoms of shock should be assumed to have internal bleeding, treated for shock, and transported immediately.

Any bleeding from the mouth, rectum, or vagina is a significant finding. Do not be misled by an apparently minor amount of external blood loss. There may be significant internal bleeding in these cases. Based on the patient's signs and symptoms, do your best to estimate the amount of blood lost.

Bleeding into the gastrointestinal tract can result in several unique signs. The color, character, smell, and volume of blood depends on the location of the bleeding and how long the blood has been in the gastrointestinal tract. Damage to the delicate gastrointestinal lining anywhere along its length will cause a number of different signs and symptoms.

Blood can enter the stomach either by swallowing or from direct damage to the stomach lining (eg, bleeding ulcers). Blood is very irritating to the stomach lining and usually causes the patient to vomit. If the patient vomits soon, the vomit will be tinged with bright red blood. If the blood remains in the stomach for a period of time, it mixes with digestive juices, turns very dark brown, and has a consistency of coffee grounds. Any time that a patient gives a history of vomiting material looking like coffee grounds or bright red blood, you should strongly suspect internal bleeding.

If the patient is bleeding into the small or large intestine, the blood will be partially digested as it passes through the gastrointestinal tract. Digested blood appears as very dark, tarry stool. If the bleeding is lower in the gastrointestinal tract, the stool may be tinged with bright red blood.

Damage to the vessels in the abdominal cavity can result in massive, difficult-to-control internal bleeding. The abdominal cavity can hold up to 10 L of extra fluid. Disruption of abdominal vessels is a common medical emergency in the elderly when a major artery in the abdomen is damaged from long-term high blood pressure. Damage to the blood vessels in the abdomen can also be the result of abdominal trauma and pelvic injuries.

Blood in the abdominal cavity can distend the abdomen. Blood is irritating to the abdominal organs and causes abdominal rigidity and tenderness. When you assess the abdomen, findings of rigidity and tenderness are very serious signs of internal bleeding.

EMERGENCY CARE FOR INTERNAL BLEEDING

As always, be sure to follow body substance isolation precautions in all cases of bleeding. Ensure that the patient has a patent airway and provide artificial ventilation if necessary. In all cases of severe bleeding, administer high-flow oxygen via a nonrebreather mask if this was not already begun during the initial assessment.

If you suspect that internal bleeding is caused by injury to an extremity, you can slow this bleeding by direct pressure and splinting the injury.

If a patient has signs and symptoms of shock, the lower abdomen is tender, and you suspect a pelvic injury, a PASG may be indicated. The PASG should

---

BOX 25-5

Signs and Symptoms of Internal Bleeding

- Signs and symptoms of shock
- Bleeding from any body orifice
- Blood-tinged vomit or feces
- Coffee ground vomit
- Dark tarry stool
- Abdominal rigidity or tenderness
- Distended abdomen

BOX 25-6

The Management of Internal Bleeding

- Follow body substance isolation precautions
- Maintain an open airway and adequate ventilation
- Treat patient for shock
- Quickly splint any suspected extremity injuries
- Apply the pneumatic antishock garment (for suspected pelvic injuries with tender abdomen and signs and symptoms of shock)
- Transport immediately

not be used if the patient has a chest injury and should be inflated only after approval by medical direction. The PASG may slow the bleeding enough so that the patient will survive to have the injury repaired surgically.

Above all, if the patient has signs and symptoms

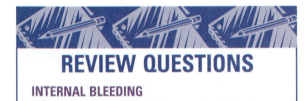

REVIEW QUESTIONS

INTERNAL BLEEDING

1. Abdominal rigidity and tenderness are possible signs of _____.

2. When do you use pneumatic antishock garments to control internal bleeding?

3. As an EMT, what can you do to decrease the internal bleeding associated with extremity injuries?

1. Internal bleeding into the abdomen
2. When the patient shows signs and symptoms of shock; lower abdominal tenderness when a pelvic injury is suspected and medical direction agrees
3. Splint the injury

of internal bleeding, transport immediately! Box 25-5 lists these signs and symptoms. Internal bleeding is extremely difficult to control and must be evaluated at the hospital. There is little that you can do in the field to stop the bleeding, so you must rapidly assess, recognize, immobilize, and transport. Box 25-6 summarizes the management of internal bleeding.

CHAPTER SUMMARY

SHOCK

Bleeding is one of the most dramatic emergencies that EMTs encounter. Blood is the fluid of life, delivering oxygen and nutrients to every cell in the body. When the cardiovascular system is unable to deliver blood to all of the body's tissues, hypoperfusion results. Hypoperfusion, otherwise known as *shock*, is a life-threatening condition that requires rapid recognition and quick intervention.

The earlier that you recognize the signs and symptoms of shock and intervene, the better chance the patient has for a full recovery. The early signs and symptoms of shock can be subtle and easily missed. You must carefully and completely assess every patient to identify the early signs and symptoms of shock. Rapid transport to the hospital is one of the most important steps in managing the patient with signs and symptoms of shock.

EXTERNAL BLEEDING

External bleeding is striking and alarming. As an EMT, you should be able to estimate the amount of blood that a patient has lost and report it to the receiving hospital. You must be adept at quickly controlling arterial, venous, and capillary bleeding by using concentrated and diffuse direct pressure, pressure points, elevation, and (as a last resort) tourniquets. Splinting and the use of the pneumatic antishock garment can also be beneficial for controlling bleeding in certain situations.

INTERNAL BLEEDING

Internal bleeding can be difficult to recognize and also very dangerous. The possibility for internal bleeding exists with any traumatic injury. The greater the forces involved in the mechanism of injury, the greater the potential for internal hemorrhage. Internal bleeding can also result from a number of medical conditions. Any bleeding from a body orifice is an important sign suggesting internal bleeding. To decrease the complications of internal bleeding, watch for the signs and symptoms of shock and transport the patient to the hospital quickly.

With a thorough knowledge of bleeding and shock, careful assessment, prompt recognition, and quick action, you can help save victims of sudden traumatic and medical emergencies.

UNITED STATES DEPARTMENT OF TRANSPORTATION NATIONAL HIGHWAY TRAFFIC SAFETY ADMINISTRATION EMT–BASIC OBJECTIVES

Check your knowledge. The National Registry of EMTs and many state EMS agencies use the objectives below to develop EMT–Basic certification examinations. Can you meet them?

COGNITIVE

1. List the structure and function of the circulatory system.
2. Differentiate between arterial, venous, and capillary bleeding.
3. State the methods of emergency medical care of external bleeding.
4. Establish the relationship between body substance isolation and bleeding.
5. Establish the relationship between airway management and the trauma patient.
6. Establish the relationship between mechanism of injury and internal bleeding.
7. List the signs of internal bleeding.
8. List the steps in the emergency medical care of the patient with signs and symptoms of internal bleeding.
9. List signs and symptoms of shock (hypoperfusion).
10. State the steps in the emergency medical care of the patient with signs and symptoms of shock (hypoperfusion).

AFFECTIVE

1. Explain the sense of urgency to transport patients that are bleeding and show signs of shock (hypoperfusion).

PSYCHOMOTOR

1. Demonstrate direct pressure as a method of emergency medical care of external bleeding.
2. Demonstrate the use of diffuse pressure as a method of emergency medical care of external bleeding.
3. Demonstrate the use of pressure points and tourniquets as a method of emergency care of external bleeding.
4. Demonstrate the care of the patient exhibiting signs and symptoms of internal bleeding.
5. Demonstrate the care of the patient exhibiting signs and symptoms of shock (hypoperfusion).
6. Demonstrate completion of a prehospital care report for patients with bleeding and/or shock (hypoperfusion).

26 SOFT-TISSUE INJURIES

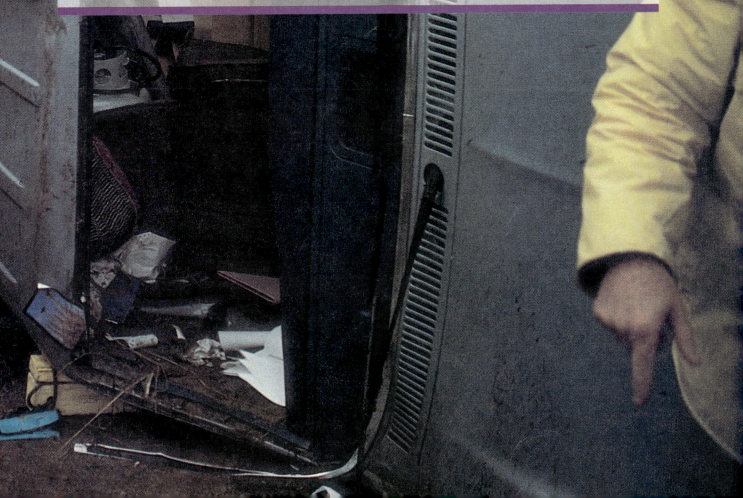

KEY TERMS

Abrasion: An open soft-tissue injury resulting from a scraping force; the epidermis is damaged.

Amputation: The removal of an appendage from the body.

Avulsion: A flap of skin that is torn or pulled loose.

Bandage: A material used to secure a dressing in place on an injury.

Contusion: A type of closed soft-tissue injury; also called a bruise.

Crush injury: An open or closed soft-tissue injury resulting from a blunt force trauma.

Dressing: A sterile material used to control bleeding and protect an open soft-tissue injury.

Evisceration: An open wound in the abdomen through which organs are protruding.

Full-thickness burn: a burn that affects all layers of the skin.

Hematoma: A closed soft-tissue injury produced by an accumulation of blood under the skin.

Laceration: A break in the skin of varying depth caused by a sharp object.

Occlusive: Referring to protection from the air; an occlusive dressing will not let air into the wound.

Partial-thickness burn: A burn that affects the epidermis and dermis.

Penetration or puncture: An open soft-tissue injury caused by an object being pushed into the skin.

Superficial burn: A burn that affects only the epidermis.

IN THE FIELD

"**A**mbulance 41, please report to 111 Fourth Avenue for a domestic dispute with unknown injuries. Police have been dispatched. No answer on the call back."

EMTs Faye and Johnny arrived at the address and parked their vehicle. "We'd better be careful with this one, Johnny," Faye said. "I was out here once before, and it could get violent." As they approached the scene, they were relieved to see law enforcement officers approaching the house. They took the trauma bag and oxygen tank and headed for the house. An officer on the front porch yelled to them that there was a woman bleeding on the floor.

From the front door, Johnny and Faye saw a woman lying on the carpet in a pool of blood, with a knife protruding from her abdomen. In the next room they heard a man yelling and fighting. "Is it okay to enter?" Faye asked the officer on the porch. "It is now, come on in," he said. They put their gloves on, checked the woman's airway for patency, and assessed her breathing. Her breaths were barely audible, and her pulse fast and weak. They knew they had to act quickly because she was showing signs and symptoms of shock. It appeared as though she had lost approximately 400 mL of blood externally and maybe more internally.

Within 5 minutes, they were ventilating the patient with 100% high-flow oxygen via bag-valve-mask and had controlled the bleeding, stabilized the impaled object, and immobilized her on a long spine board. Ambulance 41 was now en route to the nearest trauma facility.

Would you have rushed into this situation without first checking to see if the scene was safe?

Soft-tissue injuries are common and can be very dramatic. Most of these injuries are not life threatening, but some may result in severe bleeding. Soft-tissue injuries range from abrasions to serious full-thickness burns. You must be familiar with the treatment of various soft-tissue injuries to control bleeding, prevent further injury, and reduce contamination and infection.

THE SKIN

FUNCTION

The skin, the largest organ in the human body, is an important protective barrier. The skin protects the body from the environment and from bacteria, viruses, and other harmful organisms. The skin regulates body temperature by acting as insulation. The pores open or close to release or contain heat. The skin contains nerves that sense heat, cold, touch, pressure and pain, and transmit this information to the brain.

LAYERS

The skin is structured in three layers (Fig. 26-1). The outermost layer is the epidermis, which consists of dead skin cells and pores that open to the environment. Because this layer is composed of dead skin cells, injuries to only this layer usually do not cause pain or bleeding. This layer is very thin, and the most superficial injuries damage only the epidermis. The dermis is the next layer, which contains sweat and sebaceous glands, hair follicles, small blood vessels, and nerve endings. When this layer of the skin is injured, bleeding occurs and pain is felt. The deepest layer is the subcutaneous layer. If an injury is as deep as this layer, there is more bleeding and pain. This layer may also be damaged enough to expose underlying bone, muscle, or other tissue.

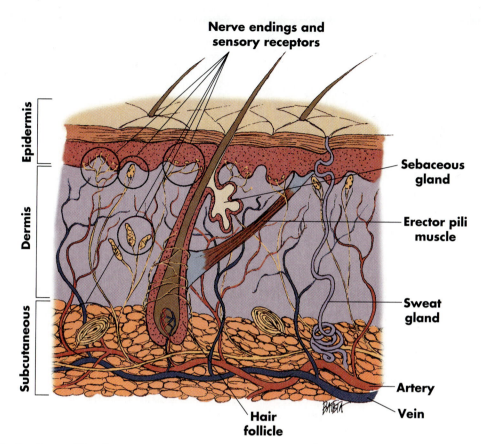

Nerve endings and sensory receptors

Epidermis

Dermis

Subcutaneous

Sebaceous gland

Erector pili muscle

Sweat gland

Artery

Vein

Hair follicle

Fig. 26-1. The three layers of the skin.

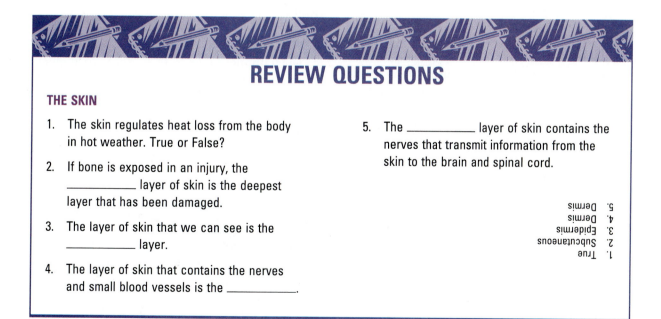

REVIEW QUESTIONS

THE SKIN

1. The skin regulates heat loss from the body in hot weather. True or False?

2. If bone is exposed in an injury, the _____ layer of skin is the deepest layer that has been damaged.

3. The layer of skin that we can see is the _____ layer.

4. The layer of skin that contains the nerves and small blood vessels is the _____.

5. The _____ layer of skin contains the nerves that transmit information from the skin to the brain and spinal cord.

1. True
2. Subcutaneous
3. Epidermis
4. Dermis
5. Dermis

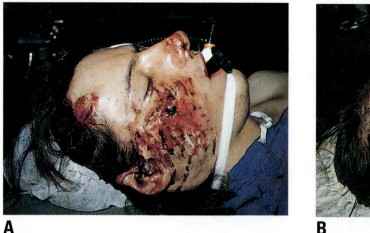 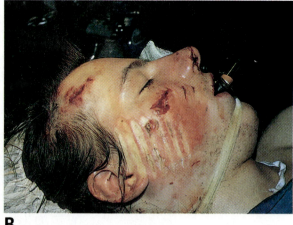

A   **B**

Fig. 26-2. Soft-tissue injuries may appear worse than they are. A, A soft-tissue injury before cleaning. B, The same injury after it has been cleaned.

INJURIES

EMTs care for many different types of soft-tissue injuries, including closed and open injuries and burns. This chapter discusses these injuries and the appropriate emergency medical care. Although these injuries may appear critical, they often require only minor emergency care (Fig 26-2A and B).

CLOSED INJURIES

With a closed soft-tissue injury, the skin remains intact and there is no external bleeding.

CONTUSION

A **contusion** is a closed soft-tissue injury in which cells are damaged in the skin and blood vessels are torn in the dermis (Fig. 26-3). This injury is commonly called a *bruise* and produces a discoloration in the skin because of the internal blood accumulation. Swelling and pain are sometimes present.

> # ALERT
> A bruise over a vital organ may mean that the organ has been damaged and internal bleeding may be present.

HEMATOMA

A **hematoma** is similar to a contusion, but there is a much larger amount of blood collected beneath the skin and more tissue damage. Larger blood vessels are injured, and 1 or more liters of blood could be lost and accumulated under the skin. With larger injuries, the signs and symptoms of hypoperfusion could be present.

CLOSED CRUSH INJURY

A **crush injury** is an injury where force is applied to an area of the body with a blunt instrument (Fig. 26-4). This mechanism of injury can produce organ damage. Internal bleeding may be severe and could lead to shock.

OPEN INJURIES

Open injuries range from abrasions to amputations. With open soft-tissue injuries, the skin is usually broken and there is external bleeding.

ABRASION

An **abrasion** occurs when the outermost layers of skin are damaged by scraping forces. Though this

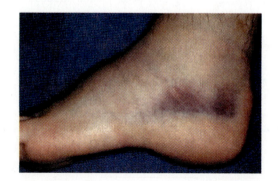

Fig. 26-3. A contusion occurring as a result of a sprained ankle.

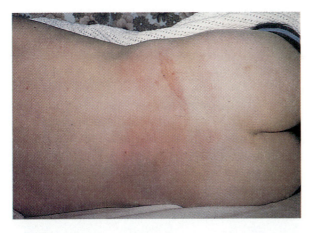

Fig. 26-4. A closed crush injury, produced when a van wheel passed over the trunk of the patient.

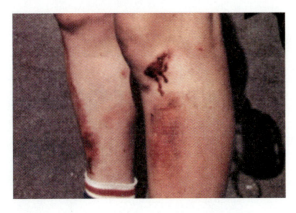

Fig. 26-5. Abrasions caused by a fall from a bicycle.

type of wound is superficial, it can be very painful. There may be little oozing of blood, though the injury usually appears red in color (Fig. 26-5).

LACERATION

A **laceration** is a break in the skin extending to a variable depth (Fig. 26-6). This injury can be linear

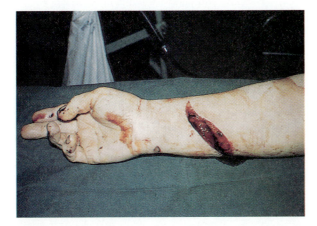

Fig. 26-6. A laceration.

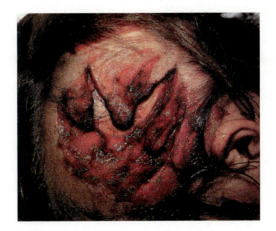

Fig. 26-7. An avulsion of the scalp over the left ear.

(regular) or stellate (irregular) and can occur alone or along with other soft-tissue injuries. These injuries are caused by a forceful impact with a sharp object, such as a knife or piece of glass. The bleeding may be severe, depending on the location and depth of the wound.

AVULSION

An **avulsion** occurs when a piece of skin or soft tissue is partially torn loose or pulled completely from the body (Fig. 26-7). This injury can happen anywhere on the body and can also be found with other types of soft-tissue injury.

PENETRATION OR PUNCTURE

A **penetration or puncture** wound is caused by an object, such as a knife or bullet, that is forced into the body (Fig. 26-8). The object may still be in the wound, may have been pulled out, or may have exited the body at another location. There may be no external bleeding because of closure of the skin around the opening when the object is pulled out,

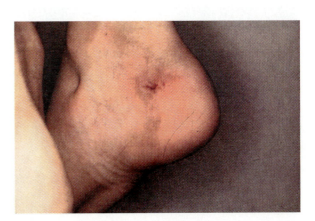

Fig. 26-8. A puncture wound caused by a dog bite.

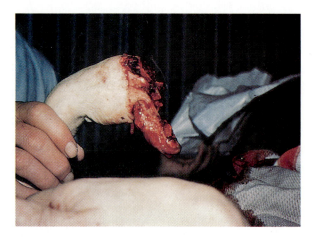

Fig. 26-9.   A hand with a nearly amputated thumb and amputated fingers.

but the internal bleeding can be severe if a blood vessel or vital organ was punctured. Gunshot wounds may involve erratic paths through the body and cause vast amounts of internal damage along with entrance and exit wounds.

AMPUTATION

An **amputation** involves the separation of an appendage from the body, such as a finger or an arm (Fig. 26-9). These injuries may be the result of great shearing forces. Massive bleeding may be present or bleeding may be limited.

OPEN CRUSH INJURY

Crush injuries may also produce an open soft-tissue injury and damage to internal organs (Fig. 26-10). Painful, swollen, deformed extremities are common, and external bleeding may be minimal or absent. Internal bleeding may be severe.

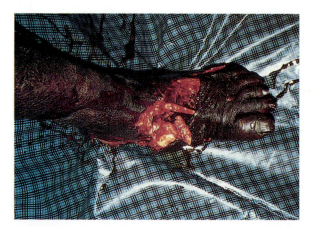

Fig. 26-10.   An open crush injury.

EMERGENCY MEDICAL CARE FOR PATIENTS WITH SOFT-TISSUE INJURIES

When providing emergency medical care to a patient with a soft-tissue injury, always follow body substance isolation precautions. Wash your hands, wear gloves, and take other precautions as required. You can never be too cautious, because even a patient with a closed injury may vomit or begin to bleed externally. After putting on gloves and taking appropriate precautions, provide the care described in Principle 26-1.

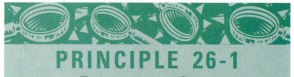

PRINCIPLE 26-1
Emergency Care for Patients With Soft-Tissue Injuries

1. Ensure a patent airway. Provide artificial ventilation with oxygen if the patient is not breathing adequately.

2. If the patient is showing signs of shock (eg, fast pulse, cool, clammy skin, and decreased level of responsiveness), treat for shock immediately by administering high-flow oxygen via a nonrebreather mask at a rate of 15 L/min and placing the patient in a supine position. Chapter 25, "Bleeding and Shock," fully describes the care of a patient in shock. Transport the patient as soon as possible, and try to keep the patient calm and quiet.

3. To manage bleeding with an open soft-tissue injury, expose the wound. Control the bleeding and minimize contamination by placing a dry sterile dressing over the wound and bandaging it in place. For serious bleeding, follow the steps outlined in Chapter 25, "Bleeding and Shock."

4. Assess the patient for a possible spinal injury and immobilize appropriately.

5. If the patient is stable and the airway is patent, you may choose to splint any painful, swollen, deformed extremity before transporting. If the patient is in shock, the extremity may be splinted en route to the receiving facility, if there is time.

ALERT
When you encounter a patient with a soft-tissue injury, always check for an exit wound, especially with penetrating injuries. An object may have passed entirely through the body.

DRESSINGS AND BANDAGES

Manage soft-tissue injuries with **dressings** and **bandages**. The purpose of the dressing is to stop the bleeding and to prevent further damage to the wound. Dressings are made of sterile material and protect the wound from further contamination and infection. The bandage is the material that secures the dressing in place.

Dressings come in many shapes and sizes (Fig. 26-11). There are universal dressings, dressings classified according to size (2 × 2, 4 × 4, 5 × 9, etc.), and adhesive and occlusive types of dressings. An **occlusive dressing** is made of nonporous material to prevent the entry of any air and usually contains an ointment that seals the dressing; a piece of plastic wrap or foil can be used as a seal. The appropriate size dressing should be used to completely cover the wound, with about 2.5 cm (1 in) extra on each side. All dressings should be sterile.

Bandages are used to secure dressings in place. Bandages do not have to be sterile and should be chosen appropriately for the area of injury (Fig. 26-12). Some bandages are self-adherent and sticky. Others are not self-adherent and require the use of adhesive tape that is placed directly over the

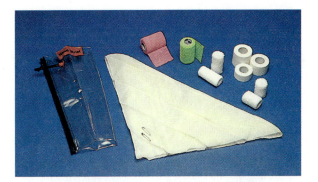

Fig. 26-12. Different types of bandages include adhesive tape, triangular bandages, gauze rolls, self-adherent bandages, and an air splint.

bandage or dressing with some pressure to help control bleeding. Gauze rolls may be wrapped around the dressing and injured extremity. A triangular bandage may also be used in this manner. An air splint can be placed around an injured extremity that has been covered with a dressing and bandage. When the splint is inflated, pressure is put on the wound (*see* Chapter 27, "Musculoskeletal

PRINCIPLE 26-2
Dressing and Bandaging

1. Follow body substance isolation precautions.
2. Expose the injured area.
3. Place a sterile dressing over the entire injury.
4. Maintain pressure to control bleeding. If bleeding is not controlled, remove the dressing to check that you are putting direct pressure on the correct site of bleeding.
5. Use a bandage to secure the dressing in place with some pressure. Assess distal skin color and circulation to assure the bandage is not too tight.
6. If the dressing becomes saturated with diffuse bleeding, add another dressing over it and secure in place. Do not remove the bottom dressing that is in contact with the wound, because that would cause the portion of the wound that had clotted to reopen. Remove the very top layers if they get too thick to provide appropriate pressure.

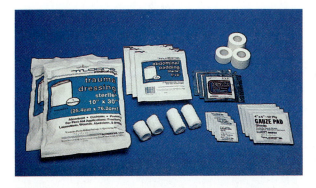

Fig. 26-11. Different sizes of dressings are used for different sizes of soft-tissue injuries, including large universal dressings, various sized gauze dressings and Vaseline gauze. Tape and bandages secure them in place.

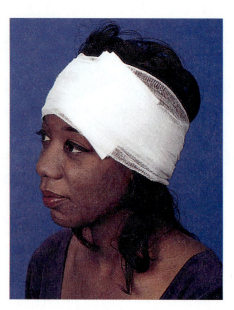

Fig. 26-13. Wrap the bandage around the head to secure the dressing.

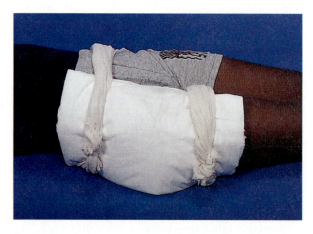

Fig. 26-15. To bandage a hip wound, secure the dressing with bandages wrapped around the waist and leg.

Care,'' for the use of splints). Principle 26-2 summarizes the steps for dressing and bandaging soft-tissue injuries.

The following are examples of how to dress and bandage some specific injured areas.

1. **Forehead**: If there is no accompanying skull injury, place a dressing over the wound and wrap the bandage around the head to secure the dressing (Fig. 26-13).
2. **Shoulder**: Wrap the bandage around the armpit and opposite shoulder (Fig. 26-14).
3. **Hip**: Secure the dressing by wrapping the bandage around the body and around the leg on the injured side (Fig. 26-15).

4. **Hand**: Wrap the bandage around the hand and the wrist in figure-8 pattern (Fig. 26-16).
5. **Joint (elbow or knee)**: Wrap the bandage around the extremity to secure the dressing. Attempt to stabilize the extremity in the position found (Fig. 26-17).

INJURIES REQUIRING SPECIAL CONSIDERATION

Some injuries require special considerations for emergency medical care. For penetrating chest injuries, an occlusive dressing should be applied to the wound and high-flow oxygen provided to the patient. The dressing is placed over the wound and sealed on all four sides, except with a sucking chest wound. A sucking chest wound is an injury to the chest when an object has penetrated the skin and lung, and air is moving into and out of the chest cavity through the wound. You may hear the sound of air going into and out of the wound as the patient breathes, and the patient may cough up red,

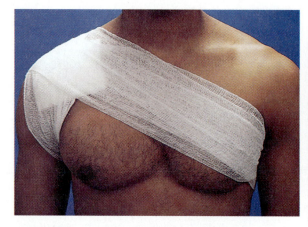

Fig. 26-14. For an injured shoulder, wrap the bandage around the armpit and opposite shoulder to secure the dressing.

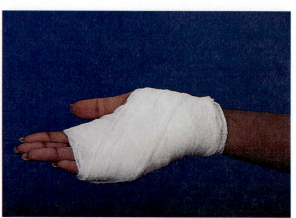

Fig. 26-16. Use a ''figure 8'' pattern to bandage a hand wound.

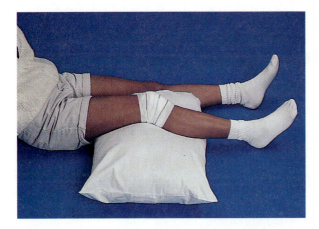

Fig. 26-17. With a wounded elbow or knee, wrap the bandage around the extremity to secure the dressing. Be sure to support the joint and stabilize it in the position found.

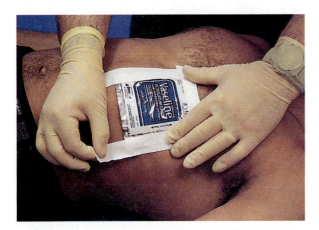

Fig. 26-18. For a sucking chest wound, use an occlusive dressing taped on three sides, leaving one side open to allow air inside the chest to escape but to prevent more air from entering. The packaging can be taped over the Vaseline gauze to secure the dressing.

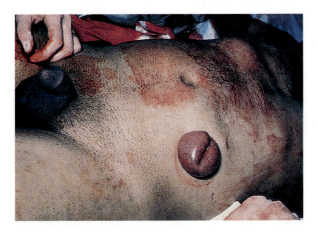

Fig. 26-19. An evisceration caused by a stabbing knife wound.

frothy blood. An occlusive dressing should be applied, but taped only on three sides. Leaving one side open will allow the air inside the chest to escape but will prevent more air from entering in through the wound (Fig. 26-18). If no spinal injury is suspected, the patient may assume a position of comfort.

An **evisceration** is an abdominal injury in which the organs are protruding through the wound, exposed to the outside environment (Fig 26-19). Technique 26-1 lists the steps of care for abdominal evisceration.

Any object that is still in the wound when you reach the patient is considered an impaled object (Fig 26-21). The care you give depends on the site of the object. An object through the cheek may be removed if it could interfere with the airway; the cheek is then dressed on both sides. An object that would interfere with chest compressions or transportation may also be removed. Objects in most other sites should be left in place and stabilized there, including an object in the cheek that does not pose a threat to the airway or an object in the chest that does not interfere with CPR compressions. If the protruding portion of the object can be cut off or shortened, stabilize it and cut or break that portion off rather than removing the whole object and risking further damage. Secure the object in place following the steps described in Technique 26-2.

Do not remove objects lodged in the eye, ear, or nose. Stabilize the object and transport the patient. An impaled object in the eye should be stabilized and bandaged. A protective covering such as a cone or a cup should be placed over the injured eye and the protruding object. The other eye should also be covered, because both eyes move together and covering the uninjured eye will help minimize the movement of the injured eye. Explain to the patient why you are covering the other eye and emphasize the patient will be safe. If the patient is very uncomfortable with both eyes covered, the uninjured eye can be uncovered.

An amputation of an extremity requires special considerations. Not only does the patient require emergency medical care, but the amputated part (if salvageable) also requires appropriate care to prevent damage and ensure the success of reattachment. Refer to Principle 26-5 for the care of an amputated part.

If the patient has a large open neck injury, air may enter the bloodstream and travel to the lungs, brain, or other vital organs and cause an air embo-

TECHNIQUE 26-1
Care of Patients With an Abdominal Evisceration

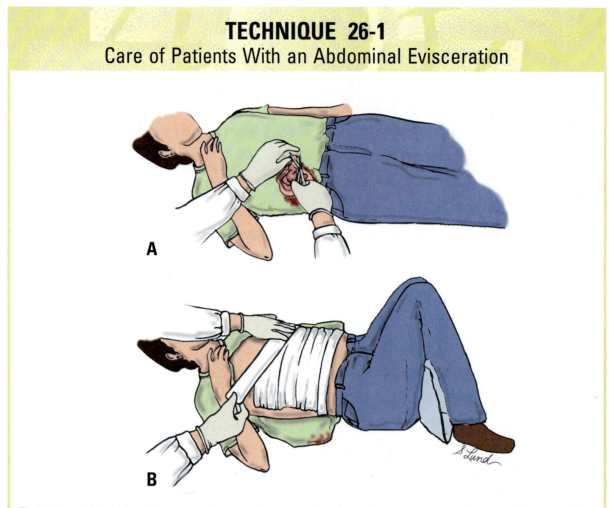

Fig. 26-20 Follow body substance isolation precautions. Do not touch or try to replace the exposed organs in the body. **A, Cut clothing away from the injured area.** Cover the organs with a sterile dressing, moistened with sterile water or saline. **B, Next, use an occlusive dressing to cover the organs and the wound to prevent air from entering and drying the wound. Secure the dressing in place. When positioning the patient, flex the knees and hips if they are uninjured and if a spinal injury is not suspected.** This will help relieve the stretching of the abdominal muscles caused when the legs are straight.

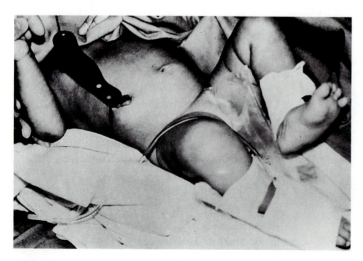

Fig. 26-21. An knife impaled in a child's abdomen.

TECHNIQUE 26-2
Care of Patients With an Impaled Object Injury

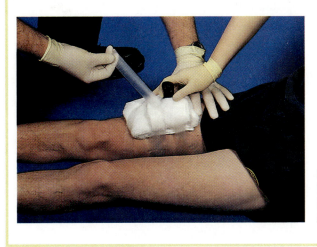

Fig. 26-22   Follow body substance isolation precautions. **Expose the wound area, control the bleeding, and place bulky dressings around the object to stabilize it. Secure the dressings in place with bandages.**

lism. Cover this wound with a sterile occlusive dressing. Do not compress the carotid artery unless it is absolutely necessary to control the bleeding. If necessary, apply direct pressure to the inferior portion of the artery. Consult medical direction for appropriate positioning of the patient.

Injuries often occur to the face and head. A soft-tissue injury to the scalp may produce significant bleeding that is difficult to stop. There are a large number of capillaries on the surface of the head. When an injury occurs, such as an abrasion or laceration, many capillaries are damaged and the bleeding often appears worse than it is. These injuries are more serious in the elderly and infants and children because blood loss has a greater effect on them. Direct pressure should be applied with a dressing and bandage to control the bleeding if there is no evidence of a skull fracture. If there is evidence of a skull fracture, apply the dressings and bandages without pressure. If there is any evidence of a spinal injury, immobilize the spine as discussed in Chapter 28, "Injuries to the Head and Spine."

Eye injuries are another common soft-tissue injury. If a patient has a foreign body in the eye, such as dust or dirt, the particle may cause irritation and could scratch the eye. The eye should be flushed with sterile saline solution using a bulb syringe, until the object is washed out. This may be done at the scene unless the patient has other life-threatening conditions. Then transport the patient to the nearest receiving facility.

If you encounter a patient who has had a chemical splashed into the eye, flush the eye with large amounts of sterile saline solution. Consult with medical direction concerning the chemical in the eye, and follow their instructions regarding continued flushing and transport to an appropriate receiving facility. Be careful to flush the water from the inside corner of the affected eye, in a direction

PRINCIPLE 26-5
Care for Patients With an Amputation

1. Follow body substance isolation precautions.
2. Control bleeding, place sterile dressings over the wound, and secure them in place.
3. Take special care to transport the amputated part with the patient so that it may be reattached. Wrap the amputated part in sterile dressings and then wrap it in plastic. Keep the amputated part cool, but do not freeze it. Do not place it directly onto ice.
4. If the patient has a partial amputation, do not complete it. Immobilize the part in place and treat the wounds.

away from the eye that was not exposed, to prevent contamination of the uninjured eye.

If the eye or eyelid is burned, both eyes should be covered with dressings moistened with sterile saline. Coverings, such as 2 × 2s or eye shields, can then be placed over the dressings.

An injury to the mouth may produce loose teeth and blood that can obstruct the airway. Examine the inside of the mouth for possible obstructions. Remove any loose teeth and foreign objects, and use dressings to put pressure on bleeding. Remove dentures if they are not secure and may obstruct the airway. Place teeth in sterile saline and transport them with the patient to the receiving facility. For injuries that go through the cheek, use dressings on the inside and outside of the cheek. A rolled dressing may be placed between the patient's cheek and teeth to hold some pressure on the wound. Do not place a dressing on the inside of the mouth unless the patient is alert and cooperative. If a spinal injury is not suspected, allow the patient to lie on the side to prevent blood or other fluid from entering the airway and causing obstruction. For suspected spinal injuries, take appropriate spinal immobilization precautions.

Injuries to the nose that cause external bleeding should be controlled like any other soft-tissue injury by placing dressings and bandages to control the bleeding. If the injury was caused by blunt trauma, be cautious and suspect a head injury. If the nosebleed is nontraumatic or the bleeding comes from inside the nose, use the methods to control bleeding described in Chapter 25, "Bleeding and Shock."

BURNS

Burns are also a type of soft-tissue injury. Burns are classified according to the depth of injury. The severity of a burn is based on the depth or degree of the burn, the percentage of body area burned, the location of the burn, whether the patient has a preexisting medical condition, and the age of the patient. To determine the severity of a burn, first determine the depth or degree of the burn.

CLASSIFICATION OF BURNS

A **superficial burn** involves only the epidermis. The skin appears red and there is pain at the burn site (Fig. 26-23A). A **partial-thickness burn** involves both the epidermis and dermis, but not the under-

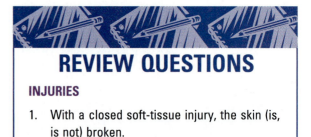

REVIEW QUESTIONS

INJURIES

1. With a closed soft-tissue injury, the skin (is, is not) broken.

2. With an open soft-tissue injury, the skin (is, is not) broken.

3. _____ soft-tissue injuries include abrasions and lacerations.

4. The EMT should always freeze an amputated part and transport it with the patient. True or False?

5. Closed soft-tissue injuries can lead to shock because they can produce _____ bleeding.

1. Is not
2. Is
3. Open
4. False
5. Internal

lying tissue. There is intense pain at the site, and blisters form. The skin is white to red in color and moist or mottled (Fig. 26-23B). A **full-thickness burn** extends through all layers of skin to the underlying tissue, including the subcutaneous layer, and may involve the muscle, bone, or other organs (Fig. 26-23C). The skin appears dry and leathery and can be white, dark brown, or charred, and feels hard to the touch. There is little or no pain at the site of the burn because of loss of sensation from nerve damage, but pain may be present at the edges where the burn is of partial thickness.

One method to calculate the percentage of body area burned is called the "Rule of Nines." For an adult, the head and neck are 9% of the body, each upper extremity is 9%, the anterior trunk (front) is 18%, the posterior trunk (back) is 18%, each lower extremity is 18% and the genitalia is 1%. Quickly estimating what sections of the body are burned and adding those sections together produce the total percentage burned. For an infant, the head and neck is 18%, each upper extremity is 9%, the

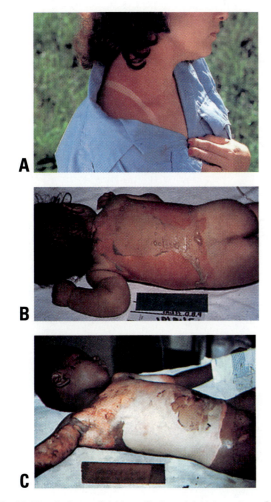

Fig. 26-23. **A,** A superficial burn. **B,** A partial-thickness burn. **C,** A full-thickness burn.

anterior trunk is 18%, the posterior trunk is 18% and each lower extremity is 14% (Fig. 26-24).

Next, determine if the patient has any critical body area burned. These critical areas are the face and upper airway, the hands, the feet, and the genitalia; also determine if the burn is circumferential (ie, wraps all the way around an extremity). Find out the history of the patient to see if there is a medical condition or illness that may make the effects of a burn worse. For example, in a patient with a respiratory disease, inhalation of smoke could worsen a respiratory problem. In a patient with an immune deficiency, the burn wounds can become infected very easily.

Consider the age of the patient, and take extra care and urgency with patients who are younger than 5 years of age or older than 55 years of age. The immune and cardiopulmonary systems at these ages function less efficiently, increasing the

risk of complications such as hypothermia or severe infection.

SEVERITY OF BURNS

Based on all the factors above, the severity of a burn can be determined. Determining that the burn is critical should prompt immediate transport. Do not stay at the scene to treat the burn. Assure a patent airway and transport the patient to the appropriate burn care facility. The patient should be placed on high-flow oxygen via a nonrebreather mask at a rate of 15 L/min or ventilated with the bag-valve-mask, if appropriate. The dressings and bandages may be applied en route.

CRITICAL BURNS

A critical burn involves the face, hands, feet, or genitalia or is associated with a respiratory injury or illness in adults, infants, and children. A burn is considered critical if it is full thickness and covers more than 10% of the body surface or partial thickness covering more than 30% of the body surface. If the burn is associated with a painful, swollen, deformed extremity or encompasses an arm, leg, or the chest, it is also considered critical. A burn considered moderate in adults is considered a critical burn in infants, children, or the elderly because their immune system is less efficient.

MODERATE BURNS

A moderate burn is a full-thickness burn covering 2% to 10% of body surface not covering the face, hands, feet, genitalia, or upper airway. A moderate burn is also a partial-thickness burn covering 15% to 30% of the body surface area for an adult. A superficial burn that covers more than 50% of the body surface area may also be considered a moderate burn. Any of these conditions in infants, children, or the elderly are considered critical burns. A partial-thickness burn covering 10%–20% of a child's body is classified as a moderate burn.

MINOR BURNS

A burn is classified as minor if it is full thickness covering less than 2% of the body surface area or partial thickness covering less than 15% of the body surface area in an adult, less than 10% of the body surface area of a child, and does not involve the face, hands, feet, genitalia, or upper airway. Box 26-1 summarizes burn classifications.

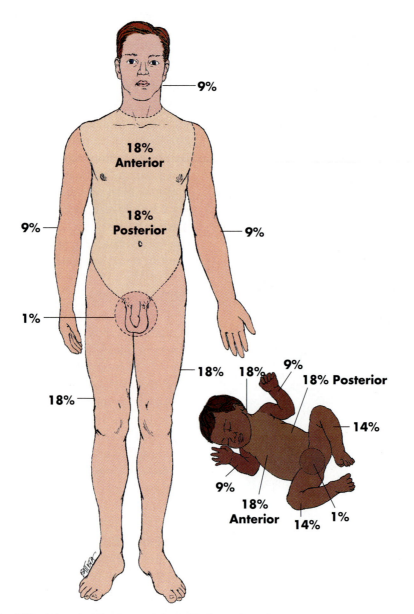

Fig. 26-24. The "Rule of Nines" for calculating the percentage of body area burned.

ALERT
Use caution with patients who have burns near the face or neck. The condition of patients who are breathing adequately can deteriorate rapidly if the throat swells as a result of heat and smoke inhalation.

ALERT
Because burned skin cannot regulate body temperature as normal skin can, patients with burns lose heat to the environment and should be kept warm.

EMERGENCY MEDICAL CARE FOR BURN VICTIMS

See Principle 26-6 for the emergency medical care for burns.

Take extra care and precaution when dealing with an infant or child with a burn. These patients have greater surface area in relationship to the total body size than an adult. This results in greater fluid

BOX 26-1

Severity of Burns

Critical

- Full and partial thickness involving face, hands, feet, and genitalia
- Circumferential
- Associated respiratory injury or painful, swollen, deformed extremity or other illness
- Full thickness > 10%
- Partial thickness > 30%
- Moderate burns in infants, children, and elderly

Moderate

- Full thickness covering 2%–10% of the body excluding the hands, feet, face, and genitalia
- Partial thickness covering 15%–30% of an adult's body or 10%–20% of a child's body
- Superficial burn covering > 50% of body

Minor

- Full thickness covering < 2% of body surface area, excluding hands, feet, face, and genitalia
- Partial thickness covering < 15% of an adult's body
- Partial thickness covering < 10% of a child's body

PRINCIPLE 26-6
Emergency Medical Care for Burn Victims

1. Take appropriate body substance isolation precautions.
2. Use room temperature water or saline to stop the burning process.
3. Remove any jewelry and smoldering clothing.
4. Continually monitor the patient's airway. An open airway could become a closed airway because of swelling caused by smoke inhalation. Apply oxygen with appropriate technique.
5. To prevent further contamination of burns, cover with a dry clean dressing. Do not use any type of lotion, ointment, or antiseptic, and do not break blisters. Follow the local protocol for applying dressings.
6. Follow local protocol for cooling small burns, for keeping the patient warm during transport, and for other emergency care for burns.
7. Transport the patient to the nearest burn facility according to the local protocol.

and heat loss. These patients are at a greater risk for shock (hypoperfusion), airway problems, and hypothermia. Make sure that the patient is covered to maintain adequate body temperature. Avoid freezing the burned area; never use cold water or ice on burns. Cool water may be used initially to cool the burn.

With burned children, always consider the possibility of child abuse because burns are a common form of this abuse. Any suspicion of abuse must be documented and reported to the receiving facility.

Chemical burns are another type of burn, occurring not from heat or fire, but from a chemical reaction. Take appropriate precautions for protection against any hazardous material. Wear gloves and eye protection, along with gowns and other gear. An industrial facility should have information on

all chemicals used at the site. This documentation describes the first aid care for that particular chemical. For any chemical burn, check that the container of the chemical is at the scene, and search for instructions on the label for managing contact burns. For a patient with a burn caused by a chemical powder, in most cases the dry powder can be brushed off and the skin flushed with large amounts of water. Dry lime should be brushed from the site, but the burn should not be flushed with water because the reaction will cause further damage. For other chemical burns, flush the site immediately and continue flushing while en route to the receiving facility. Try not to contaminate the area that is being flushed or any uninjured area; burns are open wounds that may be infected very easily.

For ingestion of a chemical, contact the local poison control center for assistance with emergency medical care procedures. Chemical containers typically include instructions on the label for management of cases of ingestion or contamination. Transport the container with the patient when possible and read the precautions on the label. Medical direction can be contacted for further information.

An electrical burn results from exposure to an electrical source. Do not attempt to remove patients from the source unless you have been educated to do so. Do not touch patients until they have been removed from the electrical source. Once the danger has been removed, administer oxygen and monitor the patient continuously for respiratory and cardiac arrest. Look for entrance and exit wounds. Be prepared with the automatic external defibrillator because cardiac arrest is a possibility. Damage from an electrical burn is often more severe than it appears externally. The electric current may have produced only small entrance and exit wounds (Fig 26-25A and B), but could have traveled a long route inside the body. Treat the injuries as you would any soft-tissue injury, but suspect internal and cardiac injury.

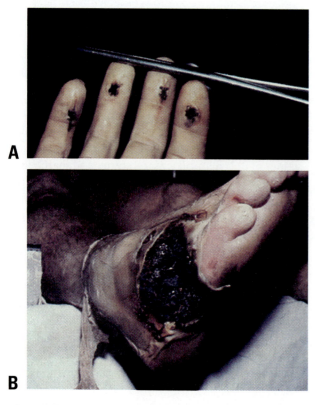

Fig. 26-25. An electrical burn. **A,** The entrance wound. **B,** The exit wound.

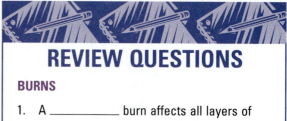

REVIEW QUESTIONS

BURNS

1. A _____ burn affects all layers of skin and may cause little or no pain at the site.

2. A burn is considered critical if:
   A. It involves the hands
   B. There is no airway compromise
   C. There are partial-thickness burns on less than 10% of the body
   D. It is a burn on the upper arm

3. To determine severity, look for the location, the percentage, the age of the patient, the depth, and _____.

4. EMTs _____ (should, should not) remove clothing from a burn patient.

5. Infants are at less risk than adults for hypothermia. True or False?

1. Full-thickness
2. A
3. Preexisting medical conditions
4. Should
5. False

CHAPTER SUMMARY

THE SKIN

The skin protects the body from the environment, bacteria, viruses, and other harmful organisms. The skin acts as insulation, regulating body temperature, sensing heat, cold, touch, and pressure, and transmitting that information to the brain.

The skin is structured in layers. The outermost layer is the epidermis. The middle layer is the dermis, which contains the nerves, blood vessels, and sebaceous glands. The innermost layer is the subcutaneous layer.

INJURIES

A closed soft-tissue injury is one in which the skin remains intact and there is no external bleeding. Contusions, hematomas, and some crush injuries are types of closed soft-tissue injuries.

Open soft-tissue injuries occur when there is a break in the skin. Abrasions, lacerations, avulsions, penetrations and punctures, amputations, and some crush injuries are examples of open soft-tissue injuries.

Emergency medical care for soft-tissue injuries includes body substance isolation precautions, adequate ventilation and oxygen when appropriate, and treatment for signs and symptoms of shock. Extremity injuries may require splinting, dressing, and bandaging. Dressings and bandages provide protection for the wound along with pressure to stop the bleeding. Dressings are sterile and are placed directly over the wound. Bandages are then used to hold the dressing in place and need not be sterile.

Other injuries require extra care; an open chest wound requires an occlusive dressing; an evisceration requires a moist occlusive dressing; an impaled object should be stabilized in place with bulky dressings; an amputation should be dressed and bandaged and the amputated part kept cool; a large open neck injury should be covered with a sterile occlusive dressing.

BURNS

Burns are classified according to their depth. The severity of a burn depends on the depth or degree of the burn, the percentage of body area burned, the location of the burn, the presence of a preexisting medical condition, and the age of the patient. A superficial burn involves only the epidermis. It is red and painful. A partial-thickness burn involves the dermis and has blisters and intense pain. A full-thickness burn extends through all layers of skin, appears white or charred, and may cause little or no pain.

Use the ''Rule of Nines'' to determine the percentage of body area burned. Critical burned areas are the hands, feet, face and upper airway, and the genitalia. Stop the burning process with water, and remove the clothes and jewelry of the patient if necessary. The patient's airway should be monitored and oxygen provided, and the burns should be covered with dry clean dressing.

A dry powder chemical should be brushed away from a burn before washing, and all other chemical burns should be flushed with large amounts of water. With dry lime, do not flush the burn with water, but brush all of the chemical from the skin. An electrical burn should be treated as a soft-tissue injury; search for exit and entrance wounds and suspect internal and cardiac injury. Do not touch the patient until removed from the electric charge. Burn patients should be kept warm.

UNITED STATES DEPARTMENT OF TRANSPORTATION NATIONAL HIGHWAY TRAFFIC SAFETY ADMINISTRATION EMT–BASIC OBJECTIVES

Check your knowledge. The National Registry of EMTs and many state EMS agencies use the objectives below to develop EMT–Basic certification examinations. Can you meet them?

COGNITIVE

1. State the major functions of the skin.
2. List the layers of the skin.
3. Establish the relationship between body substance isolation (BSI) and soft-tissue injuries.
4. List the types of closed soft-tissue injuries.
5. Describe the emergency medical care of the patient with a closed soft-tissue injury.
6. State the types of open soft-tissue injuries.
7. Describe the emergency medical care of the patient with an open soft-tissue injury.
8. Discuss the emergency medical care considerations for a patient with a penetrating chest injury.
9. State the emergency medical care considerations for a patient with an open wound of the abdomen.
10. Differentiate between the care for an open wound to the chest from an open wound to the abdomen.
11. List the classifications of burns.
12. Define superficial burn.
13. List the characteristics of a superficial burn.
14. Define partial-thickness burns.
15. List the characteristics of a partial-thickness burn.
16. Define full-thickness burn.
17. List the characteristics of a full-thickness burn.
18. Describe the emergency medical care of the patient with a superficial burn.
19. Describe the emergency medical care of the patient with a partial-thickness burn.
20. Describe the emergency medical care of the patient with a full-thickness burn.
21. List the functions of dressing and bandaging.
22. Describe the purpose of a bandage.
23. Describe the steps in applying a pressure dressing.
24. Establish the relationship between airway management and the patient with chest injury, burns, blunt and penetrating injuries.
25. Describe the effects of improperly applied dressings, splints, and tourniquets.
26. Describe the emergency medical care of the patient with an impaled object.
27. Describe the emergency medical care of a patient with an amputation.
28. Describe the emergency care of a chemical burn.
29. Describe the emergency care for an electrical burn.

PSYCHOMOTOR

1. Demonstrate the steps in the emergency medical care of closed soft-tissue injuries.
2. Demonstrate the steps in the emergency medical care of open soft-tissue injuries.
3. Demonstrate the steps in the emergency medical care of a patient with an open chest wound.
4. Demonstrate the steps in the emergency medical care of a patient with open abdominal wounds.
5. Demonstrate the steps in the emergency medical care of a patient with an impaled object.
6. Demonstrate the steps in the emergency medical care of a patient with an amputation.
7. Demonstrate the steps in the emergency medical care of an amputated part.
8. Demonstrate the steps in the emergency medical care of a patient with superficial burns.
9. Demonstrate the steps in the emergency medical care of a patient with partial-thickness burns.
10. Demonstrate the steps in the emergency medical care of a patient with full-thickness burns.
11. Demonstrate the steps in the emergency medical care of a patient with a chemical burn.
12. Demonstrate completing a prehospital care report for patients with soft-tissue injuries.

27 MUSCULOSKELETAL CARE

KEY TERMS

Angulation: An injury that is deformed (bent) at the site.

Closed injury: An injury that does not break the continuity of the skin.

Crepitation: The sound made when bone ends rub together or there is air inside the tissue.

Direct injury: An injury that results from a force that comes into direct contact with an area of the body.

Indirect injury: An injury in one body area that results from a force that comes into contact with a different part of the body.

Mechanism of injury: The force that acts upon the body to produce an injury.

Open injury: An injury that breaks the continuity of the skin.

Pneumatic splints: Devices such as air or vacuum splints that conform to the injury.

Position of function: The relaxed position of the hand or foot in which there is minimal movement or stretching of muscle.

Rigid splints: A type of splint that does not conform to the body.

Sling and swathe: Bandaging used to immobilize a shoulder or arm injury.

Traction splints: A special device used to immobilize a midfemur injury.

Twisting injury: An injury that results from a turning motion of the body in opposite directions.

IN THE FIELD

"**A**mbulance 41, we have report of a pedestrian-motor vehicle collision at the corner of Main and South Streets," announced the radio at the base. Juan, Julia, and Bob set down their dinner plates, grabbed their radios, and set off to the ambulance. Two minutes later the dispatcher called again: "Ambulance 41, an update of information: one pedestrian hit by a car, lying in the street, patient is responsive."

Approaching the scene where police were already present directing traffic, they saw the woman lying in the street and parked the ambulance. They sized up the scene and then walked toward the patient with their equipment. As they came closer, Juan said, "Look at the hood of that car!" Julia looked to see the dented hood and bumper of the car, indicating significant impact. "It must have been going pretty fast to do that much damage," she said as she picked up the pace. "We are lucky to have Bob along as a third person today."

Bob immediately put on gloves and stabilized the cervical spine, while Juan continued the initial assessment of the airway, breathing, and circulation, and placed high-flow oxygen on the patient with a nonrebreather face mask. He continued to monitor the airway to ensure no obstructions occurred from the tongue and to ensure adequate breathing. A cervical collar was placed on the patient after assessing the neck area.

Julia cut the slacks away from the legs and saw a large hematoma with swelling at the midthigh of the right leg. Knowing that bleeding from this area can be massive, she went to get the long backboard. Recognizing the need for immediate transport, the mechanism of injury, and the potential for blood loss, they immobilized the patient to a long board with pneumatic antishock garments (PASG) and moved her into the ambulance.

En route to the receiving facility, Juan completed the detailed physical examination and repeated the ongoing assessment. Juan and Julia decided not to splint the leg with a traction splint, though they consulted with medical direction and inflated the PASG. Minutes later they arrived at the receiving facility, transferred the patient to the emergency department staff, and submitted their report. Because of the EMTs' recognition of both the life-threatening situation and the need for immediate transportation, the patient's life was saved.

Would you have splinted the leg at the scene?

Musculoskeletal injuries are among the most common injuries you will encounter. Usually, these injuries are not life threatening, although some may be. Prompt identification and treatment of musculoskeletal injuries are crucial to reduce pain, prevent further injury, and minimize permanent damage.

MUSCULOSKELETAL REVIEW

The following sections briefly review the musculoskeletal system. For more detailed information, see Chapter 4, "The Human Body."

THE MUSCULAR SYSTEM

The muscular system performs several specific functions. Muscles give the body shape, protect internal organs, and provide movement. There are three different types of muscle (Fig. 27-1).

Voluntary, or skeletal, muscles are attached to bones. These muscles form the major muscle mass of the body and are controlled by the nervous system and brain. They can be contracted and relaxed at will and are responsible for movement.

Involuntary, or smooth, muscles are found in the walls of the hollow structures of the gastrointestinal tract and urinary system, as well as the

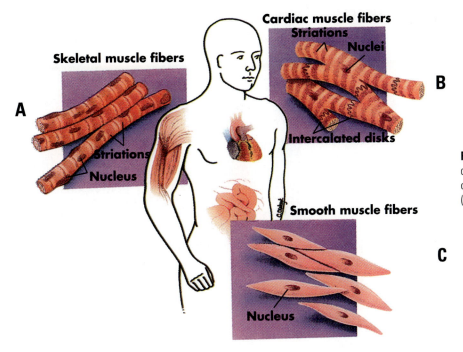

Fig. 27-1 The three types of muscles are **A**, voluntary (skeletal), **B**, cardiac muscles, and **C**, involuntary (smooth).

blood vessels and bronchi. Involuntary muscles control the flow of blood, body fluids, and other substances through these structures, and there is generally no conscious control of these muscles. They carry out the automatic muscular functions of the body and respond to stimuli such as heat or cold or the stretching produced when an organ is full.

Cardiac muscle exists only in the heart and has automaticity, the ability of the muscle to contract on its own. Cardiac muscle is involuntary muscle that has its own supply of blood through the coronary artery system. This muscle can tolerate only short interruptions of blood supply.

THE SKELETAL SYSTEM

The skeletal system helps provide body shape, protects internal organs, and assists in body movement. The skeletal system consists of the bones of the skull and face, the spinal column and thorax, the pelvis, the lower extremities, and the upper extremities. The spinal column consists of seven cervical, 12 thoracic, five lumbar, five sacral, and four coccygeal vertebrae, and the thorax consists of 12 ribs and a sternum. The lower extremities are composed of the femur (thigh), the tibia and fibula, and the tarsals, metatarsals, and phalanges, which make up the ankle and foot. The upper extremities are composed of the humerus, radius and ulna, and the carpals, metacarpals, and phalanges, which make up the wrist and hand.

Muscles and bones, together with other connec-

tive tissue, allow for body movement. Extremities move at the joints where bones are connected to other bones. There are ball-and-socket joints such as the shoulder, and there are hinge joints such as the elbow. Refer to Chapter 4, "The Human Body," for a diagram of the skeletal system.

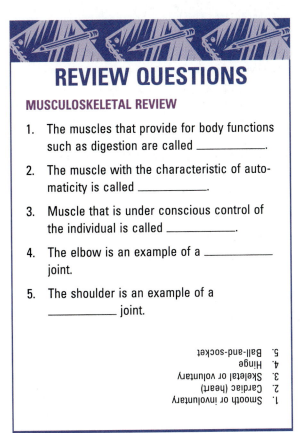

REVIEW QUESTIONS

MUSCULOSKELETAL REVIEW

1. The muscles that provide for body functions such as digestion are called _____.

2. The muscle with the characteristic of automaticity is called _____.

3. Muscle that is under conscious control of the individual is called _____.

4. The elbow is an example of a _____ joint.

5. The shoulder is an example of a _____ joint.

1. Smooth or involuntary
2. Cardiac (heart)
3. Skeletal or voluntary
4. Hinge
5. Ball-and-socket

INJURIES TO BONES AND JOINTS

Various injuries to bones and joints are described in the following sections. You must understand the various forces that can cause damage to bones. Some injuries are much more traumatic and serious than others and must be cared for as such.

The elderly are often more susceptible to bone injury because of osteoporosis, a disease in which bone matter is lost and there is greater air space within a bone. This condition is more prevalent in the elderly and makes the bones more brittle.

Immobilization in the elderly may also be complicated by arthritis. Arthritis is the inflammation of the joints and may produce an angulation that can not be straightened, such as a curvature of the spine.

MECHANISM OF INJURY

The **mechanism of injury** can help you determine the severity of the injury. Musculoskeletal injuries usually result from a force applied to an area of the body. Some injuries result from a direct force onto an area of the body, such as a **direct injury** caused by a baseball bat swung into a person's arm. The arm's injury results from direct contact with the baseball bat. Other injuries are caused by indirect forces. An example of **indirect injury** is an auto collision in which a patient's knees are thrown forward into the dashboard. The knees are directly injured from contact with the dash. The hips and pelvis are indirectly injured because the knees are pushed backward with a great force that indirectly reaches the hips and pelvis.

Some injuries are caused by twisting forces. If an extremity becomes pulled and twisted, a **twisting injury** may result from that force. For instance, a wrestler who becomes entangled in an opponent's hold may pull and twist his body. This force may produce an injury to the muscles and bones that are twisted.

Always consider the force that was involved in the cause of the injury. It takes a much greater force to injure a femur (thigh), for example, than it takes to injure the ulna (forearm) because the bone is much larger, more dense, and protected by larger muscles. Gather as much information as possible regarding the mechanism of injury, and include this in your report to the receiving facility.

BONE OR JOINT INJURIES

Musculoskeletal injuries are either open or closed. An **open injury** involves a break in the continuity of the skin and usually produces some exter-

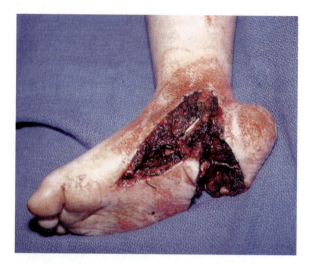

Fig. 27-2 An open injury involves a break in the continuity of the skin.

nal bleeding (Fig. 27-2). A **closed injury** does not involve a break in the skin or external bleeding, although it may produce internal bleeding (Fig. 27-3).

Various signs and symptoms are characteristic of bone or joint injuries. The area of injury may have some deformity or angulation and may be painful to move and tender to touch. If the bone ends are separated, some **crepitation** (grating) may be heard or felt during the examination, caused by the bone ends rubbing together. However, do not purposefully seek this sign, and do not try to repeat it if you note it during the assessment because it may produce further injury. The area of injury may be swollen, appearing larger than the same area on the

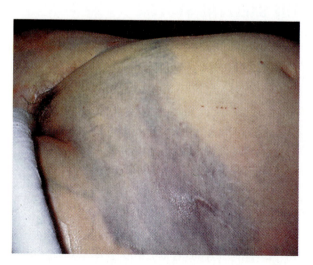

Fig. 27-3 A closed injury, such as this fractured pelvis, does not involve a break in the skin but may produce internal bleeding.

BOX 27-1

Signs and Symptoms of a Bone or Joint Injury

- Deformity or angulation
- Pain and tenderness
- Crepitation (grating)
- Swelling
- Bruising (discoloration)
- Exposed bone ends (open injury)
- Joints locked into position

other side of the body, and may be discolored. In an open bone injury, the ends of the bones that are injured may be protruding through the skin and exposed to the outside environment. With a joint injury, the joint may be locked in position and unmovable. Box 27-1 summarizes the signs and symptoms of a bone or joint injury.

EMERGENCY CARE FOR PATIENTS WITH BONE OR JOINT INJURIES

Emergency medical care for bone or joint injuries consists of both basic techniques and specialized techniques. First, always use appropriate personal protective equipment (PPE) for body substance isolation precautions before examining the patient. Even a closed injury that is not bleeding may become an open injury because of movement or pressure.

Establish a patent airway and administer high-flow oxygen to all patients as indicated. Any major bleeding or life-threatening situations should be controlled using the methods, such as direct pressure, described in Chapter 25, "Bleeding and Shock."

ALERT
Always care for life-threatening injuries before focusing on a painful, swollen, deformed extremity. Do not waste scene time on an extremity if the patient is not breathing adequately or has other threats to life!

Splint the injury appropriately to prevent movement of bone ends or fragments (described later in this chapter), and prepare the patient for transport. During transport, a cold pack may be applied to the injured area to reduce swelling and pain. An injured extremity should be elevated to reduce blood flow to that area, unless other injuries are present and would cause complications.

Monitor the patient's vital signs en route to the receiving facility. Any changes in the patient's condition or vital signs should be reported to the receiving facility.

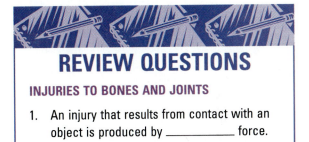

REVIEW QUESTIONS

INJURIES TO BONES AND JOINTS

1. An injury that results from contact with an object is produced by _____ force.

2. If an injury site was not directly in contact with the force that produced it, it is said to have been caused by a(n) _____ force.

3. Emergency medical care includes the application of a(n) _____ to reduce swelling.

4. An injured extremity should be _____ to reduce blood flow to the injury site.

5. A(n) _____ injury produces a break in the skin.

5. Open
4. Elevated
3. Cold pack
2. Indirect
1. Direct

SPLINTING AN INJURY

The specialized emergency medical care provided for a painful, swollen, deformed extremity includes applying a splint to immobilize the injury and prevent further damage. This chapter describes various types of splints and how they are used.

REASONS FOR SPLINTING

Splinting a painful, swollen, deformed extremity prevents movement of bone fragments, bone ends,

BOX 27-2

Reasons for Splinting

- Prevent movement of bone fragments, bone ends, or injured joints
- Minimize damage to muscles, nerves, and blood vessels
- Minimize the chance of converting a closed injury into an open injury
- Minimize the restriction of blood flow resulting from bone ends compressing blood vessels
- Minimize bleeding from damaged tissue caused by bone ends
- Minimize the pain associated with movement of bone ends
- Minimize chance of paralysis of extremities due to spinal damage

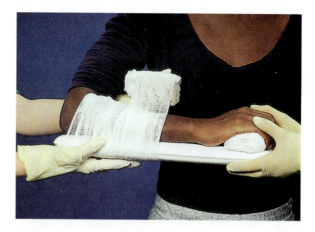

Fig. 27-4 For a hand injury, place a roll of gauze in the palm to support and immobilize the hand in the position of function.

or injured joints. The splint minimizes damage to muscles, nerves, and blood vessels caused by broken bones. Immobilization helps to prevent a closed injury from becoming an open injury. It also minimizes the restriction of blood flow resulting from bone ends compressing blood vessels and limits the bleeding caused by tissue damage from the bone ends. Splinting reduces pain by limiting the movement of bone ends. Paralysis resulting from spinal damage is also minimized. Box 27-2 summarizes the reasons for splinting.

PRINCIPLES OF SPLINTING

With all splinting techniques, always assess the patient first. Evaluate the pulse, motor function, and sensation distal to the injury both before and after applying a splint, and record the findings. A splint that is placed improperly or secured too tightly may impede circulation. If there is a change in distal circulation, loosen the splint and reassess. If the circulation does not return, the extremity may need to be resplinted.

The bones and joints above and below an injury site must be immobilized with the splint to minimize muscle movement near the injury. Before splinting, cut clothing away to expose the area and

make the splint more effective. Open injuries should be dressed and bandaged before application of the splint.

If there is a severe deformity or the distal extremity is cyanotic or lacks a pulse, the injury should be aligned with gentle traction before splinting in an attempt to regain circulation. If resistance is felt, splint the extremity in the position in which you find it. If no pulse returns distal to the injury, rapid transport is indicated to prevent possible loss of the extremity. If any bones are protruding through the skin, do not try to replace them, although they may retract when the splint is applied. Splints should be padded to prevent pressure and discomfort to the patient.

When splinting a hand or foot, immobilize it in the **position of function**. This is the most comfortable position for the hand or foot and requires the least amount of muscle use or stretching. This is the

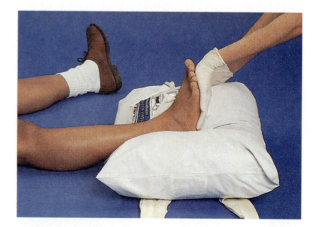

Fig. 27-5 For a foot injury, support the sole and immobilize in the position of function.

PRINCIPLE 27-1
Principles of Splinting

1. Assess pulse, motor function, and sensation distal to the injury before and after splinting, and record your findings.

2. Immobilize the joint above and below the musculoskeletal injury. If a joint injury, immobilize the bone above and below the injury.

3. Remove or cut away clothing before splinting.

4. Cover open wounds with sterile dressings before splinting.

5. Splint the injury in the position found, unless there is severe deformity or the distal extremity is cyanotic or lacks a pulse. Then attempt to align the extremity with gentle traction before splinting.

6. Do not intentionally replace protruding bones, but note them in your prehospital care report.

7. Pad the splint to prevent pressure and discomfort to the patient.

8. Splint the injury before moving the patient unless there are life-threatening situations present.

9. If in doubt whether an injury is present, apply a splint.

10. If the patient has the signs and symptoms of shock, use full-body immobilization, align the patient in the normal anatomic position on a backboard, and transport.

Without an X-ray, it is impossible to differentiate between a broken ankle and a sprain or strain; therefore, you should assume the ankle is broken. Do not waste time trying to identify the actual injury. See Principle 27-1 for the procedure for splinting.

If the patient is showing the signs and symptoms of shock, align the patient in the normal anatomic position and transport using total body immobilization, including backboard and cervical collar. Do not waste time splinting each injury separately. Chapter 28, "Injuries to the Head and Spine," describes full-body immobilization.

EQUIPMENT AND TECHNIQUES

Many types of splints are used to immobilize various musculoskeletal injuries. For all types of splints, remember the general principles previously described.

Rigid splints are nonformable splints used to support a painful, swollen, and deformed extremity and immobilize the joints or bones above and below the injury. Common examples are padded-board splints, cardboard splints, and ladder splints (Fig. 27-6). Technique 27-1 describes one method for using rigid splints.

Traction splints are used for a specific purpose. **Traction splints** are indicated for a closed painful, swollen, deformity at the midthigh (femur) when there is no joint or lower leg injury. A direct force to the femur may cause this injury. Do not use a traction splint if the injury is close to the knee or if the knee, hip, pelvis, lower leg, or ankle is injured, or if bone ends are protruding through the skin. Also do not use the traction splint if there is partial amputation or avulsion with bone separation or if the distal limb is connected only by marginal tissue such as a thin piece of skin. Traction in such cases

resting position for the hand or foot. For the hand, place a roll of gauze in the palm to support the hand, and for the foot, support the sole (Figs. 27-4 and 27-5).

Splint the injury before transporting only if there are no life-threatening situations present. If you are in doubt whether to splint an injury, splint it. Err on the side of caution. It is acceptable to splint an injury that did not need it, but it is unacceptable to fail to treat an injury that does require splinting.

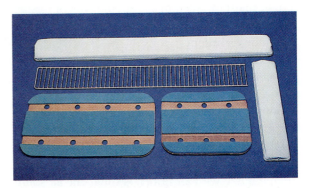

Fig. 27-6 Common types of splints include padded-board splints (*top and right*), ladder splints (*middle*), and cardboard splints (*bottom*).

TECHNIQUE 27-1
Splinting a Long Bone With a Rigid Splint

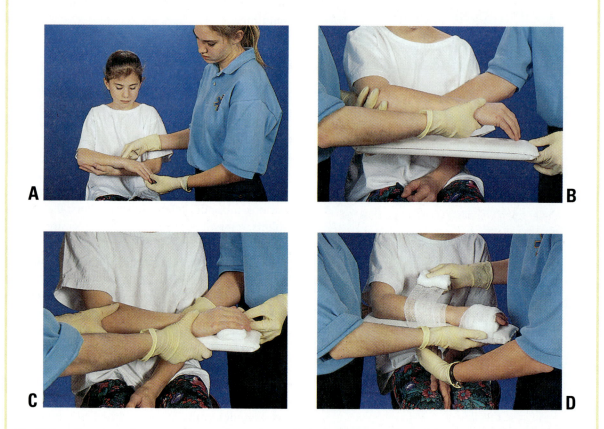

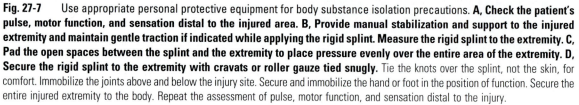

Fig. 27-7 Use appropriate personal protective equipment for body substance isolation precautions. **A, Check the patient's pulse, motor function, and sensation distal to the injured area. B, Provide manual stabilization and support to the injured extremity and maintain gentle traction if indicated while applying the rigid splint. Measure the rigid splint to the extremity. C, Pad the open spaces between the splint and the extremity to place pressure evenly over the entire area of the extremity. D, Secure the rigid splint to the extremity with cravats or roller gauze tied snugly.** Tie the knots over the splint, not the skin, for comfort. Immobilize the joints above and below the injury site. Secure and immobilize the hand or foot in the position of function. Secure the entire injured extremity to the body. Repeat the assessment of pulse, motor function, and sensation distal to the injury.

would risk separation. Technique 27-2 details the use of the Hare traction splint, one type of bipolar splint (Fig. 27-8). Other types of traction splints use different techniques; consult the directions supplied with the device.

Pneumatic splints, such as vacuum splints, are flexible, conforming splints that are used commonly with **angulated** injuries. The air splint and the PASG are other types of pneumatic splints that are used for nonangulated injuries (Fig. 27-10).

The air splint is applied to the injured area and then inflated with air until it is snug. The air splint usually has a zipper and is used primarily for injuries below the elbow and the knee. The advantages of the air splint include pressure on bleeding areas,

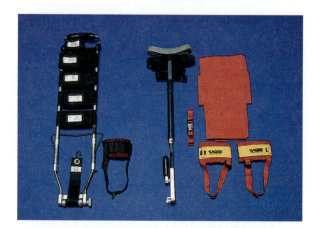

Fig. 27-8 Hare traction splint (*left*) and Sager splint (*right*).

TECHNIQUE 27-2
Use of the Hare Traction Splint

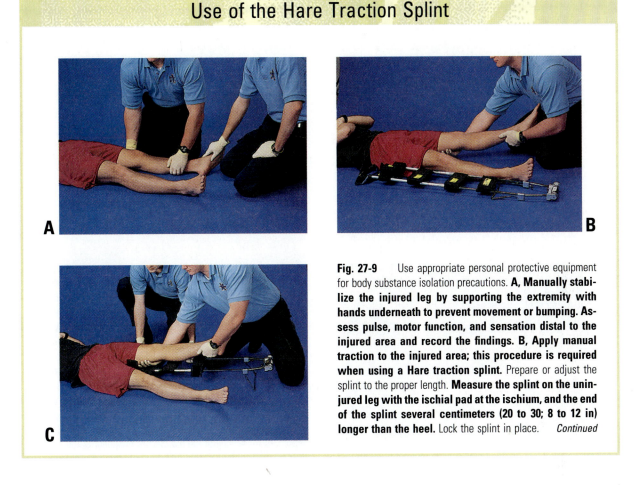

Fig. 27-9   Use appropriate personal protective equipment for body substance isolation precautions. **A, Manually stabilize the injured leg by supporting the extremity with hands underneath to prevent movement or bumping. Assess pulse, motor function, and sensation distal to the injured area and record the findings. B, Apply manual traction to the injured area; this procedure is required when using a Hare traction splint.** Prepare or adjust the splint to the proper length. **Measure the splint on the uninjured leg with the ischial pad at the ischium, and the end of the splint several centimeters (20 to 30; 8 to 12 in) longer than the heel.** Lock the splint in place.   *Continued*

comfort to the patient, and uniform contact. The disadvantage of the air splint is that air may leak from the splint or the pressure may change with changes in temperature or altitude. Air splints are difficult to clean, and the method of inflation may compromise body substance isolation precautions.

When using an air splint, cover all wounds with clean dressings before applying the splint. Place the injured extremity within the splint, and inflate the splint by blowing into the valve (Fig. 27-11). The port for the air may be cleansed with an alcohol wipe prior to inflation. Some air splints may come with an adapter and a pump to inflate them with air. This process requires two rescuers, one to support the extremity and one to apply the splint. As when applying any splint, check patient pulse, motor function, and sensation distal to the injury before and after application.

Pneumatic antishock garments can also be used as immobilization devices. They are indicated for the emergency medical care of pelvic instability and long bone injuries of the legs with signs and symptoms of shock. They are usually applied by placing them open on a long backboard and moving the patient onto them by log roll or scoop stretcher. The appropriate compartments are then inflated. For example, if the patient has a painful, swollen, deformed left femur, the PASG is inflated in the leg compartment on the side of the injury to act as an air splint. If the patient has pelvic instability and the signs and symptoms of shock, all compartments are inflated to immobilize the lower half of the body. The PASG may be used as a splint on a lower-leg injury only if the ankle is securely immobilized as well. This is possible using a pillow splint applied over the end of the PASG and around the foot and secured. As always, check pulse, motor function, and sensation distal to the injury before and after applying the PASG as a splint. Local protocols may differ and must be followed in the application of the PASG.

The vacuum splint is wrapped around the injured area, and then the air is removed with a pump so that the splint conforms to the injured area (Fig.

TECHNIQUE 27-2
Use of the Hare Traction Splint

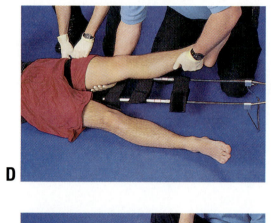

D

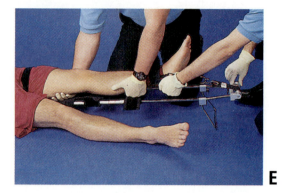

E

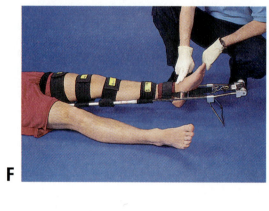

F

Fig. 27-9 *Continued* **C, Open the support straps, position the splint under the injured leg and D, position the straps as shown. Apply the proximal securing device (ischial strap). E, Apply the distal securing device (ankle hitch). Apply mechanical traction by tightening the ankle hitch to the splint. F, Position and secure the support straps.** Reevaluate the proximal and distal securing devices to ensure tightness. **Reassess the patient's pulse, motor function, and sensation distal to the injury site and record the findings.** If these findings are diminished compared with those before splinting, adjust the tension of the traction being applied. Secure the patient's torso to the long backboard to immobilize the hip. Secure the splint to the long board to prevent movement of the extremity.

27-12). The splint becomes very rigid and lacks the disadvantages of the air splint. Vacuum splints can be used with angulated injuries.

Improvised splints, such as pillows, may be used to support joint injuries and are commonly used for ankle injuries. The pillow is wrapped completely around the ankle and secured. The toes are left visible so that assessment may be made of the

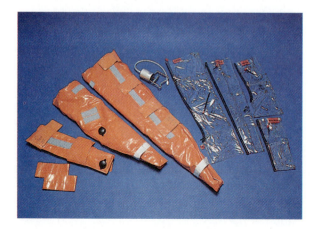

Fig. 27-10 Vacuum splints (*left*) and air splints (*right*) are commonly used pneumatic splints.

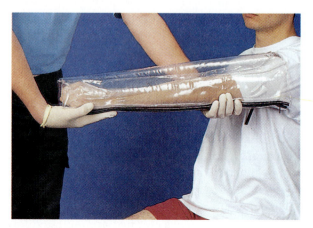

Fig. 27-11 An injured arm immobilized by an air splint.

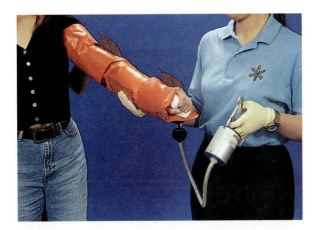

Fig. 27-12 A vacuum splint conforms to the injured area.

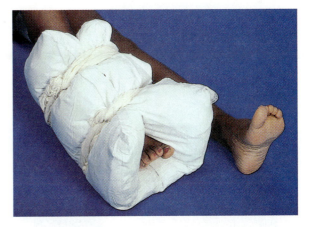

Fig. 27-13 A pillow splint is an improvised splint that provides support for an injured ankle or foot.

pulse, motor function, and sensation (Fig. 27-13). Cardboard splints may also be cut to form to an angle and then secured in place.

The **sling and swathe** is the common splinting technique for a shoulder injury. The arm is placed into the sling and the swathe is wrapped around the arm and the body so that the arm and shoulder cannot move (Fig. 27-14). The sling and swathe may be used along with other types of splints for arm injuries (Fig. 27-15 and Fig. 27-16). See Principle 27-2 for the proper method in splinting joint injuries.

ALERT
Always use properly sized splints. Some devices, such as PASG and traction splints, come in infant and child sizes. Familiarize yourself with all the available equipment provided on your ambulance and with local protocols.

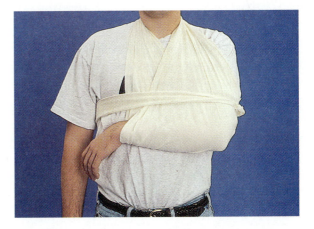

Fig. 27-14 A sling and swathe is a common splinting technique for a shoulder injury to prevent movement of the arm and shoulder.

RISKS OF SPLINTING

Using splints improperly can lead to complications. If they are not used correctly, they may cause more harm than benefit. A splint can compress nerves, tissues, and blood vessels; therefore, the pressure of the splint should be monitored continuously along with the pulse, motor function, and sensation distal to the injury. A splint applied too tightly on an extremity can reduce distal circula-

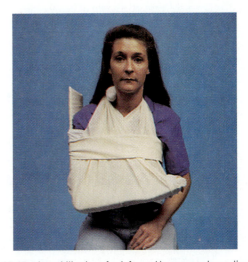

Fig. 27-15 Immobilization of a deformed humerus using a sling and swathe splint.

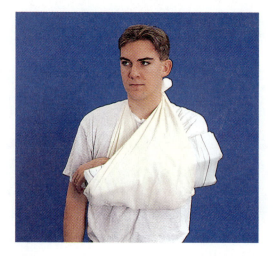

Fig. 27-16 Immobilization of an injured elbow using a sling and swathe splint.

Splinting an injury takes time. Do not delay treating or transporting a critical patient to splint an extremity injury. Splinting may be done en route or not at all if the patient has any life-threatening injuries. When moving the patient, take extreme care to keep the injury stable.

tion. An improperly applied splint can increase bleeding and tissue damage associated with the injury, cause permanent nerve damage or disability, convert a closed injury to an open injury, or increase the pain caused by excessive movement.

> ### ALERT
> **Injuries to bones and joints require splinting prior to moving the patient unless life-threatening injuries are present. In this case, splinting should be done en route to the receiving facility if possible.**

PRINCIPLE 27-2
Splinting

1. Use appropriate personal protective equipment for body substance isolation precautions.

2. Apply manual stabilization to the injured area.

3. Assess the pulse, motor function, and sensation distal to the injury.

4. Align the bones with gentle traction only if the distal extremity is cyanotic or lacks pulse and no resistance is met.

5. Immobilize the injury site with the splint.

6. Immobilize the bone above and below the injured joint. Immobilize the joint above and below the injured bone.

7. Reassess the distal pulse, motor function, and sensation and record the findings.

REVIEW QUESTIONS

SPLINTING AN INJURY

1. Always check pulse, motor function, and _____ distal to the injury before and after applying splints.

2. The injury should be splinted before transport even when the patient is not breathing. True or False?

3. The splint used for a midfemur injury is the _____ splint.

4. Splinting an injury properly should _____ (increase, decrease) the pain associated with the injury.

5. If the pulse distal to the injury is absent, _____ should be applied gently to the extremity.

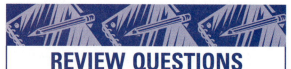

1. Sensation
2. False
3. Traction
4. Decrease
5. Manual traction

CHAPTER SUMMARY

MUSCULOSKELETAL REVIEW

The musculoskeletal system functions to give the body shape, provide for movement, and protect vital internal organs. There are three types of muscle in the human body. Voluntary, or skeletal, muscles attach bone to bone and create movement. These muscles are under voluntary control of the individual. Involuntary, or smooth, muscles are primarily found in the hollow organs of the digestive system and blood vessels and control the flow of blood and body fluids and substances through them. These muscles are not under conscious control. Cardiac muscle is the muscle of the heart and has automaticity, which is the ability to contract on its own.

The skeletal system, in conjunction with muscles, tendons, and ligaments, provides for movement, body shape, and protection. The skeleton is composed of the bones of the skull and face; the spinal column consisting of the cervical, thoracic, lumbar, sacral, and coccygeal vertebrae; the thorax (rib cage); and the lower and upper extremities. Bones are jointed primarily in two different ways: ball-and-socket joints, such as the shoulder, and hinge joints, such as the elbow or knee.

INJURIES TO BONES AND JOINTS

The mechanism of injury is important as an indication of the possible severity of the injury. A musculoskeletal injury is usually the result of a force that has been applied to an area of the body. Direct, indirect, and twisting are some types of forces that can produce injuries to the muscle and bone.

Musculoskeletal injuries can be either open or closed. Closed injuries do not break the continuity of the skin, whereas open injuries do break the skin. Excessive movement may cause a closed injury to become an open injury. Signs and symptoms of injury include deformity, angulation, pain, tenderness, grating (crepitation), swelling, bruising, exposed bone ends, and joints that are locked.

Emergency medical care of musculoskeletal injuries includes body substance isolation precautions. The airway should always be protected and assessed. High-flow oxygen is indicated for the treatment of these patients. Any major bleeding and life-threatening situations should be cared for immediately. The injured area may be elevated to reduce blood flow to that area, and cold packs may be applied to reduce swelling. Splints can be used to restrict movement and prevent further damage to the injured tissue. Never delay transport of a critical patient to splint an extremity.

SPLINTING AN INJURY

Splinting a painful, swollen, deformed extremity prevents movement of bone fragments, bone ends, or injured joints; minimizes damage to muscles, nerves, and blood vessels; minimizes the risk of converting a closed injury to an open injury; minimizes the restriction of blood flow resulting from bone ends compressing blood vessels; minimizes excessive bleeding and pain from damaged tissue caused by bone ends or fragments; and minimizes the chance of paralysis of extremities caused by spinal damage.

The principles of splinting include: assessing the pulse, motor function, and sensation distal to the injury before and after splinting the injury; manually stabilizing the joint or bone above and below the injury; removing or cutting away clothing on the extremity before splinting the injury; and covering open wounds with clean dressings. Splint the extremity in the position found, unless there is severe deformity or the distal pulse is absent, in which case use gentle traction to align the extremity before splinting. Do not intentionally replace protruding bones. Pad the splint to prevent pressure and discomfort to the patient. Splint the injury before moving unless life-threatening situations are present. If in doubt about splinting an injury, splint it. If the patient is in shock, use full-body immobilization, align in the normal anatomic position on the backboard, and transport.

Rigid splints are nonformable, such as padded-board splints. Traction splints are indicated for a closed painful, swollen, deformity at the midthigh with no joint or lower-leg injury. Do not use a traction splint if the injury is close to the knee or if there is injury to the knee, hip, pelvis, lower leg, or ankle or if the bone ends are protruding through the skin. Also do not use the traction splint if there is partial amputation or avulsion with bone separation or if the distal limb is connected only by marginal tissue.

Pneumatic splints, such as vacuum splints, are flexible, conforming splints used commonly with angulated injuries. A PASG can be used as an immobilization device also. They are indicated in the emergency medical care of pelvic instability and long bone injuries of the femur with signs and symptoms of shock.

The sling and swathe is the common splinting technique for the shoulder injury. The arm is placed into the sling, and the swathe is wrapped around the arm and the body so that the arm and shoulder cannot move. The sling and swathe can be used in conjunction with other splints for arm and elbow injuries.

Because a splint might compress nerves, tissues, and blood vessels, the pressure of the splint should be checked continually along with the pulse, motor function, and sensation distal to the injury. Excessive movement may cause or aggravate tissue, nerve, vessel, or muscle damage. Do not delay treating or transporting a critical patient to splint.

UNITED STATES DEPARTMENT OF TRANSPORTATION NATIONAL HIGHWAY TRAFFIC SAFETY ADMINISTRATION EMT–BASIC OBJECTIVES

Check your knowledge. The National Registry of EMTs and many state EMS agencies use the objectives below to develop EMT–Basic certification examinations. Can you meet them?

COGNITIVE

1. Describe the function of the muscular system.
2. Describe the function of the skeletal system.
3. List the major bones and bone groupings of the spinal column; the thorax; the upper extremities; the lower extremities.
4. Differentiate between an open and a closed painful, swollen, deformed extremity.
5. State the reasons for splinting.
6. List the general rules of splinting.
7. List the complications of splinting.
8. List the emergency medical care for a patient with a painful, swollen, deformed extremity.

AFFECTIVE

1. Explain the rationale for splinting at the scene versus load and go.
2. Explain the rationale for immobilization of the painful, swollen, deformed extremity.

PSYCHOMOTOR

1. Demonstrate the emergency medical care of a patient with a painful, swollen, deformed extremity.
2. Demonstrate completing a prehospital care report for patients with musculoskeletal injuries.

28 INJURIES TO THE HEAD AND SPINE

IN THE FIELD

"**S**quad 41, we have a call to the hockey rink on Cushings Street. Man hit with hockey stick during play, responsive, breathing, bleeding from the head." EMTs Carlos and Angie rushed to the ambulance.

Upon their arrival at the skating rink 5 minutes later, Carlos and Angie put on gloves and grabbed the oxygen, bandages, the stretcher, and the long spinal immobilization board along with cervical immobilization equipment and straps and headed toward the patient. After manually stabilizing the cervical spine, Angie took the history of what happened. The patient, Dan, responded, but his speech was slurred. Bystanders reported that he had passed out for about 3 minutes after the fall. The physical examination revealed a laceration to the forehead with bleeding, a bruise on the back of the head, and an unstable pelvis. They placed a cervical spinal immobilization device around his neck to immobilize it and placed dressings and bandages over the injury on the forehead to control bleeding.

After administering high-flow oxygen and recording Dan's vital signs, they immobilized his pelvis by placing him on the long spinal board. He was strapped in and transferred immediately to the ambulance on the stretcher. Their rapid recognition of the significant mechanism of injury led to emergency care that contributed to Dan's complete recovery and his ability to play hockey again.

Injuries to the head and spine are extremely serious and may result in severe, permanent disability or death if improperly treated or if missed in the assessment. This chapter describes how to assess a possible head or spine injury and the appropriate emergency care to give.

REVIEW OF THE NERVOUS AND SKELETAL SYSTEMS

The following sections briefly review the nervous and skeletal systems. For more extensive information about these body systems see Chapter 4, "The Human Body."

THE NERVOUS SYSTEM

The nervous system controls the voluntary and involuntary activities of the body. The nervous system is composed of the central nervous system (CNS) and the peripheral nervous system.

The CNS consists of the brain and the spinal cord. The brain is located within the cranium. The spinal cord is located within the spinal column which extends from the brain to the lumbar vertebrae. Cerebral spinal fluid (CSF) inside the spinal column and skull acts as a cushion around the brain and spinal cord.

The peripheral nervous system is made up of sensory and motor nerves. The sensory nerves carry information from the body to the brain and spinal cord. Touching something with your hand sends a message to the brain from the nerves in the hand. The motor nerves carry information from the brain and spinal cord to the body. For example, touching something hot sends a sensory nerve message to the brain, which then sends back a motor nerve message that produces a reaction of pulling the hand away from the source of the heat. Peripheral nerves extend from the spinal cord into the body to receive and send messages. Figure 28-1 diagrams the basic structures of the nervous system.

THE SKELETAL SYSTEM

The skeletal system gives the body its shape, protects internal organs, and provides for body movement. The skeletal system consists of the bones of the skull, the spinal column and thorax, the pelvis, the lower extremities, and the upper extremities.

The skull houses and protects the brain. The face is made up of the orbit of the eyes, the nasal bone, the maxilla, the mandible (lower jaw), and the zygomatic bones (cheeks).

The spinal column consists of 33 vertebrae:

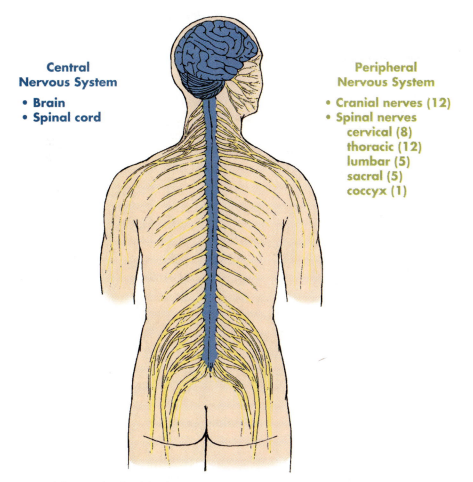

Central Nervous System
- **Brain**
- **Spinal cord**

Peripheral Nervous System
- **Cranial nerves (12)**
- **Spinal nerves**
  cervical (8)
  thoracic (12)
  lumbar (5)
  sacral (5)
  coccyx (1)

Fig. 28-1 The structures of the central and peripheral nervous system.

seven cervical (neck), 12 thoracic (upper back), five lumbar (lower back), five sacral (back wall of pelvis), and four coccygeal (tailbone) vertebrae. The spinal column surrounds and protects the spinal cord. Twelve pairs of ribs are attached to the thoracic vertebrae. Pairs 1 through 10 are attached anteriorly to the sternum (breastbone), and pairs 11 and 12 are called "floating ribs" because they do not attach to the sternum. Figure 28-2 diagrams the skeletal system.

REVIEW QUESTIONS

REVIEW OF THE NERVOUS AND SKELETAL SYSTEMS

1. If you run from a grizzly bear, the _____ nerves send the message from your brain to your legs.

2. _____ is contained around the brain and spinal cord to cushion them.

3. _____ nerves carry information from the body to the brain and spinal column.

4. The skeletal system provides for body _____, _____ and _____.

5. The ribs are attached in the posterior chest to the _____ vertebrae.

1. Motor
2. Cerebral spinal fluid
3. Sensory
4. Shape, protection, and movement
5. Thoracic

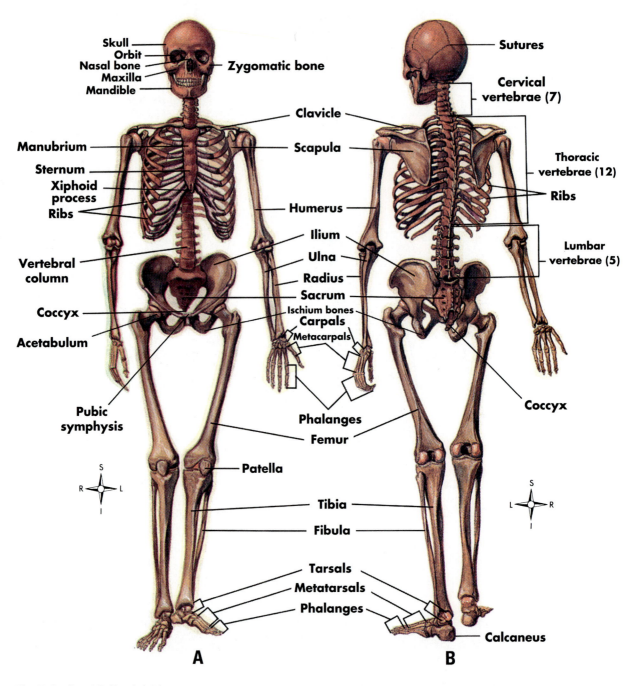

Fig. 28-2 A and B, The skeletal system.

DEVICES FOR IMMOBILIZATION

All patients suspected of having head and spinal injuries must be fully immobilized to prevent further movement of potentially injured areas. Movement could cause further damage such as becoming paralyzed. This section explains some of the immobilization devices that can be used.

CERVICAL SPINE

A **cervical spinal immobilization device,** commonly called a *cervical collar*, is indicated for any potential injury to the spine suspected because of the mechanism of injury, the patient's history, or the signs and symptoms. Cervical spinal immobilization devices are used along with short and long backboards, and usually consist of posterior and

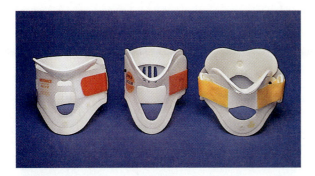

Fig. 28-3 Three types of cervical spinal immobilization devices.

anterior sections made of a rigid material. The halves are attached to each other by velcro. The anterior portion is formed to fit the chin and rest on the chest. Patients with a properly fitted immobilization device in place should not be able to turn their head side to side or up and down.

A cervical spinal immobilization device must be sized appropriately before being applied to the patient. The sizing depends on the type and design of device used (Fig. 28-3). Technique 28-1 describes how to size one type of device. An improperly sized cervical spinal immobilization device can cause further injury and can do more harm than good. An improperly fitted device either has too much space between the patient's neck and the device or is too tight. If the device is too loose, the patient's head

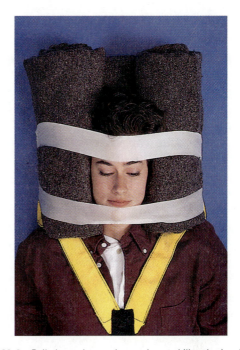

Fig. 28-4 Rolled towels may be used to stabilize the head of a patient.

may move and possibly cause further damage. A device that is too tight may obstruct the patient's airway. If no available device fits a patient, use rolled towels as a substitute for the manufactured cervical spinal immobilization device, and manually stabilize the head (Fig. 28-4). Because cervical

TECHNIQUE 28-1
Sizing a Cervical Spinal Immobilization Device

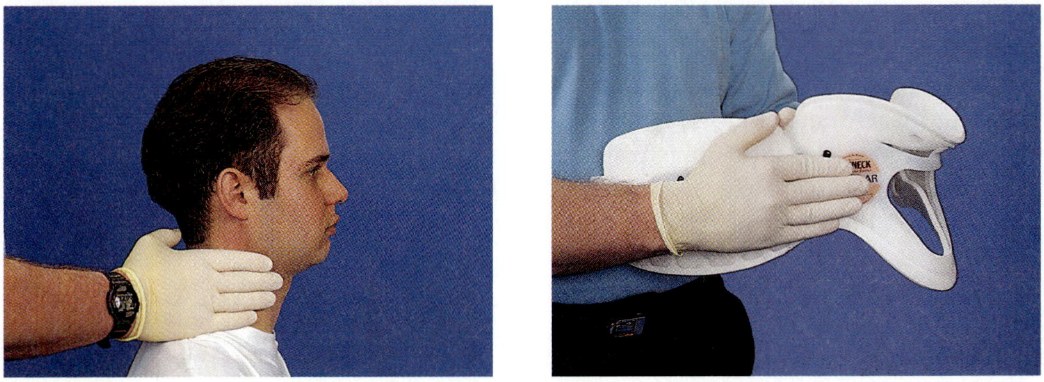

A

B

Fig. 28-5 A, Place your fingers on the patient's neck under the corner of the jawbone to determine the height (length) to the shoulder. B, Size the device to the same measurement as the patient's neck. For the device shown here, the measurement is taken under the black knob that fastens the device together.

spinal immobilization devices are sized according to their individual design, you must be familiar with the cervical spinal immobilization devices used in your service.

The width of the side of the device corresponds to the measurement of the neck. A properly fitted cervical spinal immobilization device is neither too loose nor too tight. The patient's chin should rest comfortably in the chin rest on the anterior portion of the device, and the base of the device should rest on the patient's chest. The posterior portion of the device should be fit snugly when attached to the anterior portion with the velcro straps. The patient's chin should be stable, and the head should be immobilized in the neutral position.

If the chin can slip out of the chin rest and under the device, the device is too big. If there is space between the base of the device and the patient's chest, the device is too small.

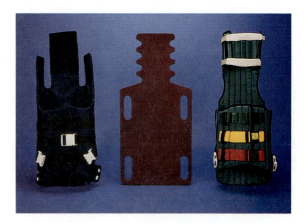

Fig. 28-6 The XP1 *(left),* short wooden backboard *(center),* and KED *(right).*

> # ALERT
> Cervical spinal immobilization devices alone do not provide adequate spinal immobilization. Manual stabilization must always be used with a cervical spinal immobilization device until the patient's body and head are secured to the long backboard.

SHORT BACKBOARDS

A **short backboard** is used for a seated patient with potential head, neck, or spinal injuries. Several different types of short board immobilization devices are used, including vest type devices and rigid short boards (Fig. 28-6). These devices provide immobilization for the head, neck, and torso from the sitting position. The techniques for applying these devices are described later in this chapter.

LONG BACKBOARDS (FULL-BODY SPINAL IMMOBILIZATION DEVICES)

Various **long backboards (full-body spinal immobilization devices)** are available (Fig. 28-7). These devices are used to immobilize the head, neck, torso, pelvis, and extremities. They immobilize patients found in lying or standing positions and are sometimes used in conjunction with short backboards

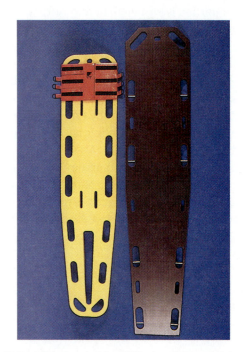

Fig. 28-7 Full-body spinal immobilization devices with the head immobilization base *(left)* and without the base *(right).*

for patients found in the sitting position. The technique for using the long board is described later in this chapter.

The correct use of all immobilization devices is very important. Devices not used correctly may actually harm the patient.

INJURIES TO THE SPINE

MECHANISM OF INJURY

The mechanism of injury refers to how the injury occurred and how much force was applied to the patient's body during the incident. By consid-

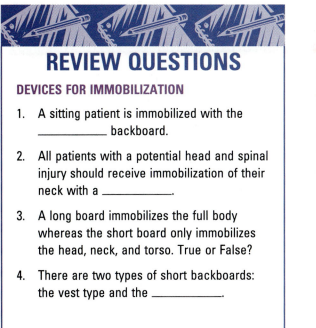

REVIEW QUESTIONS

DEVICES FOR IMMOBILIZATION

1. A sitting patient is immobilized with the _____ backboard.

2. All patients with a potential head and spinal injury should receive immobilization of their neck with a _____.

3. A long board immobilizes the full body whereas the short board only immobilizes the head, neck, and torso. True or False?

4. There are two types of short backboards: the vest type and the _____.

1. Short
2. Cervical spinal immobilization device
3. True
4. Rigid short board

ering the damage to a vehicle or the height of a fall, you can determine if the mechanism of injury involved a significant force to the patient's body. Figure 28-8 illustrates one significant mechanism of injury. In most situations, the mechanism of injury can be determined as part of the scene size-up. Box 28-1 lists some mechanisms of injury that should make you suspect that the patient may have a significant injury requiring immobilization.

Compression injuries to the spine can result from accidents such as falls, diving injuries, and motor vehicle collisions. For example, if the patient dove into a pond and hit the top of their head on a rock beneath the surface, the head could be pushed downward and could compress the spine.

Any excessive flexion, extension, rotation, or lateral bending of the spine can also cause significant injury. This type of injury is often seen in motor vehicle collisions that produce "whiplash." A person in a car that is hit from behind experiences a backward, then forward, snapping of the neck that can cause significant injury to the cervical spine.

Another type of injury to the spine is called distraction. This injury is the pulling apart of the spine, such as in a hanging victim. If the head is snapped away from the body, the spine can become separated.

Be aware of significant mechanisms of injury, and maintain spinal immobilization for all of these patients or any patient with signs and symptoms of trauma.

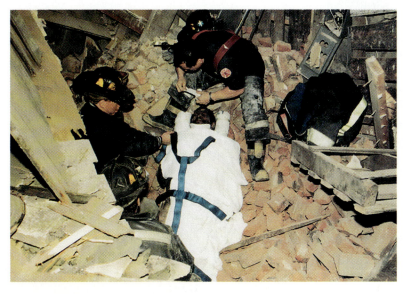

Fig. 28-8 The mechanism of injury may make you suspect that the patient has extensive injuries.

BOX 28-1

Significant Mechanisms of Injury

- Motor vehicle crash
- Pedestrian injured in vehicle collision
- Fall
- Blunt trauma to the head, chest, abdomen, or pelvis
- Penetrating trauma to the head, neck, or torso (*see* Fig. 28-9)

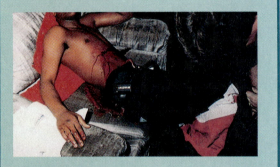

Fig. 28-9   This patient is a victim of a stabbing. The knife handle broke off, leaving the blade impaled in the victim's side.

- Motorcycle crash (*see* Fig 28-10)

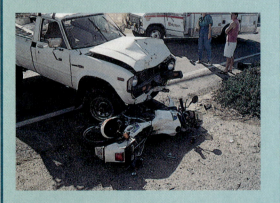

Fig. 28-10   The victims of this motorcycle crash were not wearing helmets. The driver was flown to a trauma center with serious injuries including bilateral femur fractures.

- Hanging
- Diving accident
- Any trauma resulting in unresponsive patient

ASSESSMENT

The scene size-up and the initial assessment are the first critical areas of assessment. Any injuries or associated trauma found during this time should be treated, such as any airway problems or massive bleeding. Then the focused history and physical examination may be completed. Some specific signs and symptoms should lead you to suspect a possible head or spinal injury.

SIGNS AND SYMPTOMS

Patients with spinal injuries may feel tenderness in the area of the injury or pain associated with movement of the area. However, do not ask the patient to move just to try to elicit a pain response, and do not move the patient just to test for a pain response. The patient may feel pain independent of movement or palpation along the spinal column or the extremities. The pain may be intermittent. Tell the patient not to move while you are asking questions. Stay within the patient's field of vision when talking or asking questions so that the patient does not move his/her head to look at you.

Soft tissue injuries may be associated with spinal trauma. You may palpate an obvious deformity along the spine in the injured area. The head and neck may be injured along with the cervical spine. A shoulder, back, or abdominal injury could indicate a thoracic or lumbar spine injury. Soft tissue damage to the lower extremities could indicate an injury to the lumbar or sacral spine.

Patients may feel numbness, weakness, or tingling in the extremities or may have complete loss of sensation or paralysis below the suspected level

ALERT

Spinal column or cord damage is not ruled out by the absence of pain along the spinal column or the ability to walk, move the extremities, or feel sensations. During the assessment process, you need to gather important additional information about the condition of both responsive and unresponsive patients.

of injury. These patients may also have lost control of their bowels.

RESPONSIVE PATIENTS

First complete the scene size-up. Once you are with the patient, tell the patient not to move while you ask questions. A partner can stabilize the cervical spine while you gather the history. Important questions to ask the patient are listed in Box 28-2.

Inspect and palpate for deformities, contusions, abrasions, punctures, penetrations, burns, tenderness, lacerations, and swelling (DCAP–BTLS). Assess the patient's equality of strength in the extremities. Have the patient grasp each of your hands with his/her hands (do both hands at the same time) to determine if the grasp strength is equal, and have the patient push on your hands with his/her feet to see if the strength is equal. Document all findings on the prehospital care report.

Gather pertinent information, such as what happened, what hurts, and how the patient feels, from responsive patients in a timely fashion. A responsive patient could become unresponsive at any moment.

UNRESPONSIVE PATIENTS

First complete the scene size-up. Quickly inspect the involved vehicle, equipment, or injury site for damage or other clues indicating the forces involved. Make a note of the damage done to the inside of a vehicle, such as compartment damage, a bent steering wheel, or a starred windshield, and what section of the car was damaged (front end,

side, rear). This information will help the receiving facility to determine the forces involved.

Perform the initial assessment and then rapidly inspect and palpate the patient for DCAP–BTLS. Talk to others at the scene to determine more information about the mechanism of injury and the patient's mental status before you arrived.

COMPLICATIONS

Complications that can arise in a patient with a spinal injury include inadequate breathing effort and paralysis. Take great care to immobilize the patient without excessive movement. *After every intervention, reassess the patient's vital signs and motor and sensory functions.* Any patient movement might have produced paralysis that was not previously present. Similarly, reassess a combative or uncooperative patient after any significant movement or attempted movement. Thoroughly document any changes in the patient's status.

A spinal cord injury that affects the nerves controlling the movement of the diaphragm and accessory muscles of breathing (a cervical or thoracic injury) may cause a patient to have difficulty breathing. Watch these patients closely because their breathing may need assistance.

If the patient vomits while immobilized, an airway obstruction may occur. If the patient can be suctioned, do so to clear the airway. A patient who is fully immobilized to a long board can be tilted to the side to clear the airway.

EMERGENCY MEDICAL CARE OF THE SPINE-INJURED PATIENT

Take appropriate body substance isolation precautions. For any type of extrication, wear the appropriate gear, including bunker coats, pants, and leather gloves. Establish and maintain manual in-line cervical spinal immobilization, which is described in Technique 28-2.

After the cervical spine is manually stabilized, complete the initial assessment. If needed, provide airway control and artificial ventilation while maintaining cervical in-line stabilization. Assess the pulse and motor and sensory function in all extremities. Assess the cervical region and neck for any deformities, swelling, or tenderness. You may do this assessment before placing the cervical spinal immobilization device on the patient (Technique 28-3). Otherwise, you must maintain manual stabilization and loosen the device to assess the neck region.

BOX 28-2

Important Questions for Trauma Patients

- What happened?
- Where does it hurt?
- Does your neck or back hurt?
- Can you move your fingers and toes?
- Where am I touching you now (while touching fingers and toes)?

TECHNIQUE 28-2
In-line Cervical Spinal Immobilization

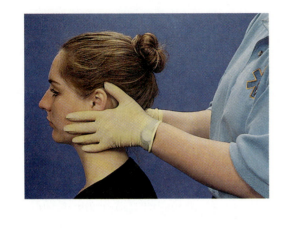

Fig. 28-11   Get into position at the top of the patient's head (with a patient lying down) or behind the patient (for a seated patient). Place your hands at the corner of the patient's jaws on both sides. Grasp the corner of the jaw and provide stabilization to the neck by wrapping your hands around the posterior portion of the neck. Place the patient's head in the neutral position in alignment with the spine. Do not attempt this positioning if the patient complains of pain, if the head is not easily moved into position, if muscle spasm occurs, or if the airways becomes compromised. A second EMT applies a cervical spinal immobilization device. Constant manual in-line stabilization should be maintained until the patient is properly secured to a backboard with the body and head immobilized.

TECHNIQUE 28-3
Application of a Cervical Spinal Immobilization Device

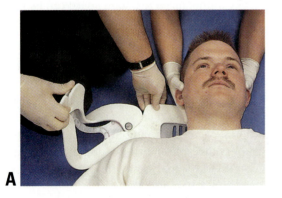
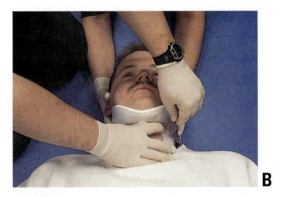

A   B

Fig. 28-12   Assess the cervical region for DCAP–BTLS, and look for tracheal deviation and jugular vein distention. Properly size the cervical spinal immobilization device as recommended by its manufacturer (*see* Technique 28-1). Apply the device to the patient without interrupting the manual stabilization. **A, Slide the posterior portion of the device under the patient's neck without lifting or moving the head or neck. B, Wrap the anterior portion of the device around the front of the patient's neck and attach the Velcro straps from both parts together to make a snug fit.** The patient's chin should rest comfortably in the device without moving the neck from the neutral position. The patient's head should not be able to turn from side to side or up and down. After the device is applied, reassess the patency of the patient's airway. Be careful not to obstruct the airway with the cervical spinal immobilization device.

TECHNIQUE 28-4
Log Roll of a Patient Found Lying Down

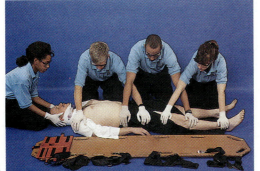

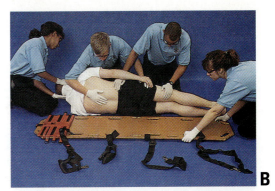

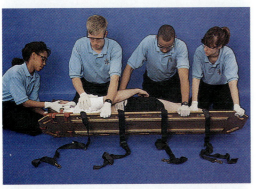

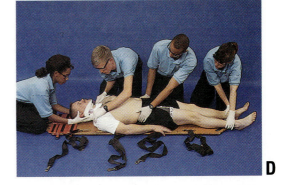

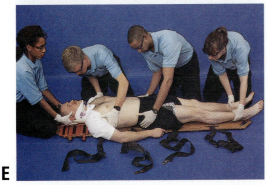

A

B

C

D

E

Fig. 28-13   A, One EMT maintains manual stabilization of the patient's head (*see* Technique 28-2) while directing all movement of the patient by the other EMTs. Another EMT should place the long spine board at one side of the patient. One to three other EMTs control the movement of the rest of the patient's body. If there is only one other EMT, he/she should take a position at the patient's torso on the opposite side of the board, reaching across the patient to support the hips and shoulders. **If there are three additional EMTs, one can support the shoulders, one can support the hips, and one can support the lower extremities. B, At the direction of the EMT at the head, the patient should be rolled toward the EMTs with a coordinated movement to keep the spine in-line.** Do not roll the patient onto an injured arm. If it is uninjured, the arm can be left at the patient's side and the patient can be log rolled onto it. The patient's posterior side should be assessed during the log roll by the EMTs at the patient's body if this procedure was not performed earlier in the initial assessment. The EMT at the torso can check the patient's back, and the EMT at the hips can check the patient's buttocks and legs for injuries. The long spinal immobilization device is then moved next to the patient by another EMT or by each of the EMTs holding the patient's body by reaching with one hand to pull the board to the patient. **C, The patient is then rolled onto the device at the direction of the EMT at the patient's head. D, If the patient must be adjusted to be centered on the board, the EMTs should hold the shoulders and hips and move the patient downward or (E) upward at the direction of the EMT at the head.** *Do not move the patient on the board by pushing him or her from the side, which creates pressure on parts of the spine.* **Always slide the patient lengthwise to maintain spinal alignment.**

A special method is used to move a lying patient onto a backboard. The **log roll** of the patient is per-formed carefully to keep the spinal column in alignment and to cause the least amount of movement to the patient. Technique 28-4 describes this procedure.

If the patient is found lying down, immobilize the patient with a long spine board. Refer to Technique 28-5 for one method of immobilizing the patient on a long backboard.

When log rolling a patient, take great care to move the patient as little as possible. During the

TECHNIQUE 28-5
Immobilization of a Lying Patient on a Long Spine Board

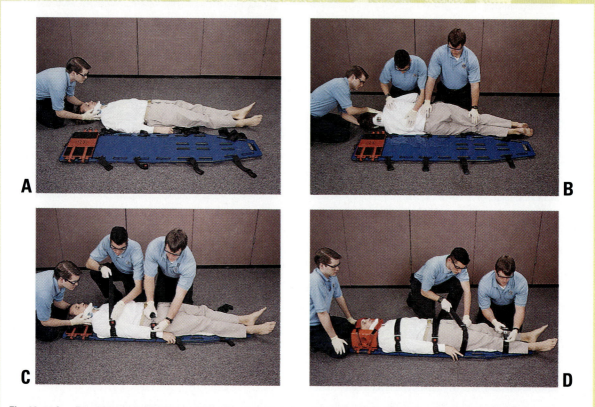

Fig. 28-14 A, **Provide manual in-line stabilization,** assess pulses, motor function, and sensation in all extremities, and record the findings on the prehospital care report. Assess the cervical area for DCAP-BTLS, and look for tracheal deviation and jugular vein distention. Size and apply a cervical spinal immobilization device. **Position the long spine board alongside the patient. Be sure that the straps are not on top of the device but have been moved to the side. B, Log roll the patient as described in Technique 28-4, assess the patient's posterior, and place the board under the patient.** Place the patient onto the board at the direction of the EMT who is maintaining manual cervical spine stabilization. Pad the spaces between the patient and the board (voids) so that the patient is supported completely. The adult patient may have voids under the neck and under the torso. The infant or child is padded under the shoulders to the toes to maintain a neutral position, compensating for the relatively large head. Be careful of extra movement during this process (place padding on the board before moving the patient there). A geriatric patient may require extensive padding because the spine may not lay smoothly on the board because of arthritis or osteoporosis. **C, Completely immobilize the torso to the board using the attached straps, and adjust them as needed. The straps should be attached straight across the body at the shoulders and hips.** Do not obstruct respiratory effort at any time by pulling the straps too tight. **D, Immobilize the patient's head to the board using the head immobilization pillows and straps designed for the long board. When the head and body are secured to the long board, the EMT holding manual in-line stabilization is relieved. Secure the patient's legs to the board proximal and distal to the knees using the attached straps, and adjust them as needed.** Reassess the pulse, motor function, and sensation in all extremities and record the findings.

TECHNIQUE 28-6
Immobilization of the Seated Patient With a Short Rigid Spine Board

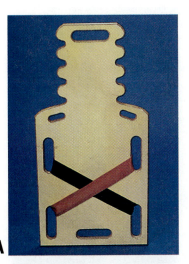

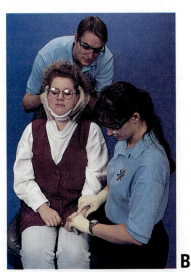

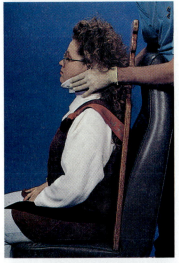

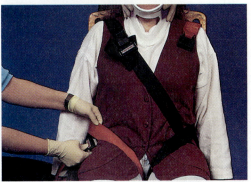

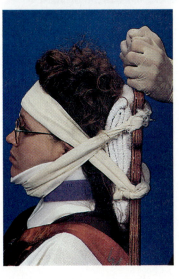

Fig. 28-15 A, Assemble the two long straps so that they form an "X" on the back of the board. The buckles should be placed through the top hole. **B,** The first EMT inspects the cervical area, while **the second EMT maintains manual cervical spinal stabilization.** A cervical spinal immobilization device is placed on the patient. **Assess the patient's distal pulses, motor function, and sensation. C,** The second EMT places the rigid spine board up between the first EMT's arms and then positions it down between the patient's back and the seat. **The hole for the strap at the top of the board should be even with the shoulder. D,** Secure the patient's torso to the board by wrapping the straps under the patient's thigh and buttocks to secure the legs and then crossing the straps over the torso. Pad under the buckles of the straps and tighten them as necessary to secure the shoulders. **E, Pad the void between the patient's head and the board as necessary.** For an infant or child, pad behind the shoulders and torso to make up for the large head. **Secure the patient's head to the board.** Secure the patient's arms, legs, and feet to prevent flailing of the extremities when extricating the patient. Reassess the distal pulses, motor function, and sensation.

TECHNIQUE 28-7
Immobilization of the Seated Patient to the Kendrick Extrication Device (KED)

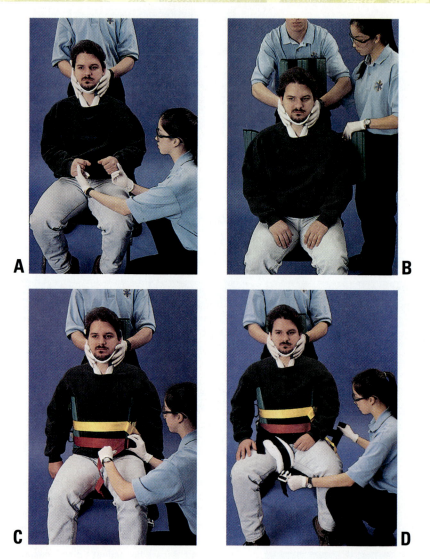

Fig. 28-16 A, The first EMT maintains manual cervical stabilization, and a cervical spinal immobilization device is placed on the patient. **Assess the patient's distal pulses, motor function, and sensation. B, The second EMT places the KED up between the first EMT's arms and then positions it down between the patient's back and the seat so that the patient's spine is centered on the device.** Pull the leg straps (white buckles) down and out of the way. The torso section of the KED should fit snugly into the patient's armpits to eliminate the possibility that the patient will slide downward when lifted. This snug fit can be achieved by gently lifting up on the side handles and vertical lift handles. **C, Secure the patient's torso to the KED by connecting the middle straps across the torso and then the lower straps across the torso. Tighten the two straps until they are snug. Do not buckle the top strap yet. D, Secure the patient's legs by placing the leg straps around each leg in a "see-sawing" motion under the patient's thigh and buttocks.** The buckles are attached to the matching buckle on the opposite side of the KED. Tighten the leg straps. Pad the void between the patient's head and the device as necessary. A pad is supplied with the KED. *Continued*

TECHNIQUE 28-7
Immobilization of the Seated Patient to the Kendrick Extrication Device (KED)

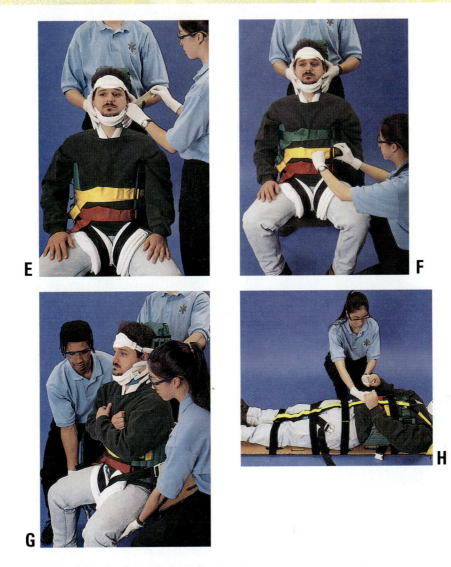

Fig. 28-16 *Continued* **E,** Secure the patient's head to the KED using the head straps. One strap wraps around the forehead and attaches to the KED, and the other strap goes under the chin and attaches to the device. **F,** Attach the top torso straps together, and tighten and readjust all straps on the KED. **G,** The patient may be lifted onto the long board. Each EMT holds with one hand onto the side-lifting handle under the patient's armpits, passing their other hands under the patient's legs at the knees and locking them together. **H,** Secure the patient to the long spine board and reassess distal pulses, motor function, and sensation.

Note: The KED should not be used in this manner for children because the patient's torso must be at least as long as the KED's torso flap is wide. Improper use may worsen a spinal injury. Always be sure that the patient's airway is not compromised or obstructed by too-tight chin straps or chest straps.

Note: This technique follows the manufacturer's recommendations. Some testing agencies may require securing all three torso straps prior to securing the head.

roll, assess the patient's posterior side for DCAP–BTLS before placing the long spine board under the patient.

Some patients may be found in a sitting position, such as a person in a car after an automobile collision. In these circumstances, the patient should be immobilized on a short spine board and then transferred to and immobilized on the long spine board. Techniques 28-6 and 28-7 describe short board immobilization procedures, including use of the **Kendrick Extrication Device (KED).**

A patient who is found self-extricated from a vehicle in a standing position with an injury to the spine should be immobilized to a long spine board by using Technique 28-8.

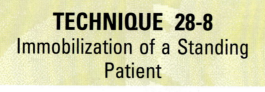

TECHNIQUE 28-8
Immobilization of a Standing Patient

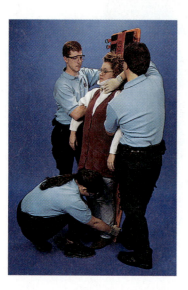

Fig. 28-17 One EMT should maintain manual cervical spine stabilization while a cervical spinal immobilization device is placed on the patient's neck. Assess the patient's distal pulse, motor function, and sensation. Position the device behind the patient. **The two EMTs on the sides of the patient reach with their hand closest to the patient under the patient's arm to grasp the board and use their hand farthest from the patient to secure the head. A third EMT is positioned facing the foot of the board.** Once this position is established, the two EMTs place their leg closest to the board behind the board and begin to tip the top backward. The EMT at the foot of the board secures the board and the patient to prevent sliding, and the board is brought to a level horizontal position. Reassess all patient distal pulses, motor function, and sensation. Secure the patient to the board as previously described in Technique 28-5.

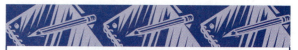

REVIEW QUESTIONS

INJURIES TO THE SPINE

1. The lying patient should be log rolled to the _____ board.

2. The standing patient cannot be immobilized from this position and must lie down first. True or False?

3. A person involved in a diving accident may experience a _____ injury to the spine, which forces the head toward the spinal column.

4. The EMT should ask trauma patients if they can move the _____ and _____ .

5. The EMT should maintain _____ cervical stabilization until the head is secured to the board.

5. Manual
4. Fingers; toes
3. Compression
2. False
1. Long

INJURIES TO THE BRAIN AND SKULL

Many injuries involving the spine also involve the brain and skull. Any patient with suspected brain and skull injuries should be completely immobilized, and a spinal injury should be suspected.

HEAD AND SKULL INJURIES

Injuries to the head may produce scalp and/or brain injuries. Wounds to the scalp often look severe because many capillary beds are located there, and even a small cut can produce major bleeding. Any bleeding on the scalp should be controlled

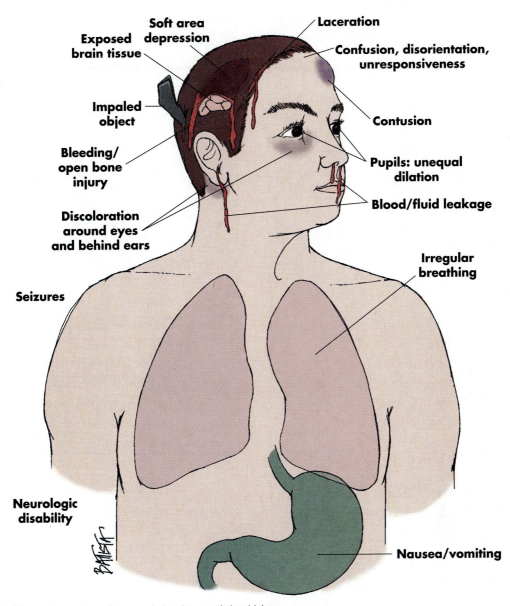

Fig. 28-18 Signs and symptoms of open and closed traumatic head injury.

with direct pressure, unless a skull fracture is suspected. Do not apply pressure to the site of a suspected skull fracture.

An injury to the skull may damage brain tissue directly or may result in bleeding inside the skull. Internal bleeding causes an increase in pressure inside the skull that can result in changes in mental status. Box 28-3 lists the signs and symptoms of closed and open traumatic head injuries (Fig. 28-18).

Other brain damage can result from nontraumatic conditions, such as blood clots, hemorrhaging, or lack of oxygen such as in a near-drowning patient. This damage can lead to altered mental status. The signs and symptoms of these conditions are similar to those of a traumatic head injury although there is no obvious mechanism of injury or evidence of trauma.

EMERGENCY MEDICAL CARE OF THE HEAD-INJURED PATIENT

Take appropriate body substance isolation precautions. The first priority with traumatic head injuries is to ensure a patent airway for the patient. Maintain the airway with high-flow oxygen and provide artificial ventilation if appropriate. Do not use the head-tilt chin-lift maneuver for the trauma patient, instead, use the jaw thrust. The initial and focused assessments and spinal immobilization should be performed on the scene, with the com-

BOX 28-3

Signs and Symptoms of a Traumatic Head Injury

- Altered mental status (best indicator of a head injury), such as confusion, disorientation, and repetitive questioning, decreasing mental status, or unresponsiveness
- Irregular breathing pattern
- Mechanism of injury such as deformity of a windshield or helmet
- Deformity to the skull or a soft area or depression upon palpation
- Blood or other fluid leaking from the ears and/or nose
- Bruising (discoloration) around the eyes
- Bruising (discoloration) behind the ears
- Neurologic disability (inability to move or feel extremity)
- Nausea and/or vomiting
- Unequal pupil size with altered mental status
- Seizure activity

Additional Signs and Symptoms of an Open Traumatic Head and Skull Injury

- Contusions, lacerations, or hematomas (bruises) on the scalp
- Penetrating injury (do not remove objects impaled in the skull)
- Exposed brain tissue
- Bleeding from the open bone injury

BOX 28-4

Emergency Medical Care for a Head Injury

- Follow body substance isolation precautions
- Maintain the patient's airway, provide high-flow oxygen, and if needed provide artificial ventilation
- Perform the initial assessment, focused history and physical examination, and spinal immobilization at the scene and the detailed physical examination during transport
- Closely monitor the airway, breathing, pulse, and mental status
- Control any bleeding
- Place a fully immobilized patient on the left side if needed to clear the airway
- Be prepared for changes in the patient's condition
- Transport immediately

long backboard can be rolled onto the left side. Be prepared for changes in the patient's condition and transport immediately. Box 28-4 summarizes the emergency medical care for the head-injured patient.

ALERT
With any head injury, the EMT should suspect a related spinal injury and provide full immobilization.

SPECIAL CONSIDERATIONS

In some instances special circumstances related to head and spinal injuries arise.

RAPID EXTRICATION

Rapid extrication of a patient is indicated in situations in which the scene is unsafe, when the

plete detailed physical examination performed en route to the receiving facility. With any head injury, suspect a spinal injury and fully immobilize the spine. The patient's airway, breathing, pulse, and mental status must be continuously monitored for deterioration.

Control any bleeding, but do not apply pressure to an open or depressed skull injury. Dress and bandage the wound as described in Chapter 26, "Soft-Tissue Injuries." If the patient vomits, place the patient on the left side to gain better control of the airway. For the immobilized patient, the entire

Although this technique does not provide adequate immobilization, there are other life-threatening dangers present in this situation and the patient must be moved.

Bring the patient's body into alignment, lower the patient carefully onto a long spine board, and remove the patient while providing manual stabilization. Transport immediately, completing the immobilization process en route. The detailed procedure for rapid extrication is described in Chapter 6, "Lifting and Moving Patients."

HELMET REMOVAL

Patients wearing helmets have special management needs. The airway and breathing must be monitored closely for changes. Whether the helmet is removed depends on the fit of the helmet, the patient's head movement within the helmet, and your access to the patient to manage airway and breathing.

There are many types of helmets, including sports helmets and motorcycle helmets (Fig. 28-19). Sports helmets are typically open anteriorly, and the airway is fairly easy to access. Motorcycle helmets can have full face shields that make it difficult to access the airway. The patency of the airway and the type of helmet are factors when deciding whether to remove the helmet.

The helmet may be left in place if there is good fit with little or no movement of the patient's head within the helmet. This tight fit is usually seen in sports helmets specially designed for the patient's head. The helmet can be left in place if the patient does not have airway or breathing problems or if removal would cause further injury to the patient. If proper spinal immobilization can be provided, the helmet may be left in place as long as you can assess and reassess the airway and breathing and

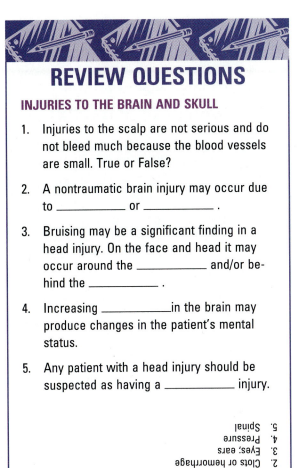

REVIEW QUESTIONS

INJURIES TO THE BRAIN AND SKULL

1. Injuries to the scalp are not serious and do not bleed much because the blood vessels are small. True or False?

2. A nontraumatic brain injury may occur due to _____ or _____ .

3. Bruising may be a significant finding in a head injury. On the face and head it may occur around the _____ and/or behind the _____ .

4. Increasing _____ in the brain may produce changes in the patient's mental status.

5. Any patient with a head injury should be suspected as having a _____ injury.

1. False
2. Clots or hemorrhage
3. Eyes; ears
4. Pressure
5. Spinal

patient's condition is unstable and warrants immediate movement and transport, or when the patient blocks access to another, more seriously injured patient. Rapid extrication is performed because of the urgency of time and the patient's condition, not because of the preference of the EMT.

ALERT
If the patient must be removed immediately because of injuries that cannot be managed in the patient's current position, a need to gain access to other more seriously injured patients, or dangers at the scene, the patient must be rapidly extricated.

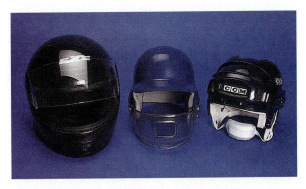

Fig. 28-19 Motorcycle and sports helmets may need to be removed from a patient.

BOX 28-5

Indications for Leaving a Helmet in Place

All conditions must be met to leave the helmet in place:

- The helmet fits well and allows little or no movement of the head within the helmet.
- The patient has no impending airway or breathing problems.
- Removal would cause further injury to the patient.
- Proper spinal immobilization can be performed with the helmet in place.
- The helmet does not interfere with your ability to assess and reassess the airway and breathing and does not interfere with the administration of oxygen.

BOX 28-6

Indications for the Removal of a Helmet

- You are unable to assess or reassess the patient's airway and breathing.
- The helmet interferes with management of the airway or breathing.
- The helmet is loose and allows for excessive patient head movement within the helmet.
- You cannot perform proper spinal immobilization due to the helmet.
- The patient is in cardiac arrest.

treat effectively with high-flow oxygen. Box 28-5 summarizes indications for leaving the helmet in place.

A helmet should be removed if you cannot assess or reassess the patient's airway and breathing or your management of the airway or breathing is restricted by the helmet. An improperly fitted helmet that allows for excessive movement of the head within the helmet is an indication for removal. If the patient is wearing football shoulder pads, they should be removed before removing the helmet. If the helmet is removed and the shoulder pads are not, the shoulders will be too high too provide for neutral positioning of the spine. If proper spinal immobilization can not be provided or if the patient is in cardiac arrest, remove the helmet. Box 28-6 summarizes the indications for helmet removal.

Technique 28-9 illustrates how to remove one type of helmet.

An alternative technique for removing the helmet is described in Technique 28-10.

Traditional commercial devices to immobilize the head to the long backboard may not be effective if the patient is wearing a helmet. Rolled towels, bulky dressings, and tape may all be used to help secure the head to the board. If spinal immobiliza-

tion cannot be adequately maintained because the helmet is in place, remove the helmet.

INFANTS AND CHILDREN

Infants and children are immobilized on a rigid board appropriate for the patient's size (short board or long board) following the procedures outlined earlier. Because various types of pediatric immobilization devices are available, you must be familiar with the devices carried on your unit. Special considerations include padding from the shoulders to the heels of the infant or child, if necessary, to maintain neutral positioning. Padding under the body raises the body but not the head. Because the head is larger, padding under the body helps maintain the in-line neutral position needed to keep the airway open. Figure 28-22A and B illustrates immobilization without and with padding.

The cervical spinal immobilization device must be sized appropriately. A device that does not fit could do more harm than good. If a properly fitting immobilization device is not available, pad under the neck, torso, and legs of the patient while maintaining manual stabilization in a neutral position. Figure 28-23 shows an example of the immobilized infant.

Remember that infants and children are less likely to cooperate with immobilization. They may actually feel more secure and reassured with good, snug, whole-body immobilization. Loose strapping or tape may encourage the child to fight.

TECHNIQUE 28-9
Removal of a Motorcycle Helmet

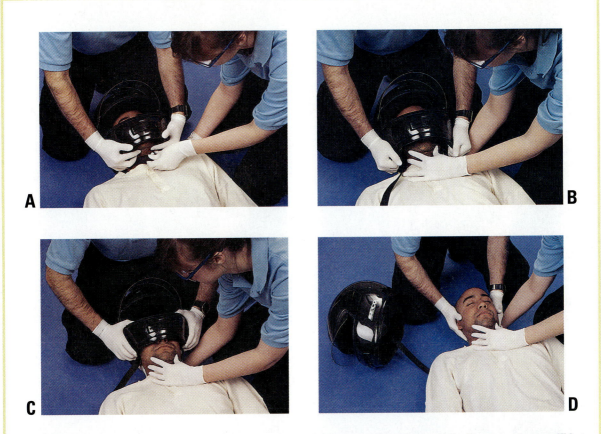

Fig. 28-20 A, One EMT stabilizes the helmet with the hands on each side of the helmet and the fingers on the mandible to prevent movement. Remove the patient's eyeglasses (if worn). **The second EMT loosens or cuts the chin strap. B, The second EMT places one hand on the mandible at the angle of the jaw and the other hand posteriorly at the occipital region. The first EMT holding the helmet pulls the sides of the helmet apart, gently slips the helmet halfway off of the patient's head, and then stops. C, The second EMT maintaining stabilization of the neck repositions and slides the posterior hand superiorly to prevent the head from falling back after complete helmet removal. D, Remove the helmet completely.** Assess the airway and proceed to complete spinal immobilization as indicated.

TECHNIQUE 28-10
Alternative Method for Removal of a Helmet

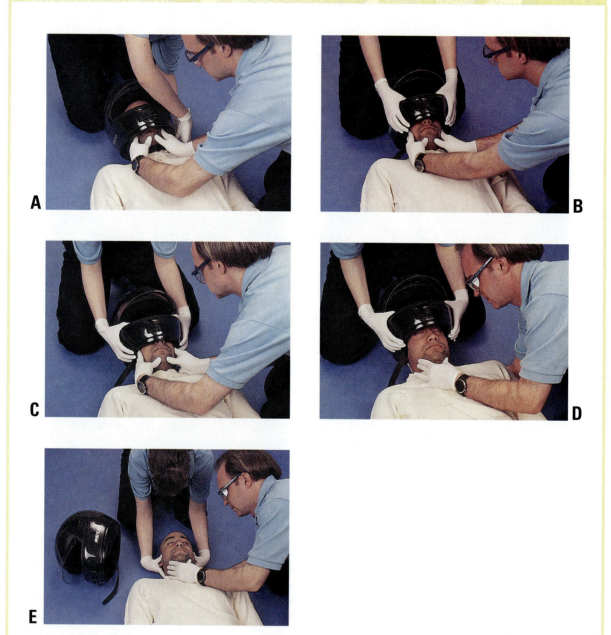

Fig. 28-21 **A, The first EMT takes a position beside the patient and stabilizes the patient's head by placing one hand on each side of the mandible and along the side of the face.** Remove the patient's eyeglasses (if worn). **The second EMT removes or cuts the chin strap. B, The second EMT pulls the sides of the helmet apart, gently slips the helmet halfway off of the patient's head, and then stops. C, The helmet is tipped forward to assist removal over the occiput. D, The first EMT repositions their hands toward the back of the patient's head to prevent the head from dropping when the helmet is removed. E, Remove the helmet completely.** Assess the airway and proceed to complete spinal immobilization as indicated.

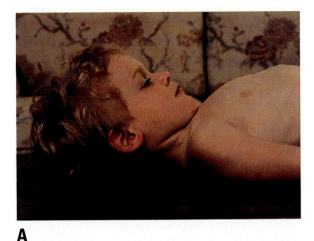
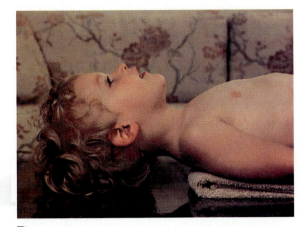

A   **B**

Fig. 28-22   A child on backboard **(A)** without padding and **(B)** with padding.

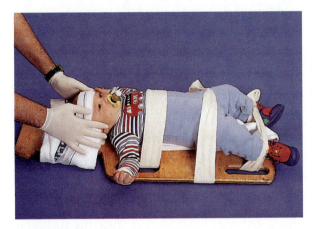

Fig. 28-23   An immobilized infant. Some agencies may also require the use of a chin strap.

GERIATRIC PATIENTS

Geriatric patients may have arthritis, a disease that may result in some joints being unable to be straightened or moved. Another disease of the elderly is osteoporosis, which affects the bones. A geriatric patient may have a curvature of the spine that cannot be straightened. These patients sometimes need additional padding in spaces between the body and the immobilization device. All spaces must be padded to provide proper support to the entire body.

CHAPTER SUMMARY

For every patient who is involved in any type of traumatic incident in which the mechanism of injury or signs and symptoms indicate a possible spinal injury, the spine must be completely immobilized. Critically injured patients may have to be moved using only rapid spinal immobilization

REVIEW QUESTIONS

SPECIAL CONSIDERATIONS

1. If the patient is wearing a form-fitted sports helmet and the airway cannot be evaluated, the helmet _____ (should, should not) be removed.

2. A patient involved in an auto accident in which gasoline is leaking around the vehicle should be _____ _____.

3. The helmet of a cardiac arrest patient should be removed. True or False?

4. The procedure for removing a helmet requires only one EMT. True or False?

5. An improperly sized cervical spinal immobilization device can cause further _____ to the patient.

1. Should
2. Rapidly extricated
3. True
4. False
5. Injury

techniques. A short backboard or spinal immobilization device is used for noncritically injured patients at the scene before moving the patient. Failure to immobilize the spine or treat the head-injured patient may lead to increased or additional patient injury. However, when patients have life threats or the scene is unsafe for the EMT, the patient is moved by a rapid extrication technique.

REVIEW OF THE NERVOUS AND SKELETAL SYSTEMS

The function of the nervous system is to control the voluntary and involuntary activities of the body. The nervous system is composed of the central nervous system (brain and spinal cord) and the peripheral nervous system (sensory and motor nerves). Sensory nerves carry information from the body to the brain, and motor nerves carry information from the brain to the body.

The skeletal system provides for body movement, body shape, and protection of internal organs. The skull houses and protects the brain. The spinal column consists of cervical, thoracic, lumbar, sacral, and coccygeal vertebrae.

DEVICES FOR IMMOBILIZATION

All patients suspected of having head and spinal injuries must be fully immobilized to prevent further movement of the injured areas. Cervical spinal immobilization devices are indicated for any suspected spine injury based on the mechanism of injury or the patient's history or signs and symptoms. The sizing of the device is important because an improperly fitted cervical spinal immobilization device can do more harm than good. Cervical spinal immobilization devices alone do not provide adequate inline immobilization. Manual stabilization must always be used with a cervical spinal immobilization device until the head and body are secured to a board.

A short backboard is indicated for a seated patient with head, neck, or spinal injuries. The short backboard provides immobilization for the head, neck, and torso. Short boards are used in conjunction with long backboards. Long backboards are recommended for immobilizing the standing or lying patient. Long boards provide immobilization to the head, neck, torso, pelvis, and extremities. Patients are log rolled from a lying position onto the long backboard. The device must be used correctly or it can cause harm to the patient.

INJURIES TO THE SPINE

The mechanism of injury is how the injury occurred, such as the damage to a vehicle or the height of a fall. If there is any doubt about the mechanism of injury, assume that the patient has significant injuries, and provide full spinal immobilization.

Compression, flexion, extension, rotation, lateral bending, and distraction are different ways that spinal injuries are caused by different mechanisms of injury.

Patients with spinal injuries may feel tenderness in the injured area or pain associated with movement. Do not ask the patient to move and do not move the patient to test for a pain response. The patient may feel pain independent of movement or palpation, and there can be obvious deformity at the site of injury. Inspect for any soft tissue damage related to the injury. The patient may feel numbness, weakness, or tingling in the extremities or may have a complete loss of sensation below the suspected injury. The ability of the patient to walk or move or the lack of pain at the injured area does not rule out the possibility of spinal injury.

With responsive patients, ask what happened, where the discomfort is, and if the patient can move and feel the hands and feet. Inspect and palpate the patient for deformities, contusions, abrasion, punctures, penetrations, burns, tenderness, lacerations, and swelling. Assess the equality of strength in the extremities.

With unresponsive patients, determine the mechanism of injury and perform an initial assessment. Attempt to obtain information from others at the scene regarding the patient's mental status before your arrival.

Spinal injuries can lead to difficulty breathing and paralysis. Constantly monitor the patient for the development of these conditions. After every intervention, reassess the patient's vital signs and motor and sensory function.

Provide manual in-line stabilization and apply a cervical spinal immobilization device to all patients suspected of having head or spinal injuries. All airway control should be done with in-line immobilization. The initial assessment should be performed and any life threats treated. The patient should have full-body spinal immobilization using the appropriate technique.

INJURIES TO THE BRAIN AND SKULL

Injuries to the head may produce scalp and/or brain injuries. These injuries may bleed heavily because the area is vascular. Damage to brain tissue or blood leaking inside the skull increases the pressure inside the skull and can result in altered mental status. Nontraumatic conditions such as blood clots, hemorrhage, or lack of oxygen to the brain may cause similar damage.

After taking body substance isolation precautions, ensure a patent airway and provide artificial ventilations if needed, while providing manual spinal stabilization. The initial and focused assessments should be performed at the scene along with immobilization and the detailed physical examination done en route to the receiving facility. The spine should be immobilized with any head injury.

SPECIAL CONSIDERATIONS

Rapid extrication of a patient is indicated in situations in which the scene is unsafe, when the patient condition is unstable and warrants immediate movement and transport, or when the patient blocks access to another, more critically injured patient.

Helmet removal is indicated when you cannot assess or reassess the airway and breathing, when the helmet does not fit securely, when proper immobilization cannot be achieved, or when the patient is in cardiac arrest. The helmet should be left in place if the airway can be secured, the patient can be immobilized, there are no airway restrictions, removal would cause further injury, and the helmet fits securely.

Infants and children can be immobilized on a rigid board of appropriate size. Infants and children may need padding from the shoulders to the heels to maintain neutral positioning of the head. The cervical spinal immobilization device must be sized appropriately to avoid further injury.

Geriatric patients may have certain diseases that affect the bones and joints. They may not be able to lay flat on an immobilization device. For this reason, additional padding may be needed to pad all spaces between the patient's body and the immobilization device to provide adequate support.

UNITED STATES DEPARTMENT OF TRANSPORTATION NATIONAL HIGHWAY TRAFFIC SAFETY ADMINISTRATION EMT–BASIC OBJECTIVES

Check your knowledge. The National Registry of EMTs and many state EMS agencies use the objectives below to develop EMT–Basic certification examinations. Can you meet them?

COGNITIVE

1. State the components of the nervous system.
2. List the functions of the central nervous system.
3. Define the structure of the skeletal system as it relates to the nervous system.
4. Relate mechanism of injury to potential injuries of the head and spine.
5. Describe the implications of not properly caring for potential spine injuries.
6. State the signs and symptoms of a potential spine injury.
7. Describe the method for determining if a responsive patient may have a spine injury.
8. Relate the airway emergency medical care techniques to the patient with a suspected spine injury.
9. Describe how to stabilize the cervical spine.
10. Discuss indications for sizing and using a cervical spine immobilization device.
11. Establish the relationship between airway management and the patient with head and spine injuries.
12. Describe a method for sizing a cervical spine immobilization device.
13. Describe how to log roll a patient with a suspected spine injury.
14. Describe how to secure a patient to a long spine board.
15. List instances when a short spine board should be used.
16. Describe how to immobilize a patient using a short spine board.
17. Describe the indications for the use of rapid extrication.
18. List steps in performing rapid extrication.
19. State the circumstances when a helmet should be left on the patient.
20. Discuss the circumstances when a helmet should be removed.
21. Identify different types of helmets.
22. Describe the unique characteristics of sports helmets.
23. Explain the preferred methods to remove a helmet.
24. Discuss alternative methods for removal of a helmet.
25. Describe how the patient's head is stabilized to remove the helmet.
26. Differentiate how the head is stabilized with a helmet compared to without a helmet.

AFFECTIVE

1. Explain the rationale for immobilization of the entire spine when a cervical spine injury is suspected.
2. Explain the rationale for utilizing immobilization methods apart from the straps on the cots.
3. Explain the rationale for using a short spine immobilization device when moving a patient from the sitting to the supine position.
4. Explain the rationale for utilizing rapid extrication approaches only when they indeed will make the difference between life and death.
5. Defend the reasons for leaving a helmet in place for transport of a patient.
6. Defend the reasons for removal of helmet prior to transport of a patient.

PSYCHOMOTOR

1. Demonstrate opening the airway in a patient with suspected spinal cord injury.
2. Demonstrate evaluating a responsive patient with a suspected spinal cord injury.
3. Demonstrate stabilization of the cervical spine.
4. Demonstrate the four-person log roll for a patient with a suspected spinal cord injury.
5. Demonstrate how to log roll a patient with a suspected spinal cord injury using two people.
6. Demonstrate securing a patient to a long spine board.
7. Demonstrate using the short board immobilization technique.
8. Demonstrate procedure for rapid extrication.
9. Demonstrate the preferred methods for stabilization of a helmet.
10. Demonstrate helmet removal techniques.
11. Demonstrate alternative methods for stabilization of a helmet.
12. Demonstrate completing a prehospital care report for patients with head and spinal injuries.

It is very rewarding to turn people on to the joys of working with kids. Half of my mission is to give medical caregivers information and confidence. The other half is to give them permission to have fun and enjoy themselves.

Lou Romig, MD, FAAP
Pediatric Emergency Medicine Attending Physician EMS Liaison Miami Children's Hospital Miami, Florida

There are two major challenges in pediatric emergency care: overcoming your own natural reaction to pediatric illness or injury, and dealing with parents. The former can be by far the easier to handle!

Laurie Romig, MD, FACEP
President, The Emergency Solutions Institute, Inc. St. Petersburg, Florida

INFANT AND CHILD EMERGENCY CARE

KEY TERMS

Adolescent: A child 12 to 18 years of age.

Blow-by oxygen: Method of oxygen delivery for infants and children without placing a mask on the face.

Central lines: Intravenous lines surgically placed near the heart for long-term use.

Child abuse: An improper or excessive action by parents, guardians, or caretakers that injures or causes harm to children.

Drowning: Death from suffocation within the first 24 hours of submersion in liquid.

Gastric tube: A tube placed directly into the stomach for feeding.

Grunting: A sound made when a patient in respiratory distress attempts to trap air to keep the alveoli open.

Infant: A child less than 1 year of age.

Nasal flaring: An attempt by the infant in respiratory distress to increase the size of the airway by expanding the nostrils.

Near drowning: Survival past 24 hours after suffocation due to submersion in liquid.

Neglect: The act of not giving attention to a child's essential needs.

Newborn: The term for an infant from birth to 1 month of age.

Preschool child: A child from 3 to 6 years of age.

Respiratory failure: A clinical condition when the patient is continuing to work hard to breathe, the effort of breathing is increased, and the patient's condition begins to deteriorate.

Respiratory distress: A clinical condition in which the infant or child begins to increase the work of breathing.

Retractions: The use of accessory muscles to increase the work of breathing, which appears as the sucking in of the muscles between the ribs and at the neck.

School-age child: A child from 6 to 12 years of age.

Secondary drowning: The rapid deterioration of respiratory status from several hours to 96 hours after resuscitation.

Shunt: A tube running from the brain to the abdomen to drain excess cerebrospinal fluid.

Sudden Infant Death Syndrome (SIDS): The sudden, unexplained death of an infant, generally between the ages of 1 month and 1 year, for which there is no discernable cause.

Toddler: A child 1 to 3 years of age.

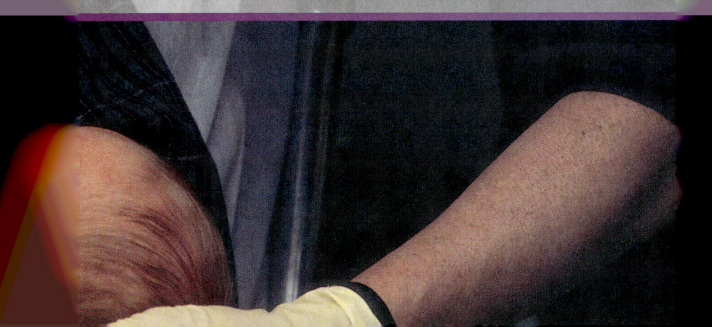

IN THE FIELD

EMTs Jorge and Sandra responded to a motor vehicle collision. En route to the scene, dispatch advised them that the incident involved two cars and that a 3-year-old child was injured. Immediately, both Jorge and Sandra felt the adrenaline starting to pump. They had no specific information about the nature of the injuries, but the thought of caring for an injured child caused anxiety. Sandra could see Jorge was thinking the same thing and reminded him that they had been well educated for this. They knew to start with the basics of airway, breathing, and circulation. They quickly reviewed the developmental characteristics of a 3-year-old. When they arrived at the scene they were both functioning well as a team, ready to take on the challenge of dealing with an injured child.

Emergency medical care providers have long been challenged by the unique aspects of caring for ill or injured infants and children. Understanding the developmental characteristics of infants and children, as well as anatomic and physiological differences, is essential for providing good patient care. These patients are significantly different from adults.

Special attention should be given to pediatric patients in areas such as airway management, oxygenation and ventilation, assessment, trauma, and near drowning. Unfortunately, as well, some children are victims of abuse and neglect. In all these instances, you must know how to deal with these difficult situations.

Finally, as an EMT you will deal with parents who have strong emotional responses when their child is ill or injured. In addition to the parents' emotional response, you must deal with your own feelings associated with caring for an ill or injured child.

DEVELOPMENTAL DIFFERENCES IN INFANTS AND CHILDREN

Developmental differences in infants and children should influence your approach to their care. Understanding these differences will help you assess and treat the ill or injured child.

NEWBORNS AND INFANTS

Newborn is the term for an infant from birth to 1 month of age, and an **infant** is a child less than 1 year of age. Infants and newborns are often less afraid of strangers and tolerate assessment and interventions fairly well (Fig. 29-1). However, they do not like to be separated from their parents. Oxygen masks may be frightening, and newborns and infants may not tolerate having masks placed directly on their faces.

Because they can lose body heat quickly, these patients must be kept warm. Try to make the environment warm. Warm your hands and stethoscope before touching the newborn or infant. A newborn or infant who is to be transported should be covered, especially the head; be careful not to cover the face or airway. Keep the surrounding air temperature warm whenever possible, even if the

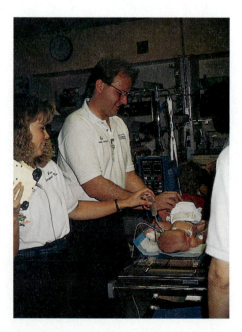

Fig. 29-1 Assessing a newborn.

temperature becomes uncomfortable for you. Heat loss in infants can cause poor circulation and increases the need for oxygen as the body tries to correct the body temperature.

Try to involve the parents in your assessment. If the situation is appropriate, allow the infant to remain on the parent's lap. As you assess a newborn or infant, examine the heart and lungs first, and the head last to prevent upsetting the infant. Try to obtain heart and lung sounds before the child becomes agitated. You can assess the respiratory rate from a distance by observing the infant and watching the effort of breathing. In addition to watching the rise and fall of the chest, note the infant's skin color, level of activity, interactions with caregivers, and use of accessory muscles to breathe.

TODDLERS

Toddlers are children from 1 to 3 years of age (Fig. 29-2). These patients may pose a challenge in their assessment and care. They do not like to be touched or separated from their parents. As you examine toddlers, remove or simply move their clothing, examine the area, and replace the clothing. It may be helpful to have the parents remove the child's clothing when possible. Many toddlers do not like to be without their clothing. Share your penlight or stethoscope with the child before using them. Examine the parent, a teddy bear, or similar object first. Like newborns and infants, they do not like the feeling of an oxygen mask.

Toddlers often think that the illness or injury is punishment for something they have done. Reassure toddlers that they are not bad and that they are not being punished. Toddlers are also afraid of

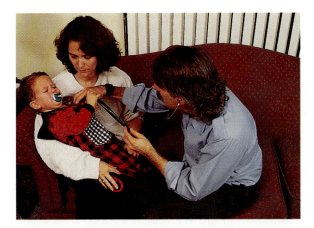

Fig. 29-2   Toddlers can be uncooperative and difficult to assess. Be patient and have the parent help while you perform the assessment.

needles and pain. If a procedure will hurt, be honest: tell them and complete the procedure quickly. Remember to keep your language simple when speaking with a toddler.

Like newborns and infants, toddlers should be examined with a trunk-to-toe-to-head approach, to build the children's confidence in you. Show children your hands and equipment as you approach. Try not to surprise them. Approach children on their own level; don't tower over them. The assessment should also be performed efficiently and quickly before children become agitated.

PRESCHOOL CHILDREN

Preschool children are from 3 to 6 years of age. Like toddlers, preschoolers do not like to be touched. They do not like to be separated from their parents or have their clothing removed. As with toddlers, remove or move the clothes, examine the child, and replace the clothing. Preschoolers also may feel suffocated by an oxygen mask.

Like toddlers, many preschoolers may think that the illness or injury is a punishment. Assure these children that you do not think they were bad. They are afraid of blood, pain, and permanent injury. If they are affected by the sight of blood, cover the area or clean it as quickly as possible. While they may not object to having their clothing removed, their modesty should be respected. Language skills in this age group allow them to give a history and to understand simple directions.

Preschoolers enjoy exploring. Your equipment may provide a convenient distraction during your examination. Talk with the patient during the assessment and always approach the painful area last.

SCHOOL-AGE CHILDREN

School-age children are 6 to 12 years of age. School-age children are more independent than toddlers and preschoolers; however, they still look to their parents for support (Fig. 29-3). In general, they are not afraid of strangers. Like preschoolers, their modesty needs to be respected, and clothing should be replaced after the area is assessed. School-age children fear blood and pain. They are also very concerned that an injury may leave them with permanent disfigurement. By keeping the parents close, you are better able to communicate with these patients. Treat these children with respect. Speak to them directly and ask them to help you. Younger school-age children often try stalling tactics when faced with a painful procedure. Try to

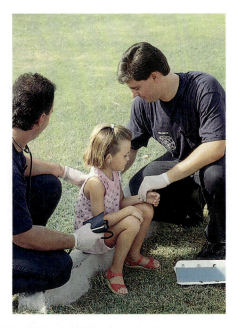

Fig. 29-3 School-age children are generally more cooperative than younger children, and need respect and protection of their modesty.

give them some control over timing of the procedure, but be firm and quickly complete the task that must be done.

ADOLESCENTS

Adolescents are 12 to 18 years of age. They may not be as mature as adults, but they should be treated as adults. Like school-age children, they are concerned about appearance and are very concerned with the possibility of permanent disfigurement and death. Respect their right to modesty and privacy. Adolescents may prefer to be assessed and questioned away from their parents or guardians. If the parents object, understand that adolescents may be less open in personal matters.

THE AIRWAY

ANATOMIC AND PHYSIOLOGICAL CONCERNS

The most important anatomical and physiological differences in infants and children relate to the airway. In general, the airways are smaller and more easily blocked by secretions and swelling. Methods of positioning the airway are different in infants and children. Do not hyperextend the neck because the airway is so flexible it may actually become occluded because of kinking.

The tongue is relatively large in relationship to the small mandible and oropharynx. This can easily cause an airway obstruction in unresponsive infants and children when they are supine. A proper head tilt-chin lift or jaw thrust maneuver can overcome this problem. Take special care not to place pressure on the soft tissues under the jaw, as this may occlude the airway.

Infants are obligate nose breathers: they do not open their mouth to breathe when their nose is occluded. Suctioning a secretion-filled nasopharynx can improve breathing problems in an infant.

Children can compensate for a breathing problem for a short period of time. Infants and children compensate by increasing the rate and effort of breathing. This increased work of breathing uses a tremendous amount of energy. After a short period of compensating, the child may experience rapid decompensation characterized by general and muscular fatigue. This is a sign of respiratory failure. Because of this, a normal respiratory rate following a fast rate may be a bad sign, especially if the child looks tired or is otherwise doing poorly. Watch for signs of mental status changes, including drowsiness, and unusual tolerance of assessment procedures and treatments such as oxygen masks.

OPENING THE AIRWAY

Chapter 7, "The Airway," describes the techniques for opening an airway using the head tilt-chin lift and the jaw thrust. Because most problems leading to the death of infants and children are related to airway difficulties, you must be knowledgeable and skilled in these techniques.

When a patient loses consciousness, the muscles relax and the tongue may fall back and occlude the airway. Because these structures are attached to the lower jaw, the airway can be opened by lifting up on the lower jaw. This can be accomplished with the head-tilt chin-lift, or when trauma is suspected, the jaw thrust without head tilt. When performing a head tilt, be careful not to hyperextend the neck. Hyperextension may occlude the small flexible airway of infants and young children. Extend the head on the neck only until the bottom of the nose points straight up. This is referred to as the "sniffing position" for infants and children. Technique 29-1 describes the steps for the head-tilt chin-lift.

When you suspect trauma, use the jaw-thrust without head tilt. With the jaw thrust maneuver, maintain the head in a neutral position, and lift the chin up and out by applying pressure to the angle of

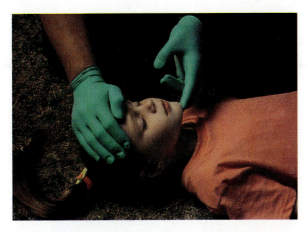

Fig. 29-4   When performing a head tilt for an infant or child, be careful not to hyperextend the neck but to use the "sniffing position."

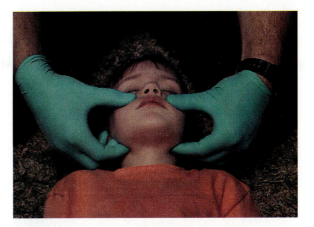

Fig. 29-5   A jaw thrust is performed using the same technique for children and adults.

the posterior jaw (Fig 29-5). Be sure to manually stabilize the spine while using this technique.

SUCTIONING

Suction may be required to clear the airway of secretions, blood, or vomit. In infants, take care not to stimulate the back of the patient's throat by touching it with the suction catheter. This stimulation can dramatically slow the infant's heart rate or cause a gag reflex or vomiting.

Suction the infant or child's airway only as deeply as you can see. In general, use a soft flexible catheter for infants and children. Measure the length of the catheter from the central incisor to the angle of the jaw. Place your finger on the catheter at this measurement. Do not insert the catheter beyond the base of the tongue. To ensure that the patient does not become deprived of oxygen, limit the suctioning to 10 to 15 seconds. Rinse the catheter and suction tubing as necessary. Be sure to preoxygenate the patient before suctioning and immediately following suctioning. When using a suction device with infants and children, the

vacuum should be limited to 80 to 120 mm Hg. Technique 29-2 describes the steps for suctioning.

Always consider the need for nasal suctioning. In infants, nasal secretions can cause significant upper airway obstruction. Mechanical suction may be used, but a bulb syringe is also simple and effective at removing nasal secretions. When using the bulb syringe, remember to squeeze out the air before inserting the tip into a nostril.

USING AIRWAY ADJUNCTS

Oropharyngeal and nasopharyngeal airways are useful in maintaining an open airway in infants and children when the head-tilt chin-lift or jaw thrust maneuvers are ineffective. They are not used for initial ventilation efforts.

OROPHARYNGEAL AIRWAY

An oral airway should be used following the head-tilt chin-lift only if the patient is unresponsive and has no gag reflex. If the oral airway is used in a patient who has a gag reflex, the patient may gag and vomit. This can seriously threaten the airway. The preferred method of inserting an oral airway in infants and children is to use a tongue depressor to insert the airway without rotating, thereby reducing the potential for damage to the soft palate. Technique 29-3 details the steps for inserting an oral airway in infants and children.

NASOPHARYNGEAL AIRWAY

The nasopharyngeal airway is less likely to stimulate vomiting than the oropharyngeal airway and is valuable for patients who are responsive but need assistance in maintaining the airway. It is very

TECHNIQUE 29-1
Head-Tilt Chin-Lift Technique

Gently lift the chin up and out. Push down on the forehead to tilt the head back. Do not close the mouth. Take special care not to hyperextend the neck (*see* Fig. 29-4).

TECHNIQUE 29-2
Suctioning

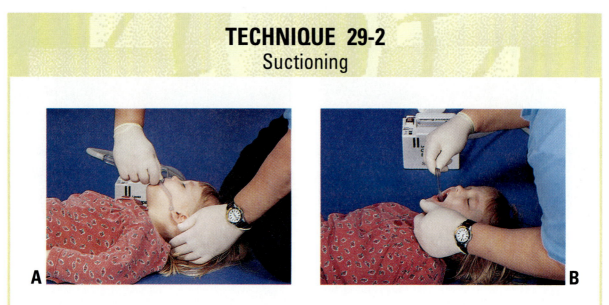

Fig. 29-6 Inspect the portable and on-board suction units at the beginning of each shift to ensure that they are working and cleaned properly. If the unit has a pressure gauge, the pump should be able to generate an 80 to 120 mm Hg vacuum. Battery-operated units should be fully charged at all times and ready for use. Follow body substance isolation precautions. Turn on the power. You will hear the motor start. Check for the presence of adequate suction by placing your thumb over the suction hose. Select and attach a catheter to the end of the suction hose. **A, Measure the distance from the central incisor to the angle of the jaw, and place your fingers at this mark. B, Insert the catheter into the mouth without suction. This makes it easier to control the tip of the catheter during insertion. You can either keep your finger off the hole in the catheter or keep the unit off while you place the catheter into the patient's mouth.** If there are copious amounts of fluid in the mouth, suction immediately upon placing the catheter into the patient's mouth. Insert the catheter until your fingertips reach the lips. This will prevent you from inserting the catheter too far. Once you have placed the catheter into the patient's mouth, apply suction by occluding the hole in the catheter or turning the unit on. Never suction for more than 10 to 15 seconds at a time. To prevent the suction catheter or tubing from becoming clogged, you can intermittently suction water to clear the line. This same technique can be used for nasal suctioning.

TECHNIQUE 29-3
Inserting the Oral Airway in Infants and Children

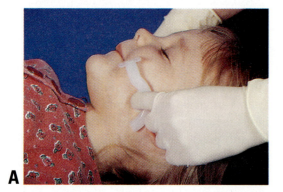
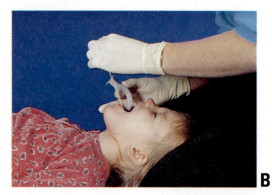

Fig. 29-7 Follow body substance isolation precautions. **A, Select the proper size airway by measuring from the corner of the patient's mouth to the angle of the jaw. B, Position yourself at the top of the patient's head. Open the patient's mouth and use a tongue depressor to move the tongue forward. Insert the airway right side up (with the tip facing toward the floor of the patient's mouth).** Advance the airway gently until the flange comes to rest on the patient's lips. Be sure not to push the tongue into the back of the throat. Ventilate the patient as needed.

TECHNIQUE 29-4
Technique for Inserting a Nasopharyngeal Airway

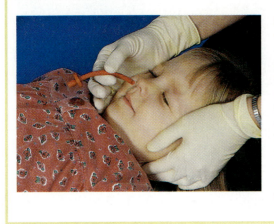

Fig. 29-8   Follow body substance isolation precautions. Select the proper size airway by measuring from the tip of the nose to the earlobe. Also consider the diameter of the patient's nostril. The nasopharyngeal airway should not be so large that it causes sustained blanching of the nostril. Lubricate the airway with a water-soluble lubricant. **Insert the airway into the nostril with the bevel toward the base of the nostril or the nasal septum. Most nasal airways are designed to be inserted into the right nostril.** Guide the airway along the floor of the nose. Advance the airway gently until the flange comes to rest at the patient's nostril. If any resistance is met, withdraw the airway. Forcing the airway may cause injury. Suction the nasal airway after insertion to remove secretions. Ventilate the patient as needed.

useful after seizures when the muscles of the throat and face relax. It should not be used in patients with head trauma. Technique 29-4 details the steps for inserting a nasopharyngeal airway.

If you cannot advance the airway in one nostril, try the other. Never force the nasal airway past or through an obstruction. Even a well-lubricated nasopharyngeal airway may be uncomfortable for the patient and may elicit a pain response. Upon insertion the patient may gag, but after it is inserted some patients may say that they feel it in the back of the throat but it is not too bothersome.

OXYGEN THERAPY

Remember that oxygen is always given to a patient who needs it, regardless of the patient's age. When deciding how to deliver oxygen to an infant or child, keep in mind developmental factors. Infants, toddlers, and preschoolers may feel that they are suffocating from wearing an oxygen mask. Never force an oxygen mask onto a child's face. The patient's struggle to avoid would increase the oxygen demand. Unless the child is in severe respiratory distress, the **blow-by oxygen** method should be used for oxygen delivery. *Blow-by oxygen* means that an oxygen delivery device is held close to the infant's or child's nose and mouth without actually being placed on the face. Often the parents can help deliver oxygen to the child. Some children may be able to assist by holding their own mask. Because

many children do not like to be separated from their parents, the parent or guardian may hold the oxygen mask or tubing near the patient's face.

BLOW-BY OXYGEN

To administer oxygen with the blow-by method, hold the oxygen tubing about 5 cm (2 in) from the patient's face. Another blow-by method is to place the tubing through a hole in a paper cup and hold the cup close to the infant's face. If a cup is not available, the tubing alone or a simple face mask may be used. The flow should be set at a rate of 5 L/min for infants and 10 L/min for children. Any greater flow rate may cause the infant to become hypothermic, as the oxygen flowing from the tubing is cool. Ideally the oxygen should be warmed if possible before administration.

Often it helps to have the family members involved in caring for the patient. This is beneficial not only to the patient but may also help the parent feel useful and part of the process of providing care. Ask the parent to assist with oxygen administration (Fig. 29-9).

NONREBREATHER MASKS

The nonrebreather mask is the preferred method for delivering oxygen to patients in prehospital settings. This is a high-flow device that can deliver up to 90% oxygen when the flow rate is set at a rate of 15 L/min and the mask is tightly sealed against the face. The nonrebreather mask stores oxygen in a reservoir bag. You should inflate this

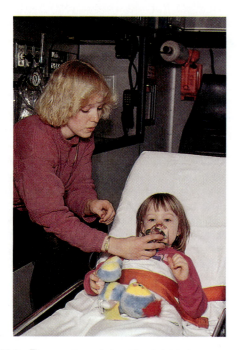

Fig. 29-9 The parent can help with administering oxygen to an infant or child.

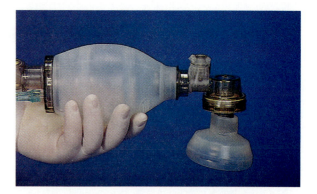

Fig. 29-10 The pop-off valve on a pediatric bag-valve-mask must be taped shut or turned off to ensure effective ventilations during pediatric resuscitation measures.

bag before you place the mask on the patient and be sure that it does not collapse completely while the patient is breathing. Be sure to select the correct sized mask for the patient. Most young children do not tolerate having a mask placed over their faces unless they have a decreased level of responsiveness.

ARTIFICIAL VENTILATIONS

When needed, provide artificial ventilation through the mouth-to-mask or bag-valve-mask method. Regardless of the method used, the tidal volume should be large enough to create a gentle chest rise. The rate for infants and children is 20 breaths per minute, or one breath every 3 seconds.

Bag-valve-mask devices are a rapid means of ventilating nonbreathing patients and may also be useful in patients with respiratory distress. To deliver a high concentration of oxygen, the bag-valve-mask must be connected to an oxygen source and have a reservoir attached.

Many pediatric bags are equipped with a pop-off valve. This valve is in place to eliminate the risk of lung injury due to high-pressure ventilation. During resuscitation attempts, the pop-off valve may hinder the delivery of adequate ventilations. If the patient has increased resistance or increased airway pressure, the pop-off valve may prevent ventilations from being effective. Increased resistance may occur in cases of an airway obstruction caused by

swelling or a foreign body. In all cases of pediatric resuscitation, the pop-off valve must be disabled. Taping the pop-off valve down is one method of disabling the valve (Fig. 29-10). Assess the adequacy of ventilation by observing an adequate rise and fall of the chest. Take care not to give strong abrupt ventilations. Allow the chest to fall before ventilating again. Try to achieve a smooth, rhythmic ventilation pattern.

When ventilating an infant or child, choose a bag-valve-mask of 450 to 750 mL. The smaller 250-mL bag may produce a tidal volume insufficient to ventilate the child. Larger bags may not provide you with a sense of resistance or delivered tidal volume. In older children and adolescents, use a bag with a volume of at least 1000 mL.

Face masks are available in a wide variety of shapes and sizes. Choose an appropriate size mask for the patient. The mask should extend from the bridge of the nose to the cleft of the chin, completely covering the mouth and nose but not putting pressure on the eyes. Excessive pressure on the eyes may cause the heart rate to decrease. Over- or under-sized masks can impede effective ventilation. If the only available mask is too large for the patient, turn the mask so that the pointed end is sealed over the chin instead of the nose. This helps maintain an adequate seal.

The mask is sealed over the patient's mouth and nose, ensuring a tight mask seal (Fig. 29-11). As the mask is held securely in place, the jaw thrust or head-tilt chin-lift should be maintained. One EMT maintains the mask seal and positioning while the other squeezes the bag.

The recommended rate of ventilation is once every 3 seconds for infants and children. As you ventilate, observe the chest for a gentle rise.

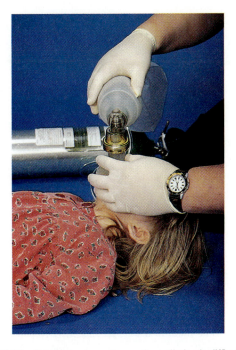

Fig. 29-11 One-person bag-valve-mask ventilation is difficult and requires much practice to perform effectively.

Another good indicator of adequate ventilation is improvement in heart rate and color. Take care to avoid over-inflation of the lungs.

Practicing these skills is essential to ensure that you stay competent with them for dealing with infants and children. Routinely practice the techniques of opening the airway, suctioning, insertion of an airway, and mouth-to-mask and bag-valve-mask ventilations.

ASSESSMENT

Once you have sized-up the scene and are prepared to assess the patient, perform an initial assessment. Assessment of infants and children requires knowledge of their developmental stages. In many cases, you can begin your assessment from a distance. Mental status, respiratory distress, and many signs and symptoms of shock can be assessed long before you touch the patient. Some patients require a trunk-to-toe-to-head approach to physical examination. Use your experience and clinical judgment to determine the order best for the patient. Always try to assess painful areas last.

In general, begin the assessment from a distance. Form a general impression of the child being well or sick based on overall appearance. Look at the patient as you enter the room. Is the child interacting appropriately with the people or items in the envi-

ronment? Does the child recognize the parents? Infants begin to recognize their parents at about 2 months of age, and failure to recognize them is an ominous sign. Is the infant or child quiet and disinterested, or is the infant or child playing with a favorite toy? Is the patient appropriately distressed or scared, or unusually quiet?

Assess mental status. Mental status changes may result in the child being uninterested in any activity or person. In some cases mental status changes may be recognized simply by the parent saying "There is something wrong." Mental status is characterized and documented in the same terms as with adults:
<u>A</u>-alert
<u>V</u>-responds to voice
<u>P</u>-responds to pain
<u>U</u>-unresponsive.

For newborns and infants, "responds to voice" means the infant turns to the parent's voice; young children typically may not obey commands.

If necessary, open the airway. Look, listen, and feel for breathing. Also look at the effort of breathing. Increased effort may be seen as nasal flaring, the use of accessory muscles, retractions, and airway noises. Evaluate the quality of the cry or speech. Determine if breath sounds are present or absent (Fig. 29-12). If necessary, administer oxygen or provide artificial ventilations. Look for equal bilateral expansion of the chest. Listen to breath sounds on each side of the chest, as far lateral as possible. Are there any associated sounds such as wheezing or stridor? As part of your respiratory assessment, assess skin color. Be alert for a dusky or bluish color to the skin. Remember that the patient may be deprived of oxygen without being cyanotic. Infants and children usually have a mottled skin color before cyanosis. Look for central cyanosis at

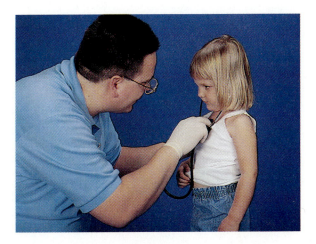

Fig. 29-12 Listening for breath sounds on a pediatric patient.

the mucous membranes and for cool extremities with a mottled color. Keep in mind that cyanosis is a late sign.

Assess circulation using the brachial and femoral pulses in infants (Fig. 29-13). In addition to heart rate, assess for quality and equality. Compare the quality of the two pulses. Any differences may be an indicator of inadequate perfusion. In children younger than 6 years of age, assess capillary refill by pressing on the skin or nailbed and counting the number of seconds until the color returns. If the infant or child is cool or cold, test capillary refill over a bony prominence in the central part of the child. Capillary refill should be less than 2 seconds. If capillary refill takes longer, the infant or child may have a perfusion problem. Assess skin color, temperature, and moisture. Assess blood pressure in children older than 3 years of age. Do not waste time attempting to get a blood pressure measurement if there are other things to do for the child.

Based on the findings from the initial assessment, you can determine the patient's priority. Infants and children with altered mental status, respiratory distress, or poor perfusion should be considered priority patients.

How you perform the focused history and physical examination or the detailed physical examination depends on the situation and the patient's age. In general this examination is often best done in a trunk-to-head approach. The components are the same as for an adult. Even though you start with the trunk, you should still assess for DCAP-BTLS. This approach provides valuable information about the patient while building the infant's or child's trust and confidence. Chapter 5, "Baseline Vital Signs and SAMPLE History," lists the average ranges of vital signs by age.

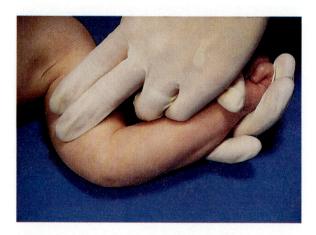

Fig. 29-13 Assessing the brachial pulse in infants.

REVIEW QUESTIONS

Match the age range for each of the following developmental categories.

1. _____ Newborn and infant
2. _____ Toddler
3. _____ Preschool
4. _____ School age
5. _____ Adolescent

   A. 3 to 6 years
   B. birth to 1 year
   C. 12 to 18 years
   D. 1 to 3 years
   E. 6 to 12 years

6. Compared to adults, the airways of infants and children are _____ and more easily _____ by secretions and swelling.

7. To open the airway of an injured child, EMTs should perform the _____.

8. When assessing infants and younger children, EMTs should start with the _____ of the body and finish with the _____.

9. Suctioning in the infant and child should be limited to:
   A. 5 to 10 seconds
   B. 10 to 15 seconds
   C. 15 to 20 seconds

10. The oral airway must be inserted by using a _____ without _____.

11. When ventilating an infant or child, you should _____ the pop-off valve.

12. Capillary refill should be assessed in infants in children less than _____ years old.

COMMON PROBLEMS IN INFANTS AND CHILDREN

This section reviews common medical emergencies. Understanding of the nature of common illnesses and their signs and symptoms helps prepare you to deal with pediatric medical emergencies in the field.

AIRWAY OBSTRUCTION

It is important to recognize the difference between partial and complete airway obstruction. If you interfere with a child's attempt to clear a partial airway obstruction, you could cause a complete obstruction. Table 29-1 highlights important comparisons of airway obstruction from foreign body and airway disease.

PARTIAL OBSTRUCTION

Partial airway obstructions are characterized by noisy respirations, sometimes with stridor or crowing. The child may be coughing. Retractions may be seen on inhalation. In general, the nailbeds and the mucous membranes are pink with signs of good peripheral perfusion because even though there is a partial obstruction, there is adequate air exchange. These infants and children are often awake and agitated. If cyanosis or altered mental status is present, there may be a complete obstruction.

Emergency Care of Patients With Partial Airway Obstruction. To assist an infant or child with a partial airway obstruction, first pay attention to positioning. Allow the child to maintain a position of comfort: assist a younger child to sit up, but do not allow the patient to lie supine, as this may worsen the obstruction. Many children will be more comfortable sitting in their parent's lap. You or a parent may offer oxygen with the blow-by method. The patient should be transported to a hospital for further evaluation. Be aware that transporting a child sitting in a parent's lap may compromise your ability to assure them safety through proper restraints. Never buckle a lap belt over both parent and child. For safety you may need to separate the parent and child; if so keep the parent restrained close and within the child's field of vision.

Make every effort to keep the child comfortable; do not agitate the child. Agitation increases the work of breathing and further complicates the situation. Perform only a limited examination. Do not assess the blood pressure because this may upset the child. If there is a deterioration in color or mental status, a complete obstruction has likely occurred.

TABLE 29-1	Comparison of Airway Obstructions from Foreign Body and Airway Illness Disease		
	PARTIAL UPPER AIRWAY OBSTRUCTION	**COMPLETE UPPER AIRWAY OBSTRUCTION**	**LOWER AIRWAY OBSTRUCTION DUE TO ILLNESS**
GENERAL APPEARANCE	Relatively well to sick	Very sick	Relatively well to very sick
WORK OF BREATHING	Increased, seen in inspiratory phase	Gasping or no effort	Increased, often seen in expiratory phase
COLOR	Normal to pale	Pale to cyanotic	Normal to cyanotic
NOISES	Inspiratory stridor or crowing. Barking cough or hoarse voice.	None, unable to cough or speak	Expiratory wheezes. Wheezy cough, hoarse voice
HISTORY	Suggestive of foreign body obstruction, cold symptoms	Suggestive of foreign body obstruction, cold symptoms	History of airway disease such as asthma or bronchitis. History of allergies

COMPLETE OBSTRUCTION

Complete airway obstruction is a life-threatening emergency. Any partial airway obstruction with altered mental status or cyanosis should be treated as a complete obstruction. Complete obstructions require immediate intervention.

Patients with complete airway obstruction cannot cry or speak. Cyanosis is often present. When complete obstruction follows partial airway obstruction, the infant's or child's efforts to clear the airway by coughing become ineffective. Increased respiratory effort is seen.

Emergency Care for the Responsive Infant With Foreign Body Airway Obstruction. Determine the presence of a complete obstruction by assessing for signs of a complete airway obstruction and assessing the environment. In some cases, the family may be suspicious of an airway obstruction if the infant or child was playing with toys with small parts or eating foods such as hot dogs or peanuts.

If the infant is unable to cry or cough effectively,

TECHNIQUE 29-5
Care for Complete Airway Obstruction in a Responsive Infant

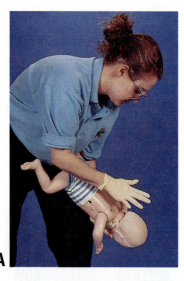

A

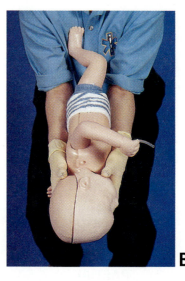

B

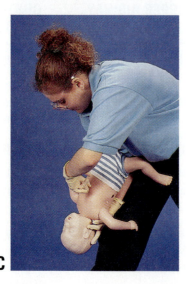

C

Fig. 29-14 Determine the presence of complete airway obstruction. **A, Support the head and body and place the infant in a position with the head lower than the trunk. With the heel of the free hand deliver up to five back blows between the shoulder blades. B, Turn the infant over. Support the head, neck, and body. C, Deliver up to five chest thrusts. Alternate back blows and chest thrusts until the obstruction is relieved or patient becomes unresponsive.**

TECHNIQUE 29-6
Care for Complete Airway Obstruction in an Unresponsive Infant

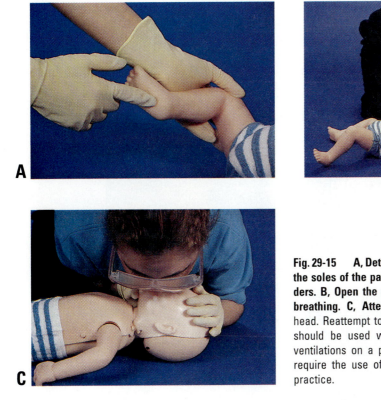

Fig. 29-15   A, Determine responsiveness by tapping the soles of the patient's feet or the patient's shoulders. B, Open the airway. Look, listen, and feel for breathing. C, Attempt to ventilate. Reposition the head. Reattempt to ventilate. *Note:* A barrier device should be used when performing mouth-to-mouth ventilations on a patient. Some agencies may also require the use of a barrier device for mannequin practice.   *Continued*

support the infant's head and neck with one hand. Support the trunk with your forearm, and hold the infant face-down with the head lower than the trunk. With the heel of your free hand, deliver up to five back blows between the shoulder blades.

If the obstruction is not relieved, support the head, turn the infant over, and again position the head lower than the trunk. Support the head with your hand and the back with your forearm. Perform up to five chest thrusts. The chest thrusts should be delivered over the lower half of the sternum using the same landmarks as for chest compressions. Be sure to avoid the xiphoid process.

Alternate the back blows and chest thrusts in rapid sequence until the obstruction is relieved or the infant becomes unresponsive. Technique 29-5 details the steps of care for complete airway obstruction in responsive infant.

Emergency Care for the Unresponsive Infant With Foreign Body Airway Obstruction. Deter-mine that the infant is unresponsive by gently tapping or shaking the shoulders. Open the airway. Assess for the presence of breathing. If the infant is not breathing, attempt to deliver two breaths. If unsuccessful, reposition the head and try again. If the attempts at breathing remain unsuccessful, deliver up to five back blows as previously described. Following the back blows, deliver up to five chest thrusts. Following each series of up to five back blows and up to five chest thrusts, open the mouth using the tongue jaw lift and inspect the oropharynx for a foreign object. If you see an object, remove it using a finger sweep. Do not perform blind finger sweeps. Repeat these steps until the obstruction is relieved. After relieving the obstruction, assess the patient for spontaneous respirations and pulse. Provide chest compressions and ventilations as needed. Follow your local transport protocol if the obstruction cannot be relieved. Even if the object is relieved, the patient should be transported

TECHNIQUE 29-6
Care for Complete Airway Obstruction in an Unresponsive Infant

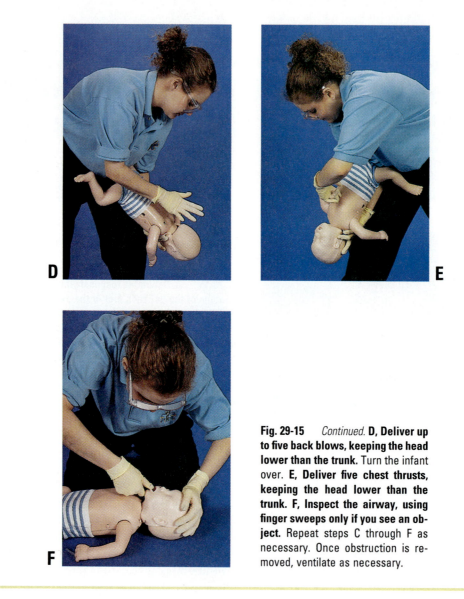

Fig. 29-15   *Continued.* **D, Deliver up to five back blows, keeping the head lower than the trunk.** Turn the infant over. **E, Deliver five chest thrusts, keeping the head lower than the trunk. F, Inspect the airway, using finger sweeps only if you see an object.** Repeat steps C through F as necessary. Once obstruction is removed, ventilate as necessary.

for evaluation of the airway. Technique 29-6 details the steps of care for complete airway obstruction in unresponsive infants.

Emergency Care for the Responsive Child With Foreign Body Airway Obstruction.   Complete airway obstructions are handled differently in children. First determine the presence of a complete airway obstruction. If a cough is ineffective or not present, you must perform the sub-diaphragmatic thrusts. Do not perform back blows. Stand or kneel behind the child and place your arms around the child's waist. Make a fist with one hand. Locate the umbilicus and the xiphoid process with the other. Position your fist on the abdomen between these two landmarks. With quick inward and upward thrusts, attempt to dislodge the obstruction. Keep in mind that it may take several series of five thrusts to relieve the obstruction. Repeat this process until the object is dislodged or the child becomes unresponsive.

If the child becomes unresponsive, assist the child to the floor. Place the child on the back. Open the mouth and attempt to visualize the obstruction. If you see an object, remove it using a finger sweep. Do not perform blind finger sweeps. If you cannot see an object, open the airway using the head-tilt chin-lift. Attempt to ventilate the child. If unsuccessful, perform abdominal thrusts. Kneel astride or next to the patient's thighs. Locate the umbilicus and the xiphoid process. Place the heel of one hand between these landmarks. Place the second hand on top of the hand resting on the abdomen. Perform up to five inward and upward thrusts. Again, the intent is to relieve the obstruction. Using the tongue jaw lift, inspect the oropharynx. If you see an object, remove it. Attempt to ventilate. If unsuccessful with your ventilation, repeat the sequence until the airway obstruction is relieved. As with infants, follow your local protocol for transporting the patient if the obstruction cannot be relieved. Technique 29-7 details the steps of care for complete airway obstruction in a responsive child.

TECHNIQUE 29-7
Care for Complete Airway Obstruction in a Responsive Child

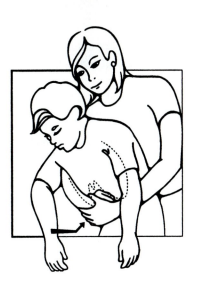

Fig. 29-16   Determine the presence of complete obstruction. **Stand or kneel behind the child. Locate landmarks for abdominal thrusts. Place fist in between landmarks.** Use quick inward and upward thrusts. Continue until the object is dislodged or the child becomes unresponsive.

Emergency Care for the Unresponsive Child With Foreign Body Airway Obstruction. Determine that the child is unresponsive. This may occur during your initial assessment or after unsuccessful attempts to clear the airway of a responsive child. Using the tongue jaw lift, quickly look for and remove any foreign object seen in the mouth. Do not perform a blind finger sweep. Open the airway and attempt to ventilate the child. If unsuccessful, reposition the child's head and reattempt the ventilation. If the airway remains obstructed, perform abdominal thrusts. Kneel astride or next to the patient's thighs. Locate the umbilicus and the xiphoid process. Place the heel of one hand between these landmarks. Perform up to five inward and upward thrusts. Using the tongue jaw lift, inspect the oropharynx. If you see an object, remove it. Attempt to ventilate. If unsuccessful, repeat the sequence until the airway obstruction is relieved. Follow local transport protocol if the obstruction cannot be relieved. Technique 29-8 details the steps of care for complete obstruction in an unresponsive child.

RESPIRATORY EMERGENCIES

The rapid recognition and treatment of respiratory emergencies in infants and children is the priority equivalent to recognition of shockable rhythms, early CPR, and early defibrillation in adults. More than 80% of all cardiac arrests in infants and children start as respiratory arrests. The two best ways to prevent unexpected death in children are to prevent injuries and to recognize and intervene early in respiratory emergencies.

EMTs must be able to recognize the difference between an upper airway obstruction and a lower airway disease that may produce similar signs and symptoms. In general, an upper airway obstruction involves a known or likely mechanism, such as the absence of a small part of a toy with which the child was playing, or the history of cold symptoms (Fig. 29-18). You should also listen for stridor on inspiration.

Often with lower airway diseases, the child has wheezing and an increased breathing effort on exhalation. Your assessment may also reveal rapid breathing without stridor or a complete airway obstruction. These children are sometimes agitated and crying. Frequently they will be coughing and may have hoarse voices. Most importantly, there is no historical or environmental evidence of a foreign body obstruction.

TECHNIQUE 29-8
Care for Complete Obstruction in an Unresponsive Child

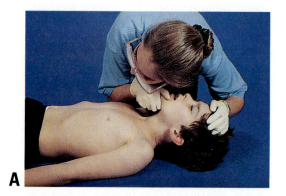
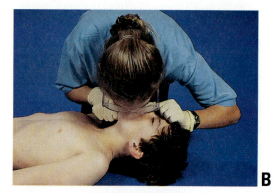
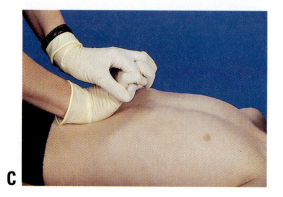
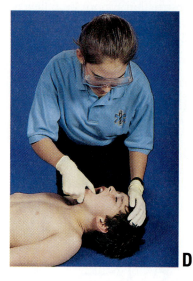

Fig. 29-17 Determine responsiveness by shaking the shoulders and calling the child's name. **A, Open the airway. Look, listen, and feel for breathing. B, Attempt to ventilate the child using a barrier device (plastic shield used here).** Reposition the child's head. Reattempt to ventilate. Kneel astride the child's legs or next to the child's thighs. Locate the landmarks for abdominal thrusts. **C, Place the heel of one hand between the landmarks. Place the other hand on top of the hand resting on the abdomen. Deliver up to five abdominal thrusts. D, Inspect the airway and perform a finger sweep only if you see an object.** Repeat steps B through D as necessary. Once the obstruction is removed, ventilate as necessary.

It is helpful to recognize the differences between early respiratory distress, respiratory failure, and respiratory arrest. The identification of early respiratory distress allows you to prevent the infant or child from deteriorating into respiratory failure or arrest.

ASSESSMENT OF RESPIRATORY PROBLEMS

Respiratory distress is a clinical condition in which the infant or child begins to experience an increased work of breathing. Infants and children increase the work of breathing at the expense of other physiologic functions. The signs and symptoms of respiratory distress include a rapid respiratory rate, nasal flaring, retractions, stridor, use of accessory muscles, lethargy, apathy, and grunting (Fig. 29-19). Often see-saw respirations may be present. This is the pronounced use of the abdomen to assist in breathing; the chest is pulled in and the abdomen is thrust out.

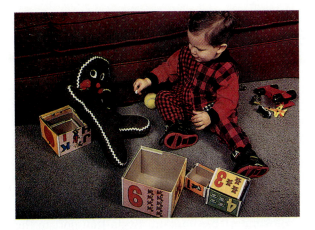

Fig. 29-18   Small removable parts that toddlers can place in their mouths, such as this button from a stuffed toy, can cause an airway obstruction.

Nasal flaring occurs as the infant tries to get more air by increasing the size of the airway by expanding the nostrils. **Retractions** are contractions of muscles to increase the ability to expand and contract the chest cavity. They appear as the sucking in of the muscles between the ribs and at the neck. Retractions occur as the effort of breathing increases. Retractions may be mild, moderate, or severe; this classification may help you determine the patient's priority. If retractions are seen only between the spaces of the ribs, called *intercostal retractions*, they are classified as mild retractions. When the muscles of the neck and the area above the clavicles are used for respiratory assistance (suprasternal and supraclavicular retractions), the retractions are classified as severe. **Grunting** is an expiratory sound made when the patient attempts to trap air to keep the alveoli open. Box 29-1 summarizes the signs of early respiratory distress.

If uncorrected, respiratory distress can progress to **respiratory failure**. In this clinical condition, the patient is continuing to work hard to breathe, and the patient's condition begins to deteriorate. As the work of breathing increases, the infant or child becomes tired and is no longer able to compensate for respiratory distress. Respiratory failure is seen in the combination of the signs and symptoms of respiratory distress with decreased peripheral perfusion, cyanosis, and mental status changes. Box 29-2 lists the signs of respiratory failure.

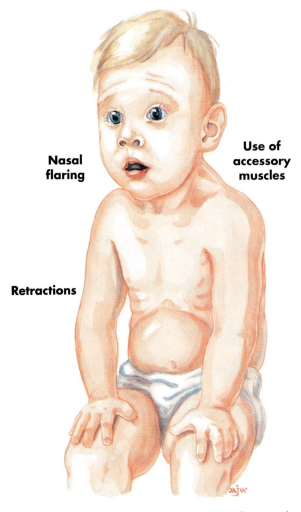

Nasal flaring

Use of accessory muscles

Retractions

Fig. 29-19   Nasal flaring, retractions, accessory muscle use, and positioning are signs of respiratory distress in children.

BOX 29-1

Signs of Early Respiratory Distress

Early respiratory distress is indicated by any of the following:

- Increased rate of breathing
- Nasal flaring
- Intercostal and supraclavicular retractions
- Mottled skin color
- Use of abdominal muscles
- See-saw respirations
- Stridor
- Wheezing
- Grunting

BOX 29-2

Signs of Respiratory Failure

Respiratory failure is the presence of any of the findings of respiratory distress along with any of the following:

- Altered mental status
- Respiratory rate over 60 or under 20 breaths per minute with signs of fatigue
- Severe retractions
- Severe use of accessory muscles
- Decreased muscle tone
- Cyanosis
- Poor peripheral perfusion

If respiratory failure is not treated, the patient will become too tired to breathe. A complete failure of the respiratory system will occur. Unlike adults, infants and children do not need to cease breathing completely before the condition is considered respiratory arrest. As the infant or child fatigues or shows signs of decompensation, you must begin more aggressive interventions. The signs of respiratory arrest are listed in Box 29-3.

EMERGENCY CARE FOR PATIENTS WITH RESPIRATORY PROBLEMS

Regardless of the origin of the patient's clinical condition, the goal is to restore effective respiratory function. The easiest way to correct this problem is

BOX 29-3

Signs of Respiratory Arrest

- Breathing rate of less than 10 per minute
- Limp muscle tone
- Unresponsive
- Slow or absent heart rate
- Weak or absent distal pulses

first to recognize the seriousness of the condition and to provide oxygen at a high concentration to all patients with respiratory problems. Act quickly and calmly to avoid upsetting the child or the parents.

Emergency Care for Patients With Respiratory Failure. In cases of respiratory failure, the patient is focused on breathing and will not resist your interventions. In these cases, you need to assist the infant's or child's ventilations.

Begin with oxygen at the highest available concentration. The child should be allowed to remain in a comfortable position. Begin transport to the hospital.

If respiratory failure progresses, you need to ventilate the child. Do this with the child in a supine position. If the child is able to struggle against being placed in this position and your efforts at ventilation, he or she does not need to be ventilated. Assisting ventilations can be an extremely difficult skill to master. Gain the confidence of the parent and child quickly. As the child begins to breathe in, seal the mask over the mouth and nose and deliver an adequate ventilation. You should be able to develop a rhythm and assist the patient's ventilations.

Emergency Care for Patients With Respiratory Arrest. In all cases of respiratory arrest, your goal is to prevent cardiac arrest. Immediately begin to ventilate the child with a bag-valve-mask connected to high-flow oxygen. Airway management and ventilation are the highest priority for these patients. Patients in respiratory arrest should be transported rapidly to a facility capable of dealing with this emergency. If the heart rate is less than 60 in an infant despite your efforts at providing artificial ventilation, begin chest compressions. If Advanced Life Support (ALS) is available in your system, request ALS back-up.

SEIZURES

Seizures result from a nervous system malfunction and are among the most common problems EMTs see in infants and children. Some infants and children have chronic seizures; others have seizures caused by an acute illness or injury. There are many types and causes of seizures, including chronic medical conditions, rapid rise of fever, infection, poisoning, low blood sugar, head injury, decreased levels of oxygen, and unknown causes. Inadequate breathing or altered mental status may occur following a seizure.

Your role as an EMT is to support the patient's vital functions. Do not worry about determining the cause of the seizure. Be alert for violent muscle contractions called *convulsions*, although not all seizures involve convulsions. Seizures may be brief or prolonged. Describe the convulsions to the medical staff at the receiving facility. Seizures themselves are rarely life-threatening but should be considered a serious emergency.

When gathering a history concerning seizures, include the following questions: Has the child had previous seizures? Does the child take antiseizure medications such as phenobarbital, tegretol, clonopin, depakene, or dilantin? If the answer to either question is yes, determine whether the medication was taken as prescribed and also whether or not this seizure is similar to previous seizures.

EMERGENCY CARE FOR PATIENTS HAVING SEIZURES

Ensure a patent airway. During the seizure, protect the patient from injury. Do not put anything in the patient's mouth. Have suction available. Following the seizure, place the patient in the recovery position if there is no possibility of spine trauma. Provide oxygen in the highest concentration available. If there is a partial airway obstruction, correct head positioning, check for a foreign body, and consider insertion of a nasopharyngeal airway. If the patient is cyanotic, ensure a patent airway and ventilate the patient artificially. Transport the patient to the hospital. Although brief seizures are usually not harmful, there may be a dangerous underlying condition. If a seizure lasts for more than 5 to 10 minutes, or if there are repeated seizures, request ALS resources, if available, because antiseizure medications may be required. If the patient has "routine" seizures and their condition returns to normal, transport may not be necessary; contact medical direction.

ALTERED MENTAL STATUS

Altered mental status is another medical condition commonly encountered in infants and children. There are many common causes of altered mental status; no one cause predominates in infants or children. Altered mental status may be caused by diabetic emergency, poisoning, seizure, infection, head trauma, decreased oxygen levels, and signs and symptoms of shock (hypoperfusion).

Altered mental status in infants and young children may be characterized by a lack of an appropri-

ate response to the environment or persons, a lack of interest in items in the environment, and a failure to recognize parents. As with adults, use the *AVPU* acronym to assess and categorize the level of responsiveness in infants and children.

EMERGENCY CARE FOR PATIENTS WITH ALTERED MENTAL STATUS

Support the patient. Do not worry about trying to determine a specific cause of the altered mental status, except by obtaining a focused history. Maintain an open airway. Place the patient in the recovery position if there is no possibility of spine trauma. Provide oxygen and have suction available. If the patient is cyanotic, ensure a patent airway and artificially ventilate.

POISONING

Poisoning is a common reason for EMS responses to infants and children. The nature and severity of poisonings vary considerably. Preschoolers often ingest a small amount of a single substance. Poisoned infants almost always have been given the toxic substance, either unintentionally or as a form of abuse. Adolescents often intentionally ingest larger amounts of substances for their psychological effects or because of emotional or psychiatric distress.

Try to identify the substance by looking for evidence at the scene and questioning the patient, family, or both. Bring any containers found at the scene to the receiving facility if possible.

In many areas, poison centers are available to assist EMTs and other healthcare workers to determine the best treatment for poisoning. This can be a valuable resource. Check your local protocol about contacting the poison center or consult with medical direction. When in doubt, contact medical direction, who can in turn contact the poison center and provide you with guidance, such as whether a known poison is likely to cause seizures or respiratory depression.

EMERGENCY CARE FOR PATIENTS WITH POISONING

As always do a scene size-up. Remember that some poisons are inhaled or absorbed through the skin, and you too could become a patient. Perform the initial assessment. Ensure patency of the airway, and administer high-flow oxygen. Be ready for vomiting, and have suction available.

Be prepared to ventilate the patient artificially. Complete the focused history and physical examination. If a poisoning patient has altered mental status, assess for signs of injury. Contact medical direction and provide as much information as possible. If the patient is responsive, be prepared for orders to administer activated charcoal orally, as described in Chapter 21, "Poisoning and Overdose." Perform ongoing assessments. Be aware that even if the patient is responsive and breathing well initially, some substances may cause the patient to become unresponsive, have a seizure, or have inadequate respirations.

FEVER

Fever is a common reason that EMTs are called to care for infants and children. There are many causes of fever. Although fever itself is not life threatening, some of its causes are. One potentially life-threatening cause of fever is meningitis. Because of the potential serious causes, fever, especially when occurring with a rash, is a potentially serious condition.

EMERGENCY CARE FOR PATIENTS WITH FEVER

Fever is defined as a temperature above 38°C (100.4°F). When you are called for an infant or child with fever, carefully observe the child while obtaining a history. Observe for alertness, motor activity and response, and irritability, and note whether the parents can console the child. Also be aware of the parent's or guardian's assessment. Ask if there is any medical history. Also ask about present illness, vomiting or diarrhea, cough, rash, and recent exposure to ill persons. A complete trunk-to-head examination should be performed.

When dealing with infants and children with a fever, follow your local transport protocols. Remove excess clothing. Be prepared to replace clothing if the child becomes too cool. Perform on-going assessments because a rapid rise in fever may lead to seizures in infants and young children. Never bathe febrile children with cold or ice water or alcohol. Such bathing may lead to shivering, which will ultimately make the temperature increase.

SHOCK

Shock (hypoperfusion) is the failure of the cardiovascular system to supply adequate oxygenated blood to the vital organs. If uncorrected, it can lead to death rapidly. Attention to assessment findings will help you identify this condition. The signs and symptoms of shock in infants and children rarely result from a cardiac problem. Common causes include dehydration from vomiting and or diarrhea, trauma, blood loss, and infection.

When assessing the infant or child, be alert for the following circulatory signs and symptoms. As the body attempts to compensate, respirations become rapid, and the skin becomes pale, mottled, cool, and clammy. The pulse becomes rapid, and peripheral pulses may be weak or absent compared with central pulses. Note that decreased blood pressure need not be present as a sign of shock. Accurate blood pressure management is difficult in children. Use all other signs of circulatory function as primary indicators of shock. Assess capillary refill in infants and children less than 6 years of age. If signs and symptoms of shock are present, capillary refill will be delayed (longer than 2 seconds). You may see mental status changes ranging from agitation and disorientation to unresponsiveness. If the child is dehydrated, there may be an absence of tears, even when crying. Another important finding is decreased urine output. Assess this by asking the parents about diaper wetting and checking the diaper.

EMERGENCY CARE FOR PATIENTS IN SHOCK

The goal in the management of the signs and symptoms of shock is to transport the patient to a facility capable of establishing vascular access and rapidly administering fluid. In some EMS systems this may be accomplished by ALS back-up; in others this requires transport to a hospital. Your actions at the scene must be rapid and organized. After completing the scene size-up, perform an initial assessment. During the initial assessment, ensure a patent airway and administer oxygen. Be prepared to ventilate artificially. Manage bleeding if present. Elevate the patient's legs several centimeters if there is no history of trauma, and keep the infant or child warm. If trauma is present or suspected, take necessary spinal immobilization precautions. Do not delay transport. The focused history and physical examination and detailed physical examination may be completed en route to the hospital, if time permits and the patient's condition allows.

NEAR DROWNING

Drowning is the third most common cause of death in children 1 to 14 years of age. **Drowning** is death from suffocation within 24 hours of submersion in liquid. **Near drowning** is survival beyond 24 hours after submersion. **Secondary drowning** is rapid deterioration of respiratory status up to 96 hours after resuscitation.

Adequate ventilation and oxygenation are the top priority in all cases of near drowning and secondary drowning. Remember that there is a possibility that the incident involved a traumatic injury, such as diving into a shallow pool and striking the head. Other considerations include the possibility of hypothermia. Any environmental (air or water) temperature less than 37°C (98.6°F) can cause hypothermia. Infants, toddlers, and preschoolers generally drown because they fall in the water. Adolescents drown primarily due to the effects of drugs or alcohol or spinal injuries resulting from diving into shallow water.

EMERGENCY CARE FOR NEAR DROWNING PATIENTS

Your own safety is most important. Water rescue is a specialized form of rescue and should only be attempted if you have specialized education. Often when you respond to the scene you find that the patient has already been pulled from the water. Priorities in caring for these patients include immobilization of the spine if trauma is suspected. Whenever possible, do this while the person is still in the water. Ensure an adequate airway. Provide oxygen, and ventilate the patient as necessary. Provide external chest compressions if indicated. Have suction ready. Because of the risk of secondary drowning, any patient involved in a near drowning incident should be transported to the hospital.

In some cases, patients have survived after extremely long immersions in very cold water. Any patient found pulseless following submersion in cold water must receive resuscitation efforts. Check the pulse for at least 1 minute; if the patient has a palpable slow pulse rate, do not perform external chest compressions.

SUDDEN INFANT DEATH SYNDROME

Sudden infant death syndrome (SIDS) is the sudden death of an infant who is generally less than 1 year of age. SIDS deaths often occur early in the morning. The death is not apparently related to anything in the infant's history and remains unexplained even after a thorough autopsy. SIDS is the leading cause of death in infants less than 1 year of age.

EMERGENCY CARE FOR SUDDEN INFANT DEATH SYNDROME VICTIMS

Unless rigor mortis, or the rigid stiffening of the muscles after death, is present, try to resuscitate the infant. Follow basic life support procedures and transport the infant to an appropriate care facility. Be especially observant of scene details and document them well. Unfortunately, some infants who seem to be victims of SIDS are actually victims of abuse. Your documentation may be critical to any investigation that is conducted.

The death of a child is very difficult for parents and healthcare professionals. Parents experience intense feelings of guilt, anger, denial, and disbelief. Their initial reaction may range from hysteria to complete silence. It is essential to allow the family to express their grief. Be careful to avoid comments that might suggest blame. Be prepared to provide emotional support to the parents. Some EMS and law enforcement agencies provide bereavement teams to help families deal with their emotional trauma. Check to see if any agencies in your area provide this service.

This is an extremely emotional event for EMTs as well. Do not hesitate to request critical incident stress debriefings for you and others involved (*see* Chapter 2, "The Well-Being of the EMT–Basic"). Communicating your feelings with one another can greatly reduce the stress.

For additional information about SIDS, contact the National Sudden Infant Death Syndrome Foundation or your local SIDS chapter.

TRAUMA

Trauma is a leading cause of death in children and adolescents. Blunt trauma is most common, but penetrating trauma is becoming more common. The injury patterns in infants and children are different from those in adults. Because the child is smaller, the traumatic forces are more generalized and may spread throughout the body rather than dissipating over a small area. Often more than one body system is involved. With the small size and the closeness of internal organs, more energy is transmitted to more organs. The bones of a child are less calcified and are more resilient. This makes the musculoskeletal system less likely to absorb the impact of trauma. In addition, there may be more significant internal damage without serious outward signs (Fig. 29-20).

REVIEW QUESTIONS

COMMON PROBLEMS IN INFANTS AND CHILDREN

1. Define respiratory distress, and list the possible signs and symptoms.

2. Define respiratory failure, and list the possible signs and symptoms.

3. Define respiratory arrest, and list the possible signs and symptoms.

4. Management of the seizure patient includes which of the following?
   1. Maintaining airway
   2. Assuring adequate ventilations
   3. Maintaining circulation
   4. Protecting the patient from the environment
      - A. 1 and 3
      - B. 2 and 4
      - C. 1, 2, and 3
      - D. All of the above

5. Management of the patient with altered mental status includes which of the following?
   1. Maintaining airway
   2. Assuring adequate ventilations
   3. Maintaining circulation
   4. Providing oxygen
      - A. 1 and 3
      - B. 2 and 4
      - C. 1, 2, and 3
      - D. All of the above

6. The primary goal in the management of poisonings includes which of the following?
   1. Administration of an antidote
   2. Administration of oxygen
   3. Inducing vomiting
   4. Maintaining ABCs
      - A. 1 and 3
      - B. 2 and 4
      - C. 1, 2, and 3
      - D. All of the above

7. Management efforts of SIDS include:
   1. Attempting to resuscitate the infant
   2. Transporting the infant to an appropriate facility
   3. Supporting the parents
   4. Telling the parents that they performed CPR incorrectly
      - A. 1 and 3
      - B. 2 and 4
      - C. 1, 2, and 3
      - D. All of the above

7. C
6. B
5. D
4. D

3. Respiratory arrest is the result of respiratory failure. Signs and symptoms: breathing rate less than 10 per minute, limp muscle tone, unresponsive, slow or absent heart rate, weak or absent distal pulses.

2. Respiratory failure is a clinical condition when the patient is continuing to work hard to breathe, the effort of breathing is increased, and the patient's condition begins to deteriorate. Signs and symptoms: respiratory rate above 60, cyanosis, decreased muscle tone, excessive use of accessory muscles, severe retractions, poor peripheral perfusion, altered mental status, grunting.

1. Respiratory distress is a clinical condition in which the infant or child begins to increase the work of breathing. Signs and symptoms: nasal flaring, intercostal retraction, supraclavicular, subcostal retractions, stridor, use of abdominal muscles, audible wheezing, grunting, increased respiratory rate.

It is critical to have properly sized equipment when caring for injured children. This includes the full range of sizes of cervical spine immobilization devices, splints, respiratory equipment, and pediatric immobilization devices.

Children are often injured in motor vehicle crashes. If infants or children are not restrained in infant or child car safety seats, they often sustain head injuries. When improperly restrained they often receive abdominal and lower spine injuries. Air bag deployment may cause facial trauma. Children may be injured as pedestrians or bicycle riders who are struck by vehicles. Children may also be injured in falls from a height, burns, or as a result of

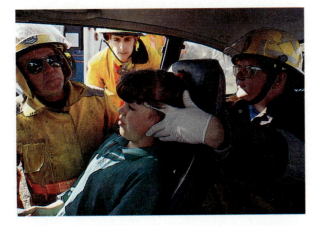

Fig. 29-20 Children involved in a trauma will often initially appear to be fine, but can deteriorate more rapidly than adults. Your treatment should therefore be based on the mechanism of injury and suspicion of internal injuries.

child abuse. The following sections describe certain common injuries and their appropriate emergency medical care.

HEAD INJURY

Head injury is the most common cause of death in pediatric trauma patients. Unfortunately, many severe injuries result in death even with the best treatment.

Children with head injuries are likely to sustain internal injuries as well. The signs and symptoms of shock in a patient with a head injury should cause you to be suspicious of other possible injuries since, with the exception of infants, an isolated head injury does not cause the signs and symptoms of shock. Vomiting is common in head injuries, and the airway must be protected. The most common cause of decreased oxygen in unresponsive head injury patients is the tongue obstructing the airway. For this reason, the jaw-thrust technique is critically important. Respiratory arrest is common secondary to severe head injuries and may occur during transport.

EMERGENCY CARE FOR PATIENTS WITH HEAD INJURY

After completing the scene size-up, proceed immediately to the initial assessment. In a patient with a head injury, ensure an open and patent airway while stabilizing or immobilizing the spine. During the initial assessment, provide oxygen and artificially ventilate the patient as needed. Be alert for vomiting and have suction ready. These patients must be immobilized on a backboard or

pediatric immobilization device using cervical immobilization. Use an appropriate sized cervical spine immobilization device, if available, and an approved head immobilization device. You may need to improvise for very small children. Pad all voids between the child's body and the spine board to immobilize the entire spine. Also pad from the shoulders to the heels to keep the neck and airway in the neutral position. Do not use sandbags to stabilize the head because the sand may shift, especially if the board needs to be turned, thus possibly moving the neck or head out of alignment.

CHEST INJURY

Suspect a chest injury based on the mechanism of injury. Children have soft, pliable ribs. When a child is injured in the chest, the resiliency of the chest wall allows the forces to be transferred to the heart, lungs, and blood vessels. There may be significant internal injuries without obvious external signs. Any abrasions or contusions present on the chest signal an increased risk of internal chest injury. Be sure to listen to breath sounds to determine if they are equal; a collapsed lung may occur due to blunt chest trauma. This injury is poorly tolerated in children.

EMERGENCY CARE FOR PATIENTS WITH CHEST INJURY

The management of chest injuries follows the accepted principles for rapid assessment and ensuring adequate oxygenation and ventilation. If you are ventilating the patient, assess the chest for adequate rise and fall as well as symmetry. These patients should be immobilized appropriately and must be transported rapidly to the appropriate facility.

ABDOMINAL INJURY

The abdomen is a common site of injury in infants and children. Often the injury is not obvious. Always suspect internal injuries when evaluating trauma patients. Always consider the possibility of an abdominal injury in a deteriorating trauma patient without external signs of trauma or blood loss. The abdomen may collect a lot of blood that cannot be seen, and it may be distended.

BURNS

For very young patients, burns are very serious. You must assess whether the burn is critical and determine whether the patient should be transported to a burn center. Respiratory involvement is the most immediate danger in many infants and children with burns. Assess the extent and nature of the burn rapidly and transport the patient to an appropriate facility.

When evaluating whether a burn is critical, keep in mind the concepts discussed in Chapter 26, "Soft-Tissue Injuries." Consider the depth of the burn, the total body surface area burned, the age of the patient, and whether there is respiratory involvement or any associated injuries. Local protocol determines which patients should be transported to a burn center. Remember that respiratory compromise is the most immediate danger to many burn victims. Always be ready to provide support for oxygenation and ventilation.

EMERGENCY CARE FOR BURN VICTIMS

Your personal safety is always a priority. Do not attempt a rescue for which you have not been educated and equipped. As soon as the patient is in a safe place, stop the burning process on the patient.

During the initial assessment, ensure airway position and patency. Use the modified jaw thrust. Suction as necessary with a large-bore suction catheter. Provide oxygen and be prepared to assist ventilations for severe respiratory distress. Ventilate infants or children in respiratory arrest artificially with a bag-valve-mask. During the focused history and physical examination, cover burned areas with dry sterile dressings (nonstick, if possible) or sterile sheets. Avoid wet dressings due to the increased risk of hypothermia. If you suspect trauma, provide spinal immobilization. Transport immediately to the appropriate facility. Do not hesitate to contact medical direction for advice.

OTHER TRAUMA CONSIDERATIONS

Pneumatic antishock garments (PASGs) are available in pediatric sizes (Fig. 29-21). Follow local medical direction for using the PASGs. Be cautious when using PASGs; use it only if it fits the child. Do not place an infant in only one leg of larger trousers. Inflation of the abdominal section may hinder breathing. Carefully consider the effect on breathing and the potential damage to internal organs before inflating the abdominal section. This decision should be made by medical direction. The potential indications for PASGs are trauma with signs of hypoperfusion and pelvic instability, with the absence of penetrating chest trauma. Check with local medical direction regarding other uses.

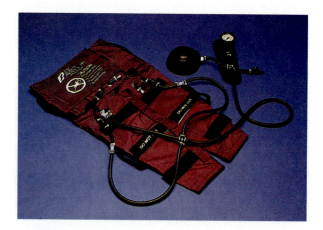

Fig. 29-21 The pediatric pneumatic antishock garment (PASG).

REVIEW QUESTIONS

TRAUMA

1. Which of the following areas is most often injured in infants and children?
   A. Head
   B. Chest
   C. Abdomen
   D. Extremities

2. When assessing an injured infant or child with deteriorating perfusion, EMTs should suspect hidden injuries in the—
   A. Head
   B. Chest
   C. Abdomen
   D. Extremities

3. If a child does not fit in the PASG, it is acceptable to wrap one leg of the PASG around the child. True or False?

4. Burns should be covered with:
   A. Occlusive dressings
   B. Burn cream
   C. Dry sterile sheets
   D. Wet sterile sheets

4. C
3. False
2. C
1. A

CHILD ABUSE AND NEGLECT

Child abuse is an improper or excessive action by parents, guardians, or caretakers that injures or causes harm to an infant or child. This includes direct physical abuse, sexual abuse, and emotional battery. Some children may also be neglected. **Neglect** is giving insufficient attention or respect to an infant or child, which may result in problems such as poor nutrition, inappropriate exposure to environmental conditions, or inadequate healthcare. Recognizing these problems depends on being aware of their signs and symptoms. It is estimated that 2.5% of all American children are abused or neglected, and the number is growing.

SIGNS AND SYMPTOMS OF CHILD ABUSE AND NEGLECT

You should be able to recognize the signs and symptoms of abuse so that you can report situations as necessary and give appropriate treatments. Box 29-4 lists the signs and symptoms of abuse. Central nervous system injuries are most lethal, such as those caused by vigorously shaking a baby. In this

---

BOX 29-4

Signs and Symptoms of Abuse

- Multiple bruises in various stages of healing
- Injury inconsistent with the mechanism described by parent or caretaker
- Mechanism of injury inconsistent with child's developmental characteristics. Examples: 2-week-old rolling off a bed, 7-month-old pulling a pot off of the stove
- Repeated calls to the same address
- Fresh burns, especially on the feet, hands, and back
- Parents or caretakers who seem inappropriately unconcerned
- Conflicting histories given by parents or caretakers
- The child being afraid to discuss how the injury occurred

BOX 29-5

Signs and Symptoms of Neglect

- Lack of adult supervision
- Malnourished appearance of child
- Unsafe living environment
- Untreated chronic illness, such as an asthmatic patient not taking medication

---

type of injury, often called "shaken-baby syndrome," there are rarely external signs of injury. Box 29-5 lists the signs and symptoms of neglect.

EMERGENCY CARE FOR ABUSED AND NEGLECTED PATIENTS

Remember that the care of the infant or child is most important. Do not accuse parents or caretakers on the scene. Accusation and confrontation delay transportation and patient care. Provide appropriate medical care based on the signs and symptoms present and bring objective information to the receiving facility.

Every state has reporting requirements for child abuse and neglect. Your report will set into motion the local agency responsible for investigating the problem. Keep in mind that your report should be objective. Include pertinent environmental findings at the scene. Document potential significant remarks from caregivers in quotation marks. Report only what you see and what you hear—<u>not</u> what you think. Take a helpful rather than vindictive approach to the parent.

INFANTS AND CHILDREN WITH SPECIAL NEEDS

New technology has allowed many ill and injured children to be discharged from the hospital to their homes or interim care facilities. As an EMT you may now see all of the following in the home: Premature babies with lung disease; babies and children with heart disease; infants and children with neurological disease; and children with chronic disease or altered function from birth.

These children are often technology-dependent. Unfortunately, instruments and machines can fail, requiring emergency medical care.

TRACHEOSTOMY TUBE

Children with respiratory problems may have a surgical opening into the trachea (tracheostomy) kept open with a tube. These patients are at risk for a variety of problems that can cause a life-threatening emergency, such as loss of oxygen supply to the tube, or the occlusion or displacement of the tube.

Tracheostomy tubes may be made of metal or plastic. In most instances the tube can be suctioned. Limit suctioning time to 10 to 15 seconds. If the tube becomes dislodged and the parents cannot replace it, the patient should be ventilated as needed with a bag-valve-mask and transported to the appropriate facility. Many children with tracheostomies have good ventilation through the stoma, even without the tube. If ventilation is needed, the first preference is to use the bag-valve-mask over the mouth and nose, manually covering the stoma. If this is unsuccessful, use a small mask and ventilate directly over the stoma while holding the mouth closed.

HOME MECHANICAL VENTILATORS

Some children are discharged home on mechanical ventilators. The parents should have been educated thoroughly in the operation of the devices. If the ventilator fails, however, and the parents cannot restart it, you should remove the child from the ventilator and administer bag-valve ventilations. The great majority of these children have tracheostomies. The bag-valve device can connect directly to the tracheostomy tube for ventilation.

CENTRAL LINES

Some children have a central line in place. **Central lines** are intravenous lines usually placed near the heart for long-term use. Complications of central lines may include a cracked line, infection, clotting, and bleeding. You may need to manage a bleeding emergency. If bleeding is present from the site of a broken or dislodged central line, follow the general principles for managing bleeding. Using sterile dressings, apply direct pressure to the site where the central line passes into the body and transport the patient to an appropriate facility. Contact medical direction if pressure fails to control the bleeding from a broken central line.

GASTROSTOMY TUBES AND GASTRIC FEEDING

Some children who cannot be fed by mouth have a surgical opening into the stomach (gastrostomy). A **gastric tube** is a tube placed through the opening directly into the stomach for feeding. The gastric tube is present in the upper left quadrant of the abdomen. If the patient is diabetic or has problems with low blood sugar, watch for possible mental status changes from missed feedings. Treat this patient as you would any infant or child with an altered mental status. Gastric tubes are often seen in children with other problems. Sometimes EMTs are called because of a dislodged gastric tube. In this case, transport the patient and watch for signs of low blood sugar from missed feedings.

SHUNTS

Some children have a central nervous system shunt in place. A common type of **shunt** is one that extends from the ventricle of the brain to the peritoneal cavity. This tube runs from the skull to the abdomen to drain excess cerebrospinal fluid. You will see the tubing buried under the skin on the side of the skull and neck and down the chest. These children often have altered mental status. Treat them as you would any other patient with altered mental status or head injury (except for immobilization). Many of these patients are prone to respiratory arrest. Because of this complication, be prepared to provide artificial ventilation.

REACTIONS TO ILL AND INJURED INFANTS AND CHILDREN

THE FAMILY'S REACTION

A child cannot be cared for in isolation from the family. Family members are likely to be emotional and require your attention also. If you conduct yourself in a caring, professional manner, you will be able to interact positively with the family. A calm, supportive interaction with the family provides a better situation for dealing with the child. Consider this simple formula: Calm parents equal a calm child; agitated parents equal an agitated child.

Family members experience anxiety because of their concern for their child's pain and their fear for the child's well-being. In parents who have had no medical education, this anxiety is often made worse by a sense of helplessness and a loss of control. Because of their anxiety and helplessness, parents may react to EMTs with anger or hysteria. Respond to the parents in a caring and compassionate manner. Reassure them but do not offer false hopes. Try to involve the parents as part of the child's care unless the medical condition requires separation.

Parents can be valuable allies in caring for an injured infant or child. Ask the parents to calm the child. They can help the child maintain a position of comfort, and they can hold the oxygen delivery device. Keep in mind that parents may not have a medical education, but they are experts on what is normal or abnormal for their children and what will have a calming effect.

THE EMERGENCY MEDICAL TECHNICIAN'S REACTION

Many EMTs experience anxiety when dispatched to a call involving an ill or injured child. This anxiety often stems from a lack of experience treating children or a fear of failure. EMTs who have children of their own often experience stress from identifying the patient with their own child. Chapter 2, ''Well-Being of the EMT-Basic,'' describes measures you can take to manage the stress resulting from these situations.

Remember that you have the skills for caring for children. Much of what you have learned about adults applies to children, but you need to remember the differences.

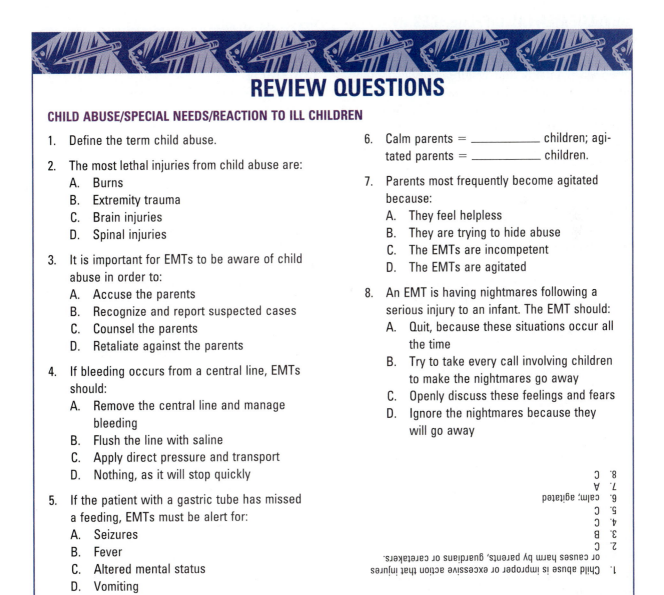

REVIEW QUESTIONS

CHILD ABUSE/SPECIAL NEEDS/REACTION TO ILL CHILDREN

1. Define the term child abuse.

2. The most lethal injuries from child abuse are:
   A. Burns
   B. Extremity trauma
   C. Brain injuries
   D. Spinal injuries

3. It is important for EMTs to be aware of child abuse in order to:
   A. Accuse the parents
   B. Recognize and report suspected cases
   C. Counsel the parents
   D. Retaliate against the parents

4. If bleeding occurs from a central line, EMTs should:
   A. Remove the central line and manage bleeding
   B. Flush the line with saline
   C. Apply direct pressure and transport
   D. Nothing, as it will stop quickly

5. If the patient with a gastric tube has missed a feeding, EMTs must be alert for:
   A. Seizures
   B. Fever
   C. Altered mental status
   D. Vomiting

6. Calm parents = _____ children; agitated parents = _____ children.

7. Parents most frequently become agitated because:
   A. They feel helpless
   B. They are trying to hide abuse
   C. The EMTs are incompetent
   D. The EMTs are agitated

8. An EMT is having nightmares following a serious injury to an infant. The EMT should:
   A. Quit, because these situations occur all the time
   B. Try to take every call involving children to make the nightmares go away
   C. Openly discuss these feelings and fears
   D. Ignore the nightmares because they will go away

8. C
7. A
6. calm; agitated
5. C
4. C
3. B
2. C
1. Child abuse is improper or excessive action that injures or causes harm by parents, guardians or caretakers.

If infants and children are rarely seen in your EMS practice, staying prepared is important. Practice using the special equipment for children, and practice examining patients. Often a local pediatrician can assist you in refining your skills. Observe normal children of all ages. Finally, consider every patient encounter with an infant or child as a learning experience. Remember that most of the children using EMS are not gravely ill or injured, and you will be able to help them. Allow yourself to appreciate the time you spend with your smallest patients.

CHAPTER SUMMARY

DEVELOPMENTAL DIFFERENCES IN INFANTS AND CHILDREN

EMTs must understand the developmental differences in infants and children. Understanding these differences help EMTs assess and provide emergency care for infants and children. The groupings are related to age and include newborns and infants, toddlers, preschool children, school-age children, and adolescents.

THE AIRWAY

Anatomic and physiological concerns related to the airway are the most important. In general, the airways in infants and children are smaller and more easily obstructed than those in adults. Positioning the airway is different; take caution not to hyperextend the neck because this may occlude the airway. The tongue is relatively large in infants and young children, and it occupies a proportionally larger amount of space. Proper positioning is important in these patients.

Opening the airway is accomplished by using the head-tilt chin-lift or the jaw thrust technique. Suctioning may be necessary to remove secretions. Limit the vacuum to 80 to 120 mm Hg, and avoid stimulation of the back of the patient's throat with the suction catheter.

Airway adjuncts may be used to assist in maintaining an open airway. The preferred method of inserting the oral airway is using a tongue blade. Nasopharyngeal airways may be used in responsive patients but should not be used when head trauma is suspected.

OXYGEN THERAPY

Oxygen therapy should always be considered. Provide oxygen in the highest concentration available. If the use of a mask upsets the infant or child, the blow-by method is acceptable.

With the exception of airway positioning, ventilating an infant or child with a mouth-to-mask or a bag-valve-mask device is the same as the procedure for adults. If pop-off valves are present, they should be deactivated.

ASSESSMENT

Assessment of the infant or child begins from a distance. Use your general impression to decide if the child is sick or well. In general, use a trunk-to-toe-to-head approach in infants and young children. Keep in mind the developmental characteristics for the child's age.

COMMON PROBLEMS IN INFANTS AND CHILDREN

The first priority when dealing with ill infants and children is airway and breathing. The leading cause of death in infants and children is an uncorrected respiratory problem. EMTs must be able to recognize the difference between an airway obstruction caused by a potential foreign body and that caused by respiratory diseases. Follow the proper sequence for relieving a foreign body airway obstruction.

Lower airway diseases are characterized by wheezing and increased effort on exhalation, use of accessory muscles, and nasal flaring. To treat these patients, ensure an open airway and provide a high concentration of oxygen.

Respiratory failure is the next step in the progression of respiratory distress. Respiratory failure is characterized by an increased or decreased respiratory rate, cyanosis, decreased muscle tone, and mental status changes. For these patients, airway positioning and oxygen administration should be top priorities. Respiratory arrest is the final stage of respiratory distress. Ventilations may be absent or inadequate. Ensure airway patency and provide ventilation with a bag-valve-mask.

Other medical emergencies in infants and children include fever, poisoning, signs and symptoms of shock, and seizures. In general, EMTs provide care that supports the vital functions. Ensure an open airway, have suction available, and support ventilation. Request ALS back up when available and appropriate. Consult medical direction for additional interventions.

TRAUMA

Trauma is a leading cause of death for children and adolescents. The pattern of injury is different from that in adults. Because of the smaller body size, multiple body systems may be involved. Management of injuries is similar to that for adults, but it is important to use appropriately sized equipment. Vehicular trauma, burns, and falls are the most common causes of childhood trauma. Head injuries are common. Never assume that the signs and symptoms of shock are caused by an isolated head injury. Look for hidden injuries as well. A chest injury should be suspected based on the mechanism of injury. It is possible to have a significant chest injury without obvious external signs. Abdominal injures are common and are often hidden. Suspect an abdominal injury in any trauma patient who is deteriorating without obvious external injury. Always expect vomiting in trauma patients; immobilize them and be prepared to turn the board on its side if vomiting occurs.

CHILD ABUSE AND NEGLECT

EMTs must be aware that child abuse and neglect do occur and must be able to recognize the signs and symptoms to identify potential abuse or neglect. You should remain objective and provide appropriate medical care and transportation. Understand and follow your local reporting procedures and requirements.

INFANTS AND CHILDREN WITH SPECIAL NEEDS

Infants and children are often cared for at interim care facilities and at home with the aid of special technologies. EMTs should have a basic understanding of these devices. Work first with the parents to correct problems associated with these devices. Consult medical direction as needed for advice.

REACTIONS TO ILL AND INJURED INFANTS AND CHILDREN

Both family members and EMTs may have strong emotional responses when confronted by ill and injured children. Recognize that this may occur and conduct yourself in a calm, professional, and reassuring manner.

Realize that most of your EMT skills for adults also apply to infants and children. Take time to gain additional experience and knowledge related to infants and children. Use every opportunity to provide care to an infant or child as a learning experience.

UNITED STATES DEPARTMENT OF TRANSPORTATION NATIONAL HIGHWAY TRAFFIC SAFETY ADMINISTRATION EMT–BASIC OBJECTIVES

Check your knowledge. The National Registry of EMTs and many state EMS agencies use the objectives below to develop EMT–Basic certification examinations. Can you meet them?

COGNITIVE

1. Identify the developmental considerations for the following age groups:
   - infants
   - toddlers
   - pre-school
   - school age
   - adolescent
2. Describe differences in anatomy and physiology of the infant, child, and adult patient.
3. Differentiate the response of the ill or injured infant or child (age specific) from that of an adult.
4. Indicate various causes of respiratory emergencies.
5. Differentiate between respiratory distress and respiratory failure.
6. List the steps in the management of foreign body airway obstruction.
7. Summarize emergency medical care strategies for respiratory distress and respiratory failure.
8. Identify the signs and symptoms of shock (hypoperfusion) in the infant and child patient.
9. Describe the methods of determining end organ perfusion in the infant and child patient.
10. State the usual cause of cardiac arrest in infants and children versus adults.
11. List the common causes of seizures in the infant and child patient.
12. Describe the management of seizures in the infant and child patient.
13. Differentiate between the injury patterns in adults, infants, and children.
14. Discuss the field management of the infant and child trauma patients.
15. Summarize the indicators of possible child abuse and neglect.
16. Describe the medical-legal responsibilities in suspected child abuse.
17. Recognize need for EMT–Basic debriefing following a difficult infant or child transport.

AFFECTIVE

1. Explain the rationale for having knowledge and skills appropriate for dealing with the infant and child patient.
2. Attend to the feelings of the family when dealing with an ill or injured infant or child.
3. Understand the provider's own response (emotional) to caring for infants or children.

PSYCHOMOTOR

1. Demonstrate the techniques of foreign body airway obstruction removal in the infant.
2. Demonstrate the techniques of foreign body airway obstruction removal in the child.
3. Demonstrate the assessment of the infant and child.
4. Demonstrate bag-valve-mask artificial ventilations for the infant.
5. Demonstrate bag-valve-mask artificial ventilations for the child.
6. Demonstrate oxygen delivery for the infant and child.

OPERATIONS

As an EMT, you may be faced with situations that tax your resources and seem almost overwhelming. The keys to any successful operation are always preparation, planning, and practice.

Captain Eugene V. McCarthy
Paramedic Coordinator
Los Angeles County Fire Department
Los Angeles, California

IN THIS DIVISION

DIVISION SEVEN

30 AMBULANCE OPERATIONS

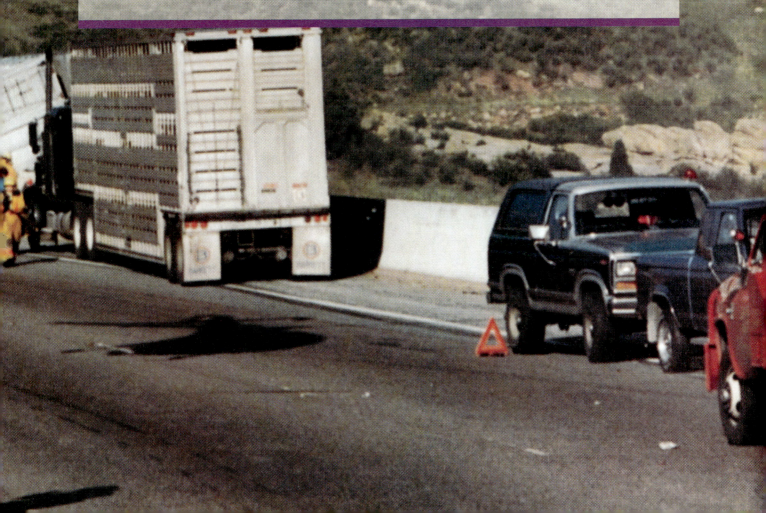

KEY TERMS

Decontamination: The use of physical or chemical means to remove, inactivate, or destroy blood-borne pathogens on a surface or item so that it can no longer transmit infection.

Disinfectant: The process of killing microorganisms on a surface or item. High-level disinfection destroys all microorganisms except large numbers of bacterial spores; it is used for equipment that has contacted mucous membranes. Intermediate-level disinfection destroys the tuberculosis bacteria, most viruses, and fungi, but it does not destroy bacterial spores; it is used for disinfecting surfaces that contact intact skin and have been visibly contaminated with body fluids. Low-level disinfection destroys most bacteria and some fungi and viruses, but not tuberculosis or bacterial spores; it is used for routine cleaning or removing of soiling when no body fluids are visible.

Due regard: The principle that a reasonable and careful person in similar circumstances would act in a way that is safe and considerate for others, such as an ambulance providing enough notice of approach to prevent a collision.

Escort: Another emergency vehicle, such as a police car, that accompanies the ambulance to the scene or from the scene to the receiving facility.

Infection control: Measures EMTs take to help prevent the transmission of infection from patients to EMTs, from one patient to another, and from EMTs to patients.

Sterilization: A disinfecting process that destroys all microorganisms including bacterial spores, used for instruments that penetrate the skin or contact normally sterile areas of the body during invasive procedures.

IN THE FIELD

The shift was about to begin for the EMTs Jane and Roy. They arrived at the station a few minutes early to prepare for their workday. In the past, they sometimes began a shift without adequate time to check the equipment, but this time they planned ahead. Roy began to inventory the medical supplies, checking that there were adequate supplies for an emergency call and that the battery-operated equipment was functioning properly. He completed the automated external defibrillator checklist and recorded the amount of oxygen in the main and portable cylinders. At the same time, Jane was inspecting the mechanics of the vehicle. She completed the daily checklist, recording fluid levels, checking tire pressure, and assuring that all lights and warning devices were functioning properly.

With the vehicle check complete, Jane and Roy stored their personal protective equipment and checked to see that the street maps were available. They reported to dispatch that they were in service and available. As they headed to the kitchen for a glass of orange juice, the radio interrupted: "Unit 37 Respond to 1818 Elm Street . . . unknown problem; patient is unresponsive, unknown if breathing." As they returned to the unit, they were confident they were prepared for the call.

Just as competent patient care skills are critical, nonmedical operational skills are equally important. As an EMT, you need a solid understanding of the skills required for all phases of an ambulance call, as well as an understanding of your roles and responsibilities in each phase. As you read this chapter, please remember that it is intended only as an overview of ambulance operations. You should seek additional educational programs in emergency vehicle operations and assistance from your EMS service.

PHASES OF AN AMBULANCE CALL

A typical EMS response consists of nine stages or phases: 1) preparation for the call; 2) dispatch; 3) en route to the scene; 4) arrival at the scene; 5) transferring the patient to the ambulance; 6) en route to the receiving facility; 7) arrival at the receiving facility; 8) en route to the station; and 9) the postrun phase. Each phase blends into the next, but you have a clear role in each.

PREPARATION FOR THE CALL

Preparation for the call refers to the phase before an ambulance call, during which you prepare to respond. This is the phase that allows you to check that all equipment is completely stocked in the emergency vehicle (Fig. 30-1), that the unit is mechanically sound (Fig. 30-2), and that you are mentally and physically prepared to respond to an emergency call.

As an EMT, you have a responsibility to yourself, your family, your partner, and your patient to be mentally and physically fit to respond to any emergency call. This includes a proper diet and exercise as described in Chapter 2, "The Well-Being of the EMT–Basic." In addition to your physical and mental status, you must remain prepared to respond through skills and knowledge learned and maintained in your initial EMT program and continuing education programs.

Continuing education is extremely important in emergency medical services, and you should attend as many additional classes as possible. Discussing operations and patient care experiences with other EMTs is also beneficial. Prehospital emergency care is a dynamic field that continually evolves along with trends and advances in medicine. You must remain flexible and open to new ideas and procedures while progressing in your career.

The emergency vehicle must also be prepared to respond to any call, and must always be stocked

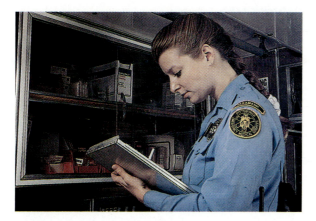

Fig. 30-1 Check all medical supplies and equipment in the ambulance to make sure the vehicle is completely stocked.

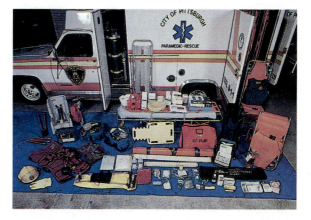

Fig. 30-3 The ambulance should be well stocked with a variety of equipment and supplies for all emergencies.

with medical and nonmedical supplies. Your EMS system along with state and local regulations dictates what specific equipment is required in the vehicle (Fig. 30-3). Most EMS services stock the typical emergency vehicle with a wide range of basic medical supplies (Box 30-1).

Besides medical supplies, certain nonmedical supplies are required for the safe and efficient operation of an EMS unit. Many states and local governments mandate specific safety equipment and personal protective equipment that EMS services should have on the unit. This equipment includes gloves, gowns, masks, and protective eye wear. Some services require EMTs to respond to automobile crashes or hazardous materials scenes.

If your system is required to respond to these situations and you have the education, special personal protective equipment should be available in your unit. EMTs responsible for rescue efforts should carry a complete set of turnout gear including bunker pants, a turnout coat, leather gloves, a helmet, and protective eye wear.

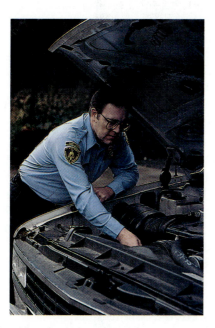

Fig. 30-2 All mechanical systems of the unit should be checked.

BOX 30-1

Emergency Vehicle Equipment

- Basic supplies
- Patient transfer equipment
- Airways
- Suction equipment
- Artificial ventilation devices
- Oxygen administration equipment
- Cardiac compression equipment
- Basic wound care supplies
- Splinting supplies
- Childbirth supplies
- Medications
- Automated external defibrillator

Note: Box 30-1 is only a suggested minimum list for a typical emergency vehicle. State and local policy may require additional specific supplies.

As violence has become more common in our society, it has also become a significant reality for EMTs in many areas. In some locations, EMTs may decide to wear additional protective equipment such as ballistic vests. Federal, state, and local regulatory agencies may require that additional personal protective equipment be made available.

Other beneficial nonmedical supplies and equipment include local street maps, preplanned routes, DOT Emergency Response Guidebooks, binoculars, and patient care reports. As an EMT, you should be familiar with your response area, including a basic knowledge of traffic patterns, one-way streets, and alternate routes to receiving facilities.

Inspect the ambulance at the beginning of your shift to ensure that it is in proper working condition, and that all equipment and materials necessary to respond to emergencies are functional and available for use. You or a maintenance crew designated by the agency should ensure adequate levels of fuel, motor oil, and engine coolant. Batteries must be charged and brakes checked. Daily evaluation of the vehicle should also include inspection of the tires for wear and adequate pressure. Also test all lights on the vehicle (headlights, emergency warning devices, stop lights, back-up lights, turn signals) to be sure that there are no burned-out bulbs. The driver should test both the siren and horn. The windshield should be clean inside and out, and the windshield wipers should be inspected because they are crucial for visibility in some situations.

Check that all seat belts, door locks, and latches are functioning properly, and test the communications system to guarantee contact with dispatch. For the comfort of the patient and crew, check the heating, cooling, and ventilation systems in the vehicle. The crew member assessing these items should replenish any low fluid levels, according to service protocol. The EMS crew should report any mechanical difficulties in the vehicle to maintenance personnel, which are then addressed following the local or service protocol.

EMS personnel should be available to respond to an emergency call at any time. The recommended minimum staffing for an ambulance is one EMT in the patient compartment and one qualified to drive the emergency vehicle. Some services require two EMTs in the patient compartment. Review the local policies and requirements in your area to be certain your service meets minimum staffing requirements.

DISPATCH

Dispatch is a critical phase of an emergency response. Many dispatch centers have a central access number, often "911". If this access number is not available in your area, a specific number is usually available for the public to reach the EMS system. The communication center is staffed 24 hours a day with personnel who may be able to provide medical instructions to the caller before the EMTs arrive. This system allows the family, friend, or bystander to begin emergency medical care while help is en route. In addition, many dispatch centers have preplanned response policies that allow the dispatcher to use a computer-assisted dispatch program or cardex system to determine what units to dispatch and to give the units a mode of response based on patient information.

Once the dispatcher notifies you of a response, you must have specific information. This information depends on your particular communications center and the caller providing the information. Usually you are informed of the location and the nature of an illness or the mechanism of injury. In some systems, the dispatcher provides the caller's name, location, and call-back number. Additional information may be available at the time of dispatch or become available while you are en route, including the exact location of the patient (eg, third-floor apartment), the number of patients, the severity of injuries or illness, the patient's age, the patient's level of responsiveness and respiratory status, and any other special problems or complications at the scene, including hazards and safety issues.

Dispatch information should also alert you to the possible need for additional public safety personnel such as firefighters or law enforcement officials.

EN ROUTE TO THE SCENE

To respond to the request for help, you must reach the scene safely. Use common sense, but also consciously remind yourself not to run to the vehicle (or later at the scene) because of the risk of injury. When you get into the emergency vehicle, be sure to put on your safety belt (Fig. 30-4). As outlined in Chapter 14, "Communications," you should notify the dispatch center that you are responding to the call. Record the essential information from dispatch and keep this information available for review as you respond.

Some states require EMTs to take an emergency vehicle operator's course or a defensive driving

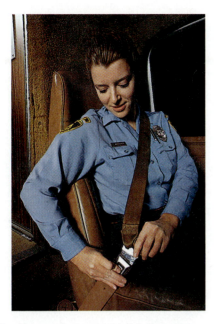

Fig. 30-4 Always wear your seat belt in the vehicle.

course before they are able to drive the emergency vehicle. Even if your state or municipality does not require this, EMS experts highly recommend that you seek this additional education on your own. Box 30-2 lists the characteristics of a good emergency vehicle operator.

Driving the unit safely is extremely important for the well-being of the ill or injured patient. If a vehicle crash injures you or another crew member en route, another emergency has been created, causing help to arrive slower to the original patient. The cost of injuries and damage to equipment can be disastrous for everyone including EMS services and the injured EMT or crew and their families.

As an added safety measure to keep you, the crew, and other passengers safe, everyone in the vehicle, including the patient compartment, should always wear safety belts. This protection may save your life and is often a state law.

In addition to safety belts, emergency vehicle operators should be familiar with the vehicle in general (eg, the amount of time required to stop the vehicle; its turning radius; and the location of blind spots). Other vehicles and drivers respond in different ways to weather and road conditions. Always be aware of changing weather and road conditions and make adjustments accordingly.

The use of red lights and sirens is a privilege reserved for only true emergencies. Not all EMS responses are true emergencies. When using the emergency warning devices such as lights and siren, exercise caution and good judgement. Remember that not all drivers immediately yield the right of way to an emergency vehicle. Many people panic when they see an emergency vehicle overtaking them with lights flashing and sirens wailing. They may begin to drive in a very unpredictable manner. You should be alert to this situation. It may be difficult for some other drivers to hear the sirens with their windows closed, air conditioning on, or stereo playing. As the driver of an emergency vehicle, you are responsible for knowing and following all state and local regulations regarding the use of emergency warning devices. The local EMS service, local police, state police, or highway patrol can provide copies of these regulations and answer any questions you may have. You should be aware of the dangers associated with the use of red lights and sirens, and their overuse and misuse. Remember that headlights are often the most visible warning devices on your unit.

BOX 30-2

Characteristics of a Good Emergency Vehicle Driver

- Physically fit
- Mentally fit
- Able to perform under stress
- Positive attitude concerning your abilities and limitations
- Tolerant of other drivers and able to anticipate their reactions

---

ALERT

As the driver of an emergency vehicle, you are responsible for knowing and following all state and local regulations regarding the use of emergency warning devices.

You must be fully aware of state regulations regarding the operation of the emergency vehicle. This knowledge includes recognizing and adhering to the posted speed limit. As well, most states do not permit ambulances to pass school buses that are boarding or dropping off students. (This procedure is typically indicated by the use of flashing red lights.)

Use your preplanned routes and comprehensive street maps when responding to an emergency. When responding or transporting a patient to the hospital, select the best route based on weather, traffic patterns, and road conditions. You should also have an alternate route planned in case of unforeseen conditions.

In a multiple-vehicle response, all drivers must be aware of possible points of conversion, where two or more emergency vehicles may seek the right-of-way at an intersection simultaneously. The consequences of striking another emergency vehicle en route to a call can be disastrous. When multiple units are responding, radio the other units to inform them of your approach to a major intersection where you may converge. Your local EMS protocol and policies may address this issue.

An additional key safety issue involves **escorts**. Escorts are extremely dangerous because most drivers do not anticipate a second emergency vehicle and tend to move after the first vehicle has passed them. In the rare instances when an escort is necessary, consider not using lights or sirens on either vehicle or use alternate or opposite siren tones, always provide a safe following distance, and anticipate the same hazards as in multiple-vehicle responses.

The most important aspect of driving the emergency vehicle is to have **due regard** for others. Due regard means that a reasonable and careful person in similar circumstances would act in a manner that is safe and considerate of others. Due regard requires that you give adequate notice of your approach to prevent a collision. As a driver of an emergency vehicle, it is your responsibility to understand and follow state and local regulations regarding vehicle stopping, procedures at red lights, stop signs and intersections, speed limits, direction of traffic flow, and specified turns. Many factors contribute to emergency vehicle crashes (Box 30-3).

Accidents at intersections are by far the most common types of crashes. Many of these incidents occur because motorists arrive at an intersection as the light changes and do not stop. Always come to a complete stop at all intersections. Try to make eye contact with drivers of other vehicles before going

---

BOX 30-3

Factors Contributing to Emergency Vehicle Crashes

- Excessive speed
- Reckless driving
- Failing to obey traffic signals or posted speed limits
- Disregarding traffic rules and regulations
- Failing to heed traffic warning signals
- Inadequate dispatch information
- Escorts
- Multiple-vehicle response
- Failure to anticipate the actions of other drivers

---

through an intersection. Other causes of crashes include multiple responding vehicles following too closely and obstructed visibility at the intersection. By following the guidelines for safe vehicle operations and receiving additional education in the operation of an emergency vehicle, you can usually avoid a costly mishap.

While traveling to the scene, the EMT not operating the vehicle should obtain additional information from the dispatcher to help in your scene size-up. This is also a good time to assign personnel to specific duties and consider any special equipment needs. Preplanning now may save time at the scene. This time may also be used to decide what equipment to take with you initially and to prepare it. If you are responding to a motor vehicle crash, for example, you should prepare a long board and straps, assorted cervical collars, and the head immobilization device. Also decide at this time who will stabilize the patient's spine and who will perform the assessment.

Before beginning patient care, you must consider your arrival at the scene carefully. The first step is to position the unit. Position the unit primarily for safety and secondly for departure from the scene. Safety considerations include parking uphill or upwind from any hazardous substance, and at least 30 m (100 ft) from any wreckage. Local policy dictates whether to park the unit in front of or beyond the wreckage.

Position the vehicle to allow safe loading of the patient and easy departure from the scene. Use the parking brake, and turn on the warning lights to alert other vehicles of your presence. At night, avoid blinding other drivers approaching the scene by turning off the headlights unless they are needed to illuminate the scene.

ARRIVAL AT THE SCENE

Upon your arrival at the scene, notify the dispatch center and record the time, as described in Chapter 15, "Documentation." Remember to size up the scene before approaching; this is an opportunity to protect yourself from harm. If there is a potential for violence or if the scene is unsafe, wait for law enforcement assistance before approaching. Consider the need for body substance isolation precautions, and assess the scene for hazards. Is the vehicle parked in a safe location? Is it safe to approach the patient? Does the patient need to be moved immediately because of any hazards?

Next, note the mechanism of injury or the nature of the illness. If there are more patients than you and your crew can handle, request additional help and begin triage. If there is only one patient, begin your initial assessment with the general impression. Despite the number of patients, be sure to record the time of arrival at the patient's side.

All of your actions at the scene should be rapid and organized, remembering the ultimate goal of safe and efficient patient transport. Once you have completed the initial assessment, you will have determined a patient priority. After providing all necessary emergency medical care, prepare the patient for transport to the nearest facility.

TRANSFERRING THE PATIENT TO THE AMBULANCE

Using the principles you learned in Chapter 6, "Lifting and Moving Patients," transfer the patient to the vehicle for transport. After performing all critical interventions, assure that all dressings and bandages or splints, if used, are secure. Cover the patient to provide protection from the weather, and secure the patient to the appropriate lifting and moving device.

Often family members request to ride to the hospital with the patients, especially if the patients are infants or children. Local policies determine your procedure. If family members accompany a patient to the hospital, they should be informed of the service's policies and procedures for passengers and helped to the seat they will occupy while en route to the hospital. Be sure all passengers wear their safety belts.

EN ROUTE TO THE RECEIVING FACILITY

Once the patient is loaded into the transporting vehicle, the vehicle operator and all passengers should secure their safety belts. The driver should notify dispatch that the unit is departing the scene, and state the destination. The time should be recorded. The driver and the EMT caring for the patient should determine a response mode for transport to the hospital based on the patient's condition.

During the transport to the receiving facility, you would typically perform the detailed and ongoing patient assessments, as described in the patient assessment Chapters 10 through 13. Evaluate all interventions that you have used to establish that they remain effective. Take additional recordings of vital signs at appropriate intervals, noting any changes and trends. Notify the receiving facility of the patient's condition and estimated time of arrival to the facility (Fig. 30-5). Reassure the patient that they are receiving the best possible care. Begin to complete the prehospital care report, if the patient's condition permits.

AT THE RECEIVING FACILITY

PATIENT TRANSFER

Notify dispatch as you arrive at the receiving facility. Transfer the patient to the appropriate room designated by the staff at the receiving facility. Provide a brief report to the receiving facility staff. This report should contain all pertinent information (*see* Chapter 14, "Communications"). Restock the ambulance and complete the prehospital care report, following local procedures. All crew members should wash their hands and perform any other infection control measures as necessary. Many crews have one person document while the remaining crew members complete restocking of the ambulance. A copy of the prehospital care report should be left with the patient's chart to become part of the permanent medical record (*see* Chapter 15, "Documentation").

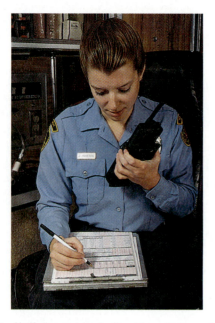

Fig. 30-5 Notify the receiving facility of the patient's condition and the estimated time of arrival.

CLEANING AND DISINFECTING

Before reporting your availability for the next prehospital call, clean and disinfect the vehicle. All supplies used during patient care should be restocked as necessary. Bag any supplies or equipment that must be disinfected at the station to prevent further contamination of the unit.

You have a risk of exposure to communicable diseases on every emergency call. Learn and use the decontamination procedures in your service area. It is the joint responsibility of you and your service to have adequate knowledge and skills for proper disinfection.

You may come in contact with body fluids and airborne diseases that are potentially infectious. To minimize the risk of infection, you must know how to protect yourself from these diseases. The practice of **infection control** prevents the transmission of infection from patients to you, from one patient to another, and from you to other patients. As stated in Chapter 2, "The Well-Being of the EMT–Basic," you must practice body substance isolation precautions whenever appropriate.

In addition to body substance isolation precautions, cleaning and decontamination measures are necessary for the ambulance and the equipment. *Decontamination* is the use of physical or chemical means to remove, deactivate, or destroy blood-borne pathogens on a surface or item so that they can no longer transmit infection, and so the surface or item is considered safe for handling, use, or

disposal. This definition, from the *Code of Federal Regulations*, describes decontamination as it relates to blood-borne pathogens.

Before using decontamination procedures, clean all equipment used in an emergency call. Cleaning begins with the removal of all dirt, tissue, and debris from the equipment or area to be decontaminated. Scrub the area or item with soap and water. If an area or object is not cleaned first, it may not be adequately disinfected when you use the chemical agents described below. Linens and uniforms are cleaned by laundering them when contaminated, following local protocol.

The Centers for Disease Control (CDC) have identified four levels of decontamination. These four levels are: sterilization; high-level disinfection; intermediate-level disinfection; and low-level disinfection. Sterilization destroys all microorganisms including bacterial spores. It is used for instruments that penetrate the skin or contact normally sterile areas of the body during invasive procedures. It is a process that involves steam pressure, a gas process, or immersion in an approved chemical agent for a prolonged period.

High-level disinfection destroys all microorganisms except large numbers of bacterial spores. It is used for equipment that has contacted mucous membranes. It uses a process of hot water pasteurization in which articles are placed in water at 176 to 212°F for 30 minutes. High-level disinfection can also be accomplished by soaking the item in an approved chemical agent for 10 to 45 minutes, the time depending on the agent manufacturer's recommendation. This process should be used on all nondisposable airway devices.

Intermediate-level disinfection destroys the tuberculosis bacteria, most viruses, and fungi, but does not destroy bacterial spores. It should be used for disinfecting surfaces that contact intact skin and that have been visibly contaminated with body fluids. It is performed by wiping the area with a disinfectant or chemical germicide that kills tuberculocidal bacteria, a commercially available germicide, or 1:100 chlorine bleach to water solution. Use intermediate disinfection procedures with equipment such as the AED, immobilization devices such as the KED or XP1, and stretchers.

Low-level disinfection destroys most bacteria and some fungi and viruses—but not tuberculosis or bacterial spores. It should be used for routine cleaning or removing of soiling when no body fluids are present. Low-level disinfection is

TABLE 30-1	Care of Specific Contaminated Equipment

Cleaning procedure key
1, Dispose; 2, Cleaning (Golden Glo); 3, *Disinfection (1:100 bleach and water solution); 4, High-level disinfection (Cidex); 5, Launder

ARTICLE	PROCEDURE	ARTICLE	PROCEDURE

Airways (ET tubes, Oropharyngeal, Nasopharyngeal)	1	Oxygen equipment
		    Cannulas and masks
		    Humidifiers, regulators, tanks
			
			1
			2

Backboards	2	Penlights	1 or 2
Emesis basins	1	Pocket masks	1 or 4
Bite sticks	1	Restraints	2
Blood pressure cuffs	2	Resuscitators (BVM)	1
Bulb syringe	1	Scissors	3
Cervical collars	1 or 2	Splints	2
Dressings and paper products	1	Stethoscope	2
Drug boxes	3	Stretcher	3
Electronic equipment	3	Stylets	1 or 4
HEPA respirator	1**	Suction unit (collection jars)	3
KED	3	Suction catheters	1
Laryngoscope or blades	4	Uniforms	5
Linens	1 or 5	Firefighter protective equipment	5
MAST suit	3		
Needles and syringes	1		

* Bleach and water solution; mix fresh daily
** Dispose of when white area appears gray

performed by wiping the surface with an approved hospital disinfectant.

Follow the specific cleaning and disinfection policies and procedures used in your EMS system. Table 30-1 describes the specific cleaning and disinfectant procedures commonly used for most equipment and supplies used in prehospital care.

EN ROUTE TO THE STATION

When returning to the station, notify dispatch of your status. At this time you can also critique the call with your crew. Discuss those elements of the call that went well and those areas that could be improved. This critique should be handled in a positive manner, with constructive advice given as needed. This time period also allows the crew an opportunity to prepare emotionally and mentally for the next call.

POSTRUN PHASE

If the vehicle needs fueling or other mechanical work, this should be handled at this phase. All paperwork from the call should be filed as required by your service. Any supplies that could not be replaced at the facility should now be restocked. Any additional disinfection procedures should be completed, and any equipment that it is air drying from previous disinfection and cleaning should be replaced.

AIR MEDICAL TRANSPORT

Air medical transportation should be considered when the patient's condition warrants and significant time can be saved, or when patients must be transported to specialty care facilities (eg, trauma centers, burn centers, neonatal centers and other tertiary care facilities). Helicopters fly in a direct route from the scene to the hospital at speeds averaging 120 mph, bypassing traffic congestion and barriers on the ground. The important issues involve when to use air medical transport, how to set up and use landing zones, and maintaining safety.

USE OF AIR MEDICAL TRANSPORT

Helicopter transport has become a standard of care for certain medical emergencies and traumatic injuries in many areas. The decision to request air medical transport should be made in consultation

BOX 30-4

Situations for Possible Air Medical Transport

Mechanism of Injury Considerations

- Vehicle rollover in which there are unrestrained passengers
- A pedestrian struck by a car at a speed of greater than 10 mph
- A fall of greater than 4.5 m (15 ft)
- A motorcyclist thrown from the motorcycle at a speed of greater than 10 mph
- A collision causing the death of an occupant in the same vehicle
- Ejection of a patient from the vehicle

Time and Distance Considerations

- Ground transport time of more than 15 minutes, even if the ground transport time to a local hospital without a trauma center is less than the air transport time to a trauma center
- The patient is entrapped and extrication will take longer than 15 minutes
- The resources of local ground units are limited, and transporting the patient to the trauma center by ground would deprive the area of available EMTs
- The patient's condition would benefit from the rapid delivery of definitive care

with the medical director. You may have guidelines that determine when to request a helicopter, or this decision may be made at the time of the individual situation. Remember that aircraft do have some limitations: they cannot fly in certain weather conditions, and they require maintenance, both scheduled and unscheduled, that may preclude their use at a time when you need them.

In general, consider using air medical transport for patients experiencing certain mechanisms of injury. In addition, consider the time and distance to a treatment center. Box 30-4 lists the specifics for these criteria. These guidelines are not inclusive and should be further discussed with the medical director and air medical care provider. Become familiar with the policies of your local air medical care provider.

LANDING ZONES

Once you have determined the need for air medical transport, you should follow certain guidelines. Identify one communications person. This person should have a good sense of direction, be familiar with the area around the landing zone, and not be directly involved in patient care. The communications officer should then contact the air medical dispatch center. Be sure to give the following essential information to the communications center: unit calling and call sign, radio frequency, number of aircraft needed, location of the incident, and prominent landmarks in the area.

A landing zone should be set up. Ideally, the landing zone should be 30 m by 30 m (100 ft by 100 ft), and minimally, 18 m by 18 m (60 ft by 60 ft). It should be free from debris, obstruction, and hazards such as overhead wires, fences, trees, or loose objects. Ideally the ground should not slope (Fig. 30-6). The person setting up the landing zone should mark each corner with an independent lighting system. Flares, light sticks, or cones that are adequately secured, or emergency vehicles with headlights pointing to the center of the landing

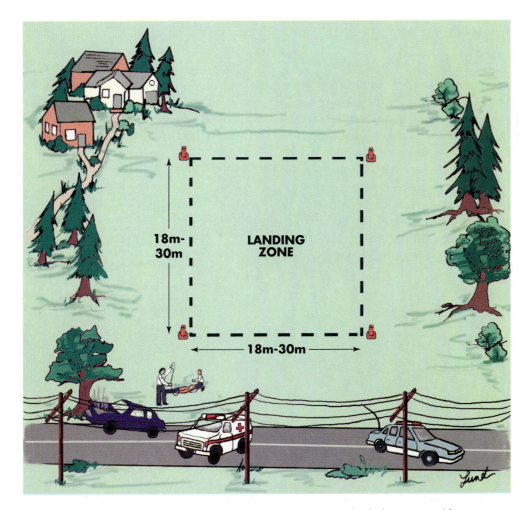

Fig. 30-6 A landing zone should be set up in an area clear of obstructions such as overhead wires, trees, and fences.

zone all make good markers. If vehicles are used, remember to turn headlights off at night as the helicopter descends into the landing zone, to avoid blinding or distracting the pilot.

The communications officer should notify the pilot when the aircraft is heard or seen. Before the aircraft arrives, provide descriptive landmark information. Good landmarks include water or radio towers, schools, tennis courts, swimming pools, high power lines, and major road intersections. You can direct the pilot to the landing zone using the clockface method. The pilot is always facing the twelve o'clock position (Fig. 30-7). If you are facing the aircraft and it is heading toward you, and you see the aircraft to the right of the landing zone, you would report that the landing zone is at the three o'clock position. Provide the pilot with a brief but detailed description of the landing zone, such as a field, road, or construction site, and the type of surface, such as grass, concrete, gravel, or dirt. Also, give boundary information such as trees, buildings, wires, fences, and towers. Information regarding the location of power lines is extremely important. Make attempts to illuminate any potential hazards.

SAFETY

Safety around an aircraft is everyone's responsibility. If the flight crews in your area provide a continuing education course regarding aircraft operations and safety, try to attend this course.

Most safety considerations around helicopters are based on common sense. Cover your eyes to protect yourself from flying particles such as dust and gravel. Always stay a safe distance from the helicopter when the blades are turning. Even when the blades have stopped turning, keep vehicles 9 m (30 ft) from the landing zone, and keep crowds 30

m (100 ft) away. Avoid running or smoking in or around the landing zone.

No one should approach the aircraft unless directed by the pilot or medical crew. If directed, you should approach only from the front of the aircraft in the view of the pilot. The tail rotor of a helicopter is often low to the ground and spinning so fast that it is nearly impossible to see. Whether or not the helicopter engine is running, all personnel should avoid the tail section. Movement in the landing zone and around the aircraft should occur only within the nine o'clock to three o'clock positions (Fig. 30-8), which is the pilot's area of vision. Never take a short cut under the body, the rear section, or the tail boom. If you are helping the flight crew, do not operate any of the aircraft doors. The flight crew is responsible for opening and closing all doors and latches.

When approaching the helicopter, stay low. Unexpected wind gusts may change the height of the blade unexpectedly. Use caution when carrying equipment to the aircraft. Approaching the helicopter carrying any equipment over your head, even if you duck low, is extremely dangerous and should be avoided. Loose equipment and hats may be blown off by the wind from the rotor blades and should be secured or avoided. If the pilot parks the aircraft on a slope, always approach from the downhill side since the main rotor blade will be lower to the ground on the uphill side (Fig. 30-9).

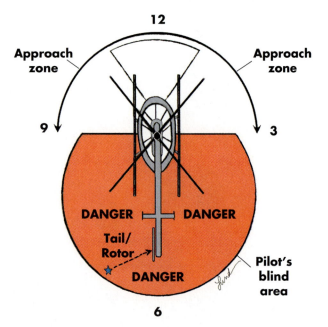

Fig. 30-8 All movement around the helicopter should be within the "nine o'clock" to "three o'clock" position.

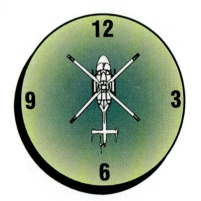

Fig. 30-7 In the clockface method of providing directions to EMS helicopters, the pilot faces the 12 o'clock position.

Always follow the directions of the flight crew regarding approach to and departure from the aircraft.

Remember that the pilot may choose a different route of departure based on winds and obstacles. The departure may require that the helicopter be turned when still close to the ground. As the aircraft prepares for departure, all personnel and equipment should be clear of the landing zone.

Many organizations and agencies can provide additional information regarding EMS helicopters, including the Association of Air Medical Services, the National Association of EMS Pilots, and your local EMS air medical provider.

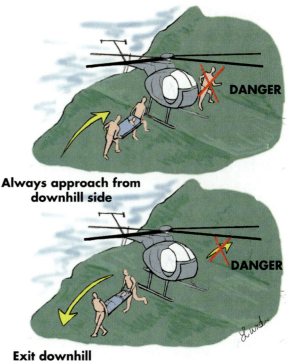

Always approach from downhill side

Exit downhill side

Fig. 30-9 If the pilot lands on a slope, approach the aircraft from the downhill side. It is very dangerous to approach from the uphill side.

REVIEW QUESTIONS

AIR MEDICAL TRANSPORT

1. Which of the following is not an essential element of information to provide the communications center?
   A. Patient name
   B. Ground contact name and call sign
   C. Frequency
   D. Location of incident

2. Which of the following is not a consideration for calling for air medical transport?
   A. Distance
   B. Cost
   C. Time
   D. Mechanism of injury

3. Who has the responsibility for safety around an aircraft?
   A. The pilot
   B. The flight crew
   C. The EMT on the ground
   D. All of the above

4. What is the minimum size for a landing zone?
   A. 7.5 m by 7.5 m (25 ft by 25 ft)
   B. 15 m by 15 m (50 ft by 50 ft)
   C. 18 m by 18 m (60 ft by 60 ft)
   D. 30 m by 30 m (100 ft by 100 ft)

1. A
2. B
3. D
4. C

CHAPTER SUMMARY

PHASES OF AN AMBULANCE CALL

The nine phases of a typical EMS response are: 1) preparation for the call; 2) dispatch; 3) en route to the scene; 4) arrival at scene; 5) transferring patient to the ambulance; 6) en route to the receiving facility; 7) at the receiving facility; 8) en route to the station; and 9) postrun.

Your roles and responsibilities depend on the phase of the call. The first phase allows you to prepare for the call and check the vehicle for medical equipment and mechanical readiness. Dispatch is an opportunity to gain information regarding the call. En route to the scene is the travel time to the scene and preplanning for the actions at the scene. Upon arrival, you size-up the scene to ensure the well-being and safety of the EMS crew. Remember that your actions at the scene should be organized with the goal of transport in mind. En route to the receiving facility, perform a detailed physical examination if necessary and ongoing assessments. This is also the time to provide noncritical interventions. Arrival at the receiving facility permits you to provide for a continuum of care by providing the hospital staff with a brief verbal and detailed written report. During the return to the station you can discuss all aspects of the call and share with your crew any thoughts regarding your performances. Finally, the postrun phase is a time to disinfect equipment, restock the vehicle, and prepare for the next response.

AIR MEDICAL TRANSPORT

Air medical transport is becoming the standard of care for some critically ill and injured patients. Considerations for the use of air medical transport include the mechanism of injury and the time and distance to the receiving facility. The set-up of a landing zone and communication should be delegated to persons not directly involved in patient care. The landing zone should be clear of debris and wires. Give the pilot as much information as possible.

Safety around the aircraft is the responsibility of everyone. Avoid running and smoking in and around the landing zone. The main rotor blades may dip as low as 4 feet from the ground. The tail rotor is spinning at a speed that makes it nearly invisible. Always approach the aircraft from the nine-to-three o'clock positions and only when directed by the flight crew. Never walk near the tail rotor or under the tailboom. Follow the instructions of the flight crew regarding safety around the aircraft.

UNITED STATES DEPARTMENT OF TRANSPORTATION NATIONAL HIGHWAY TRAFFIC SAFETY ADMINISTRATION EMT–BASIC OBJECTIVES

Check your knowledge. The National Registry of EMTs and many state EMS agencies use the objectives below to develop EMT–Basic certification examinations. Can you meet them?

COGNITIVE

1. Discuss the medical and nonmedical equipment needed to respond to a call.
2. List the phases of an ambulance call.
3. Describe the general provisions of state laws relating to the operation of the ambulance and privileges in any or all of the following categories:
   - Speed
   - Warning lights
   - Sirens
   - Right-of way
   - Parking
   - Turning
4. List contributing factors to unsafe driving conditions.
5. Describe the considerations that should be given to:
   - Request for escorts
   - Following an escort vehicle
   - Intersections
6. Discuss "Due Regard For Safety of All Others" while operating an emergency vehicle.
7. State what information is essential in order to respond to a call.
8. Discuss various situations that may affect response to a call.
9. Differentiate between the various methods of moving a patient to the unit based upon injury or illness.
10. Apply the components of the essential patient information in a written report.
11. Summarize the importance of preparing the unit for the next response.
12. Identify what is essential for completion of a call.
13. Distinguish among the terms cleaning, disinfection, high-level disinfection, and sterilization.
14. Describe how to clean or disinfect items following patient care.

AFFECTIVE

1. Explain the rationale for appropriate report of patient information.
2. Explain the rationale for having the unit prepared to respond.

31 GAINING ACCESS

KEY TERM

Extrication: The process of removing a patient from entanglement in a motor vehicle or other situation in a safe and appropriate manner.

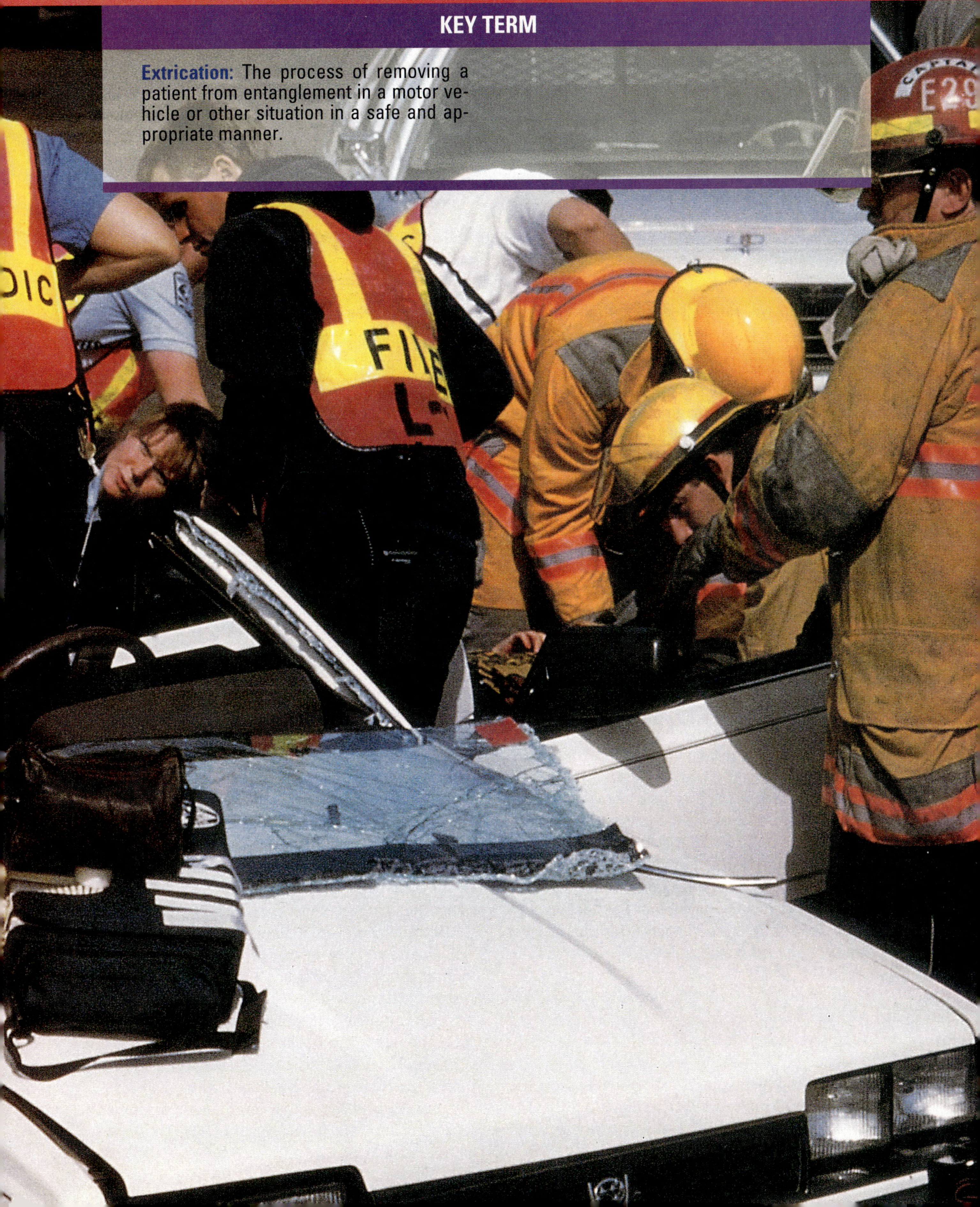

IN THE FIELD

EMTs Tony and Tami responded in their ambulance to a motor vehicle accident. There was a report of entrapment, and dispatch reported that a rescue unit was also on the way. Upon their arrival at the scene, Tony and Tami sized-up the scene. They observed a single car that had collided with a utility pole, and the driver still inside the vehicle. There were no wires down, and the vehicle did not appear to be leaking any fluids. The scene appeared to be safe, but Tami and Tony noted broken glass around the vehicle.

As they were putting on their turn-out gear, the rescue company arrived. The rescuers approached as Tony and Tami headed toward the car with their medical kit and spinal immobilization equipment. The car doors were locked and did not open when Tony tried them. The patient inside appeared unresponsive. Tami assessed the vehicle and saw that simple access was not possible. Because the vehicle was badly damaged, rescue with special equipment was required.

The rescue company first stabilized the vehicle. Because the patient inside was unresponsive, Tony and Tami wanted to gain access quickly. The rescue company broke a window, and Tami crawled into the car. As she began to assess and treat the patient, Tony prepared the equipment to remove the patient from the car. At the same time, the rescue commander ordered the rescue workers to use power tools to pry open the twisted metal door of the wreckage.

By coordinating their efforts with the rescue team, Tami and Tony were able to evaluate, immobilize, and transport the patient to the hospital quickly.

EMTs respond to many situations involving motor vehicle collisions or other situations in which a patient may be trapped (Fig. 31-1). Personal safety is very important in these situations. An EMT who is injured not only is unable to help the patient but requires additional EMS or rescue resources. In some EMS systems, EMTs are required to have special knowledge and education in rescue techniques. In other systems, rescue is handled by fire service, special rescue, or law enforcement personnel (Fig. 31-2). Therefore, you must become familiar with the system used in your area and seek additional education as necessary. This chapter provides an overview of the safety equipment EMTs use at rescue scenes and the medical aspects of extrication.

FUNDAMENTALS OF EXTRICATION

Extrication is the process of removing a patient from entanglement in a motor vehicle or other situation in a safe and appropriate manner. In some situations extrication must be preceded by removing objects from around the patient to access the patient and provide a path from the vehicle or other structure. This process, often called *disentanglement*, usually involves the use of special equipment. In many EMS systems, such rescues are the responsibility of specially educated EMTs. In other areas, rescue services are provided by specially educated firefighters or law enforcement personnel. In all systems, however, EMTs respond to situations that require extrication. Therefore, it is important to understand the role of EMS personnel at crash scenes, industrial accidents, structure collapses, and other settings of entrapment.

Depending on your system, you may be responsible for rescue. Regardless of your rescue responsibilities, however, everyone's actions at a rescue scene must follow a chain of command. In some systems, an incident management system coordinates the emergency efforts involving extrication. Chapter 32, "Overviews: Special Response Situations" discusses incident management systems.

The incident commander coordinates the efforts of both medical and rescue personnel (Fig. 31-3), as

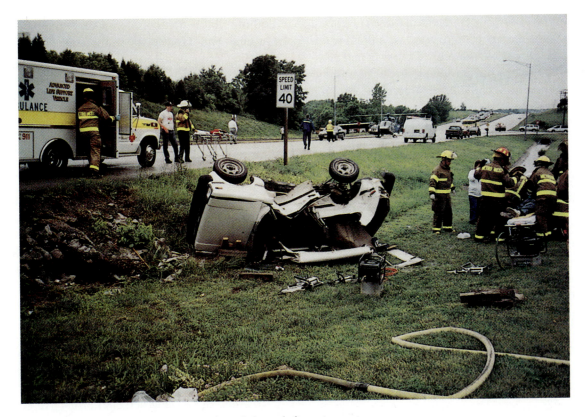

Fig. 31-1 EMTs often provide medical care to patients during and after entrapment.

well as those responsible for patient transport. Teamwork is important in these operations. Extrication depends on the knowledge, skill, and equipment of rescue personnel, just as medical care depends on your knowledge, skill, and equipment. You cooperate with the rescuers, but rescue activities should not interfere with your patient-care activities.

All critical emergency care should be provided

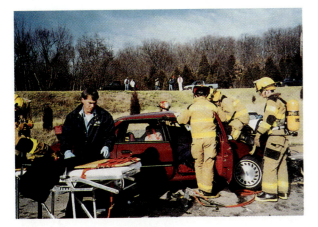

Fig. 31-2 In some areas, EMTs work with specially educated teams to rescue patients from entrapment.

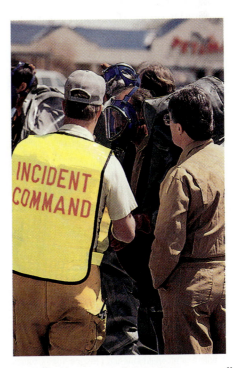

Fig. 31-3 The incident commander coordinates rescue efforts by medical and rescue personnel.

before and during the extrication. If a rescue crew is performing the extrication, work with them to ensure that the patient is removed in a way that minimizes the risk of further injury. In all cases of entrapment, critical patient care precedes extrication unless delay would endanger the life of the patient, EMTs, or rescuers, in which case extrication is done immediately. While the rescue crew works, prepare the equipment necessary to remove the patient and begin to initiate care such as assessment, bleeding control, and oxygen therapy.

This same principle applies for EMTs who also perform as rescue personnel. Provide all critical patient care before and during the extrication. Patient care precedes extrication unless an emergency move is necessary. Rescue EMTs must cooperate with medical EMTs to ensure that the patient is removed in a way that minimizes the risk of further injury.

SAFETY AND EQUIPMENT

When a patient must be extricated, your safety is the first priority, followed by the safety of the patient and bystanders.

PERSONAL SAFETY

Personal safety is always your number one priority. This rule applies to all workers involved in rescue activities or medical care. Wear protective clothing that is appropriate for the situation. The National Fire Protection Administration (NFPA) and the Occupational Safety and Health Administration (OSHA) have guidelines for personal safety equipment that many EMS services follow when purchasing equipment.

EMTs who respond to motor vehicle collisions or who are involved in rescue operations should have at least the following personal protective equipment:

- Impact-resistant protective helmet with ear protection and chin strap.
- Protective eyewear. Ideally the protective eyewear has an elastic strap and vents to prevent fogging. The shield on a helmet is not considered protective eyewear.
- Light-weight, puncture-resistant "turn-out" coat.
- Leather gloves.
- Boots with steel insoles and steel toes.

Most EMTs also use light-weight, puncture-resistant turn-out pants (Fig. 31-4).

In addition to using personal protective equipment, take body substance isolation precautions. As described in Chapter 2, "The Well-Being of the EMT–Basic," body substance isolation precautions are required any time you may come in contact with blood or other body fluids.

PATIENT SAFETY

Once the safety needs of both medical and rescue personnel are met, consider the safety of the patient and bystanders. Explain the extrication process to patients, including the sounds they will hear. Cover patients with blankets or tarps to pro-

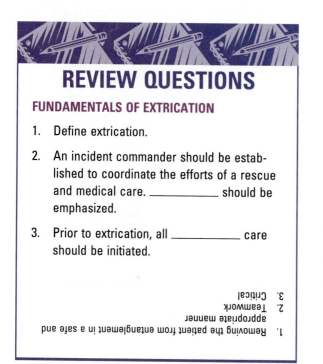

REVIEW QUESTIONS

FUNDAMENTALS OF EXTRICATION

1. Define extrication.

2. An incident commander should be established to coordinate the efforts of a rescue and medical care. _____ should be emphasized.

3. Prior to extrication, all _____ care should be initiated.

1. Removing the patient from entanglement in a safe and appropriate manner
2. Teamwork
3. Critical

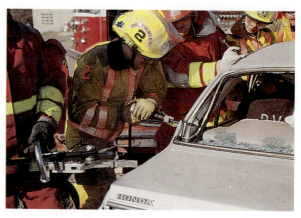

Fig. 31-4 In rescue situations, EMTs should use personal protective equipment.

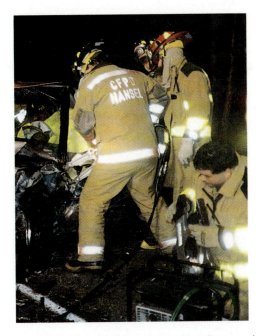

Fig. 31-5 The patient should be protected from glass, metal, and other hazards during the disentanglement process.

tect against broken glass, sharp metal, and other hazards (Fig. 31-5), as well as to keep them warm.

Bystanders and uninvolved people should be kept clear of the scene. The presence of curious onlookers at the scene increases the risk of additional injuries (Fig. 31-6).

OTHER SAFETY ISSUES

Motor vehicle accidents and other cases of entrapment may involve hazardous materials, which could prevent you from gaining access to the patient. Be familiar with your system's hazardous materials response guidelines and hazardous materials plan. For additional information on hazardous materials, see Chapter 32.

Also be alert for the possibility of fire at an accident scene. To reduce this risk, turn off the ignition of the vehicle and prevent smoking at the scene (Fig. 31-7). Unless you have had special education in vehicle firefighting, do not attempt to extinguish a fire. With a small fire, you may be able to use a fire extinguisher to stop the fire from spreading. Again, attempt this only if you have the proper knowledge, skills, and equipment.

In addition to the risk of fire, there is a risk of electric shock from downed power lines. Only utility or rescue workers who are educated in the handling of live power lines should approach downed power lines to secure them. If victims are inside a vehicle, advise them to remain inside the vehicle. If you cannot approach the vehicle because of downed power lines, try to talk to the patient through a loud speaker system, such as the vehicle radio's public address system. As described in Chapter 8, "Scene Size-Up," if the scene is unsafe, either make it safe or do not enter it. If you cannot make it safe yourself, request the appropriate agency to respond.

Unstable vehicles also pose a problem for rescuers and EMTs. As you are caring for an injured patient, the balance of the vehicle may change, causing the unstable vehicle to shift and roll or fall

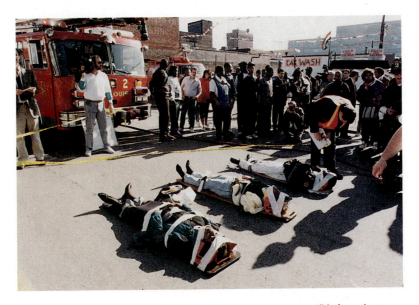

Fig. 31-6 A safe zone should be established at the rescue scene, and only those persons responsible for patient care or extrication should be in the inner circle.

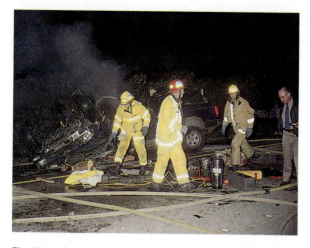

Fig. 31-7 Safety measures such as turning off the car ignition can prevent a car fire.

vehicle, or unsafe acts by the rescuers or EMTs. This person can also cycle in new rescuers when others become fatigued.

ACCESSING THE PATIENT

Accessing, or getting to the patient, may be simple or complex. Simple access does not require the use of rescue equipment and can be performed by all EMTs. Complex extrication requires additional

and potentially injure you or other personnel. Before entering a crashed vehicle, assess its stability (Fig. 31-8). Assist the rescue workers to ensure that the vehicle is stabilized before caring for the patient.

A rescue scene always must be managed. In addition to an incident commander, if enough personnel are present, a safety officer should be appointed. A person who is not directly involved in the rescue or patient care should have this responsibility. This person should be an objective observer and should watch for safety issues and additional hazards that the rescue workers may not be able to see, such as development of fires, movement of the

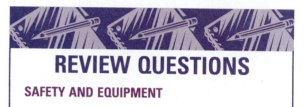

REVIEW QUESTIONS

SAFETY AND EQUIPMENT

1. The first priority at a vehicle accident is
   _____.

2. List five items of personal protective equipment needed for a crash scene.

3. List at least three potential hazards at the scene of a vehicle accident.

1. Personal safety
2. Helmet, eye protection, turn-out coat, leather gloves, and toe boots
3. Hazardous materials, fire, electrical lines, unstable vehicles

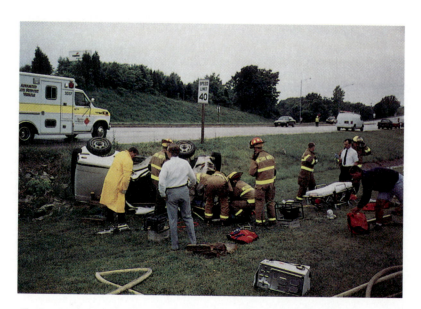

Fig. 31-8 Be sure every effort has been made to secure vehicle stability before entering. Continue to assess the vehicle's stability throughout the extrication process.

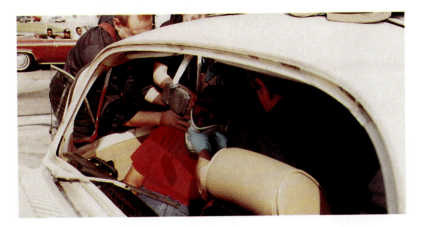

Fig. 31-9 Simple access does not require the use of mechanical tools.

education, skills, and equipment. If you are interested or required to become a rescue technician, you should investigate the variety of available programs that provide this additional education. Different basic rescue courses deal with vehicle rescue and the use of ropes and self-contained breathing apparatus. In addition, special rescue programs include water rescue, trench rescue, and high-angle rescue. Check with your instructor or service about the availability of these courses.

Even though simple access to the patient does not require the use of rescue equipment, you should always wear protective clothing when working at a scene that may pose a hazard. First, try to open the vehicle's doors. If possible, have the patient unlock a locked door or roll down a window (Fig. 31-9). Upon your arrival at the scene, if the damage to the vehicle suggests you may have difficulty accessing the patient, you may first call for additional help and then attempt these simple methods of access. If you succeed at gaining access, you can then cancel the request for the rescue crew or use them as needed to help move the injured patient.

Nonrescue EMTs should work with local rescue workers to gain an understanding of the extrication process. This will allow you to explain what is happening to the patient and help reduce the patient's anxiety.

REMOVING THE PATIENT

Once you have gained access to the patient, you should extricate or remove the patient. Chapter 28, "Injuries to the Head and Spine," describes the techniques and equipment to use in removing the patient. When removing the patient, maintain spinal immobilization at all times. Move a patient without spinal immobilization only in situations when the patient, EMTs, or rescuers are in danger if the patient is not moved immediately.

> ### ALERT
> **Move patients without spinal immobilization only when danger is present. Immobilize all other patients with spinal injuries prior to movement.**

Complete the initial assessment and provide critical interventions before removing the patient. Except in a situation that requires rapid extrication, ensure that the spine is immobilized using a short spine board or other immobilization device (Fig. 31-10).

Before removing the patient from the vehicle, ensure sufficient personnel are present to move the patient. Remember to pick up the patient rather than the immobilization device, unless the device is designed to be lifted. Before starting to move the patient from the vehicle, be sure that you have sufficient personnel. Choose the path of least resistance, protect the patient from hazards, ensure an open airway, and maintain spinal immobilization.

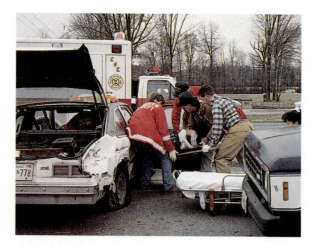

Fig. 31-10 Except in cases of emergency moves, immobilize the patient's spine before removal.

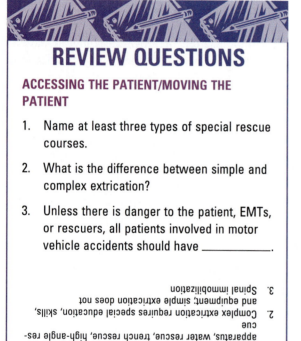

REVIEW QUESTIONS

ACCESSING THE PATIENT/MOVING THE PATIENT

1. Name at least three types of special rescue courses.

2. What is the difference between simple and complex extrication?

3. Unless there is danger to the patient, EMTs, or rescuers, all patients involved in motor vehicle accidents should have _____.

1. Vehicle rescue, rope rescue, self-contained breathing apparatus, water rescue, trench rescue, high-angle rescue
2. Complex extrication requires special education, skills, and equipment; simple extrication does not
3. Spinal immobilization

CHAPTER SUMMARY

FUNDAMENTALS OF EXTRICATION

Extrication is the process of freeing a patient from entanglement. This process may require disentanglement by specially educated rescue EMTs or rescue technicians. An incident commander should coordinate the efforts of everyone responsible for extrication and the EMTs responsible for medical care. Teamwork is important. Assess the patient and provide critical care before and during the extrication. Work with the rescue crew to ensure that the patient is removed in a way that minimizes further injury to the patient.

SAFETY AND EQUIPMENT

Personal safety is the number one priority for both rescue and nonrescue EMTs. Wear protective clothing appropriate for the situation, and take the appropriate body substance isolation precautions. Perform a scene size-up. Situations requiring extrication may involve hazardous materials. Also be alert for the potential of fire at a crash scene and the risk of electrical shock from downed power lines. Unstable vehicles also pose a problem. If the scene is unsafe, make it safe or do not enter.

ACCESSING THE PATIENT

Accessing the patient may be simple or complex. Special education programs are necessary for rescue EMTs and rescue technicians to learn complex access techniques. Once you access the patient, perform an initial assessment, immobilize the spine, and perform any interventions.

Simple access to the patient does not require the use of equipment. Try all the vehicle doors, or have the patient unlock a locked door or roll down a window.

REMOVING THE PATIENT

Once extrication procedures have been completed, remove the patient. Complete the initial assessment. Provide only critical interventions before moving the patient. Before moving the patient from the vehicle, ensure that there are sufficient personnel to move the patient safely.

UNITED STATES DEPARTMENT OF TRANSPORTATION NATIONAL HIGHWAY TRAFFIC SAFETY ADMINISTRATION EMT–BASIC OBJECTIVES

Check your knowledge. The National Registry of EMTs and many state EMS agencies use the objectives below to develop EMT–Basic certification examinations. Can you meet them?

COGNITIVE

1. Describe the purpose of extrication.
2. Discuss the role of the EMT–Basic in extrication.
3. Identify what equipment for personal safety is required for the EMT–Basic.
4. Define the fundamental components of extrication.
5. State the steps that should be taken to protect the patient during extrication.
6. Evaluate various methods of gaining access to the patient.
7. Distinguish between simple and complex access.

KEY TERMS

Extrication sector: The sector in the incident management system responsible for dealing with extrication of patients who are trapped at the scene. This responsibility includes rescue, the initial assessment, and sorting patients for transport to the treatment sector.

Hazardous material: Any substance or material that can pose an unreasonable risk to health, safety, or property.

Incident management system: A system for coordinating procedures to assist in the control, direction, and coordination of emergency response resources.

Material Safety Data Sheets: Information sheets required by the US Department of Labor that list properties and hazards associated with chemicals and compounds to assist in management of incidents involving them.

Placard: An information sign with symbols and numbers to assist in identifying the hazardous material or class of material.

Staging sector: The sector in the incident management system that coordinates with the transportation sector for the movement of vehicles to and from the transportation sector.

Support or supply sector: The sector in the incident management system responsible for obtaining additional resources including disposable supplies, personnel, and equipment for other sectors.

Transportation sector: A sector of the incident management system that coordinates resources including receiving hospitals, air medical resources, and ambulances.

Treatment sector: The sector in the incident management system that provides care to patients received from the triage and extrication sector.

Triage: A method of categorizing patients into treatment or transport priorities.

Triage sector: An optional sector in the incident management system that prioritizes patients for treatment and transport.

IN THE FIELD

"**U**nit 37, respond to the intersection of State Route 24 and Elm Street," the dispatcher requested over the radio. "Motor vehicle crash with injuries." The EMTs hurried to their response vehicle, buckled up, and departed the station. Alberto contacted dispatch en route for additional information. Dispatch reported that a tanker truck had struck a minivan. Jane and Alberto realized the potential for a hazardous materials situation because of the tanker truck and for a multiple casualty situation because of the potential number of passengers in a minivan.

Approximately one quarter of a mile from the scene Jane stopped the ambulance to look at the scene. There were visible signs of a hazardous materials spill, and with binoculars Jane saw a placard on the tanker truck identifying it as carrying flammable materials. Alberto notified dispatch, gave a brief report, and requested the hazardous materials team to respond. The EMTs waited for the arrival of the hazardous materials team, continuing to observe the situation from a distance.

On arrival of the hazardous materials team, an incident management system was established. Once it was determined safe to enter the scene, Jane and Alberto initiated triage of the patients in the minivan and the driver of the tanker truck. Because an incident management system was established early, the hazard was contained, all patients in the minivan and the truck were successfully rescued and treated, and the EMTs avoided dangerous contact with hazardous materials.

As an EMT, you may encounter a number of special response situations. As technology changes and chemists and scientists develop new chemicals that may be harmful and toxic, EMTs are even more likely to encounter hazardous materials situations. Proper education is important for your safety and well-being and that of the public in such situations.

Multiple casualty situations, in which there are more patients than EMTs at a scene, are another area that requires special knowledge and skills. In such situations you need to understand the reasons for and methods of sorting patients and prioritizing their care.

In both of these instances an incident management system can be beneficial. The incident management system has been developed to provide structure and guidance in managing such special response situations.

These topics fall under the umbrella of what is usually called *disaster planning and response*. This chapter provides only an overview of hazardous materials, incident management systems, and triage. Before being assigned to a special response team, you would require additional education in these areas.

HAZARDOUS MATERIALS

A **hazardous material** is any substance or material that can pose an unreasonable risk to health, safety, or property. Because there is a great chance that you will be involved in a hazardous materials incident during your emergency medical services (EMS) career, you should, at a minimum, attend a First Responder Awareness Level education program. Ideally, all EMTs should be educated at least to the First Responder Operations Level because EMTs respond to the scene of hazardous materials incidents. This education involves approaching hazardous materials in a manner safest for everyone involved (Box 32-1).

EXTENT OF THE PROBLEM

The issue of hazardous materials is an everyday concern and problem. Although some may think of hazardous materials only in terms of transportation incidents such as vehicle crashes, in reality many household chemicals, pesticides, and other compounds found in the home and industrial sites may cause a hazardous materials situation. A patient's home may have carbon monoxide leaking from the

BOX 32-1

Hazardous Materials First Responder Awareness Level

The First Responder Awareness Level education program is designed for those individuals who are likely to witness or discover a hazardous materials incident and to institute an emergency response plan. First Responders at this awareness level should be able to demonstrate:

- An understanding of what hazardous materials are and the risks associated with them.
- An understanding of the potential outcomes of a hazardous materials incident.
- The ability to recognize the presence of hazardous materials.
- An understanding of one's role in an agency's response plan.
- An understanding of the need for additional resources.

SAFETY CONCERNS

In all hazardous materials situations, your primary concern should be safety. Safety concerns include your own well-being and that of other crew members, patients, bystanders, and the community.

Knowledge of what is involved and what to do is necessary for successful and safe management of hazardous materials situations. While traveling to the scene of a hazardous materials incident, obtain as much additional information as you can from dispatch. This gathering of information is the start of your investigation into the scope of the problem. The United States Department of Transportation (USDOT) publishes a reference to assist in identifying and managing hazardous materials, the *Emergency Response Guidebook*, (Fig. 32-2) which lists hazardous materials and the appropriate emergency procedures. This book should be in every response vehicle to help you identify potential hazards. It can be a great resource for you until more highly educated help arrives. Always remember the scene size-up rule: If the scene is not safe, make it safe, otherwise do not enter. In a hazardous materials scene, you usually require the expertise of a highly educated hazardous materials team to make the scene safe. Do not enter the scene unless you are educated to handle hazardous materials and have skills for use of the necessary equipment.

APPROACHING THE SCENE

Once you suspect the scene may involve hazardous materials, because of either dispatch information or physical clues, follow these important safety guidelines as you approach the scene:

heating system, a patient may use an oven cleaner in a poorly ventilated room, or chlorine gas may leak at a local municipal swimming pool. Anytime there is a spill or leak of chemicals, there is a potential for a hazardous materials incident (Fig. 32-1). Anytime EMTs, the public, or the environment is at risk, there is a hazardous materials situation.

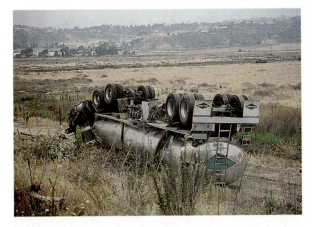

Fig. 32-1 Any spill of chemicals can become a hazardous materials incident.

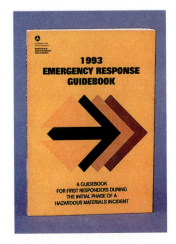

Fig. 32-2 The *Emergency Response Guidebook.*

- Approach the scene from an uphill and upwind direction.
- Isolate the area.
- Avoid contact with the area.
- Be alert for unusual odors, clouds, and leakage.
- Remember that some chemicals are odorless.
- Do not drive the response vehicle through leakage or vapor clouds.
- Keep all personnel and bystanders a safe distance from the scene.
- Approach the scene with extreme caution. Do not rush into a situation that may harm you. You cannot help others if you become a patient yourself. Until you know what the material or situation is, you cannot help.

ALERT

EMTs must not enter a hazardous materials scene unless properly educated to deal with the situation and properly protected. Approach only as close as you can without risking personal safety, but do not actually enter the scene.

INFORMATION RESOURCES

Once the scene has been recognized as a hazardous materials incident, if you are educated and required to deal with decontamination issues, you should work at identifying the extent of the problem. At the site of a vehicle crash, try to determine if the vehicle is occupied and the size and shape of the container of hazardous materials. If the hazardous materials scene does not involve a vehicle, identifying the container by shape and size is also important. This information may allow the hazardous materials team to make an early identification of the materials involved. Often hazardous materials are identified by a **placard** (Fig. 32-3). The placard may also have a four-digit identification number to help you identify the material or class of material. Check the *Emergency Response Guidebook* for any placard numbers. Shipping papers, if you can safely locate and retrieve them without personal risk, are also a valuable resource. Shipping papers are typically located in the passenger compartment of the

vehicle, with the driver. Some vehicles have a special compartment for the shipping papers. Shipping papers are not usually retrievable without the use of protective equipment.

Check the *Emergency Response Guidebook* for suggested interventions you may be able to perform before the specially educated team arrives. Most interventions beyond safety precautions around the scene usually require a minimum educational level at the First Responder Operations Level as well as protective equipment (Box 32-2).

When responding to hazardous materials incidents at industrial or business locations, also try to locate the **Material Safety Data Sheets (MSDS)**. The Department of Labor requires these information sheets to be present for all chemical products used

BOX 32-2

First Responder Operations Level

The First Responder Operations Level education program is designed for those individuals who are likely to respond to a hazardous materials incident with the intent of protecting persons, property, or the environment from the effects of the incident. These responders are educated to respond in a defensive fashion, not to stop the release of the hazardous material. Operations Level Responders should be able to demonstrate:

- Knowledge of the basic hazard and risk-assessment techniques.
- How to select and use proper personal protective equipment provided to the First Responder.
- An understanding of basic hazardous materials terms.
- The ability to perform basic control, containment, and/or confinement operations.
- The ability to implement basic decontamination procedures.
- An understanding of the relevant standard operating procedures and termination procedures.

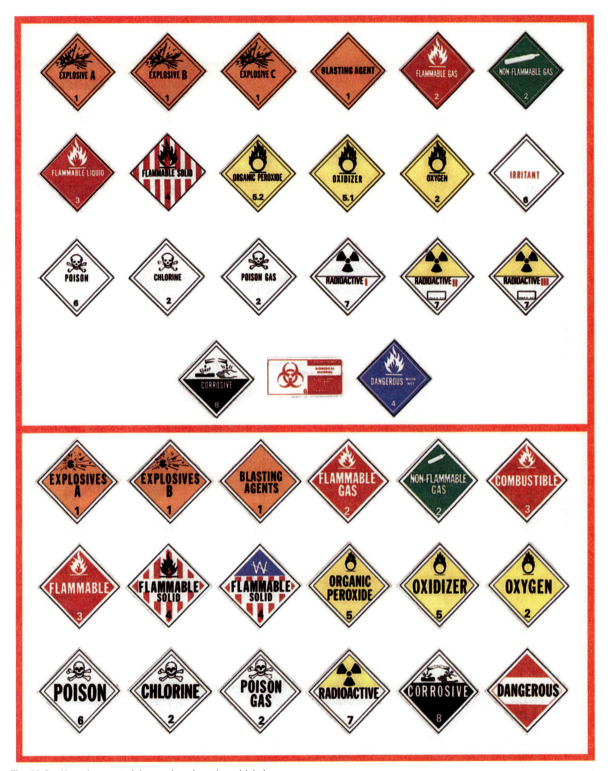

Fig. 32-3   Hazardous materials warning placards and labels.

or stored in the United States. MSDS list properties and hazards of chemicals and compounds to help manage situations involving them. MSDS are required to be displayed in a strategic and obvious location in the industrial or business location. These sheets can give you additional information about the potential health hazards of the chemical or compound. If a hazardous materials incident is located in an industrial plant, another valuable resource may be an industrial hazardous materials response team within the plant.

An additional available resource is the Chemical

Transportation Emergency Center (CHEMTREC) which is a service of the Chemical Manufacturers Association. This public service agency can provide immediate on-line advice to emergency personnel at the scene of hazardous materials incidents. CHEMTREC operates 24 hours per day, 7 days a week, and can be reached through an emergency phone number (1-800-424-9300). It is recommended that you contact CHEMTREC as soon as possible during the incident. When you call, be prepared to provide as much information as possible regarding the incident including the name of the substance, its identification number, and a description of the incident.

These are only some of the available resources. In general, do not rely on only one source of information when dealing with a hazardous materials incident. Other resources include poison centers and medical direction.

The Occupational Safety and Health Administration (OSHA) and the National Fire Protection Administration have guidelines for public safety personnel, including EMS, related to hazardous materials. Part 1910.120, 29 Code of Federal Regulations regulates the safety and health of employees in any emergency response to incidents involving hazardous substances. NFPA 473, Professional Competence for EMS Personnel Responding to Hazardous Materials Incidents, identifies the competencies required of EMS personnel who respond to hazardous materials incidents. Note that your initial EMT education program may not include the necessary components to meet these competencies. Therefore, if you are assigned to a unit responsible for hazardous materials responses, seek out and gain additional education in this area.

PROCEDURES

In general, follow the procedures below whenever dealing with a hazardous materials incident. Remember that although a patient may be involved, your care of the patient in most cases cannot begin until the situation has been determined to be safe or has been decontaminated by the hazardous materials team.

1. Approach the scene with extreme caution. Do not make the situation worse by becoming a victim.
2. Identify the hazards. Use all available resources, including placards, shipping papers, and knowledgeable bystanders. Assess each piece of information, and consult the most recent edition of the *Emergency Response Guidebook*. Follow those guidelines to avoid risk to yourself, the crew, and bystanders.
3. Assure safety around the scene. Do not enter the immediate hazard zone, and do whatever is possible to isolate the area and ensure the safety of the people and the environment. Isolate any bystanders who have been contaminated on the scene during attempts to render assistance before you arrived. Move and keep all bystanders and crew away from the scene. Do not block the entrance or exit of any equipment needed on the scene.
4. Obtain additional help. CHEMTREC, a local hazardous materials team, medical direction, and other agencies can be valuable resources during this incident.
5. Decide whether it is safe to enter the scene. Any potential rescue efforts regarding lives or property must be weighed against the possibility that you too may become a victim. If you are not part of a special response team for hazardous materials, do not enter the scene. Do not walk through leakage, and do not touch spilled material. Avoid inhaling any fumes, smoke, or vapors. Do not assume that fumes, smoke, or vapors are safe just because they are odorless. Remember that not all chemicals have an odor.

EDUCATION FOR EMERGENCY MEDICAL SERVICES RESPONDERS

There are five recognized levels of education for hazardous materials responders. These levels were created by the OHSA as mandated by the Superfund Amendments and Reauthorization Act of 1986. The five levels as identified in Part 1910, 29 Code of Federal Regulations are:

1. First Responder Awareness
2. First Responder Operations
3. Hazardous Materials Technicians
4. Hazardous Materials Specialist
5. On-Scene Incident Commander

Every EMT should be educated at least to the First Responder Awareness level. This level is designed for those individuals who are likely to discover a hazardous materials incident. State and local polices and regulations may require additional education. EMTs wanting to become more involved in this area should seek additional education programs, such as to the other four levels of education listed above.

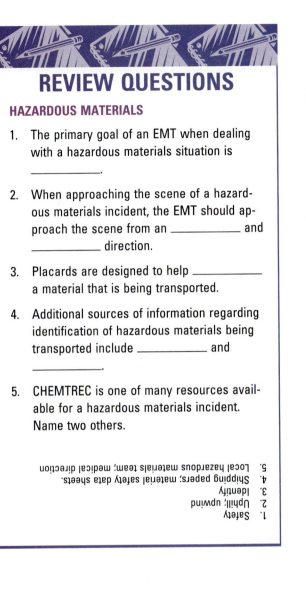

REVIEW QUESTIONS

HAZARDOUS MATERIALS

1. The primary goal of an EMT when dealing with a hazardous materials situation is
_____.

2. When approaching the scene of a hazardous materials incident, the EMT should approach the scene from an _____ and _____ direction.

3. Placards are designed to help _____ a material that is being transported.

4. Additional sources of information regarding identification of hazardous materials being transported include _____ and _____.

5. CHEMTREC is one of many resources available for a hazardous materials incident. Name two others.

1. Safety
2. Uphill; upwind
3. Identify
4. Shipping papers; material safety data sheets.
5. Local hazardous materials team; medical direction

INCIDENT MANAGEMENT SYSTEMS

An **incident management system** is a coordinated system of procedures to assist in the control, direction, and coordination of emergency response resources. This system has been developed to allow for smooth operations at the scene of an emergency regardless of its size. Incident management systems provide an orderly method for communications and decision making. Incident management systems also make communications and interactions among different agencies more efficient.

Incident management systems are established by local and state agencies. They involve the resources of various public safety and public services agencies. The incident management system may involve law enforcement, fire departments, EMS

agencies, local hospitals, and support services such as the Red Cross, Salvation Army, health department, and public works departments.

STRUCTURE OF RESPONSIBILITIES

In an incident management system, a plan has already been defined to manage any major incident. The first step is declaring that a major incident exists. Box 32-3 lists some situations in which a major incident may be declared. This list is not all inclusive, and you should follow your local protocol for declaring a major incident. Because the incident management system can be beneficial in many situations, you should not be reluctant to declare a major incident when appropriate.

Once a major incident has been declared, a commander or incident manager is identified. Usually the incident plan determines who assumes the initial command. This person must be familiar with the incident management system, the available resources, and operations procedures. An effective incident commander is a valuable resource during a major incident. There should be only one incident commander, and the commander should be clearly identified on the scene. The command position may be transferred to a more knowledgeable person arriving at the scene.

During major incidents, several sectors are established, each with unique responsibilities. These sectors are organized after an incident commander is established. Not all sectors are established for all

BOX 32-3

Situations in Which to Declare a Major Incident

- Situations requiring a great demand on resources, equipment, or personnel.
- Any hazardous materials situation.
- Any situation requiring special fire, rescue, law enforcement, or EMS resources. These special resources also includes multiple extrications and use of EMS helicopters.
- Any situation in which you are unsure whether the incident management system is needed.

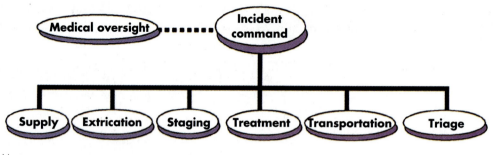

Fig. 32-4 Incident management system structure.

incidents (Fig. 32-4). Many versions of an incident management system are possible, using various sectors. In general, there are seven recognized EMS sectors:

1. Incident command
2. Extrication
3. Treatment
4. Transportation
5. Staging
6. Supply (support)
7. Triage

Each sector has a leader or sector officer. EMTs may be called on by the incident commander to become sector officers. Education programs are available for learning the different roles and responsibilities involved. Participation in disaster drills also helps EMTs become proficient in these areas. The sector officer does not perform specific tasks but coordinates the sector overall and delegates the specific roles to individuals within the sector. You are encouraged to seek additional education about incident management systems and multiple casualty incidents.

The **extrication sector** is responsible for disentanglement of patients who are trapped at the scene. This responsibility includes rescue, the initial assessment, and triaging patients for transport and treatment. Only initial assessments and treatments for potential life threats are performed within the extrication sector. All other treatment is deferred to the treatment sector.

The **treatment sector** provides additional care as patients are received from the extrication and triage sector. Within this sector, initial assessments are repeated and focused history and physical examinations are performed. In the treatment sector, patients may be further divided into additional priorities, as described in the triage section later in this chapter.

The **transportation sector** coordinates activities with the incident commander regarding the available resources of receiving hospitals, air medical resources, and ambulances. The arrival and departure of vehicles transferring patients are coordinated in the staging sector. A record of patients transported and their destinations is maintained by the transportation sector.

The **staging sector** is necessary for large incidents. The staging sector coordinates with the transportation sector for the movement of vehicles to and from the scene. This sector also coordinates with the news media and other agencies such as the Red Cross, the Salvation Army, and other disaster relief agencies. In some cases, the critical incident stress debriefing teams are staged here.

The **support or supply sector** is responsible for obtaining additional resources including additional disposable supplies, personnel, and equipment for other sectors. This sector coordinates the resources of medical facilities and incoming responding units. In addition, the supply sector officer coordinates with the transportation sector officer to obtain additional supplies from local facilities.

The **triage sector** is an optional sector. All personnel in the extrication and treatment sectors should continuously reassess patients to determine priorities for care. In some incidents, the incident commander may establish a triage sector to work closely with the extrication and treatment sectors to continuously reevaluate patients.

Each sector should be clearly defined, with appropriate sector officers designated. Commercially available kits including flags and color-coded vests often assist with this process of identifying personnel. Radio communications should be kept to a minimum and are typically reserved for the sector officers and incident commander. Preplanning for using the incident management system along with practice drills help reinforce the principles and allow for better operations when the situation requires use of an incident management system.

ROLE OF THE EMERGENCY MEDICAL TECHNICIAN

Your role in the incident management system depends in part on the point at which you arrive at the incident. EMTs arriving first may act as the incident commander or triage sector officer until additional help arrives. EMTs at the scene are typically assigned to a particular role in one of the sectors. Once the full incident management system is operational, report to the staging area for assignment on your arrival at the scene. Once assigned, report to the sector officer for specific assigned duties. After completing assigned specific tasks, report back to the sector officer for additional instructions. All decisions must be cleared through the incident commander. Individual decisions or actions by EMTs are not allowed in these situations. Although as an EMT you are educated to act independently, in a multiple casualty situation it is important that you follow the instructions of the sector officer and incident commander.

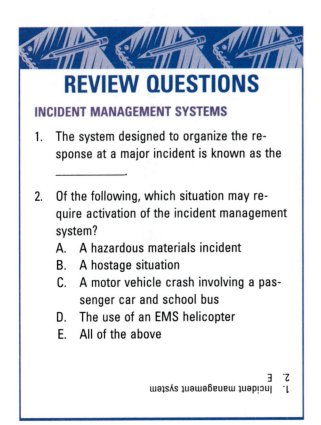

REVIEW QUESTIONS

INCIDENT MANAGEMENT SYSTEMS

1. The system designed to organize the response at a major incident is known as the

    _____ .

2. Of the following, which situation may require activation of the incident management system?
    A. A hazardous materials incident
    B. A hostage situation
    C. A motor vehicle crash involving a passenger car and school bus
    D. The use of an EMS helicopter
    E. All of the above

1. Incident management system
2. E

MULTIPLE CASUALTY SITUATIONS

A multiple casualty situation is an incident involving more patients than the responding unit can safely and efficiently handle. In general, these situations require activation of the incident management system.

TRIAGE

In a multiple casualty situation, patient triage is a priority. **Triage** is a method of categorizing patients into treatment and transport priorities. There are generally three priority levels, from highest to lowest. A tagging system is typically used to assist in designating the category of each of the patients. Through the use of color-coded or numbered tags, patients are placed into one of the triage categories (Fig. 32-5). Box 32-4 lists the conditions that fall into each of these categories.

Some tagging systems place deceased patients in a fourth category. Become familiar with your local priorities and triage tagging system.

PROCEDURES

In general, the EMS provider most knowledgeable of patient assessment and intervention who arrives on the scene first becomes the triage officer. Immediately during the scene size-up, additional help should be requested. The triage officer rapidly performs an initial assessment of all patients. Care is not provided during triage, except for correction of immediate life threats, such as opening the airway or managing major bleeding.

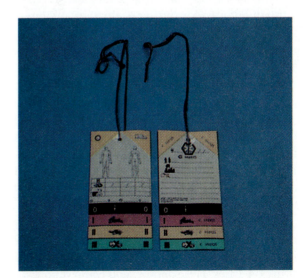

Fig. 32-5 METTAG Triage cards.

BOX 32-4

Triage Priorities

Highest Priority

- Airway or breathing difficulties
- Uncontrolled or severe bleeding
- Decreased or altered mental status
- Severe medical problems
- Signs and symptoms of shock (hypoperfusion)
- Severe burns with airway compromise

Second Priority

- Burns without airway compromise
- Multiple or major bone or joint injuries
- Back injuries with or without spinal cord damage

Lowest Priority

- Minor bone or joint injuries
- Minor soft-tissue injuries
- Prolonged respiratory arrest
- Cardiopulmonary arrest
- Death

The triage officer rapidly moves through the patients, doing an initial assessment and using triage tags to assign patients in treatment categories. As patients are assessed and tagged, they are moved to a treatment area for further evaluation and intervention. From the treatment area the patient is moved to a transportation area for transport. Transport decisions are based on patient priority, the receiving hospital's capabilities and capacity, and transportation resources.

Once all patients have been triaged, the triage officer reports to the incident commander. Often the triage officer remains in that position and continues to triage and update patient priorities based on available resources, or the triage officer may receive a new assignment.

The triage process forces EMTs to make difficult decisions. You may wish to practice using triage tags to be prepared when a true multiple casualty situation arises. For example, you could simply select one day a month and use triage tags on all patients in all calls just to practice. The important skill in triage is to be able to quickly prioritize patients to give the greatest amount of care, keeping in mind available resources, to allow the greatest amount of treatment to be provided to the greatest number of patients.

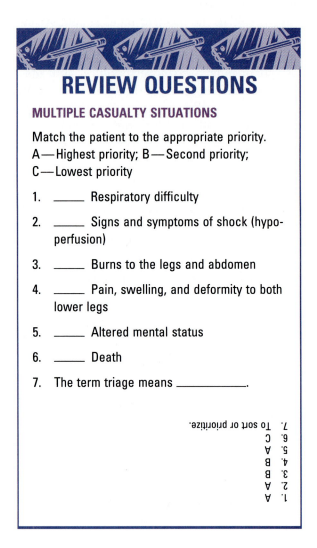

REVIEW QUESTIONS

MULTIPLE CASUALTY SITUATIONS

Match the patient to the appropriate priority.
A—Highest priority; B—Second priority;
C—Lowest priority

1. _____ Respiratory difficulty

2. _____ Signs and symptoms of shock (hypoperfusion)

3. _____ Burns to the legs and abdomen

4. _____ Pain, swelling, and deformity to both lower legs

5. _____ Altered mental status

6. _____ Death

7. The term triage means _____.

7. To sort or prioritize.
6. C
5. A
4. B
3. B
2. A
1. A

CHAPTER SUMMARY

HAZARDOUS MATERIALS

Hazardous materials are a common problem today. Your primary responsibility in hazardous materials incidents is your own safety and well-being and that of the crew, patients, bystanders, and the environment. Unless you are specifically educated to deal with hazardous materials situations, you must protect the scene and wait for additional help to arrive. A number of resources are available to identify and provide guidance when dealing with hazardous materials. These resources include placards, shipping papers, the USDOT *Emergency Response Guidebook*, and CHEMTREC. You should become familiar with all of these resources. EMTs are recommended to be educated at least to the OSHA First Responder Hazardous Materials Awareness Level.

In a hazardous materials situation, approach the scene with extreme caution, identify the hazard, assure safety around the scene, do whatever is possible to isolate the area, and ensure the safety of the people and the environment, and move and keep all bystanders and crew away from the scene. Obtain additional help, do not walk through leakage, and do not touch spilled material. Avoid inhaling fumes, smoke, or vapors.

INCIDENT MANAGEMENT SYSTEMS

Hazardous materials situations generally require activation of the incident management system. This system coordinates resources to deal with incidents efficiently and effectively. A single incident commander is established to oversee the various sectors. In general there are seven recognized sec-

tors: Incident command, Extrication, Treatment, Transport, Staging, Supply, and Triage. Each sector has a leader or sector officer. Once assigned to a specific area, EMTs complete their assigned tasks and report to the sector officer.

MULTIPLE CASUALTY SITUATIONS

Another incident requiring activation of the incident management system is a multiple casualty situation. These situations can occur when there are more patients than the responding unit can safely and effectively deal with. The first and most knowledgeable EMT on the scene begins triage, categorizing patients according to their injury into one of three categories. This is accomplished by rapidly performing an initial assessment of each patient and indicating the priority of each with a triage tag. This decision-making process allows the most patients to be treated and transported using available resources.

This chapter does not educate EMTs to deal with every situation but is an overview only. You should seek additional knowledge and skills through continuing education programs, practice drills, and experience.

Check your knowledge. The National Registry of EMTs and many state EMS agencies use the objectives below to develop EMT–Basic certification examinations. Can you meet them?

COGNITIVE

1. Explain the EMT–Basic's role in a call involving hazardous materials.
2. Describe what the EMT–Basic should do if there is reason to believe that there is a hazard at the scene.
3. Describe the actions that an EMT–Basic should take to ensure bystander safety.
4. State the role the EMT–Basic should take until appropriately trained personnel arrive at the scene of a hazardous materials situation.
5. Break down the steps to approaching a hazardous situation.
6. Discuss the various environmental hazards that affect EMS.
7. Describe the criteria for a multiple-casualty situation.
8. Evaluate the role of the EMT–Basic in the multiple-casualty situation.
9. Summarize the components of basic triage.
10. Define the role of the EMT–Basic in a disaster operation.
11. Describe basic concepts of incident management.
12. Explain the methods for preventing contamination of self, equipment, and facilities.
13. Review the local mass casualty incident plan.

PSYCHOMOTOR

1. Given a scenario of a mass casualty incident, perform triage.

ADVANCED AIRWAY

Our rural ambulance service often has extended transport times and limited personnel. We can be an hour or more from the nearest hospital. In these circumstances, proper airway management becomes especially important. BLS, or basic life support, techniques will often get you by, but when securing an airway of a critical or unstable patient is necessary, we have to be able to do it. We don't have any other options. When BLS techniques aren't enough, advanced airway skills can make a life or death difference.

**Mark Polakoff, RN,
NREMT-B**
*Red Lodge Volunteer
Ambulance Service
Red Lodge, Montana*

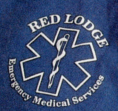

IN THIS DIVISION

33 **ADVANCED AIRWAY TECHNIQUES**

33 ADVANCED AIRWAY TECHNIQUES

KEY TERMS

Apices of the lungs: The tops of the lungs, lying just under the clavicles bilaterally.

Apneic: A term referring to patients who are not breathing.

Bases of the lungs: The bottoms of the lungs, lying approximately at the level of the sixth rib.

Carina: The point at which the trachea divides into the two main-stem bronchi.

Compliance: A measure of the elasticity of the lungs.

Direct laryngoscopy: The process of placing an endotracheal tube into the trachea while visualizing the glottic opening with a laryngoscope.

Endotracheal tube: A tube placed into the trachea to increase the delivery of oxygen to the lungs and decrease the possibility of aspiration.

Epigastrium: The area over the stomach.

Extubation: The removal of a tube.

Gastric distention: The accumulation of air in the stomach, which places pressure on the diaphragm, making artificial ventilation difficult and increasing the possibilty of vomiting.

Glottic opening: The anatomic space between the vocal cords, leading to the trachea.

Laryngoscope: An instrument used to visualize the airway during endotracheal intubation.

Main-stem bronchi: The two main branches to the lungs from the trachea.

Murphy's eye: A small hole in the side of an endotracheal tube that provides a passage of air if the tip of the tube becomes clogged.

Nasogastric tube: A tube placed through the nose, down the esophagus, and into the stomach.

Orotracheal intubation: The process of inserting an endotracheal tube through the mouth.

Pulse oximetry: A process of measuring the amount of oxygen carried in the blood.

Self-extubation: The patient's intentional or unintentional removal of a tube.

Sternal notch: The anatomic notch created by the clavicles and the sternum.

Stylet: A bendable device placed in the endotracheal tube, giving it rigidity and enabling it to hold a shape.

Vallecula: The anatomic space between the base of the tongue and the epiglottis.

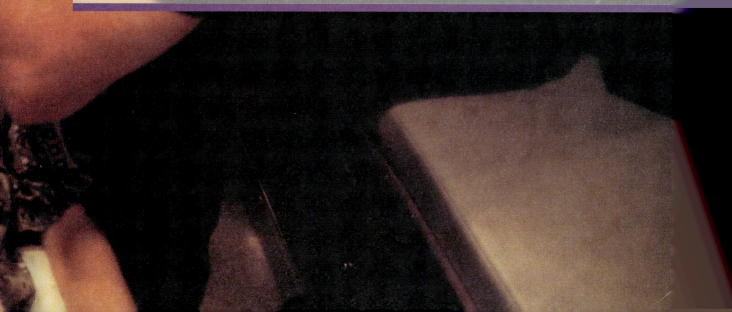

IN THE FIELD

Medic 5 was dispatched to the home of Mr. and Mrs. Bothwell after Mrs. Bothwell called 911 and said that her 61-year-old husband had just collapsed on the front lawn. He had been raking leaves. She was not sure whether he was breathing.

When Medic 5 arrived with EMTs Luan, Kim, and Mike, a neighbor had already begun cardiopulmonary resuscitation (CPR). Luan ventilated Mr. Bothwell using the mouth-to-mask technique, while Kim performed the Sellick maneuver to reduce the possibility of gastric distention and regurgitation. Mike applied the automated external defibrillator, but no shock was indicated. As the neighbor continued chest compressions, Luan hyperventilated the patient as Mike prepared to intubate.

Mike assembled his equipment and donned a mask and goggles. He chose a #3 curved blade and placed the 8-mm endotracheal tube into Mr. Bothwell's trachea in 11 seconds. When they connected the bag-valve device to the tube, no sounds were heard over the stomach, and the chest rise and breath sounds were equal bilaterally. Mike secured the tube.

The crew continued with intervals of CPR and reassessment. After ventilating the patient with 100% oxygen through the endotracheal tube for a few minutes, the semiautomatic defibrillator indicated 'shock advised.' After the third defibrillation, Kim checked for a pulse—and found one. They transported the patient to the local hospital. When they arrived, Mr. Bothwell had a pulse rate of 84 and a blood pressure of 110 by palpation. The emergency physician said that oxygenating him well probably made the difference in patient survival.

The airway management techniques described earlier in this book are the foundation of respiratory care and the first step in controlling the airway of emergency patients. In some EMS systems, EMT-Basics can perform additional skills to manage the airway. To learn the more advanced material in this chapter, you first should have practiced and become proficient in the airway skills described in Chapter 7, "The Airway."

SELLICK MANEUVER

During normal inhalation, the contraction of the diaphragm and intercostal muscles causes the chest cavity to expand and pull fresh air into the lungs. When a patient is not breathing, you must support respiration by providing positive pressure ventilations. All artificial ventilation techniques—including bag-valve-mask, oxygen-powered breathing device, and pocket mask—"push" air into the patient's lungs, rather than allowing it to be "pulled" in naturally.

When air is pushed into the mouth and nose, it enters both the lungs and the stomach. Therefore, during artificial ventilation, the stomach fills with air, a condition called **gastric distention.** The stomach does not inflate with air during normal inhalation.

As the stomach distends during artificial ventilation, upward pressure on the diaphragm increases, making ventilation difficult. Gastric distention is a problem particularly for infants and children. The stomach can only hold so much before the trapped air, partially digested food, and gastric juices come up through the esophagus and out through the mouth. This passive regurgitation is a tremendous threat to the airway.

PURPOSE

The Sellick maneuver was originally developed to decrease the risk of passive regurgitation in the operating room when patients are paralyzed and intubated before surgery. The Sellick maneuver can be used in prehospital settings in unresponsive patients who have no gag reflex. Performing the

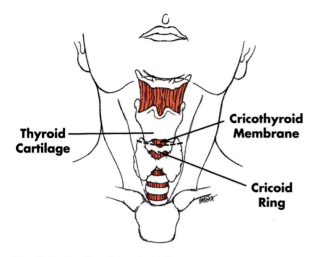

Fig. 33-1 Location of the cricoid ring.

TECHNIQUE

To perform the Sellick maneuver, place your thumb and index finger on the sides of the midline on the cricoid ring. Exert firm pressure posteriorly (Fig. 33-2). This process collapses the esophagus between the cricoid ring and the cervical spine without compromising the airway. Because the cricoid ring is the only upper airway structure that is a complete ring, it is the only place that you can exert posterior pressure without risk to the airway.

Maintain continuous pressure until the patient's airway is protected with an endotracheal tube because patients often vomit when pressure is released. Do not begin the Sellick maneuver if you cannot maintain it during resuscitation.

Sellick maneuver reduces gastric distention and helps prevent passive regurgitation during artificial ventilation.

ANATOMIC LOCATION

It is very important to perform the Sellick maneuver in the proper anatomic location at the cricoid ring. The cricoid ring is inferior to the cricothyroid membrane. The easiest way to find the cricoid ring is to palpate the depression just below the thyroid cartilage (Adam's apple). This depression is the cricothyroid membrane. The cricoid ring is the bump immediately inferior to this depression (Fig. 33-1).

> ### ALERT
> Proper location of the cricoid ring is critical for performing the Sellick maneuver safely. Posterior pressure anywhere other than on the cricoid ring will compromise the airway and may cause damage to other airway structures.

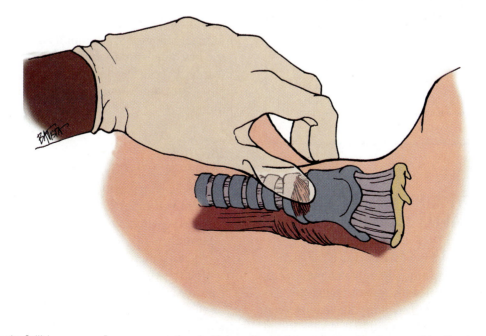

Fig. 33-2 In the Sellick maneuver, firm pressure on the cricoid ring collapses the esophagus without compromising the airway.

SPECIAL CONSIDERATIONS

It may be difficult to locate the proper landmarks for the Sellick maneuver in some people. Obese patients may have layers of fat that make locating airway structures difficult. The thyroid cartilage is less prominent in women, children, and infants. If you cannot locate the proper landmarks, it is best not to use the Sellick maneuver. Because the trachea in younger patients is softer and more pliable, excessive pressure is more likely to cause tracheal obstruction in infants and children.

An obvious disadvantage of this technique is the need for a third EMT during artificial ventilation. Once an EMT establishes posterior pressure in the Sellick maneuver, that person should not let go until an endotracheal tube is in place. Be sure that you have enough help before you decide to use the Sellick maneuver.

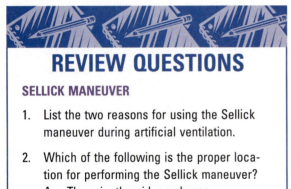

REVIEW QUESTIONS

SELLICK MANEUVER

1. List the two reasons for using the Sellick maneuver during artificial ventilation.

2. Which of the following is the proper location for performing the Sellick maneuver?
   A. The cricothyroid membrane
   B. The thyroid cartilage
   C. The Adam's's apple
   D. The cricoid ring

1. Reduce gastric distention, reduce the possibility of passive regurgitation
2. D

ADVANCED AIRWAY MANAGEMENT OF ADULTS

Proper management of the airway is the highest priority in managing any patient. You have already learned some critical skills for managing the airway. In some areas of the country, EMT-Basics can control the airway with additional, sophisticated skills. Advanced airway skills do not, however, re-place the need to master the basic skills described in earlier chapters. All of these skills require continual practice to maintain proficiency.

To family members or bystanders, some advanced airway procedures may seem painful, brutal, or undignified. Whenever possible, you should explain the importance of proper delivery of oxygen to the patient.

OROTRACHEAL INTUBATION

The best way to control the airway is to place a tube, an **endotracheal tube**, directly into the trachea. The endotracheal tube, with its inflatable cuff, creates a tight seal between the ventilation device and the trachea, creating a closed system between the ventilation device and the lungs. With an endotracheal tube you can control how much air is delivered to the patient's lungs (Fig. 33-3) and prevent gastric distention. **Orotracheal intubation** is the process of inserting an endotracheal tube through the patient's mouth and into the trachea.

PURPOSE

The endotracheal tube creates an airtight connection between the bag-valve device and the patient's lungs. Placing this tube into the trachea is the most effective way to manage a patient's airway and is the best way to ventilate an **apneic** patient who has no gag reflex. Patients are apneic if they are not breathing.

Endotracheal intubation has some major advantages for apneic patients. Endotracheal intubation minimizes the risk of aspiration and allows for better oxygen delivery to the lungs. Endotracheal intubation provides complete control of the airway and allows for suctioning of the trachea and bronchi.

INDICATIONS

There are four situations in which to consider endotracheal intubation in prehospital settings:
1. When you cannot ventilate an apneic patient.
2. When a patient is unresponsive to any painful stimuli.
3. When a patient has no gag reflex or coughing.
4. When a patient cannot protect the airway (such as in cardiac arrest or unresponsiveness).

Follow your local protocol, because individual medical directors may have different specific indications for endotracheal intubation.

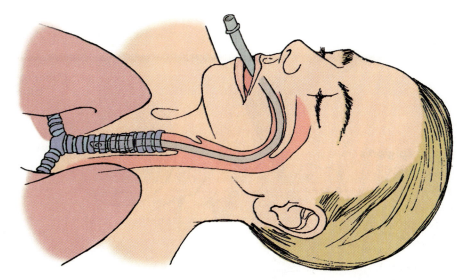

Fig. 33-3 The endotracheal tube provides control of the patient's airway and is the best way to manage an apneic patient without a gag reflex.

EQUIPMENT

Because airway procedures expose you to body fluids, use body substance isolation precautions when you perform advanced airway techniques.

The endotracheal tube is a hollow tube that is open on both ends. At one end, a 15-mm adapter allows for attachment to a bag-valve device. The other end is beveled and is placed into the patient's airway. There is a small hole, a **Murphy's eye**, on the side of the tube across from the bevel. The Murphy's eye decreases the chance of obstruction if the tip of the tube becomes blocked.

About 3 cm from the distal end of the tube is an inflatable cuff that holds about 5 to 10 mL of air and is inflated against the walls of the trachea to provide an airtight seal. The airtight seal ensures that all of the air delivered into the tube reaches the lungs, decreasing the possibility of gastric distention and aspiration. The cuff is inflated by injecting air with a 10-mL syringe through a valve. The small "pilot balloon" also inflates to verify that the cuff has been inflated (Fig. 33-4).

Before you insert an endotracheal tube into the trachea, test the cuff for leaks. Do this by inflating the balloon and gently squeezing it to be sure that it holds air. Once you have tested the cuff, deflate it and reattach the syringe so that you can quickly reinflate the cuff after the patient is intubated.

Endotracheal tubes come in a wide variety of sizes. The most important consideration when

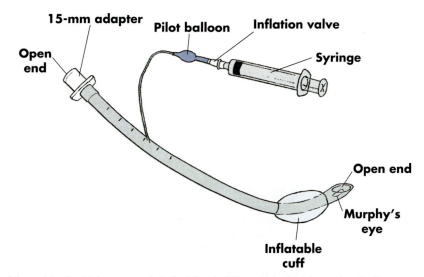

Fig. 33-4 The cuff of the endotracheal tube ensures that all of the air delivered into the tube reaches the lungs.

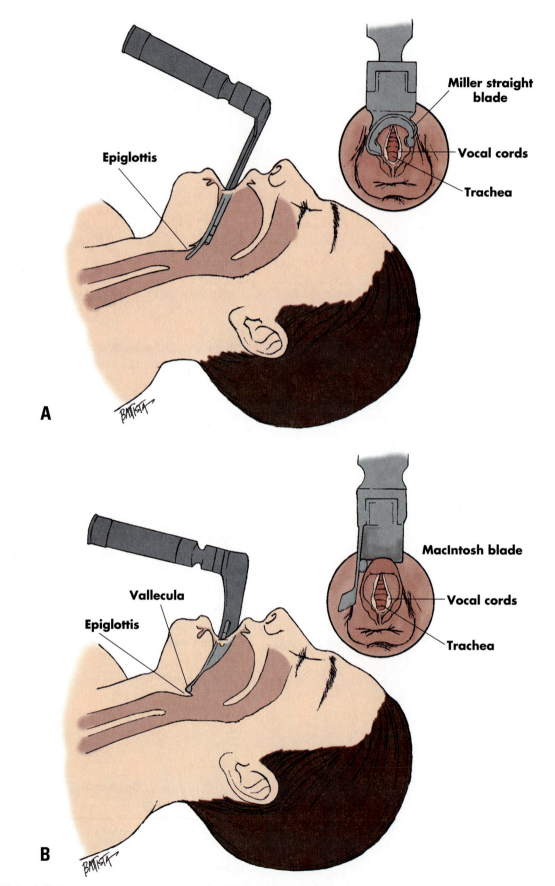

Fig. 33-5   **A**, The Miller straight blade is used to lift the epiglottis to allow visualization of the glottic opening and vocal cords. **B**, The MacIntosh curved blade is inserted into the vallecula to lift the epiglottis out of the way to allow visualization of the airway.

selecting a tube size is to consider the diameter of the patient's trachea. As a general rule, adult men usually require an 8- to 8.5-mm internal diameter endotracheal tube. The average adult woman usually requires a 7- to 8.0-mm internal diameter endotracheal tube. In an emergency, a 7.5-mm tube will work for almost any adult patient. The length of the tube for adults is 33 cm, which is marked along the barrel of the tube as centimeters from the tip.

The endotracheal tube is made from flexible material, which makes it difficult to control the tip of the tube while inserting it into the airway. To alleviate this problem, a malleable piece of metal, a **stylet**, is inserted into the tube to make it stiff and hold its shape during the procedure.

To place an endotracheal tube into the trachea, you must be able to see the **glottic opening**. The tool that you use to see into the airway is a **laryngoscope**. The laryngoscope's handle contains batteries to power its light. A locking bar at the end of the handle fastens the blade to the handle.

The blade goes into the patient's mouth. There are two main blade types, straight and curved, called *Miller* and *MacIntosh*, respectively. Both types come in four sizes. The tip of the straight blade is used to lift the epiglottis out of the way to allow you to visualize the glottic opening and the vocal cords (Fig. 33-5A). The tip of the curved blade is placed into the **vallecula**. Lifting on the vallecula lifts the epiglottis out of the way and enables you to visualize the airway (Fig. 33-5B). For an adult patient, the choice of blade is largely a personal preference and a straight blade is usually used for infants and young children.

Once you have selected the blade, lock it into the handle by matching the notch of the blade onto the locking bar of the handle. Lifting the blade into the perpendicular position locks it into place and turns on the light (Fig. 33-6). Before you use the laryngoscope, be sure that the light is bright and steady, white, and tightly screwed in place. Always carry spare batteries and extra bulbs.

After you have placed the endotracheal tube, you must secure it in place. Specially designed securing devices are available, or you can use tape (Fig. 33-7). Be sure that your medical director has approved the device and technique you use. A bite block or an oral airway should always be placed into patients' mouths after intubation so that they do not bite on the tube if they later become responsive.

You need to have two other pieces of equipment ready before you intubate: a suction unit and towels. Suction must be immediately available to clear fluid or debris from the mouth. Two or more folded towels may be very helpful to properly position a nontrauma patient for intubation.

TECHNIQUES OF INSERTION

The most common method of intubation is by **direct laryngoscopy**. In this technique, you use the laryngoscope to lift the airway structures out of the way to visualize the glottic opening. Watch the tube as it passes through the vocal cords. Intubation by direct laryngoscopy is a very effective intubation technique (Technique 33-1).

Different techniques are used to intubate patients. All of them should follow the same general principles of intubation (Principle 33-1).

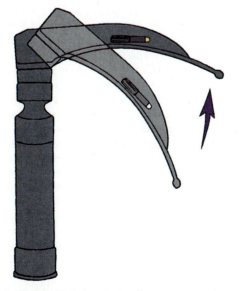

Fig. 33-6 Locking the blade into the handle.

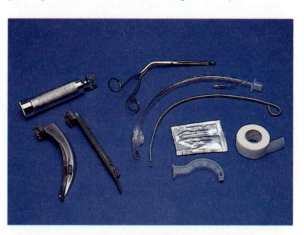

Fig. 33-7 Intubation equipment including laryngoscope handle, Macintosh curved blade, Miller straight blade, Magill forceps, endotracheal tube, stylet, lubrication packets, OP airway, and tape.

TECHNIQUE 33-1
Intubation by Direct Laryngoscopy

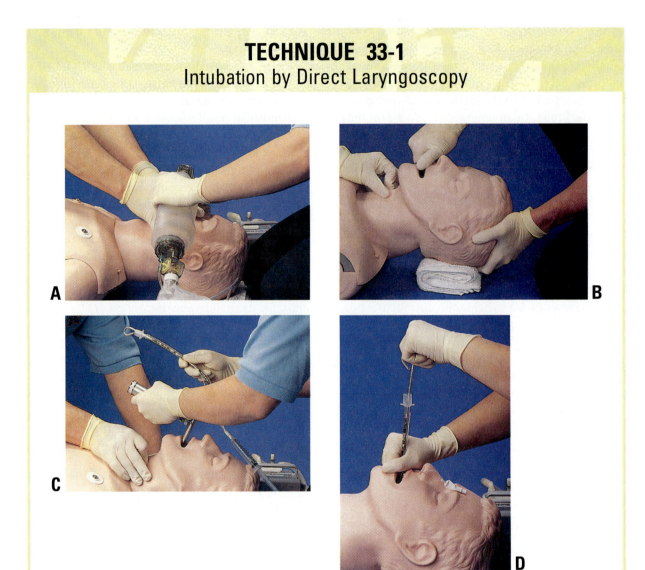

Fig. 33-8   Follow body substance isolation precautions. (Body fluids may be splashed while performing airway procedures.) **A, Assure adequate ventilation with 100% oxygen.** Before you attempt advanced airway procedures, you must ensure that the basic airway techniques being used are adequate. Assemble and test all equipment. Select the appropriate type of blade and the proper size blade. Connect the blade to the handle and check the light (bright, white, steady, tight). Select the proper size endotracheal tube. Lubricate the stylet (for easy removal) and the end of the endotracheal tube with a small amount of water-soluble lubricant. Insert the stylet into the tube. The stylet must not extend beyond the tip of the tube. It is best if the end of the stylet is kept 0.25 inch away from the cuff or the proximal end of Murphy's eye. Check the cuff to ensure that it holds air, and leave the syringe attached. Most people find that forming the endotracheal tube into a "hockey stick" shape makes it easier to properly place the tube. Prepare the securing device or tape. **Hyperventilate the patient at a rate of 24 breaths per minute, ideally for at least 2 minutes. Your partner should preoxygenate the patient because the patient will not be ventilated during intubation. Remember that two EMTs should perform ventilation with the bag-valve-mask when possible. B, Align the patient's head. If no trauma is suspected, tilt the patient's head, lift the chin, and place a folded towel under the patient's head.** If trauma is suspected, have a partner stabilize the patient's head in the neutral position. **While one EMT ventilates and aligns the patient's head, another EMT should perform the Sellick maneuver.** Cricoid pressure will decrease the possibility of vomiting. **C, Hold the laryngoscope handle in your left hand, insert the blade into the right corner of the mouth, and sweep the tongue up and to the left.** The tip of the curved blade is placed into the vallecula; the tip of the straight blade is used to directly lift the epiglottis. **Lift the tongue with the laryngoscope, and visualize the glottic opening and the vocal cords. Lift the laryngoscope up and away from the patient, taking great care to avoid pressure on the teeth. Insert the endotracheal tube with your right hand.** Insert the tube through the glottic opening until the cuff just passes the vocal cords. Note the markings on the tube at the upper teeth or gumline. Remove the laryngoscope blade, and extinguish the light. Do not let the light continue to burn because it may burn out or become hot. Do not let go of the tube until placement is verified and the tube is secured. **D, Remove the stylet.** *Continued*

TECHNIQUE 33-1
Intubation by Direct Laryngoscopy

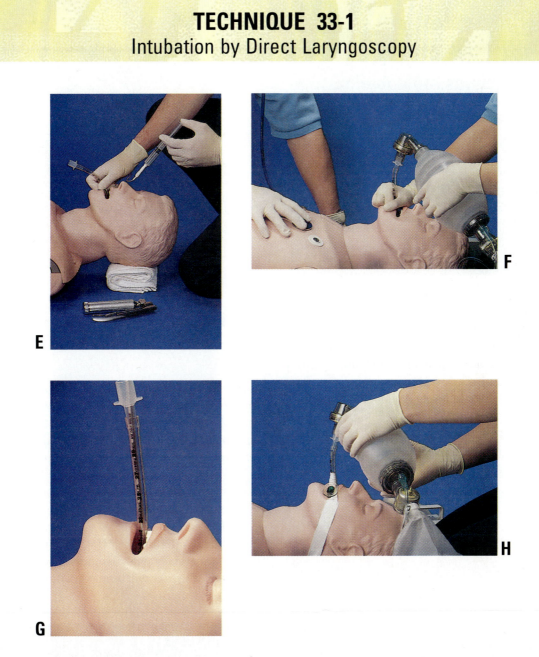

Fig. 33-8 *Continued* **E, Inflate the cuff with 5 to 10 mL of air. An airtight seal now has been created. F, Ventilate the patient, and confirm proper tube placement.** Watching the tube pass through the vocal cords is the best way to be certain that you have placed the tube properly. Listen with a stethoscope over the **epigastrium** during the first ventilation (you should not hear any gurgling sounds). **Listen to the left and right apices of the lungs (these sounds should be equal).** Listen to the left and right **bases of the lungs** (these sounds should be equal). Consider using other methods of confirming correct tube placement:

- improvement of heart rate, skin color, and general patient condition
- equal chest rise and fall during ventilation
- carbon dioxide detectors
- **pulse oximetry**
- improvement in the patient's mental status

G, Note the markings on the tube at the upper teeth or gumline and record this information. H, Secure the tube and place an oral airway (or bite block) into the mouth to prevent the patient from biting on the tube. Continue to ventilate at an age-appropriate rate.

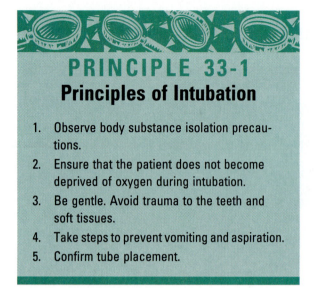

PRINCIPLE 33-1
Principles of Intubation

1. Observe body substance isolation precautions.
2. Ensure that the patient does not become deprived of oxygen during intubation.
3. Be gentle. Avoid trauma to the teeth and soft tissues.
4. Take steps to prevent vomiting and aspiration.
5. Confirm tube placement.

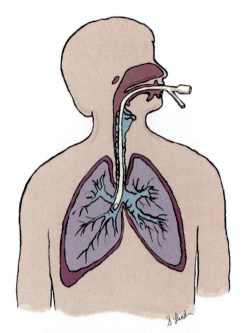

Fig. 33-9 Because the right bronchus is larger and straighter than the left, right main-stem intubation is more likely.

If you do not hear breath sounds or if you hear gurgling in the stomach while ventilating the patient, you most likely have placed the tube into the esophagus. In this case, you must immediately deflate the cuff and remove the tube. The patient should be hyperventilated for 2 to 5 minutes before you reattempt intubation. If you are not able to intubate the patient on the next attempt, continue ventilating and transport the patient to the hospital.

ALERT
An unrecognized esophageal intubation is fatal. You must confirm correct tube placement immediately after you intubate. If there is any question that the tube is not in the trachea, remove the tube immediately and ventilate the patient.

If you hear breath sounds on only one side, you have most likely inserted the tube too far and it has come to rest in one of the main-stem bronchi. Because the right bronchus is larger and straighter than the left, right main-stem intubation is more likely than left (Fig. 33-9). If you hear breath

sounds only on one side, place your stethoscope on the silent side. Deflate the cuff and slowly withdraw the tube while continuing to ventilate until you hear breath sounds. Then compare the right and left breath sounds to ensure that they are equal before reinflating the cuff. Being familiar with the distances shown in Box 33-1 helps ensure you have inserted the tube the correct distance.

As the patient is moved, the tube may be dislodged inadvertently. Securing the tube with tape or a commercially available device will minimize the chance the tube will be moved. Be careful not to

BOX 33-1

Distance From Front Teeth to Airway Landmarks in the Average Adult

- 15 cm from the front teeth to the vocal cords
- 20 cm from the front teeth to the **sternal notch**
- 25 cm from the front teeth to the **carina**
- 22 cm from the front teeth to the tip of a properly positioned endotracheal tube

move the tube in or out of the mouth. Prevent movement of the tube by placing your hand on the tube at the patient's mouth to hold it in place. Reassess breath sounds following every major move (such as from the scene to the ambulance, from the ambulance to the receiving hospital, or if the patient moves from combativeness or a seizure). Continue to reevaluate the tube placement frequently, even after the tube is secured. The placement of the endotracheal tube also should be reassessed with any changes in the patient's condition.

COMPLICATIONS

Endotracheal intubation must be performed carefully because improper technique can lead to serious complications. The most common complication is trauma to the teeth or soft tissues of the airway. Because some of the instruments used are made of metal, improper technique can cause damage to the teeth, lips, tongue, gums, and other airway structures.

While you are in the process of intubating, the patient is not receiving oxygen. Never let a nonbreathing patient go for more than 30 seconds without a breath for any reason—including intubation. During intubation, the patient's pulse should be continuously monitored. Stimulation of the airway during intubation may slow the heart rate.

Because patients occasionally vomit during intubation attempts, observe body substance isolation precautions while intubating. If the tube is placed too far into the airway, it will go into one of

> ### ALERT
> **Never take more than 30 seconds to intubate or the patient may become profoundly deprived of oxygen.**

the bronchi (usually the right main-stem bronchus, because it is larger and straighter). If the tube goes into either of the **main-stem bronchi**, only one lung will be ventilated. In this case the cuff should be deflated and the tube pulled back slowly until breath sounds are heard in both lung fields equally.

The most dangerous problem with intubation is misplacement of the tube. If the tube is accidentally placed into the esophagus, no oxygen will reach the lungs and the patient will die unless the tube is immediately removed (Fig. 33-10). Misplacement can occur if you do not watch the tube pass through the vocal cords and into the trachea or if the tube becomes dislodged during movement. To ensure that a misplaced endotracheal tube does not go unnoticed, constantly evaluate the chest rise, breath sounds, and general condition of an intubated patient. Anytime that an intubated patient's condition changes, immediately check the tube's placement. Moving the patient is the most common cause of accidental **extubation** in infants and children.

Box 33-2 summarizes the possible complications of intubation.

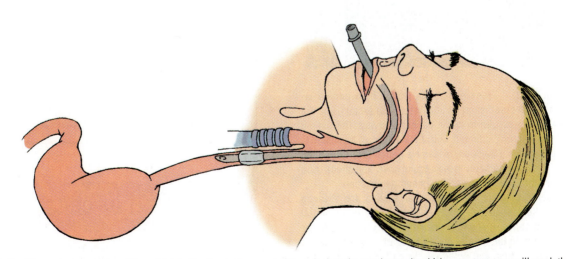

Fig. 33-10 The most dangerous problem of intubation is misplacement of the tube into the esophagus, in which case no oxygen will reach the lungs and the patient will die unless the tube is immediately removed.

BOX 33-2

Complications of Intubation

- Esophageal intubation
- Chipped teeth and trauma to soft tissue (eg, lips, tongue, gums, etc.)
- Decreased heart rate
- Hypoxia, the lack of oxygen to the body's tissues, from prolonged intubation attempts
- Main-stem intubation
- Vomiting
- **Self-extubation**

TRACHEAL SUCTIONING

In addition to improving ventilation, endotracheal intubation allows suctioning of the trachea. Tracheal suctioning can be a life-saving skill for a

TECHNIQUE 33-2
Tracheal Suctioning

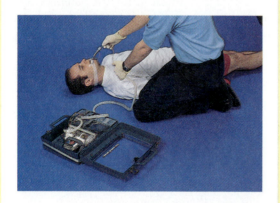

Fig. 33-11 Preoxygenate the patient by hyperventilation at 24 breaths per minute. When you suction, you are removing oxygen from the patient's airway. The patient must be preoxygenated, and suctioning must be limited to 10 seconds. Check and assemble equipment. Attach the soft suction catheter to the suction hose, and check to be sure that the suction unit is generating suction.
Insert the suction catheter without suction, and advance it to the desired location. The suction catheter is inserted to the carina—about 25 cm in the average adult. **Cover the hole in the side of the catheter to start the suction. Apply suction, and withdraw the catheter in a twisting motion.**

patient who is otherwise difficult to ventilate because of fluid in the trachea or bronchi (Technique 33-2). Because the suction catheter enters the trachea, observe sterile technique.

The indications for tracheal suctioning are:

1. Secretions seen coming out of the endotracheal tube.
2. Poor **compliance** while ventilating.

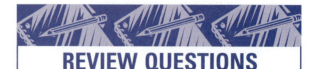

REVIEW QUESTIONS
ADVANCED AIRWAY MANAGEMENT OF ADULTS

1. List the four purposes for endotracheal intubation.

2. Which of the following is the most common complication of endotracheal intubation?
   A. Tooth and soft tissue trauma
   B. Vomiting
   C. Self-extubation
   D. Bradycardia

3. What should you do if you hear breath sounds only on the right side following endotracheal intubation?

4. What should you do if two attempts to intubate a patient have been unsuccessful?

5. Endotracheal attempts should be limited to _____ seconds, and tracheal suctioning should be limited to _____ seconds.

5. 10, 30.
4. Begin transport while ventilating the patient with basic life support techniques.
3. Deflate the cuff and slowly withdraw the tube while listening to the silent side of the chest. Stop withdrawing the tube when sounds occur, reinflate the cuff, and secure the tube.
2. A
1. Completes control of the airway, minimizes the risk of aspiration, allows for better oxygen delivery to the lungs, allows for deeper suctioning.

ADVANCED AIRWAY MANAGEMENT OF CHILDREN AND INFANTS

The airway is a high priority in the management of any patient, but it is even more important for infants and children. Many of the life-threatening emergencies in pediatric patients are respiratory or airway problems. Careful attention to the airway and breathing of infants and children can prevent many catastrophic emergencies.

NASOGASTRIC TUBES

Because children rely heavily on the diaphragm for breathing, gastric distention can make it very difficult to ventilate a pediatric patient. When gastric distention occurs, you can release the trapped air by inserting a long tube down the esophagus into the stomach. This tube is usually inserted through the nose and is a **nasogastric tube**.

A nasogastric tube is used to decompress the stomach and the proximal bowel of air in intubated or unintubated patients. In hospital settings, nasogastric tubes are also used for relieving bowel obstructions, for gastric lavage (removing poisons or blood from the upper gastrointestinal tract), for administering medications or nutrition (tube feeding), and for diagnosing and treating trauma patients.

The primary indication for using a nasogastric tube in prehospital settings is an inability to artificially ventilate the infant or child because of gastric distention. If you are treating an unresponsive child who will require ventilation for an extended period of time, you should consider inserting a nasogastric tube before gastric distention interferes with ventilation. Box 33-3 lists the equipment for nasogastric tube insertion.

BOX 33-4

Complications of Nasogastric Tube Insertion

- Tracheal insertion
- Nasal trauma
- Vomiting
- Passage of the tube into the cranium if the patient has a skull fracture
- Tube curling up in the back of the patient's throat

Box 33-4 lists the possible complications of nasogastric tube insertion in an infant or child. Technique 33-3 describes the procedure for insertion of nasogastric tube in an infant or child.

ALERT

Do not attempt nasogastric tube insertion if the patient has major facial, head, or spinal trauma.

OROTRACHEAL INTUBATION

Because many emergencies in pediatric patients are caused by respiratory difficulties, airway management of the infant or child is a very high priority and may include endotracheal intubation.

ANATOMIC AND PHYSIOLOGICAL CONSIDERATIONS

The anatomy of the airway in infants and children is different in several ways from the airway of adults. The most obvious difference is the size of airway structures. The smaller diameter of the airway in infants and children increases the likelihood of obstruction from small items, fluid, or swelling. A child's tongue is proportionally larger and takes up more space in the mouth than an adult's tongue (Fig. 33-13). Opening the airway to lift the tongue, therefore, is extremely important when managing the pediatric airway.

The cricoid ring is less developed and less rigid in infants and younger children. The cricoid ring is

---

BOX 33-3

Equipment for Nasogastric Tube Insertion

- Proper sized nasogastric tube

Newborn/infant	8 Fr
Toddler/preschooler	10 Fr
School age child	12 Fr
Adolescent	14-16 Fr

- 20-mL syringe
- Water-soluble lubricant
- Emesis basin
- Tape
- Stethoscope
- Suction unit and suction catheters

TECHNIQUE 33-3
Insertion of Nasogastric Tube in an Infant or Child

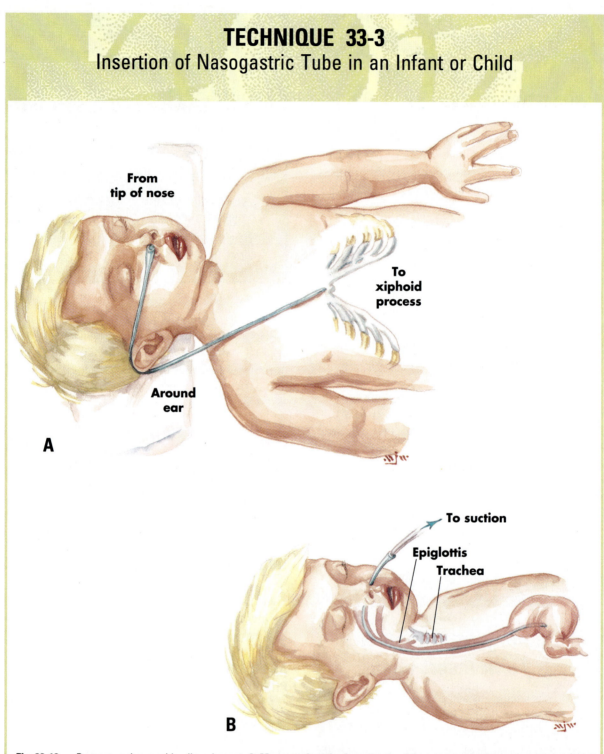

Fig. 33-12 Prepare and assemble all equipment. **A, Measure the tube from the tip of the nose, around the ear, to the xiphoid process and note the cm marking at the nostril.** Lubricate the distal end of the tube. If trauma is not suspected, place the patient in the supine position with the head turned to the left side. Pass the tube along the nasal floor until you insert it to the cm marking previously noted. There are two ways to check the placement of the tube: 1) Place the syringe at the end of the tube, and withdraw the stomach contents; and 2) Listen for gurgling over the stomach while injecting 10 to 20 mL of air into the tube. **B, Aspirate stomach contents by attaching the tube to suction.** Tape the tube securely to the nostril.

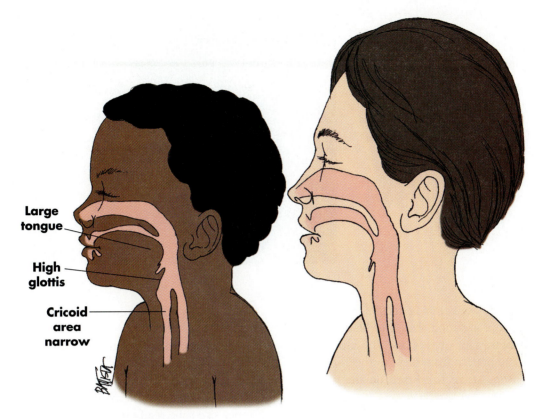

Fig. 33-13 Comparison of the adult and child airways.

also the narrowest portion of the airway in infants and children. Because of the narrow cricoid ring, cuffs are not needed on endotracheal tubes to provide a seal. Uncuffed endotracheal tubes generally are used in patients less than 8 years of age.

Infants' and children's heads are proportionally larger than adults, with more of the skull projecting behind the neck. When they lie flat on the back, the head is forced into a flexed position. This position quickly compromises the airway and requires immediately placing the child in the neutral position, with the head tilted slightly back so that the nose points directly upward.

The trachea and vocal cords in children are higher and lie more anteriorly than in adults. For this reason the straight blade usually is used for intubating infants and children.

INDICATIONS

Endotracheal intubation of the infant or child is used in the following situations:
1. Prolonged artificial ventilation is needed, making gastric distention likely.
2. Artificial ventilation cannot be achieved by any other method.
3. The patient is apneic.

4. The patient is unresponsive, without a cough or a gag reflex.

EQUIPMENT

The equipment for intubating pediatric patients is the same as for adults but must be sized properly.

Bag-valve-masks come in a variety of sizes. Be careful to use the proper size bag and mask for the individual patient. Make sure that the patient's chest rises and falls with each ventilation and that all pop-off valves are disabled.

A straight laryngoscope blade is preferred in infants because it provides greater displacement of the tongue and directly lifts the relatively large epiglottis out of the way. This displacement results in better visualization of the glottic opening and the vocal cords.

A curved blade is sometimes used in older children because it has a broader base and flange, which provide better displacement of the tongue. The curved blade is placed into the vallecula to allow for visualization of the glottic opening and the vocal cords.

As discussed earlier, proper endotracheal tube size is critical for infants and children. There are a number of ways to select the proper size tube. A

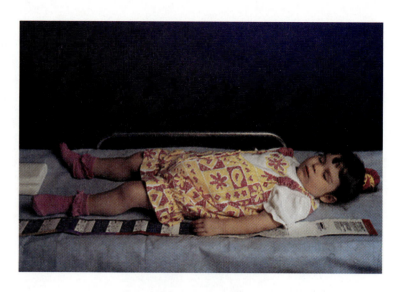

Fig. 33-14 The Braslow tape device measures the patient from head to toe and calculates the proper tube size.

chart or tape device is most effective. Most charts list the appropriate tube sizes and blade size for various patient ages or weights. The tape device measures the patient from head to toe and calculates the proper tube size based on the patient's length (Fig. 33-14).

In general, newborns and small infants need a 3- to 3.5-mm tube, and 4.0-mm tubes are used in children up to 1 year of age. The formula (16 + age ÷ 4) is an excellent guide for tube size selection in children over 2 years of age.

In emergency situations, it can be difficult to remember a formula, and a chart may not be immediately available. Do not delay intubation to look for a chart. Anatomic clues can help you determine the correct size tube. The size of the patient's little finger and the inside diameter of the nostril are both good indicators of the size of a pedi-

atric patient's airway and can be used to size the endotracheal tube.

When preparing to intubate a child, it is a good idea to have tubes ready that are one size larger and one size smaller than you anticipate using. If your original estimate is off, you will then have the proper size tube ready to use.

Most pediatric endotracheal tubes have one or more black rings near the distal tip of the tube that identifies the optimal depth of insertion of the tube. The vocal cord marker helps ensure that the tip of the tube is placed halfway between the vocal cords and the carina (Fig. 33-15). Follow manufacturer recommendations for specific ring placement. Table 33-1 lists average distances from the teeth and gumline to the midtrachea.

Just as with adults, you should insert a lubricated stylet into the tube before intubation and

TABLE 33-1	Distances From Teeth/Gumline to Midtrachea
AGE	**DISTANCE**
6 months–1 year	12 cm
2–4 years	14 cm
4–6 years	16 cm
6–10 years	18 cm
10–12 years	20 cm

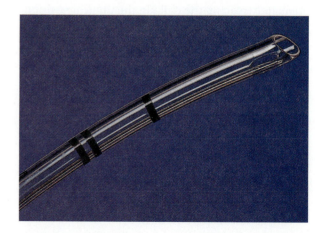

Fig. 33-15 Some pediatric endotracheal tubes have a vocal cord marker to ensure that the tip of the tube is placed halfway between the cords and the carina.

form it into a "hockey stick" shape. Be sure to use a water-soluble lubricant on the tube before insertion. You should also prepare a securing device and have a suction unit available before intubation.

TECHNIQUES OF INSERTION

The principles of intubation for pediatric patients are the same as for adults. Because of anatomic differences, however, some of the techniques are slightly modified. Technique 33-4 describes the procedure for intubation of an infant or child.

ALERT
Assume that there is a problem with the endotracheal tube anytime an intubated patient's condition suddenly deteriorates. Reassess chest rise, breath sounds, and vital signs immediately.

Recognizing a misplaced endotracheal tube is more difficult in infants and children. Breath sounds are less reliable because sounds from the stomach and chest may be transmitted across the small chest. You must rely on multiple parameters, including continuous assessment of the patient's vital signs and general condition. When in doubt, it may be beneficial to revisualize the glottic opening to ensure that the tube is properly positioned.

The management of esophageal and main-stem intubation for pediatric patients is exactly the same as for adults. If the tube is placed properly but inadequate lung expansion occurs, there are five possible causes:

1. The tube is too small, and a large air leak is present at the subglottic area. This condition can be assessed by listening at the neck with a stethoscope. If air is leaking and the patient has inadequate lung expansion, the tube must be removed and replaced with a larger one. Consider a cuffed tube if the patient is over 8 years of age.
2. The pop-off valve on the bag-valve-mask has not been disabled. Pop-off valves should be disabled by taping them down.
3. There is a leak or malfunction in the bag-valve device or a kink in the endotracheal tube. If the bag-valve-mask is malfunctioning, use another one. Check as much of the tube as you can see, and make sure the tube is not bent.
4. Inadequate tidal volume is being given with ventilations. Ventilate with more volume or use a bigger bag-valve device.
5. The tube is blocked with secretions. If endotracheal suctioning does not relieve the obstruction, remove and replace the tube.

COMPLICATIONS

The complications of endotracheal intubation are the same for infants and children as for adults. Because of the anatomic and physiological differences, however, complications are more common.

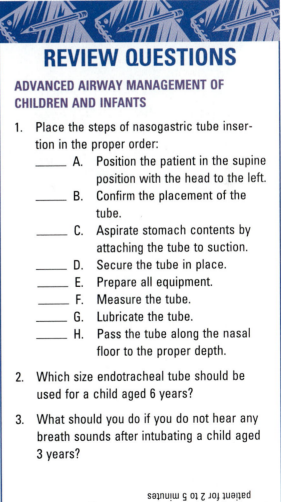

REVIEW QUESTIONS

ADVANCED AIRWAY MANAGEMENT OF CHILDREN AND INFANTS

1. Place the steps of nasogastric tube insertion in the proper order:
   - _____ A. Position the patient in the supine position with the head to the left.
   - _____ B. Confirm the placement of the tube.
   - _____ C. Aspirate stomach contents by attaching the tube to suction.
   - _____ D. Secure the tube in place.
   - _____ E. Prepare all equipment.
   - _____ F. Measure the tube.
   - _____ G. Lubricate the tube.
   - _____ H. Pass the tube along the nasal floor to the proper depth.

2. Which size endotracheal tube should be used for a child aged 6 years?

3. What should you do if you do not hear any breath sounds after intubating a child aged 3 years?

1. E, F, G, A, H, B, C, D
2. 5.5 mm
3. Immediately withdraw the tube and hyperventilate the patient for 2 to 5 minutes.

TECHNIQUE 33-4
Intubation of Infant or Child

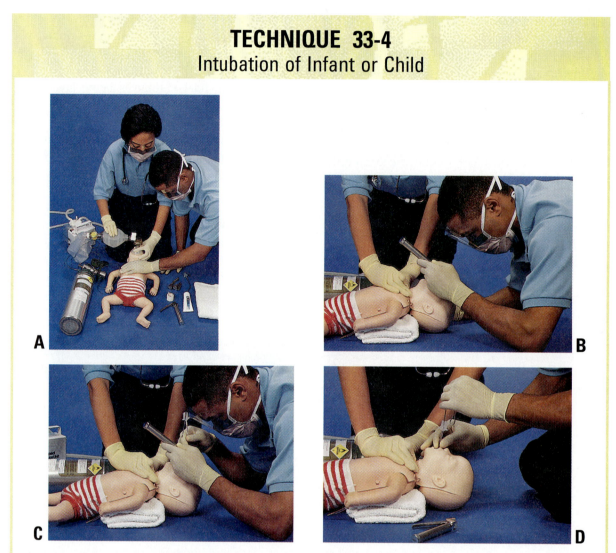

Fig. 33-16   Follow body substance isolation precautions. (Body fluids may be splashed while performing airway procedures.) **A, Ensure adequate ventilation with 100% oxygen.** Before any attempt at advanced airway procedures, ensure that the basic techniques being used are adequate. Assemble and test all equipment. Select the appropriate and proper size blade. Connect the blade to the laryngoscope handle and check the light (bright, white, steady, tight). Select the proper size endotracheal tube, and lubricate and insert a stylet. Prepare the securing device or tape. Hyperventilate the patient at an age-appropriate rate. Your partner should preoxygenate the patient because the patient will not be ventilated during the intubation process. **B, Align the patient's head.** If no trauma is suspected, tilt the patient's head and lift the chin. **Infants may require a towel under the upper back to raise the shoulders approximately 2.5 cm.** If trauma is suspected, have a partner hold the patient's head in the neutral position during the intubation. **Perform the Sellick maneuver. Cricoid pressure decreases the possibility of vomiting.** Continuously monitor the heart rate during any intubation attempt. Bradycardia is a sign of oxygen deprivation in pediatric patients. Mechanical stimulation of the airway during intubation also can cause the heart rate to slow. If the heart rate slows, stop the intubation attempt and re-ventilate the patient. **Hold the laryngoscope in your left hand, insert the blade into the right corner of the mouth, and sweep the tongue up and to the left.** The tip of the curved blade is placed into the vallecula (in a child); the tip of the straight blade is used to lift the epiglottis (in an infant). **C, Lift the tongue with the laryngoscope, visualize the glottic opening and the vocal cords. Lift the laryngoscope up and away from the patient, taking great care to avoid pressure on the teeth.** Very little force is required to intubate pediatric patients. **Insert the lubricated endotracheal tube with your right hand.** Insert the tube until the mark at the tip is placed just past the vocal cords. Note the markings on the tube at the upper teeth or gumline. Remove the laryngoscope blade, and extinguish the light. Do not let the light continue to burn because it may burn out or become hot. Do not let go of the tube until it is secured. **D, Remove the stylet.**   *Continued*

TECHNIQUE 33-4
Intubation of Infant or Child

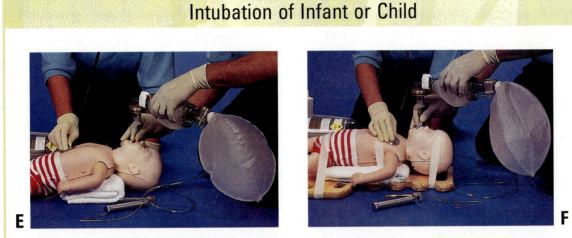

Fig. 33-16 *Continued* **E, Ventilate the patient, and confirm correct tube placement.** Watching the tube pass through the cords is the best way to confirm tube placement. Watch for equal chest rise because breath sounds can be misleading in pediatric patients. **Listen with a stethoscope over the epigastrium during the first ventilation (you should not hear any gurgling sounds). F, Listen to the left and right apices of the lungs (these sounds should be equal).** Listen to the left and right bases of the lungs (these sounds should be equal). Listen at the sternal notch. Consider the use of other methods of tube confirmation:

- improvement of heart rate, skin color, and general patient condition
- equal chest rise and fall during ventilation
- carbon dioxide detectors
- pulse oximeter
- improvement in the patient's mental status

Secure the tube, and place an oral airway into the mouth to prevent the patient from biting on the tube. Note the distance that the tube is inserted, and continue to ventilate at an age-appropriate rate. **Secure the patient to an appropriate device to minimize movement of the head that could dislodge the tube.** Reassess tube placement after every major move or any adverse change in the patient's condition.

The pediatric patient's heart rate depends heavily on oxygenation, and a slow heart rate is often a response to being deprived of oxygen. Avoid prolonged attempts at intubation. The mechanical stimulation of the airway may also slow the heart rate due to a reflex of the nervous system. If the heart rate falls, immediately stop your intubation attempt and reventilate.

Because the distance from the vocal cords to the carina is very short, the risk of main-stem intubation is greater in pediatric patients. Likewise, tube displacement can easily occur with movement of the patient or the tube. Just as in adults, vomiting, self-extubation, and trauma are complications of endotracheal intubation.

Ventilating too forcefully can collapse the lung of an intubated pediatric patient. Be careful to ventilate evenly and gently, looking for chest rise. Being gentle and using proper technique throughout the intubation procedure decreases the possibility of complications.

CHAPTER SUMMARY

SELLICK MANEUVER

The Sellick maneuver is used to decrease gastric distention and lower the risk of passive regurgitation during artificial ventilation. It is performed by placing your thumb and index fingers on the lateral portions of the cricoid ring and pushing firmly posteriorly.

ADVANCED AIRWAY MANAGEMENT OF ADULTS

Basic airway skills are the foundation of good airway management. In some systems, EMT-Basics can perform additional skills to control the airway. Orotracheal intubation provides complete control of the airway because it prevents gastric distention, reduces the risk of aspiration, provides better oxygenation to the lungs, and provides a route for tracheal suctioning. Tracheal suctioning can be a life-saving procedure to remove fluid from the trachea and bronchi.

ADVANCED AIRWAY MANAGEMENT OF CHILDREN AND INFANTS

Many of the threats to life in infants and children involve compromise of the airway or respiratory system. Nasogastric tubes are used in prehospital settings to decompress gastric distention, which can severely affect breathing in children. The benefits and indications of endotracheal intubation are the same for infants and children as for adults. Although the principles of endotracheal intubation are the same, the technique is slightly modified to accommodate anatomic and physiological differences.

Check your knowledge. The National Registry of EMTs and many state EMS agencies use the objectives below to develop EMT–Basic certification examinations. Can you meet them?

COGNITIVE

1. Identify and describe the airway anatomy in the infant, child, and the adult.
2. Differentiate between the airway anatomy in the infant, child, and the adult.
3. Explain the pathophysiology of airway compromise.
4. Describe the proper use of airway adjuncts.
5. Review the use of oxygen therapy in airway management.
6. Describe the indications, contraindications, and technique for insertion of nasal gastric tubes.
7. Describe how to perform the Sellick maneuver (cricoid pressure).
8. Describe the indications for advanced airway management.
9. List the equipment required for orotracheal intubation.
10. Describe the proper use of the curved blade for orotracheal intubation.
11. Describe the proper use of the straight blade for orotracheal intubation.
12. State the reasons for and proper use of the stylet in orotracheal intubation.
13. Describe the methods of choosing the appropriate size endotracheal tube in an adult patient.
14. State the formula for sizing an infant or child endotracheal tube.
15. List complications associated with advanced airway management.
16. Define the various alternative methods for sizing the infant and child endotracheal tube.
17. Describe the skill of orotracheal intubation in the adult patient.
18. Describe the skill of orotracheal intubation in the infant and child patient.
19. Describe the skill of confirming endotracheal tube placement in the adult, infant and child patient.
20. State the consequences of and the need to recognize unintentional esophageal intubation.
21. Describe the skill of securing the endotracheal tube in the adult, infant, and child patient.

AFFECTIVE

1. Recognize and respect the feelings of the patient and family during advanced airway procedures.
2. Explain the value of performing advanced airway procedures.
3. Defend the need for the EMT–Basic to perform advanced airway procedures.
4. Explain the rationale for the use of a stylet.
5. Explain the rationale for having a suction unit immediately available during intubation attempts.
6. Explain the rationale for confirming breath sounds.
7. Explain the rationale for securing the endotracheal tube.

PSYCHOMOTOR

1. Demonstrate how to perform the Sellick maneuver (cricoid pressure).
2. Demonstrate the skill of orotracheal intubation in the adult patient.
3. Demonstrate the skill of orotracheal intubation in the infant and child patient.
4. Demonstrate the skill of confirming endotracheal tube placement in the adult patient.
5. Demonstrate the skill of confirming endotracheal tube placement in the infant and child patient.
6. Demonstrate the skill of securing the endotracheal tube in the adult patient.
7. Demonstrate the skill of securing the endotracheal tube in the infant and child patient.

ATLAS OF TRAUMA INJURIES

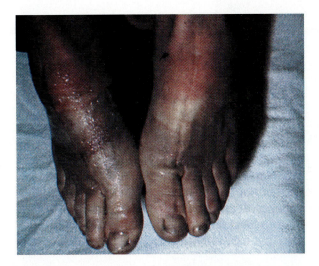

Fig. AT-1   A local deep cold injury during thawing.

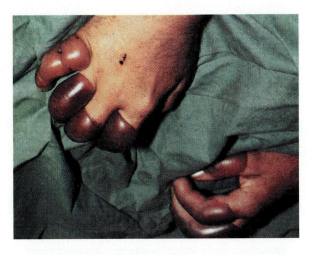

Fig. AT-3   A superficial local cold injury 2 days after the injury occurred.

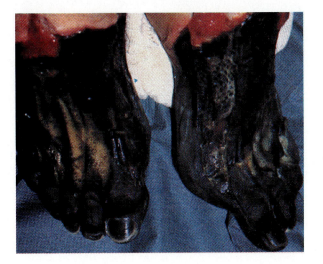

Fig. AT-2   The same injury examined approximately 1 week later.

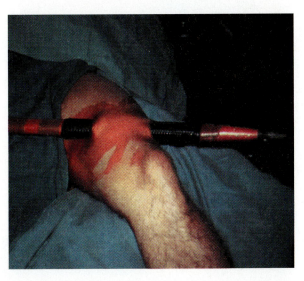

Fig. AT-4   A penetrating injury resulting from a fall onto an ice axe.

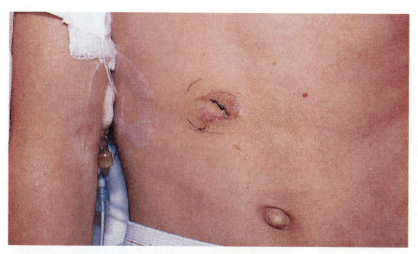

Fig. AT-5 A contusion and laceration to the upper right quadrant caused by a bicycle handlebar.

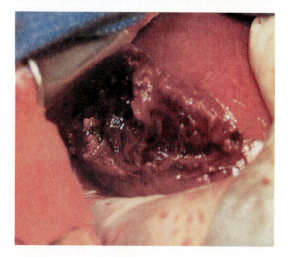

Fig. AT-6 A large laceration to the liver caused by the same handlebar as the injury in Fig. AT-5.

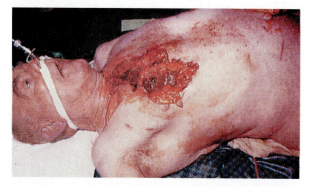

Fig. AT-8 A large wound, through which the lung is visible, that was caused by an industrial accident.

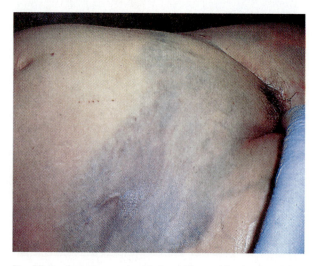

Fig. AT-7 Contusions and pelvic instability resulting from a pelvic fracture. Severe internal bleeding should be suspected here.

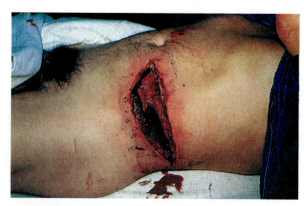

Fig. AT-9 A large wound caused by a broken power saw.

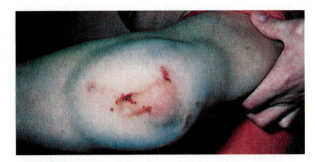

Fig. AT-10   Injury of the elbow joint caused by a fall.

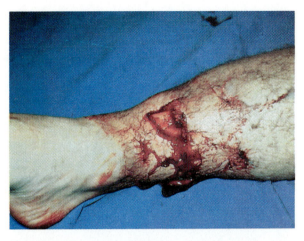

Fig. AT-13   An open injury of the lower leg with protruding bone ends.

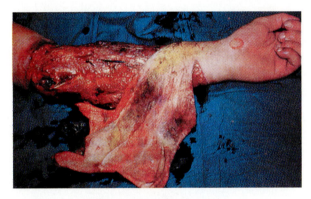

Fig. AT-11   Extensive soft-tissue injury to the forearm skin, caused when the limb was run over in the road.

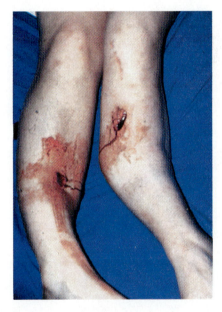

Fig. AT-14   Open injuries of both legs.

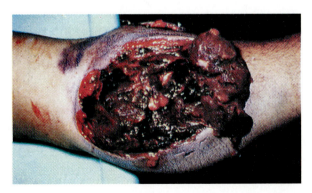

Fig. AT-12   An exit wound caused by a shotgun fired at close range.

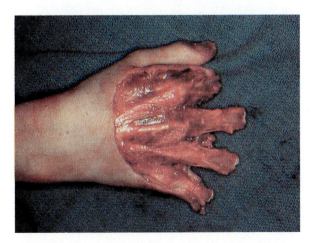

Fig. AT-15   Avulsion injury of the hand caused by a farm equipment accident.

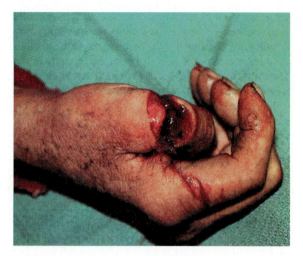

Fig. AT-16   Near amputation of the thumb.

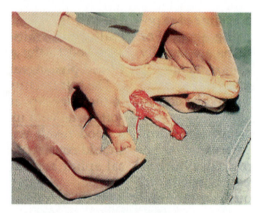

Fig. AT-17   Degloving injury of the finger in Fig. AT-18.

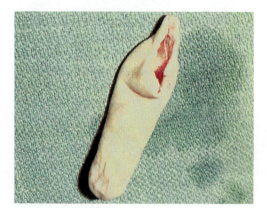

Fig. AT-18   Degloved portion of finger in Fig. AT-17.

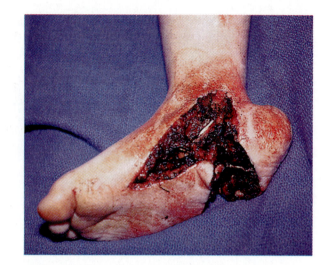

Fig. AT-19   Soft-tissue injuries to a 2-year-old's foot following a lawn mower accident.

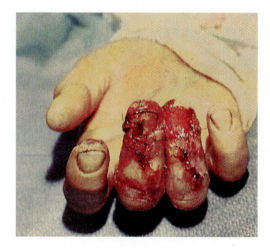

Fig. AT-20   A crush injury of the fingers.

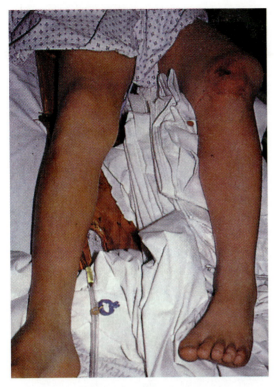

Fig. AT-21   A deformed distal femur.

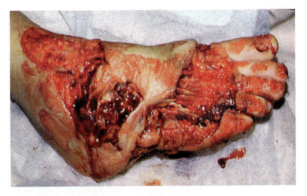

Fig. AT-23   A crush injury caused when the pedal of a bicycle was broken off by a car. The patient made a good recovery.

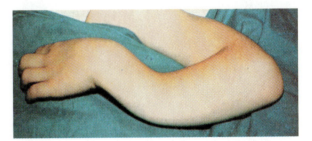

Fig. AT-24   An angulated deformity of the forearm.

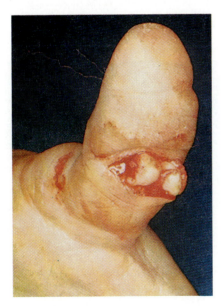

Fig. AT-22   Open joint injury of the thumb.

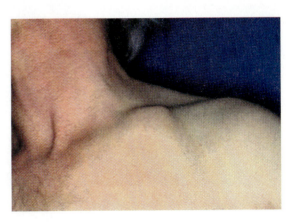

Fig. AT-25   A clavicular fracture with obvious deformity.

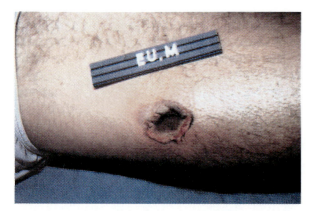

Fig. AT-26   Lightning entrance wound on the thigh.

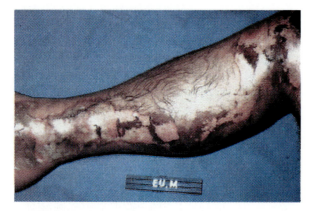

Fig. AT-27   Lightning exit wound of the lower leg.

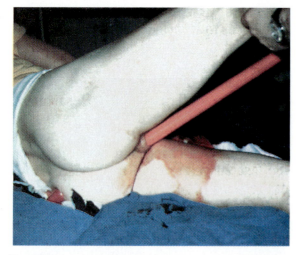

Fig. AT-28   A skier with a penetrating injury from a slalom stick.

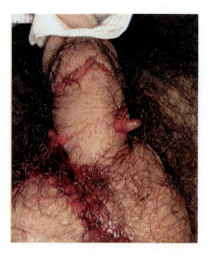

Fig. AT-29   Lacerations of the penis resulting from a direct kick during a soccer game.

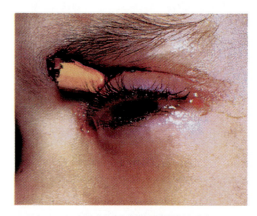

Fig. AT-30   Penetrating trauma caused by a pencil.

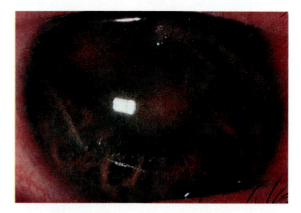

Fig. AT-31   Blood in the anterior chamber of the eye caused by a blow from a squash ball.

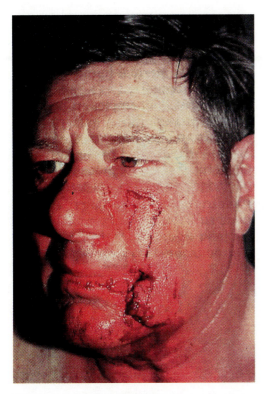

Fig. AT-32 A horse bite on the face.

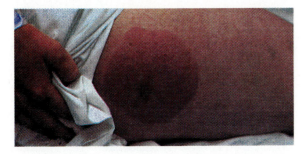

Fig. AT-33 A brown recluse spider bite after 48 hours.

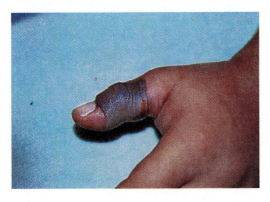

Fig. AT-34 Moderate rattlesnake envenomation.

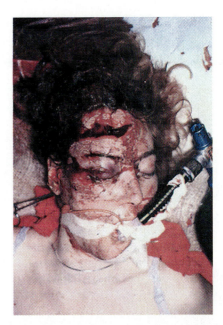

Fig. AT-35 Severe head injury with substantial blood loss, resulting from multiple massive blows.

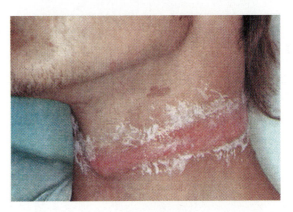

Fig. AT-36 A rope burn on the neck of a motor trialist who ran off of the circuit into a boundary rope.

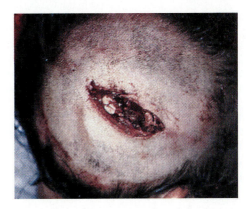

Fig. AT-37 An open head injury with exposed brain tissue.

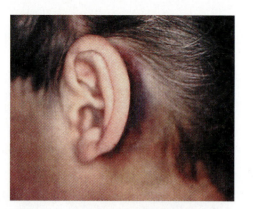

Fig. AT-38   Bruising behind the ears is an indicator of injury to the base of the skull.

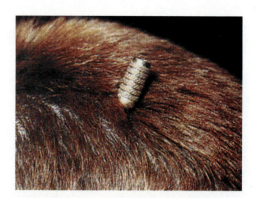

Fig. AT-40   A dart partially embedded in the head.

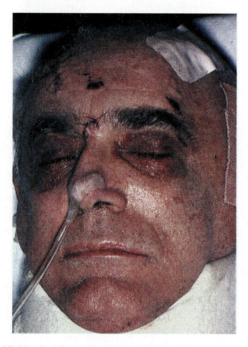

Fig. AT-39   Bruising under the eyes is also an indicator of injury to the base of the skull.

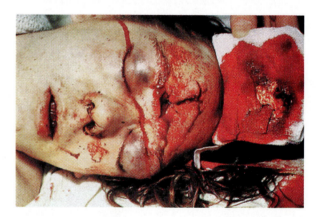

Fig. AT-41   An open head injury with some brain matter visible on the gauze pad. This patient made a good recovery in all respects.

Figs. AT-1, AT-2, AT-3, AT-4, AT-13, AT-14, AT-26, AT-27, AT-28 From Vallatton J, Dubas F: *Color Atlas of Mountain Medicine,* London, England, 1991, Wolfe Medical Publications.

Figs. AT-5, AT-6, AT-7, AT-19, AT-21, AT-30 From Nakayama: *A Color Atlas of Pediatric Surgery,* New York, 1992, Gower.

Figs. AT-8, AT-9, AT-10, AT-11, AT-12, AT-23, AT-24, AT-41 From London, PS: *A Colour Atlas of Diagnosis After Recent Injury,* Ipswich, England, 1990, Wolfe Medical Publications.

Figs. AT-15, AT-16 From Moylan JA: *Principles of Trauma Surgery,* New York, 1992, Gower.

Figs. AT-35, AT-37, AT-38, AT-39, AT-40 From Teddy, Anslow: *Pocket Picture Guide to Head Injuries,* Hong Kong, 1989, Gower.

Figs. AT-17, AT-18, AT-20, AT-32 From Grossman JA: *Atlas of Minor Injuries and Repairs,* London, England, 1992, Gower.

Figs. AT-22, AT-25, AT-29, AT-31, AT-36 From Williams JG: *Color Atlas of Injury in Sport,* ed 2, Chicago, 1990, Yearbook Medical Publishers.

Figs. AT-33, AT-34 From Auerbach PS: *Management of Wilderness and Environmental Emergencies,* ed 3, St. Louis, 1995, Mosby.

APPENDIX A

JOB DESCRIPTION FOR THE EMERGENCY MEDICAL TECHNICIAN – BASIC

CAREER REQUIREMENTS

Responds to emergency calls to provide efficient and immediate care to the critically ill and injured, and transports the patient to a medial facility.

After receiving the call from the dispatcher, drives the ambulance to address or location given using the most expeditious route, depending on traffic and weather conditions. Observes traffic ordinances and regulations concerning emergency vehicle operation.

Upon arrival at the scene of crash or illness, parks the ambulance in a safe location to avoid additional injury. Prior to initiating patient care, the EMT–Basic will also "size-up" the scene to determine that the scene is safe, the mechanism of injury or nature of illness, total number of patients, and to request additional help if necessary. In the absence of law enforcement, creates a safe traffic environment, such as the placement of road flares, removal of debris, and redirection of traffic for the protection of the injured and those assisting in the care of injured patients.

Determines the nature and extent of illness or injury and establishes priority for required emergency care. Based on assessment findings, renders emergency medical care to adult, infant, and child, medical and trauma patients. Duties include, but are not limited to, opening and maintaining an airway, ventilating patients, and cardiopulmonary resuscitation, including use of automated external defibrillators. Provide prehospital emergency medical care of simple and multiple system trauma such as controlling hemorrhage, treatment of shock (hypoperfusion), bandaging wounds, and immobilization of painful, swollen, deformed extremities. Medical duties include assisting in childbirth, management of respiratory, cardiac, diabetic, allergic, behavioral, and environmental emergencies, and suspected poisonings. Searches for medical identification emblem as a clue in providing emergency care. Additional care is provided based upon assessment of the patient and obtaining historical information. These interventions include assisting patients with prescribed medications, including sublingual nitroglycerin, epinephrine autoinjectors, and hand-held aerosol inhalers. The EMT–Basic will also be responsible for administration of oxygen, oral glucose, and activated charcoal.

Reassures patients and bystanders by working in a confident, efficient manner. Avoids mishandling and undue haste while working expeditously to accomplish the task.

Where a patient must be extricated from entrapment, assesses the extent of injury and gives all possible emergency care and protection to the entrapped patient and uses the prescribed techniques and appliances for safely removing the patient. If needed, radios the dispatcher for additional help or special rescue and/or utility services. Provides simple rescue service if the ambulance has not been accompanied by a specialized unit. After extrication, provides additional care in triaging the injured in accordance with standard emergency procedures.

Complies with regulations on the handling of the deceased, notifies authorities, and arranges for protection of property and evidence at scene.

Lifts stretcher, placing in ambulance and seeing that the patient and stretcher are secured, and continues emergency medical care.

From the knowledge of the condition of the patient and the extent of injuries and the relative locations and the staffing of emergency hospital facilities, determines the most appropriate facility to which the patient will be transported, unless otherwise directed by medical direction. Reports directly to the emergency department or communications center the nature and extent of injuries, the number being transported, and the destination to assure prompt medical care on arrival. Identifies assessment findings which may require communications with medical direction for advice and for notification that special professional services and assistance be immediately available upon arrival at the medical facility.

Constantly assesses patient en route to emergency facility, administers additional care as indicated or directed by medical direction.

Assists in lifting and carrying the patient out of the ambulance and into the receiving facility.

Reports verbally and in writing their observation and emergency medical care of the patient at the emergency scene and in transit to the receiving facility staff for purposes of records and diagnostics. Upon request, provides assistance to the receiving facility staff.

After each call, restocks and replaces used linens, blankets, and other supplies, cleans all equipment following appropriate disinfecting procedures, makes careful check of all equipment so that the ambulance is ready for the next run. Maintains ambulance in efficient operating condition. Ensures that the ambulance is clean, washed, and kept in a neat, orderly condition. In accordance with local, state, or federal regulations, decontaminates the interior of the vehicle after transport of patient with contagious infection or hazardous materials exposure.

Determines that vehicle is in proper mechanical condition by checking items required by service management. Maintains familiarity with specialized equipment used by the service.

Attends continuing education and refresher training programs as required by employers, medical direction, licensing, or certifying agencies.

Meets qualifications within the functional job analysis.

APPENDIX B

CONTINUING EDUCATION AND ITS IMPORTANCE IN LIFELONG LEARNING

This curriculum is designed to provide the student with the essentials to serve as an EMT–Basic. The 110-hour time constraint of this program as recommended by the national emergency medical services community during the 1990 NHTSA *Consensus Workshop on Emergency Medical Services Training Programs* necessitates the need for enrichment and continuing education in order to bring the student to full competency. As an entry-level medical education program, we understand that a laborer who works with his hands and even a craftsmen who works with his hands and head may be achievable within the 110-hour time limit constraint, but an artist who works with this hands, head, and heart cannot be achieved within these constraints. We strongly urge employers and service chiefs to integrate new graduates into specific orientation training programs.

It is important to understand that this curriculum does not provide students with extensive knowledge in hazardous materials, blood-borne pathogens, emergency vehicle operations, or rescue practices in unusual environments. These areas are not core elements of education and practice as identified in the *National EMS Education and Practice Blueprint.* Identified areas of competency not specifically designed within the EMT–Basic: National Standard Curriculum should be taught in conjunction with this program as a local or state option.

APPENDIX C

Cardiopulmonary Resuscitation (CPR) Review for Adults, Children, and Infants

	OBJECTIVES	ACTIONS		
		Adult (over 8 yrs)	**Child (1 to 8 yrs)**	**Infant (under 1 yr)**
A -- Airway	1. Assessment: Determine unresponsiveness	Tap or gently shake shoulder.		
		Ask "Are you okay?"		Observe
	2. Position patient	Turn on back as unit, supporting head and neck.		
	3. Open airway	Open airway with head-tilt/chin-lift.		
B -- Breathing	4. Assessment: Determine breathlessness	Maintain open airway. Place ear over mouth, observing chest. Look, listen, feel for breathing (3-5 sec).		
	5. Give two rescue breaths	Seal mouth-to-mouth with barrier device or bag-valve device.		Seal mouth-to-mouth/nose with barrier device.
		Give two rescue breaths 1.5 - 2 sec each.	Give two rescue breaths 1-1.5 sec each.	
		Observe chest rise. Allow lung deflation between breaths.		
C -- Circulation	6. Assessment: Determine pulselessness	Feel for carotid pulse (5-10 sec); maintain head-tilt/chin-lift.		Feel for brachial pulse; maintain head-tilt/chin-lift
	7. If pulseless, begin chest compressions. a. Landmark check b. Hand placement	Place two hands on lower third of sternum. Depress 1.5 to 2 inches.	Place heel of one hand on lower third of sternum. Depress 1 to 1.5 inches.	Place 2-3 fingers on sternum, 1 finger's width below nipple line. Depress 0.5 - 1 inch.
	c. Compression rate	Give 80-100 compressions per minute.	Give at least 100 compressions per minute	
CPR Cycles	8. Compressions to breaths	Give 2 breaths every 15 compressions.	Give 1 breath every 5 compressions	
	9. Number of cycles	4	20	
	10. Reassessment	Feel for carotid pulse		Feel for brachial pulse
		If there is no pulse, resume CPR.		
Entrance of second rescuer		Compression rate for two-rescuer CPR is 80-100 per min; the compression ratio is 5 chest compressions to 1 breath.		
Option for pulse return		If no breathing, give rescue breaths.	Give 1 breath every 5 sec (12/minute)	Give 1 breath every 3 sec (20/minute).

GLOSSARY

Abandonment: Termination of care without the patient's consent and without making any provisions for continuing care at the same or a higher level.

Abnormal behavior: A behavior exhibited by a person that is outside of the norm for the situation and is socially unacceptable; this behavior may result in harm to the person or to others.

Abortion: Medical term for any delivery or removal of a human fetus before it can live on its own.

Abrasion: An open soft-tissue injury resulting from a scraping force; the epidermis is damaged.

Absorbed toxin: A toxin that enters the body through the skin.

Accessory muscles: The additional muscles used to facilitate breathing in a person in respiratory distress.

Acetabulum: The socket of the hip joint.

Acromion process: The tip of the shoulder.

Activated charcoal: A medication that medical direction may authorize for management of poisoning caused by an ingested toxin.

Administrative information: The elements of the minimum data set related to the prehospital care call.

Adolescent: A child 12 to 18 years of age.

Adrenaline: A hormone that helps prepare the body for emergencies.

Advance directives: Orders from patients and their physicians regarding what care should be provided or withheld in certain emergency situations.

Air embolism: An abnormal presence of air in a blood vessel that obstructs the flow of blood.

Airway: The respiratory system structures through which air passes.

Allergen: A substance that causes an allergic response.

Allergic reaction: An exaggerated immune response in an individual to any substance.

Altered mental status: A state of mind that is not normal for the patient; a condition in which the patient is not oriented to person, place, or time (not necessarily all three together).

Alveoli: The air sacs in the lungs where gas exchange takes place.

Amniotic sac: The membrane forming a closed, fluid-filled sac around a developing fetus.

Amputation: The removal of an appendage from the body.

Anatomic position: Position in which the patient is standing upright and facing forward, with palms facing forward.

Angina: The discomfort felt when the heart does not receive enough oxygen. It is commonly experienced after exertion, and the patient usually feels better with rest.

Angulation: An injury that is deformed (bent) at the site.

Anterior: A directional term meaning toward the front; also called *ventral*.

Anterior chamber: The chamber of the eye between the cornea and the iris.

Anterior axillary line: Located near the cavity beneath the junction of the arm and shoulder containing the axillary artery and vein; a part of the brachial plexus of nerves, many lymph nodes, and fat and areolar tissue; armpit.

Aorta: The major artery of the body.

APGAR score: A method of evaluation of an infant's physical condition at 1 and 5 minutes after birth.

Apices of the lungs: The tops of the lungs, lying just under the clavicles bilaterally.

Apneic: Patients who are not breathing.

Arteries: Blood vessels that carry blood away from the heart.

Arteriole: The smallest branch of an artery.

Assault: Threatening or attempting to inflict offensive physical contact.

Asystole: A cardiac rhythm (or lack of rhythm) that produces no electrical or mechanical activity within the heart.

Atria: The two chambers of the heart that receive blood and pump it to the ventricles.

Automaticity: The ability of cardiac muscle to contract on its own.

Avulsion: A flap of skin that is torn or pulled loose.

Backboard: A device used to maintain immobilization of the head, neck, and torso.

Bag-valve-mask (BVM): A common ventilation device consisting of a self-inflating bag, a one-way valve, a mask, and an oxygen reservoir.

Bandage: A material used to secure a dressing in place on an injury.

Base station: A radio transceiver located at a stationary site such as a hospital, mountain top, dispatch center, or other public safety agency.

Bases of the lungs: The bottoms of the lungs, lying approximately at the level of the sixth rib.

Battery: Offensive touching of a person without the person's consent.

Behavior: The manner in which a person acts or performs.

Behavioral emergency: A situation in which a person exhibits abnormal behavior that is unacceptable or intolerable to the person, family members, or the community.

Bilateral: A directional term used when describing the right and left sides of the body relative to each other.

Bilaterally: On both the right and left sides of the body.

Birth canal: The lower part of the uterus and the vagina.

Blood pressure: A measure of the pressure exerted against the walls of the arteries.

Bloody show: The expulsion of the mucous plug, sometimes mixed with blood, as the cervix dilates; often occurs at the beginning of labor.

Blow-by oxygen: Method of oxygen delivery for infants and children without placing a mask on the face.

Body mechanics: The principles of effective movement used in lifting and moving patients.

Body substance isolation (BSI) precautions: Measures taken to prevent EMTs from coming in contact with any body fluid.

Brachial arteries: The primary arteries to the upper extremities.

Breath sounds: The sound of air moving in and out of the lungs.

Breech presentation: The presentation of the baby's feet or buttocks first in delivery.

Bronchi: The two major branches of the trachea into each lung.

Capillaries: The smallest blood vessels in the body where the exchange of oxygen and nutrients for carbon dioxide and other waste occurs.

Capillary refill: A measure of the perfusion of the skin; decreased capillary refill is a good indicator of shock in patients under 6 years of age; measured as the amount of time required to refill the capillary bed after applying and releasing pressure on a fingernail.

Cardex system: A system of dispatch that allows the EMS dispatcher to select the most appropriate unit and to provide callers with prearrival instructions.

Cardiac muscle: Muscle of the heart, with the unique property of being able to contract on its own.

Carina: The point at which the trachea divides into the two main-stem bronchi.

Carotid arteries: The primary arteries to the head.

Carpals: The tiny bones in the wrist.

Central lines: Intravenous lines surgically placed near the heart for long-term use.

Central nervous system (CNS): The division of the nervous system containing the brain and the spinal column.

Central pulse: A pulse point in or near the trunk.

Cephalic presentation: The presentation of the baby's head first in delivery.

Cerebrospinal fluid (CSF): Fluid surrounding the brain and spinal cord that acts as a cushion.

Cervical spinal immobilization device: A device used to maintain immobilization of the head and neck; commonly called a *cervical collar*.

Cervical vertebrae: The vertebrae in the neck.

Cervix: The lower part of the uterus.

Caesarean section: A surgical delivery in which the muscles of the abdomen are cut and the baby is delivered through the abdomen.

Chemical name: A precise description of a drug's chemical composition.

CHEMTREC: The Chemical Transportation Emergency Center, a service of the Chemical Manufacturers Association, a public service agency that can provide immediate on-line advice to emergency personnel at the scene of hazardous materials incidents.

Child abuse: An improper or excessive action by parents, guardians, or caretakers that injures or causes harm to children.

Chronic: Refers to something occurring as a repeating event, present for a prolonged period of time, such as chronic illness.

Circumferential pressure: Pressure put around the circumference of an extremity to control bleeding.

Clavicle: The anterior bone in the shoulder girdle; also called the *collar bone*.

Closed injury: An injury that does not break the continuity of the skin.

Coccyx: Fused vertebrae that form the tailbone.

Communication: The transmission or exchange of information, ideas, and skills through language, body movements, gestures, and expressions.

Compliance: A measure of the elasticity of the lungs.

Compression injury: A type of injury causing bones to be pushed together.

Conduction: The transfer of heat directly from one object to another.

Continuous quality improvement: A systematic review of the EMS system to assess the quality of care given.

Contraindication: A situation in which a medication should not be used.

Contusion: A type of closed soft-tissue injury; also called a *bruise*.

Convection: The transfer of heat to moving air or liquid.

Cranium: The skull.

Crepitation: A grating or crackling sound or sensation, such as that caused when fractured ends of bone move against each other.

Cricoid ring: A firm cartilage ring just inferior to the lower portion of the larynx.

Critical incident: Any situation that causes an emergency worker to experience unusually strong emotional reactions and that interferes with their ability to function immediately or at some time in the future.

Critical incident stress debriefing (CISD): A debriefing process conducted by a team of peer counselors and mental health professionals to help emergency workers deal with their emotions and feelings after a critical incident.

Crowing: A long, high-pitched sound made when breathing in; indicates a respiratory problem.

Crowning: The stage when the head of the baby is seen at the vaginal opening.

Crush injury: An open or closed soft-tissue injury resulting from a blunt force trauma.

Cyanotic: Bluish discoloration of mucous membranes and skin caused by hypoperfusion of tissues.

DCAP–BTLS: Acronym standing for the eight components of assessment: Deformities, Contusions, Abrasions, Penetrations or Punctures, Burns, Tenderness, Lacerations, and Swelling.

Decontamination: The use of physical or chemical means to remove, inactivate, or destroy blood-borne pathogens on a surface or item so that it can no longer transmit infection.

Dermis: The middle layer of the skin containing blood vessels, nerves, and sebaceous glands.

Detailed physical examination: The complete methodical head-to-toe evaluation of the patient.

Diabetes mellitus: A disease that prevents insulin from being produced. Without insulin, the body can not break down sugar into usable forms of energy.

Diaphoresis: Profuse sweating.

Diaphragm: The large, dome-shaped muscle that separates the thoracic from the abdominal cavities; used in breathing.

Diastolic blood pressure: Measurement of the pressure in an artery while the ventricles are at rest.

Direct injury: An injury that results from a force that comes into direct contact with an area of the body.

Direct laryngoscopy: Placing an endotracheal tube into the trachea while visualizing the glottic opening with a laryngoscope.

Direct medical direction: Medical direction in which the physician speaks directly with EMTs in the field; also referred to as *on-line medical direction*.

Disinfecting: The process of killing microorganisms on a surface or item. High-level disinfection destroys all microorganisms except large numbers of bacterial spores and is used for equipment that has contacted mucous membranes. Intermediate-level disinfection destroys the tuberculosis bacteria, most viruses, and fungi, but it does not destroy bacterial spores; it is used for disinfecting surfaces that contact intact skin and have been visibly contaminated with body fluids. Low-level disinfection destroys most bacteria and some fungi and viruses, but not tuberculosis or bacterial spores, and it is used for routine cleaning or removing of soiling when no body fluids are visible.

Distal: A directional term meaning away from the trunk.

Distal pulse: A pulse taken away from the center of the body, such as at the wrist.

Distraction injury: A type of spinal injury produced by a pulling force such as a hanging.

Domestic dispute: A form of violence that results from a family argument and may result in abuse of spouse or children.

Dorsalis pedis arteries: Arteries leading to the feet.

Dose: The amount of the medication that should be administered.

Dressing: A sterile material used to control bleeding and protect an open soft-tissue injury.

Drowning: Death from suffocation within the first 24 hours of submersion in liquid.

Drug: Any substance that alters the body's functioning when taken into the body.

Due regard: The principle that a reasonable and careful person in the circumstances would act in a way that is safe and considerate for others, such as an ambulance providing enough notice of approach to prevent a collision.

Duty to act: Legal obligation that certain personnel, either by statute or function, have a responsibility to provide patient care when the opportunity presents itself.

Electrodes: Remote pads that are attached to the defibrillator with lead wires and attached to the patient to monitor the electrical activity within the heart.

Electrolytes: Electrically charged particles that are dissolved in a solution, such as plasma.

Emancipated minors: Children who are free from parental care and responsibility and therefore have control over their own lives and are free to make their own decisions; legally considered to be an adult.

Emergency medical dispatcher: EMS dispatcher who has received special education for giving medical care instructions to patients or others over the phone before the EMTs arrive.

Emergency Medical Services (EMS) System: A system of many agencies, personnel, and institutions involved in planning, providing, and monitoring emergency care.

Emergency Medical Technician (EMT): The generic term for a prehospital emergency care provider educated at least to the EMT–Basic level.

Emergency move: Moving a patient when there is an immediate danger to the patient or crew members if the patient is not moved, or when life-saving care cannot be given because of the patient's location or position.

EMT–Basic: A basic prehospital life support provider trained to the NHTSA guidelines for EMT–Basic.

EMT–Intermediate: An EMT with additional education in one or more advanced techniques such as vascular access and intubation.

EMT–Paramedic: An EMT with additional education to the level of full advanced life support.

Encoders and decoders: A part of a series of digital radio equipment that allows the user to block out radio transmissions not intended for that unit.

Endotracheal (ET) tube: A tube placed into the trachea to increase the delivery of oxygen to the lungs and decrease the possibility of aspiration.

Epidermis: The outermost layer of the skin.

Epigastrium: The area over the stomach.

Epiglottis: The flaplike structure that prevents food and liquid from entering the trachea during swallowing.

Epistaxis: Bleeding from the nose.

Error of commission: A situation in which an EMT provides improper care.

Error of omission: A situation in which an EMT fails to provide care that is required by usual standards of care.

Escort: Another emergency vehicle, such as a police car, that accompanies the ambulance to or from the scene to the receiving facility.

Evaporation: The transfer of heat that occurs when a liquid changes into a gas.

Evisceration: An open wound in the abdomen through which organs are protruding.

Expressed consent: Condition in which the patient agrees to the treatment plan and gives the EMT permission to proceed, while understanding any risks associated with the treatment.

Extrication: The process of removing a patient from entanglement in a motor vehicle or other situation in a safe and appropriate manner.

Extrication sector: The sector in the incident management system responsible for dealing with extrication of patients who are trapped at the scene. This includes rescue, the initial assessment, and sorting patients for transport to the treatment sector.

Extubation: The removal of a tube.

Febrile: Having a fever, a body temperature above normal.

Femoral arteries: The primary arteries to the lower extremities.

Femur: The long bone of the thigh.

Fetus: An unborn, developing baby.

First Responder: An individual in a position that includes providing initial medical assistance in an emergency.

Floating ribs: The lower ribs that extend laterally from the vertebrae.

Fontanelle: The soft spots on an infant's head created by incomplete skull bone fusing.

Fowler's position: Position in which the patient is lying on the back with an approximately 45° bend at the hips.

Full-thickness burn: A burn that affects all layers of the skin.

Gag reflex: A reflex that causes the patient to retch when the back of the throat is stimulated; this reflex helps unresponsive patients protect their airways.

Gastric distention: The accumulation of air in the stomach; places pressure on the diaphragm, making artificial ventilation difficult and increasing the possibility of vomiting.

Gastric tube: A tube placed directly into the stomach for feeding.

General impression: The EMT's immediate assessment, in the first few seconds, of the environment and the patient's chief complaint.

Generic name: The name of a medication listed in the *US Pharmacopeia,* the official name assigned to the medication. The generic name is usually a simple form of the chemical name.

Glottic opening: The anatomic space between the vocal cords, leading to the trachea.

Glottis: The passageway into the trachea from the pharynx.

Glucose: A form of sugar that is converted into usable energy.

Greater trochanter: The top of the femur where it joins the pelvis.

Grunting: Respirations that sound like the patient is grunting when attempting to breathe. The sound comes from the airway and is not intentional; indicates a respiratory problem.

Gurgling: A liquid sound during breathing; indicates a respiratory problem.

Hazardous materials: Materials that pose a threat or unreasonable risk to life, health, or property if not properly controlled during manufacture, processing, packaging, handling, storage, transportation, use, and disposal.

Heart rate: The number of times the heart beats per minute.

Hematoma: A closed soft-tissue injury produced by accumulation of blood under the skin.

Hemoglobin: The chemical that carries oxygen in the blood and releases it when it reaches the tissues.

Hemorrhagic shock: Hypoperfusion that results from bleeding.

History: A concise and inclusive set of information EMTs gather about the patient.

Hormones: Body chemicals secreted by glands in the endocrine system that regulate body activities and functions in many body systems.

Humerus: The bone of the upper arm.

Hyperthermic: The condition in which the body temperature is above normal (98.6°F or 37°C).

Hypoglycemia: Low level of sugar in the blood.

Hypoperfusion: The state that results when cells are not perfused adequately; oxygen and nutrients are not delivered and there is an inadequate removal of metabolic waste products.

Hypothermic: The condition in which the body temperature is below normal (98.6°F or 37°C).

Hypovolemic shock: Hypoperfusion that results from an inadequate volume of blood.

Hypoxia: Decreased oxygen supply to an area of tissue.

Idiopathic: Arising spontaneously from an obscure or unknown cause.

Iliac wings: The anteriosuperior tips of the pelvis.

Implied consent: Condition in which EMTs have legal permission to provide treatment to a person who is mentally, physically, or emotionally unable to provide expressed consent or otherwise able to agree to treatment when treatment is needed due to a serious or life-threatening injury or illness. Care is given on the assumption that the patient would ask for and agree to treatment if able to.

Incident management system: A system for coordinating procedures to assist in the control, direction, and coordination of emergency response resources.

Indication: The condition for which a medication may be used.

Indirect injury: An injury in one body area that results from a force that comes into contact with a different part of the body.

Indirect medical direction: Any direction provided by physicians that is not direct, including system design, protocol development, education, and quality improvement; also referred to as *off-line medical direction*.

Infant: A child less than 1 year of age.

Infection control: Measures EMTs take to help prevent the transmission of infection from patients to EMTs, from one patient to another, and from EMTs to patients.

Inferior: A directional term meaning toward the bottom of the body.

Ingested toxin: A toxin that is consumed orally.

Inhalation: A route of administration for medications in the form of a fine mist or a gas that are absorbed by the capillaries of the lungs.

Inhaled toxin: A toxin that is breathed into the lungs where it is absorbed into the bloodstream.

Injected toxin: A toxin that enters the body through a puncture in the skin.

Insulin: A hormone that is crucial for the body's use of sugars.

Insulin dependent: A diabetic patient who requires injections of insulin for the body to use sugar. Not all diabetics require insulin injections.

Intercostal muscles: Muscles located between the ribs that move with breathing.

Involuntary: Referring to a bodily activity that is not controlled consciously by the person.

Involuntary muscle: Smooth muscle of internal hollow organs that is not under conscious control of the individual.

Ischemia: A decreased oxygen supply to an area of tissue.

Ischium: A lower bone in the pelvis; the posterior hip.

Jaw thrust: A method of opening the airway by displacing the jaw forward; used instead of the head-tilt chin-lift in patients with suspected spinal injury.

Joints: The location where bones come together to provide for movement.

Jugular vein distention (JVD): Abnormal enlargement of the veins on the sides of the neck.

Kendrick Extrication Device (KED): A type of short board used to immobilize a seated patient.

Labored respirations: An increase in the effort expended to breathe.

Laceration: A break in the skin of varying depth caused by a sharp object.

Laryngectomy: A surgical procedure in which the larynx is removed.

Laryngoscope: An instrument used to visualize the airway during endotracheal intubation.

Larynx: The voice box, or *vocal cords*, consisting of bands of cartilage that vibrate when we speak.

Lateral: A directional term meaning away from the midline.

Ligaments: Fibrous tissue that binds together joints and bones and cartilage.

Log roll: A method used to move a lying patient onto a long board.

Long board (full body spinal immobilization device): A device used to maintain immobilization of the head, neck, torso, pelvis, and extremities.

Lumbar vertebrae: The vertebrae that support the weight of the head and trunk in the lower back.

Main-stem bronchi: The two main branches to the lungs from the trachea.

Mandible: The jaw bone.

Manubrium: The superior one-third of the sternum.

Material Safety Data Sheets: Information sheets required by the United States Department of Labor that list properties and hazards associated with chemicals and compounds to assist in management of incidents involving them.

Maxilla: One of the pair of large bones that form the upper jaw.

Mechanism of action: How a medication affects the body.

Mechanism of injury: The event or forces that caused the patient's injury.

Meconium: Fetal stool that may be present in the amniotic fluid.

Medial: A directional term meaning toward the midline.

Medial malleolus: The rounded bottom part of the tibia at the ankle joint.

Medical direction: The process of physicians ensuring that EMT care given to ill or injured patient is medically appropriate; also called medical oversight or medical control.

Metacarpals: The bones of the hand.

Midclavicular line: An imaginary line parallel to the long axis of the body and passing through the midpoint of the clavicle on the anterior surface of the body.

Midaxillary line: An imaginary line that extends vertically from the armpits to the ankles, dividing the body into anterior (front) and posterior (back) halves.

Midclavicular line: Each of two imaginary lines that divide the clavicles (collar bones) in two and extend down the trunk through each nipple.

Midline: An imaginary line through the middle of the body that starts at the top of the head and goes through the nose and the umbilicus.

Minimum data set: The essential elements of patient and administrative data required for accurate and complete prehospital data collection.

Miscarriage: Spontaneous delivery of a human fetus before it is able to live on its own.

Motor function: Testing the ability to move.

Motor nerves: Nerves that send information from the brain to the body.

Multitiered response system: A system in which EMS responses to calls involve basic and advanced levels; may include First Responders, EMTs, paramedics, and other healthcare professionals. Various levels of healthcare professionals may arrive at the scene or meet en route to facilities to provide patient care.

Murphy's eye: A small hole in the side of an endotracheal tube that provides a passage of air if the tip of the tube becomes clogged.

Muscle: Tissue that provides for body shape and movement; there are voluntary, involuntary, and cardiac muscles.

Nasal bones: A collection of bones that create the nose.

Nasal cannula: A device for delivering oxygen from tubing that has holes that blow oxygen directly into the patient's nostrils.

Nasal flaring: An attempt by a patient in respiratory distress to increase the size of the airway by expanding the nostrils.

Nasogastric tube: A tube placed through the nose, down the esophagus, and into the stomach.

Nasopharyngeal airway: A flexible tube of rubber or plastic that is inserted into the patient's nostril to provide an air passage.

Nasopharynx: The part of the pharynx behind the nose.

National EMS Education and Practice Blueprint: A consensus document that establishes a core content for the scope of practice for the four levels of prehospital care providers.

Nature of illness: The patient's description of the chief complaint, or why EMS was called.

Near drowning: Survival past 24 hours after suffocation due to submersion in liquid.

Neglect: The act of not giving attention to a child's essential needs.

Negligence: Failure to act as a reasonable, prudent EMT would under similar circumstances.

Newborn: The term for an infant from birth to 1 month of age.

Noisy respirations: Any noise coming from the patient's airway; indicates a respiratory problem.

Nonrebreather mask: A high-flow device for delivering oxygen to the patient.

Nonurgent move: A patient move used when there is no present or anticipated threat to the patient's life and care can be administered.

Normal respirations: Respirations occurring without airway noise or effort from the patient, usually occurring at a rate of between 12 and 20 breaths per minute for adult patients.

Occlusive: Referring to protection from the air; an occlusive dressing will not let air into the wound.

Olecranon process: The end of the ulna at the elbow joint.

Ongoing assessment: The final step of the patient assessment process; repeats the initial and focused assessment during transport.

Open injury: An injury that breaks the continuity of the skin.

OPQRST: Acronym for eliciting patient information: Onset, Provocation, Quality of pain, Radiation, Severity, and Time.

Orbits: Bones that form the eye sockets.

Oropharyngeal airway: A curved piece of plastic that goes into the patient's mouth and lifts the tongue out of the oropharynx.

Oropharynx: The part of the pharynx behind the mouth.

Orotracheal intubation: The process of inserting an endotracheal tube through the mouth.

Palliative: Refers to something that eases symptoms without curing the underlying problem, such as to diminish pain.

Palpate: Physical examination technique using pressure of the hand or fingers on the surface of the body, especially to determine the condition (as of size or consistency) of an underlying part or organ.

Paradoxical motion: An abnormal movement of the chest wall during inspiration and exhalation, in which the affected portion moves opposite the unaffected portion.

Paralysis: The inability to move an area of the body because of a nervous system problem.

Partial-thickness burn: A burn that affects the epidermis and dermis.

Patella: The bone on the anterior surface of the knee joint; also called the *kneecap*.

Patient information: The elements of the minimum data set related to the patient's clinical condition and the emergency medical care provided.

Patient narrative: The section of a prehospital care report that allows EMTs to write a standard medical format and include additional information.

Penetration or puncture: An open soft-tissue injury caused by an object being pushed into the skin.

Perfusion: The process of circulating blood to the organs, delivering oxygen, and removing wastes.

Perineum: The area of skin between the vagina and anus.

Peripheral: Pertaining to the extremities.

Peripheral nervous system: The network of sensory and motor nerves outside the skull or spinal cord.

Peripheral pulse: A pulse point in an extremity.

Phalanges: The bones of the fingers or toes.

Pharmacology: The science of drugs and study of their origin, ingredients, uses, and actions on the body.

Pharynx: The part of the airway behind the nose and mouth, divided into two regions: the nasopharynx and the oropharynx.

Placard: An information sign with symbols and numbers to assist in identifying the hazardous material or class of material.

Placenta: The fetal and maternal organ through which the fetus absorbs oxygen and nutrients and excretes wastes; attached to the fetus via the umbilical cord.

Plantar: Referring to the bottom of the foot.

Plasma: The fluid portion of the blood.

Platelets: Blood component that plays an important role in blood clotting.

Pneumatic antishock garment (PASG): An inflatable, pressurized garment used to immobilize an unstable pelvis when hypotension is present; can also be used to splint painful, swollen, deformed lower extremities.

Pneumatic splints: Devices such as air or vacuum splints.

Position of function: The relaxed position of the hand or foot in which there is minimal movement or stretching of muscle.

Posterior: A directional term meaning toward the back; also called *dorsal*.

Posterior tibial arteries: Arteries leading to the feet.

Postictal state: A patient condition after a seizure in which the patient seems asleep and almost unresponsive.

Power grip: A hand position that provides maximum force to the object being lifted, using a maximum surface area of the hands; the fingers and palm come into complete contact with the object.

Prehospital care report: A form used to document the events occurring during a patient encounter, including the minimum data set of patient and administrative information.

Preschool child: A child from 3 to 6 years of age.

Presenting part: The part of the fetus that appears at the vaginal opening first.

Pressure point: A place in an extremity where a major artery lies close to a bone; used with direct pressure and elevation to stop bleeding in an arm or leg.

Prolapsed cord: Situation in which the umbilical cord delivers through the vagina before any other presenting part.

Prone: Positional term meaning the patient is lying flat on the stomach.

Provocation: Refers to something that induces a physical reaction.

Proximal: A directional term meaning toward the trunk.

Psychotic: Refers to behavior by a person who has lost touch with reality.

Pulse: The pressure wave felt in an artery when the left ventricle contracts.

Pulse oximetry: A process of measuring the amount of oxygen carried in the blood.

Quality improvement (QI): A system for continually evaluating and improving the care provided within an EMS system.

Radial arteries: The primary arteries to the hands.

Radiation: The loss of heat, in the form of infrared energy, to cooler surroundings.

Radius: The lateral bone in the forearm.

Rapid assessment: The quick evaluation of the patient which is accomplished in 60 to 90 seconds; it can be performed with both trauma and medical patients.

Rapid extrication: The technique used to move a patient from a scene quickly when absolutely necessary.

Reactive to light: Referring to pupil constriction when exposed to a penlight.

Reasonable force: The force necessary to keep a person from injuring him- or herself or others.

Recovery position: The left lateral recumbent position for a patient to maintain an open airway by allowing secretions to drain by gravity and prevent the tongue from occluding the posterior aspect of the mouth.

Red blood cells: The blood cells that contain hemoglobin.

Remote console: Controls the base station radio; used by the dispatcher.

Repeater: A remote receiver that receives a transmission from a low-power portable or mobile radio on one frequency and then transmits the signal at a higher power, often on another frequency.

Respiratory distress: A clinical condition in which the patient begins to increase the work of breathing.

Respiratory failure: A clinical condition when the patient is continuing to work hard to breathe, the effort of breathing is increased, and the patient's condition begins to deteriorate.

Response mode: A decision regarding the use of lights and sirens for an emergency response.

Retractions: The use of accessory muscles to increase the work of breathing, which appears as the sucking in of the muscles between the ribs and at the neck.

Rigid splints: A type of splint that does not conform to the body; immobilizes from two sides.

Route of administration: The way the medication is administered to the patient.

Sacral vertebrae: Fused vertebrae that form the back of the pelvis.

SAMPLE History: Acronym for history of Signs and Symptoms, Allergies, Medications, Pertinent history, Last oral intake, and Events leading to the illness.

Scapula: The posterior bone in the shoulder girdle.

Scene size-up: The evaluation of the entire environment for possible risks to yourself, crew members, patients, or bystanders.

School-age child: A child from 6 to 12 years of age.

Scope of practice: The range of duties and skills EMTs are allowed to and supposed to perform when necessary.

Secondary drowning: The rapid deterioration of respiratory status from several hours to 96 hours after resuscitation.

Seizure: Rapid discharge of nerve cells in the brain, typically causing muscular contractions that create erratic movements of the body or an otherwise unexplained change in mental status.

Self-extubation: The patient's intentional or unintentional removal of a tube.

Sensation: The ability to feel a touch against the skin.

Sensory nerves: Nerves that send information from the body to the brain.

Shallow respirations: Respirations that have low volumes of air in inspiration and expiration.

Shock: Inadequate tissue perfusion; also called *hypoperfusion*.

Shock position: Position in which in the patient is lying flat on the back, bent at the hips with feet lifted approximately 12 inches.

Shunt: A tube running from the brain to the abdomen to drain excess cerebrospinal fluid.

Sign: Any medical or trauma condition that can be observed and identified in the patient.

Skeletal muscles: Muscles attached to bones, used in movement.

Sling and swathe: Bandaging used to immobilize a shoulder or arm injury.

Smooth muscles: Muscles in the walls of tubular structures.

Snoring: A sound that indicates the patient is unable to keep the airway open; the tongue is falling back into and partially obstructing the upper airway.

Splints: Devices used to immobilize a musculoskeletal injury.

Staging sector: The sector in the incident management system that coordinates with the transportation sector for the movement of vehicles to and from the transportation sector.

Standard of care: The minimum acceptable level of care readily provided within a general area.

Sterilization: A disinfecting process that destroys all microorganisms including bacterial spores; used for instruments that penetrate the skin or contact normally sterile areas of the body during invasive procedures.

Sternal notch: The anatomic notch created by the clavicles and the sternum.

Sternum: The breastbone.

Stimulant: A drug that increases the metabolism of the body.

Stress: Bodily or mental tension caused by a physical, chemical, emotional, or other factor.

Stridor: A harsh sound heard during breathing (usually inhalation) that indicates an upper airway obstruction.

Stylet: A bendable device placed in the endotracheal tube to give it rigidity and enable it to hold a shape.

Subcutaneous layer: The deepest layer of skin.

Sublingual route: Putting a medication under the patient's tongue.

Suction devices: Device used to suction secretions and fluids from the mouth and oropharynx of unresponsive patients.

Sudden infant death syndrome (SIDS): The sudden, unexplained death of an infant, generally between 1 month and 1 year of age, for which there is no discernable cause.

Superficial burn: A burn that affects only the epidermis.

Superior: A directional term meaning toward the top of the body.

Supine: Positional term meaning the patient lying flat on the back.

Support or supply sector: The sector in the incident management system responsible for obtaining additional resources including disposable supplies, personnel, and equipment for other sectors.

Sutures: Joints between the skull bones.

Symptom: Any nonobservable condition described by the patient.

Systolic blood pressure: Measurement of the pressure in an artery when the ventricles are contracting.

Thermoregulatory emergency: Any emergency involving a change in the temperature of the body.

Thoracic vertebrae: The vertebrae that attach to the ribs in the upper back.

Thorax: The bone structure composed of 12 pairs of ribs and the sternum.

Thyroid cartilage: A structure of the larynx that forms the "Adam's Apple."

Tibia: The shin bone; the main weight-bearing bone of the lower leg.

Tidal volume: The volume of air per breath.

Toddler: A child 1 to 3 years of age.

Toxin: Any substance that produces adverse effects when it enters the body; all poisons are toxins.

Trachea: The windpipe.

Tracheal stoma: An permanent artificial opening in the trachea.

Tracheostomy: A procedure in which an artificial permanent opening is made into the trachea.

Traction splints: A special device used to immobilize a midfemur injury.

Trade name: The name assigned by the company that sells a medication. Trade names are copyrighted and carry the copyright symbol ®.

Transceiver: A radio with transmit and receive capabilities.

Transportation sector: The sector in the incident management system that coordinates resources including receiving hospitals, air medical resources, and ambulances.

Treatment sector: The sector in the incident management system that provides care to patients received from the triage and extrication sector.

Trendelenburg position: Position in which the patient is lying flat on the back, on an incline, with feet elevated approximately 12 inches above the head.

Trending: The process of comparing serial recordings of a patient's vital signs or other assessments to note changes.

Triage: A method of categorizing patients into treatment or transport priorities.

Triage sector: An optional sector in the incident management system that prioritizes patients for treatment and transport.

Twisting injury: An injury that results from a turning motion of the body in opposite directions.

Ulna: The medial bone of the forearm.

Umbilical cord: The cord that connects the placenta to the fetus.

Umbilicus: Belly button.

Urgent move: A patient move used when the patient's condition may become life-threatening.

Uterus: The female reproductive organ in which a baby grows and develops.

Vagina: The canal that leads from the uterus to the external opening in females.

Vallecula: The anatomic space between the base of the tongue and the epiglottis.

Vasoconstriction: The contraction of the smooth muscles of blood vessels.

Veins: The vessels that carry blood toward the heart.

Ventricles: The larger chambers of the heart; the left ventricle pumps blood to the body, and the right to the lungs.

Ventricular fibrillation: A chaotic electrical rhythm in the ventricles. There is no ventricular contraction or pumping of blood through the heart, and therefore no pulse.

Ventricular tachycardia: Three or more heart beats in a row at 100 beats or more per minute, originating in the ventricles and overriding the normal pacemaker of the heart. In this state the atria and ventricles do not work together; a pulse may or may not be present.

Venule: The smallest branch of a vein.

Vertebrae: The bones of the spinal column.

Voluntary: Referring to bodily activity that is controlled consciously by the person.

Voluntary muscle: Skeletal muscle under conscious control of the individual.

Wheezing: A high-pitched whistling sound usually caused by constriction of the smaller airways or bronchioles; indicates a respiratory problem.

White blood cells: Blood cells that are a main part of the body's defense against infection.

Xiphoid process: The part of the sternum that extends from the posterior end.

Zygomatic arches: Relating to the region of the zygoma (area of the skull on the front side of the face below the eye).

Zygomatic bones: Bones that form the cheek bones.

REFERENCES AND RECOMMENDED READINGS

Emergency Care and Transportation of the Sick and Injured, ed 5, Rosemont, Ill., 1993, American Academy of Orthopaedic Surgeons.

Advanced Cardiac Life Support Provider, Dallas, 1994, American Heart Association.

Textbook of Pediatric Advanced Life Support, Dallas, 1994, American Heart Association.

Auf der Heide E: *Disaster Response: principles of preparation and coordination*, St. Louis, 1989, CV Mosby.

Barkin R, editor: *Pediatric Emergency Medicine Concepts and Clinical Practice*, St. Louis, 1992, Mosby-Year Book.

Beck RK: *Pharmacology for Prehospital Emergency Care*, ed 2, Philadelphia, 1994, FA Davis.

Berelson B, Stiener GA: *Human Behavior: an inventory of scientific findings*, New York, 1964, Harcourt Brace Jovanovich.

Bevelacqua AS: *Prehospital Documentation*, Englewood Cliffs, 1992, Brady.

Bledsoe B, *et al*: Paramedic Emergency Care, ed 2, Englewood Cliffs, 1994, Brady.

Bronstein and Currance: *Emergency Care for Hazardous Materials Exposure*, St. Louis, 1994, Mosby Lifeline.

Brown-Nixon C: *Documentation, the Credibility Skill*, Lake Worth, 1989, EES Publications.

Kidd S, Czajkowski J: *Carbusters!*, Naples, 1990, American Safety Video Publishers.

Caroline N: *Emergency Care in the Streets*, ed 3, Boston, 1987, Little, Brown and Company.

Stock YN: *Basic Pharmacology for Nurses*, ed 10; edited by Clayton BD, St. Louis, 1993, Mosby-Year Book.

Code of Federal Regulations, 40 CFR, part 311, Washington, 1981, Office of the Federal Registrar, National Archive and Records Services, General Services Administration.

Code of Federal Regulations, 49 CFR, 173.500, parts 100–177, Washington, 1981, Office of the Federal Registrar, National Archive and Records Services, General Services Administration.

Code of Federal Regulations, 29 CFR, part 1910, Washington, 1989, Office of the Federal Registrar, National Archive and Records Services, General Services Administration.

Dernocoeur KB: *Streetsense Communication, Safety and Control*, Englewood Cliffs, 1990, Prentice Hall.

Grant HD, *et al*: *Emergency Care*, ed 6, Englewood Cliffs, 1994, Brady/Prentice Hall.

Hafen BQ, Karren KJ: Prehospital Emergency Care and Crisis Intervention, ed 4, Englewood Cliffs, 1992, Brady/Morton/Prentice Hall.

Heckman, J: *Emergency Care and Transportation of the Sick and Injured*, ed 5, Rosemont, Ill., 1992, American Academy of Orthopaedic Surgeons.

Henry MC, Stapleton ER: *EMT Prehospital Care*, Philadelphia, 1992, WB Saunders.

Judd RL, Ponsell DD: *First Responder*, ed 2, St. Louis, 1988, CV Mosby.

Klein, *et al*: *Emergency Vehicle Driver Training*, 1991, Federal Emergency Management Agency and the United States Fire Administration.

Krebs D, *et al*: When Violence Erupts, St. Louis, 1990, CV Mosby.

Kuehl, A: *Out-of-hospital Systems and Medical Oversight*, St. Louis, 1994, Mosby-Year Book.

London PS: *Color Atlas of Diagnosis After Recent Injury*, Philadelphia, 1990, Mosby-Year Book.

National Association of Emergency Medical Services Physicians: Air Medical Dispatch: guidelines for scene response. *Prehospital and Disaster Medicine*, vol 7(1):75–78, 1992.

National Association of Emergency Medical Services Physicians; National Association of State Emergency Medical Services Directors: Use of Warning Lights and Siren in Emergency Medical Vehicle Response and Patient Transport, vol 9(2):63–66, 1994.

National Traffic Highway Safety Administration: *Technical Assessment Standards*, Washington, 1994.

National Registry of EMTs: National Registry Skill Evaluation Sheets, 1994, Columbus, Ohio.

Pediatric Advanced Life Support (PALS) Plus, St. Louis, 1992, American Safety Video Publishers-Mosby Lifeline.

Prehospital Trauma Life Support Committee of the National Association of Emergency Medical Technicians, in cooperation with the Committee on Trauma of the American College of Sugeons: *PHTLS: basic and advanced prehospital trauma life support*, St. Louis, 1994, Mosby-Year Book.

Prehospital Trauma Life Support Committee of the National Association of Emergency Medical Technicians, in cooperation with the Committee on Trauma of the American College of Surgeons: *PHTLS: basci and advanced prehospital trauma life support*, ed 3, 1994, Mosby Lifeline.

Sanders MJ: *Mosby's Paramedic Textbook*, St. Louis, 1994, Mosby Lifeline.

Silent War Infection Control for Emergency Responders, Fort Collins, Colo., OnGUARD and Emergency Resources.

Simon J, Goldberg A: *Prehospital Pediatric Life Support*, St. Louis, 1989, Mosby-Year Book.

Tate P, Seely RR, Stephens TD: *Understanding the Human Body*, St. Louis, 1994, Mosby-Year Book.

The Crimes Code of Pennsylvania, 1993, Gould Publications.

Thibodeau GA, Patton KT: *Anatomy and Physiology*, ed 2, St. Louis, 1993, Mosby-Year Book.

Trenholm S, Jensen A: *Interpersonal Communication*, Belmont, Calif., 1988, Wadsworth Publishing.

United States Department of Transportation: *Emergency Response Guidebook*, Washington, D.C., 1993.

US Department of Transportation, National Highway Traffic Safety Administration, Emergency Medical Technician–Basic: National Standard Curriculum, Washington, DC, 1994, US Government Printing Office.

PHOTO CREDITS AND ACKNOWLEDGMENTS

Division Openers: Photographer Vincent Knaus

Chapter 1 Opener: Photographer Colin Williams

Fig. 1-2: US Department of Transportation, National Highway Traffic Safety Administration, Emergency Medical Technician–Basic: National Standard Curriculum, Washington, DC, 1994, US Government Printing Office

Fig. 1-4: Courtesy of the National Registry of EMTs, Columbus, Ohio

Chapter 2 Opener: Courtesy of William Greenblatt

Fig. 2-6: HEPA-TECH Foam Mask; a product of *uvex*.

Table 2-1: From the Centers for Disease Control: Guidelines for Prevention of Transmission of Human Immunodeficiency Virus and Hepatitis B Virus to Healthcare and Public Safety Workers. *MMWR* 1989;38(S-6):35.

Chapter 3 Opener: Photographer Colin Williams

Fig. 3-1: US Department of Transportation, National Highway Traffic Safety Administration, Emergency Medical Technician–Basic: National Standard Curriculum, Washington, DC, 1994, US Government Printing Office

Fig. 3-3: Courtesy of EMS Data Systems Inc., Phoenix, Arizona

Fig. 3-5: Courtesy of the State of Virginia Department of Health, Office of Emergency Medical Services, Richmond, Virginia

Fig. 3-7: Courtesy of Medic Alert®

Chapter 4 Opener: Photographer James Silvernail

Figs. 4-8, 4-9, and 4-11: From London PS: *A Colour Atlas of Diagnosis After Recent Injury*, Ipswich, England, 1990, Wolfe Medical Pulications.

Fig. 4-10: From Williams JG: *Color Atlas of Injury in Sport*, ed 2, Chicago, 1990, Yearbook Medical Publishers.

Figs. 4-12 and 4-13: From Sanders MJ: *Instructor's Resource Kit to Accompany Mosby's Paramedic Textbook*, St. Louis, 1995, Mosby Lifeline. (Illustrator, Mark Wieber).

Figs. 4-15, 4-16, and 4-19: Modified from Thibodeau: *Anatomy and Physiology*, ed 2, St. Louis, 1993, Mosby. (Illustrator, Rolin Graphics)

Fig: 4-17: From Sanders MJ: *Mosby's Paramedic Textbook*, St. Louis, 1994, Mosby Lifeline. (Illustrator, Christine Oleksyk)

Fig. 4-21: From Thibodeau: *Anatomy and Physiology*, ed 2, St. Louis, 1993, Mosby. (Illustrator, David Mascaro Associates)

Fig. 4-23: From Sanders MJ: *Mosby's Paramedic Textbook*, St. Louis, 1994, Mosby Lifeline.

Fig. 4-24: From Tate, Seeley, and Stephens: *Understanding the Human Body*, St. Louis, 1994, Mosby. (Illustrator, David Mascaro Associates)

Fig. 4-26: From Tate, Seeley, and Stephens: *Understanding the Human Body*, St.Louis, 1994, Mosby. (Illustrator, Christine Oleksyk)

Fig. 4-27: From Tate, Seeley, and Stephens: *Understanding the Human Body*, St. Louis, 1994, Mosby. (Illustrator, Rolin Graphics)

Fig. 4-33: From Tate, Seeley, and Stephens: *Understanding the Human Body*, St. Louis, 1994, Mosby. (Illustrator, Joan Beck)

Chapter 5 Opener: Photographer Colin Williams

Table 5-1: Sheehy SB: Emergency Nursing: Principles and Practice, ed 3, St. Louis, 1992, Mosby.

Fig. 5-1: From Thelan: *Critical Care Nursing*, ed 2, St. Louis, 1994, Mosby.

Fig. 5-2: From Aehlert: *PALS Study Guide*, St. Louis, 1994, Mosby Lifeline. (Illustrator, Kim Battista)

Fig. 5-13: Courtesy of the City of St. Louis Emergency Medical Services, St. Louis, Missouri

Chapter 6 Opener: Photographer Vincent Knaus

Fig. 6-16: Ambulance Cot; a product of Ferno Washington, Inc.

Fig. 6-17: Folding Emergency Stretcher; a product of Ferno Washington, Inc.

Fig. 6-18: Folding Scoop Stretcher; a product of Ferno Washington, Inc.

Fig. 6-19: Reeves Stretcher; a product of Reeves Mfg.

Fig. 6-20: Basket Stretcher; a product of Ferno Washington, Inc.

Fig. 6-21: Stair Chair; a product of Dynamed

Fig. 6-22: Long backboard; a product of Ferno Washington, Inc.

Fig. 6-23: Emergency Wood Back/Spine Board; a product of Moore Medical Corporation; KED, Ferno Washington, Inc.; XP1, Medical Specialties, Inc.

Fig. 6-25: Photographer Colin Williams

Fig. 6-26: Courtesy of JA Preston Corp., Lifeseat

Chapter 7 Opener: Photographer Thomas E. Cooper

Fig. 7-2: From Thompson: *Mosby's Clinical Nursing*, ed 3, St. Louis, 1993, Mosby.

Fig. 7-5: Oxygen Regulators; products of Veri-Flow Corp. and Life Support Products, Inc.

Figs. 7-7, 7-8, and 7-9: Oxygen Masks and Nasal Cannula; products of Hudson RCI

Figs. 7-10 and 7-11: From Cummins: *Handbook of ACLS Scenarios*, St. Louis, 1995, Mosby Lifeline. (Illustrator, Kim Battista)

Fig. 7-13: Oropharyngeal airways; products of Hudson RCI (green)

Fig. 7-17: Nasopharyngeal airway (red); a product of Rusch

Figs. 7-18 and 7-26: From Aehlert: *ACLS Quick Review Study Guide*, St. Louis, 1994, Mosby Lifeline. (Illustrator, Kim Battista)

Fig. 7-21: Portable suction units; products of Laerdal and SS Cort.

Fig. 7-22: V-vac; a product of Laerdal

Fig. 7-32: From Sanders MJ: *Mosby's Paramedic Textbook*, St. Louis, 1994, Mosby Lifeline.

Fig. 7-33: From London PS: *A Colour Atlas of Diagnosis After Recent Injury*, Ipswich, England, 1990, Wolfe Medical Publications.

Chapter 8 Opener: Photographer Vincent Knaus

Figs. 8-1A and 8-3: Photographer James Silvernail

Figs. 8-1C and 8-7A: Photographer Ronald Olshwanger

Fig. 8-2: *uvex* Highflyer safety glasses and HEPATECH; products of *uvex* Safety. Barrier TM Personal Protection Kit; a product of Johnson and Johnson

Figs. 8-5 and 8-8: Photographer William Greenblatt

Fig. 8-7B: Photographer Kenneth Hines

Chapter 9 Opener: Photographer Vincent Knaus

Chapter 10 Opener: Photographer Colin Williams

Fig. 10-1: Photographer Ronald Olshwanger

Chapter 11 Opener: Photographer Peter Escobedo

Fig. 11-1: Photographer Ronald Olshwanger

Fig. 11-5: Courtesy of the City of St. Louis Emergency Medical Services, St. Louis, Missouri

Fig. 11-6: Photographer William Greenblatt

Fig. 11-7: Photographer Colin Williams

Chapter 12 Opener: Photographer Peter Escobedo

Chapter 13 Opener: Photographer Vincent Knaus

Chapter 14 Opener: Photographer Peter Escobedo

Fig. 14-1: Photographer Colin Williams

Fig. 14-2: Portable hand-held and mounted radio units; products of BK (Bendix King) Radio, Inc.

Fig. 14-4: Courtesy of the Maryland Institute for Emergency Medical Services System, Baltimore, Maryland

Fig. 14-5: Photographer Colin Williams

Fig. 14-7: Courtesy of the Center for Emergency Medicine, Pittsburgh, Pennsylvania

Chapter 15 Opener: Photographer Vincent Knaus

Fig. 15-1: Courtesy of the Center for Emergency Medicine, Pittsburgh, Pennsylvania

Figs. 15-2, 15-3, 15-4, and 15-5: Courtesy of EMS Data Systems, Inc., Phoenix, Arizona

Chapter 16 Opener: Image ©1995 Photo Disc, Inc.

Fig. 16-2: Proventil®; a registered trademark of Schering, a wholly owned subsidiary of Schering Plough Corporation, Kenilworth, New Jersey; Ventolin®; a registered trademark of Allen and Hanburys, Division of Glaxo, Inc., Research Triangle Park, North Carolina

Fig. 16-3A: Liqui-char®; a registered trademark of Jones Medical Industries, Inc., St. Louis, Missouri

Fig. 16-3B: Glutose®; a registered trademark of Paddock Laboratories Inc., Minneapolis, Minnesota

Fig. 16-3D: Proventil®; a registered trademark of Schering, a wholly owned subsidiary of Schering Plough Corporation, Kenilworth, New Jersey

Fig. 16-3E: Nitro-Lingual® is a registered trademark of Rhone-Poulenc Rorer Pharmaceuticals, Inc., Collegeville, Pennsylvania; Nitro-Stat®; a registered trademark of Parke Davis, Division of Warner Lambert Co., Morris Plains, New Jersey

Fig. 16-3F: EpiPen®; a registered trademark of Center, Division of EM Industries, Inc., Port Washington, New York

Chapter 17 Opener: Courtesy of the City of St. Louis Emergency Medical Services, St. Louis, Missouri.

Fig. 17-3: Photographer Lou Ellen Romig, MD

Fig. 17-5: From James and Studdy: *A Color Atlas of Respiratory Diseases*, London, England, 1993, Wolf Medical Publications.

Fig. 17-6: Photographer Colin Williams

Fig. 17-7: Proventil®; a registered trademark of Schering, a wholly owned subsidiary of Schering Plough Corporation, Kenilworth, New Jersey

Fig. 17-9: Ellipse®; a registered trademark of Allen and Hanburys, Division of Glaxo, Inc., Research Triangle Park, North Carolina; Proventil®; a registered trademark of Schering, a wholly owned subsidiary of Schering Plough Corporation, Kenilworth, New Jersey

Chapter 18 Opener: Photographer Vincent Knaus

Fig. 18-1: From Thibodeau: *Structure and Function of the Human Body*, ed 9, St. Louis, 1992, Mosby. (Illustrator, Christine Oleksyk)

Fig. 18-5: Nitro-Linqual®; a registered trademark of Rhone-Poulenc Rorer Pharmaceuticals, Inc., Collegeville, Pennsylvania; Nitro-Stat®; a registered trademark of Parke Davis, Division of Warner Lambert Co., Morris Plains, New Jersey

Table 16-2

Fig. 18-7: Automatic external defibrilators; products of Laerdal and PhysioControl

Fig. 18-8: From Huszar: *Basic Dysrythmias*, St. Louis, 1994, Mosby Lifeline.

Fig. 18-9: From Grauer: *ACLS Certification Preparation*, St. Louis, 1993, Mosby Lifeline.

Fig. 18-10: Automated external defibrillator; a product of Laerdal, Inc.

Fig. 18-11B: Automated external defibrillator; a product of Physio Control, Inc.

Fig. 18-13: Reproduced with permission. *Textbook of Advanced Cardiac Life Support*, 1994, Copyright American Heart Association.

Chapter 19 Opener: Photographer Peter Escobedo

Fig. 19-1: Insta-glucose®; a product of ICN

Chapter 20 Opener: Photographer Peter Escobedo

Fig. 20-2: From Sanders MJ: *Mosby's Paramedic Textbook*, St. Louis, 1994, Mosby Lifeline. (Courtesy of Gary Quick, MD)

Fig. 20-4: EpiPen®; a registered trademark of Center, Division of EM Industries, Inc., Port Washington, New York

Chapter 21 Opener: Courtesy of the City of St. Louis Emergency Medical Services, St. Louis, Missouri

Fig. 21-2: Photographer William Greenblatt

Figs. 21-4 and 21-7: Courtesy of the St. Louis Zoo, St. Louis, Missouri

Figs. 21-5 and 21-6: From Auerbach PS: *Management of Wilderness and Environmental Emergencies*, ed 3, St. Louis, 1995, Mosby. (Courtesy of the University of Indiana Medical Center)

Fig. 21-8: From Auerbach PS: *A Medical Guide to Hazardous Marine Life*, ed 2, St. Louis, 1991, Mosby.

Fig. 21-10: Liqui-char®; a registered trademark of Allen and Hanburys, Division of Glaxo, Inc., Research Triangle Park, North Carolina; Actidose-Aqua®; a registered trademark of Paddock Laboratories, Inc., Minneapolis, Minnesota

Chapter 22 Opener: Photographer Thomas Cooper

Figs. 22-2 and 22-3: From Grossman JA: *Color Atlas of Minor Injuries and Repairs*, London, England, 1993, Gower.

Fig. 22-6A,B, and C: From Auerbach PS: *Management of Wilderness and Environmental Emergencies*, ed 3, St. Louis, 1995, Mosby.

Fig. 22-6B: Courtesy of John Williamson, MD

Chapter 23 Opener: Photographer Peter Escobedo

Fig. 23-1: From London PS: *A Colour Atlas of Diagnosis After Recent Injury*, Ipswich, England, 1990, Wolfe Medical Publishing, Ltd.

Fig. 23-2: From Krebs: *When Violence Erupts*, St. Louis, 1990, Mosby.

Figs. 23-3 and 23-4: From Sanders MJ: *Mosby's Paramedic Textbook*, St. Louis, 1994, Mosby Lifeline.

Chapter 24 Opener: Courtesy of the City of St. Louis Emergency Medical Services, St. Louis, Missouri

Fig. 24-1: From Thibodeau: *Structure and Function of the Human Body*, ed 9, St. Louis, 1992, Mosby. (Illustrator, Barbara Cousins)

Table 24-1: From Aehlert: *Pediatric Advanced Life Support Study Guide*, St. Louis, 1994, Mosby Lifeline.

Fig. 24-3: From Thibodeau: *Structure and Function of the Human Body*, ed 9, St. Louis, 1992, Mosby. (Photographer, Lennart Nilsson)

Fig. 24-6: From Sanders MJ: *Mosby's Paramedic Textbook*, St. Louis, 1994, Mosby Lifeline.

Fig. 24-17: From Al-Azzawi A: *Color Atlas of Childbirth and Obstetric Techniques*, London, England, 1990, Wolfe Medical Publishing, Ltd.

Fig. 24-19: Reproduced with permission. *Textbook of Pediatric Advanced Cardiac Life Support*, 1988, Copyright American Heart Association as seen in Aehlert: *Pediatric Advanced Life Support Study Guide*, St. Louis, 1994, Mosby Lifeline.

Chapter 25 Opener: Photographer William Greenblatt

Chapter 26 Opener: Photographer Colin Williams

Figs. 26-2, 26-4, 26-6, 26-9, 26-10, and 26-19: From London PS: *A Colour Atlas of Diagnosis After Recent Injury*, Ipswich, England, 1990, Wolfe Medical Publishing Ltd.

Figs. 26-3, 26-5, and 26-8: From Williams: *Color Atlas of Injury in Sport*, ed 2, Chicago, 1990, Yearbook Medical Publishers.

Fig. 26-7: From Grossman JA: *Atlas of Minor Injuries and Repairs*, London, England, 1992, Gower.

Fig. 26-11: Trauma dressings, abdominal dressings, gauze pads, and tape; products of Moore Medical Corporation; vaseline gauze strips; a product of Sherwood Medical

Fig. 26-12: Self-adherent bandages; a product of 3M; all others are products of Moore Medical Corp.

Fig. 26-21: From Eichelberger MR: *Pediatric Trauma*, St. Louis, 1993, Mosby.

Fig. 26-23A: Judd RL, Posnell DD: *Mosby's First Responder Textbook*, ed 2, St. Louis, 1988, Mosby.

Figs. 26-23B and C: Courtesy of St. Johns Mercy Medical Center, St. Louis, Missouri

Fig. 26-25: From Sanders MJ: *Mosby's Paramedic Textbook*, St. Louis, 1994, Mosby Lifeline.

Chapter 27 Opener: Courtesy of the Maryland Institute for Emergency Medical Services, Baltimore, Maryland.

Fig. 27-1: From Tate, Seely, and Stephens: *Understanding the Human Body*, St. Louis, 1994, Mosby. (Illustrator, Christine Oleksyk)

Figs. 27-2 and 27-3: Nakayama: *A Color Atlas of Pediatric Surgery*, New York, 1992, Gower.

Fig. 27-6: Ladder splint, padded board splints, and cardboard splints; products of Moore Medical Corp.

Fig. 27-8: Sager traction splint; a product of Minto Research and Development; Fernotrac traction splint; a product of Ferno Washington, Inc.

Fig. 27-10: Air splints; a product of Moore Medical Corp.; vacuum splints; a product of Medical Devices, Inc.

Fig. 27-15: From Sanders MJ: *Mosby's Paramedic Textbook*, St. Louis, 1994, Mosby Lifeline.

Chapter 28 Opener: Photographer Peter Escobedo

Fig. 28-2: From Thibodeau: *Anatomy and Physiology*, ed 2, St. Louis, 1990, Mosby.

Fig. 28-3: Stifneck® Extrication collar; a registered trademark of Laerdal; Philadelphia Flat 2-piece collar; a product of Philadelphia Cervical Collar Co.; Vertabrace collar; a product of Jobst

Fig. 28-6: Emergency Wood Back/Spine Board; a product of Moore Medical Corp.; KED; a product of Ferno Washington Inc.; XP1; a product of Medical Specialties, Inc.

Fig. 28-7: Plastic Backboard; a product of Moore Medical Corp.; Wooden Backboard, Head Block, Block System; products of Fleming (Iron Duck)

Fig. 28-8: Photographer William Greenblatt

Fig. 28-9: Photographer Ronald Olshwanger

Fig. 28-10: Photographer Colin Williams

Fig. 28-22: Prehospital Trauma Life Support Committee of the National Association of Emergency Medical Technicians, in cooperation with the Committee on Trauma of the American College of Surgeons: *PHTLS: basic and advanced prehospital trauma life support*, St. Louis, 1994, Mosby.

Chapter 29 Opener: Photographer Colin Williams

Fig. 29-1: Courtesy of St. Louis Children's Hospital

Fig. 29-3: Photographer Colin Williams

Figs. 29-4 and 29-5: From Aehlert: *Pediatric Advanced Life Support Study Guide*; St. Louis, 1994, Mosby Lifeline.

Fig. 29-16: ASVP: *Pass CPR*, Naples, 1994, Mosby.

Fig. 29-21: Pediatric trauma airpant; a product of Life Support Products

Chapter 30 Opener: Photographer Thomas Cooper

Table 30-1: From West: *Care of Specific Contaminated Equipment*, Fairfax County Fire/Rescue Department, Fairfax, Virginia, as it appeared in West: *The Infectious Disease Handbook*, 1994, American Conference of Governmental Industrial Hygenists, Inc.

Fig. 30-7: Courtesy of Stat Helicopter, Pittsburgh, Pennsylvania

Chapter 31 Opener: Photographer Colin Williams

Figs. 31-1, 31-2, 31-5 and 31-8: Photographer James Silvernail

Fig. 31-3: Photographer Thomas E. Cooper

Figs. 31-6 and 31-9: Photographer William Greenblatt

Fig. 31-7: Photographer Colin Williams

Fig. 31-10: Courtesy of the Maryland Institute for Emergency Medical Services System, Baltimore, Maryland.

Chapter 32 Opener: Photographer William Greenblatt

Fig. 32-1: Photographer Colin Williams

Fig. 32-2: The United States Department of Transportation: *Emergency Response Guidebook*, Washington, DC, 1990.

Fig. 32-3: From Bronstein: *Mosby's Emergency Care for Hazardous Material Exposure*, St. Louis, 1988, Mosby Lifeline.

Fig. 32-5: Courtesy of Mettag Products, Starke, Florida

Chapter 33 Opener: Photographer Colin Williams

Figs. 33-1 and 33-14: From Aehlert: *Pediatric Advanced Life Support Study Guide*; St. Louis, 1994, Mosby Lifeline. (Illustrator, Kim Battista)

Fig. 33-2: From Cummins: *Handbook of ACLS Scenarios*, St. Louis, 1995, Mosby. (Illustrator, Kim Battista)

Fig. 33-14: Broselow resuscitation tape; a product of Armstrong

Appendix A and Appendix B: US Department of Transportation, National Highway Traffic Safety Administration, Emergency Medical Technician–Basic: National Standard Curriculum, Washington, DC, 1994, US Government Printing Office.

Appendix C: Modified from: Sanders MJ: Mosby's Paramedic Textbook, St. Louis, 1994, Mosby Lifeline.

Cover photography: Colin Williams, Thomas Cooper, Vincent Knaus, William Greenblatt.

INDEX

Items for note are *italics* for illustrations and boxed material and *t* for tables.